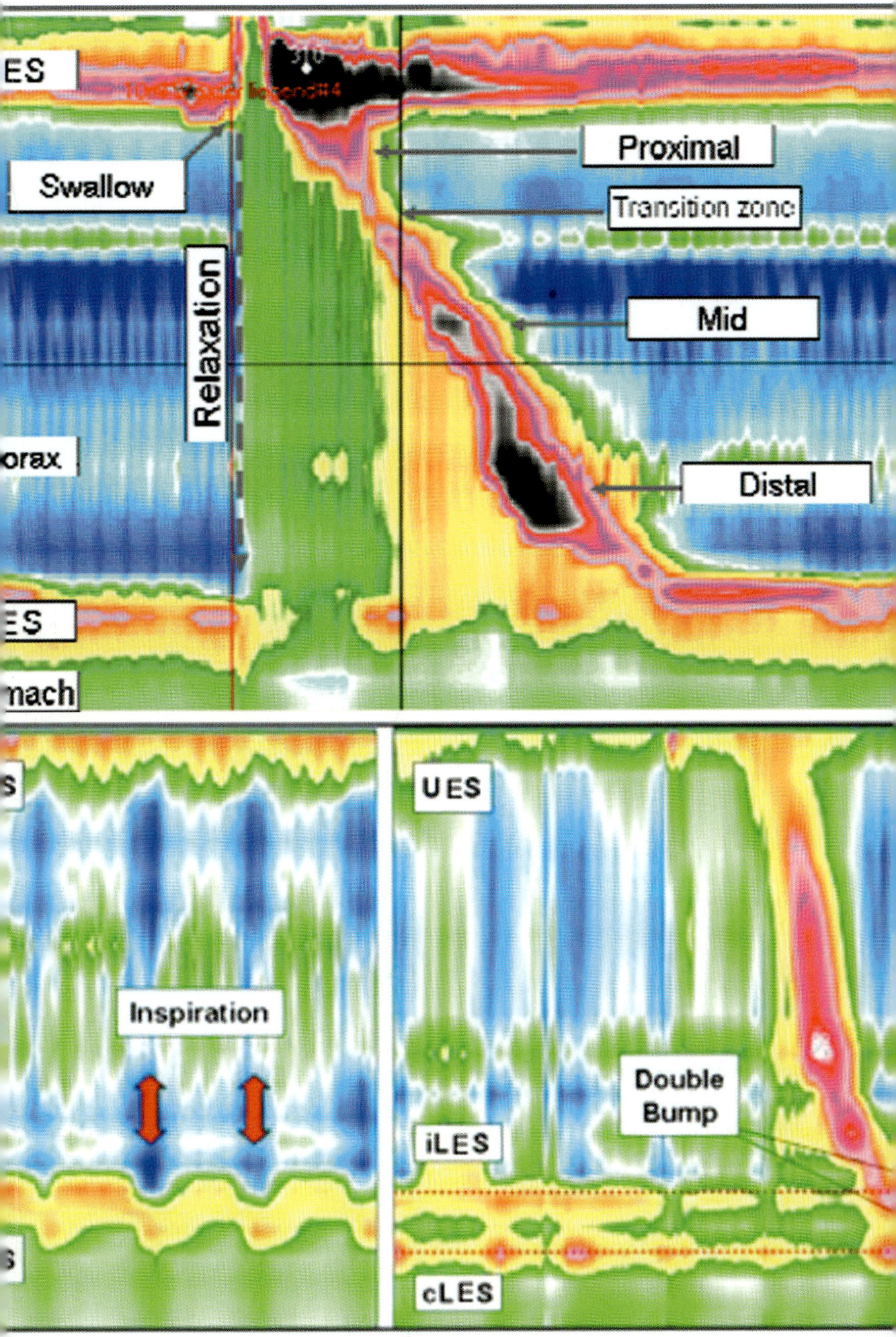

Swallow
Proximal
Transition zone
Relaxation
Mid
Distal
Inspiration
UES
Double Bump
iLES
cLES

ISBN 978-2-7420-0721-9

Éditions John Libbey Eurotext
127, avenue de la République, 92120 Montrouge, France
Tél: 01 46 73 06 60
E-mail: contact@jle.com
Site internet: http://www.jle.com

John Libbey Eurotext Limited
42-46 High Street
Esther, Surrey, KT 10 9QY
United Kingdom

o(eso

the esophagus

The Foregut

Function - Dysfunction

Robert Giuli
Carmelo Scarpignato
Charles J. Lightdale
Editors

John Libbey EUROTEXT

PREVIOUS BOOKS of O.E.S.O.

- 1985: *Cancer of the esophagus*. 135 questions.
  Paris: Maloine, 430 p.
  R. Giuli Ed.
- 1988: *Benign lesions of the esophagus and cancer*. Answers to 210 questions.
  Paris: Springer Verlag, 850 p.
  R. Giuli, R.W. McCallum Eds.
- 1991: *Primary motor disorders of the esophagus*. 450 questions - 450 answers.
  Paris: John Libbey Eurotext, 1 220 p.
  R. Giuli, R.W. McCallum, D.B. Skinner Eds.
- 1994: *The esophageal mucosa*. 300 questions - 300 answers.
  Paris: Elsevier, 1 200 p.
  R. Giuli, G.N.J. Tytgat, T.R. DeMeester, J.-P. Galmiche Eds.
- 1998: *The esophagogastric junction*. 420 questions - 420 answers.
  Paris: John Libbey Eurotext, 1 600 p.
  R. Giuli, J.-P. Galmiche, G.G. Jamieson, C. Scarpignato Eds
- 2003: *Barrett's esophagus*. 250 questions - 250 answers.
  Paris: John Libbey Eurotext, 860 p.
  R. Giuli, J.R. Siewert, D. Couturier, C. Scarpignato Eds
- 2006: *The duodenogastroesophageal reflux*. 125 questions - 125 answers.
  Paris: John Libbey Eurotext, 530 p.
  R. Giuli, C. Scarpignato, J.-M. Collard, J.E. Richter Eds

Editors

Robert Giuli, MD, FACS, FCCP
Professor of Surgery
Executive Director of OESO
Paris, France

Carmelo Scarpignato, MD, DSc (Hons), PharmD (*h.c.*), FRCP (London), FCP, FACG
Professor of Pharmacology & Therapeutics
Associate Professor of Gastroenterology
School of Medicine & Dentistry
University of Parma
Parma, Italy

Charles J. Lightdale, MD
Professor of Clinical Medicine
Gastroenterology - Gastrointestinal Endoscopy
Columbia University
New York, USA

Preface

It may be difficult to imagine a better time than today to be involved in both basic and clinical research on esophageal disease. Indeed, this is an exciting era for both basic scientists, who can see their ideas being put into clinical practice, and for clinicians who can offer their patients increasingly effective means for both diagnosis and therapy.

Knowledge concerning esophageal pathophysiology has until recently lagged far behind that of the pathophysiology of other portions of the gastrointestinal (GI) tract for reasons that still remain unclear. Yet, it is the fact that, at least until the last few decades, interest in the esophagus was primarily based on pathologic anatomy. Even today, much remains to be learnt on the pathophysiology of esophageal disease.

The recent development of methods of studying both morphology and function of the esophagus has resulted in a better understanding of normal and abnormal esophageal patterns with a corresponding improvement in treatment, which is now physiologically, rather than anatomically based. As customary, the World OESO Congresses are planned to provide each time a thorough analysis of a specific topic in esophageal disease.
The 8th World Congress of OESO was devoted to the **Foregut: Function and Dysfunction** to emphasize the complex interaction between the esophagus and the other portions of the upper GI tract, either in maintaining physiological function or in triggering esophageal disease. The choice is a timely one because recent investigations have allowed new insights into the pathophysiology of these complex interactions to be gained. It is indeed becoming clear that there are intriguing pathophysiological abnormalities that account for upper GI symptoms and that more targeted therapy is needed to address the unmet clinical needs. Within this framework, specific sessions were devoted to disorders of secretion, of motility as well as of nutrition with a special emphasis on recent advances.

Unlike some of the other publications, this volume does not merely represent the proceedings of an International Congress. With its now established and successful format, it collects the answers to 130 key questions, offered by 110 basic scientists and clinicians from the World over, all of whom have personally contributed to the topic, in order to provide a glimpse of what may lie ahead.
We trust that the careful reader will appreciate the in-depth answer to a question he or she is asking for. This easily to read format will allow the practicing and busy physician to keep up efficiently with advances in diagnosis and therapy in this rapidly evolving field.

We wish to express our deep appreciation to the Chairmen, Speakers and participants. The high level of their scientific contributions to the Congress has made this book possible. This book is proof that there are many dedicated scientists and clinicians that have given their best efforts to the study of esophageal diseases. We are indebted to all of them for having provided us with excellent manuscripts, despite the many calls on their time.
This book is their book.

This volume would have never gone to press without the careful and dedicated work of Mrs Catherine Cahn at Book Editing Department of John Libbey Eurotext, Paris, and without the educational support of the Janssen-Cilag, European Pariet® Team.
In addition, we owe so much to the OESO Administrative Assistant, Ms Michèle Liegeon, for her outstanding job of managing papers, corresponding with authors and following every stage of editorial work.
Finally, our sincere gratitude goes to "our" Publisher for having supported the publication of "OESO book series" over the years.

Robert Giuli, MD, FACS, FCCP
Professor of Surgery
Director, Executive Committee, OESO Foundation
OESO Executive Director

Carmelo Scarpignato, MD, FRCP, FACG
Professor of Pharmacology & Therapeutics
Associate Professor of Gastroenterology
OESO Secretary General

Colour plates

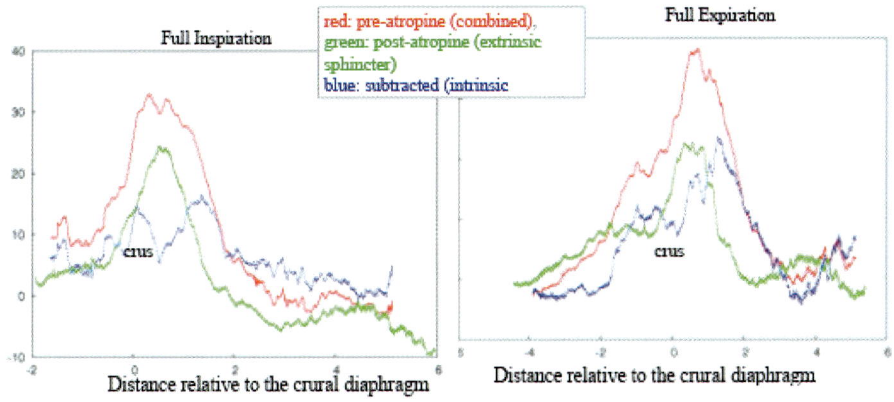

Figure 2. The combined high-pressure zone and its extrinsic and intrinsic components for both the full inspiration (FI on left) and full expiration respiratory (FE on right) states in 15 normal control subjects. The red line represents the pre-atropine pressure curve (combined external and internal sphincters). The green line represents the post-atropine pressure curve (the extrinsic sphincter). The blue line represents the pre-atropine minus the post-atropine subtraction curve (the intrinsic sphincter components). Note that in both the subtraction curves (full inspiration and full expiration) there are two peaks. The distal peak represents the gastric sling fiber/clasp fiber complex and the proximal curve represents the LES. (**See page 11**).

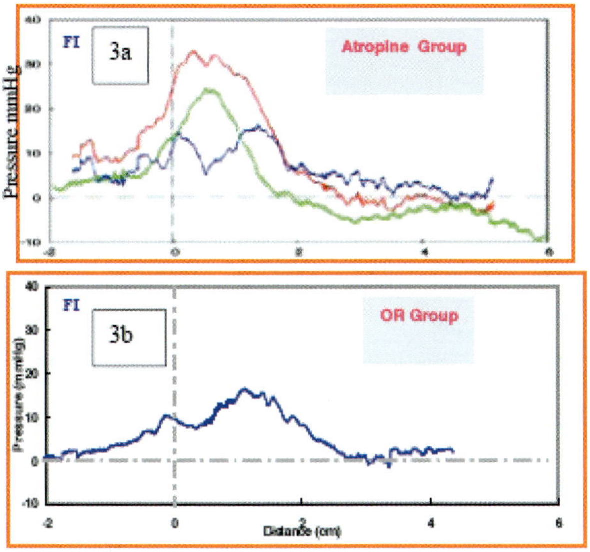

Figure 3. a. This graphs show the ensemble averaging of the normal control group who were evaluated pre- and post-atropine. **b.** This graphs show the ensemble averaging of seven patients undergoing crural diaphragm paralysis (OR group). This graph represents the residual pressure profiles only from the intrinsic sphincter components. Comparing these curves with the normal control atropine group pressure curves in blue, the same two peaks in both full inspiration) is demonstrated at the same relative geographic location with respect to the right crural diaphragm. Therefore, the results from crural diaphragm paralysis are consistent with localization of the intrinsic esophageal sphincter components using smooth muscle ablation with atropine in normal control subjects. The distal peaks represent the pressure profile from the gastric sling fiber/clasp fiber complex while the proximal peaks represent the pressure profile from the intrinsic LES. (**See page 13**).

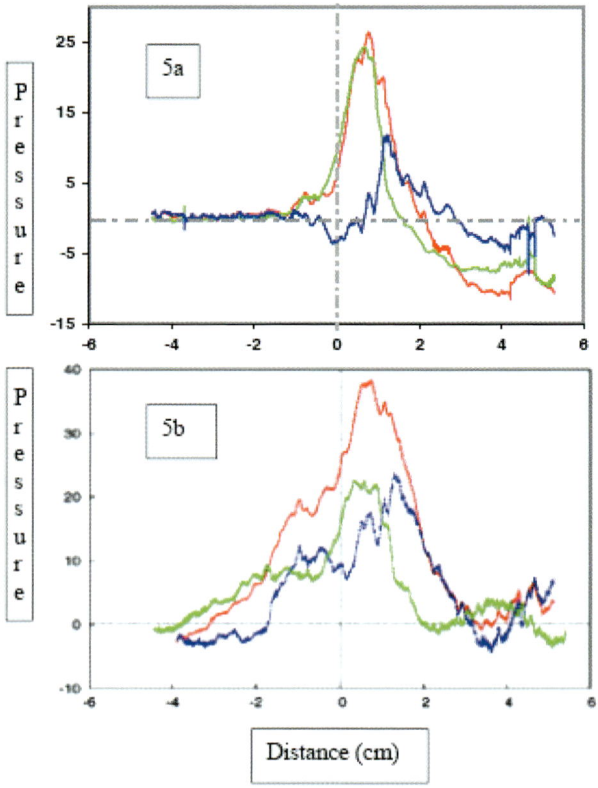

Figure 5. In GERD patients **(a)** the subtraction curves between the pre- and post-atropine pressure profiles demonstrated that the distal peak (gastric sling fiber/clasp fiber pressure profile) was totally absent in both full inspiration (FI, left graph) and full expiration (FE, right graph). The proximal peak representing the LES was present in the same axial position relative to the right crural diaphragm as in the normal volunteers **(b)**. Note: red curve represents pre-atropine pressure; green curve represents post-atropine pressure; blue curve represents post-atropine subtracted from preatropine pressures, to extract the intrinsic sphincter contribution to the GEJ high pressure zone. The vertical dashed line represents the start of the crural diaphragm, used as an axial reference mark. (**See page 15**).

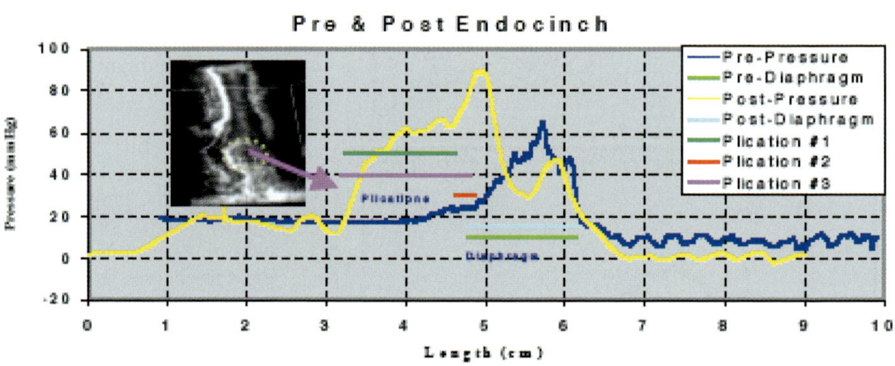

Figure 6. This picture shows the pressure profiles through the GEJ high pressure zone pre- and post-EndoCinch in a patient with GERD referenced to the right crural diaphragm. Note, the blue curve represents the pre-the EndoCinch pressure profile, while the yellow curve represents the post-EndoCinch pressure profile. The horizontal lines represent the locations of the endoscopic plications (red, pink and green lines), and the right crural diaphragm (light blue, and light green lines) located by ultrasound imaging. (**See page 15**).

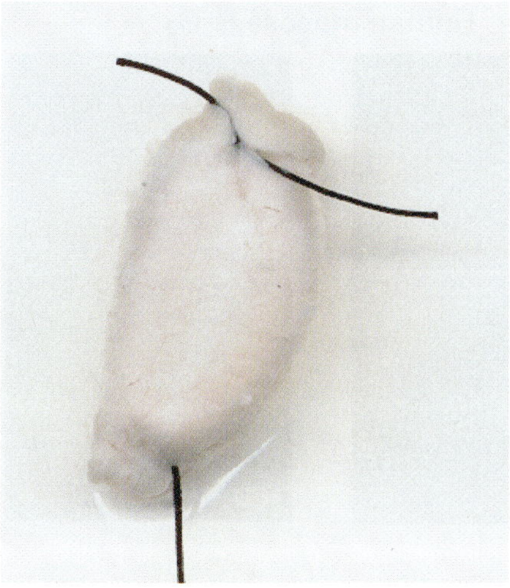

Figure 1. We produced an *in vitro* model of esophageal inflammation using an esophageal mucosa tube tied at both ends. The tube was created by removing the muscle layers from the esophagus by sharp dissection at the level of the submucosa. It had the squamous epithelium on the inside and the submucosa on the outside. HCl or Kreb's buffer was injected inside the tube, which was then kept in oxygenated Kreb's buffer at 36°C for 3 hours. (1 ml Kreb's buffer/100 mg mucosa). After 3 hours the supernatant outside the tube was collected and analyzed or used to incubate circular muscle strips. (**See page 68**).

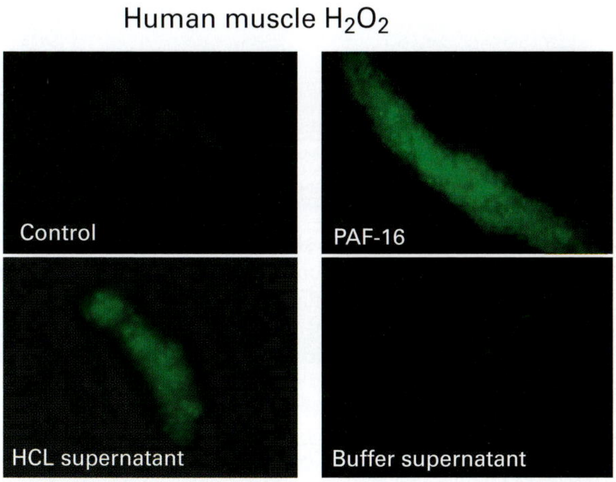

Figure 18. Rhodamine fluorescence in muscle cells enzymatically isolated from esophageal circular muscle layer as a probe for measurement of intracellular ROS. Dihydro-rhodamine (DHR 123) enters the cells as a freely permeable dye which, when oxidized, is converted to rhodamine 123, which is not membrane permeable. Rhodamine 123 is a common laser dye, which is excitable at 488 detectable at 515 nm, under confocal microscopy. Rhodamine 123 fluoresces when exposed to reactive oxygen species (ROS), including H_2O_2. ROS levels were low in normal esophageal smooth muscle cells (Control) and were not affected by supernatant of normal Krebs' treated mucosa (Buffer supernatant). In contrast incubating normal smooth muscle cells with supernatant of HCl (pH 5.8)-filled mucosa (HCl supernatant), or with PAF-16, visibly increased cytoplasmic ROS, confirming the data in *Figure 17*, and indicating that PAF induced-fluorescence is most likely a reflection of NADPH-dependent production of H_2O_2. (**See page 74**).

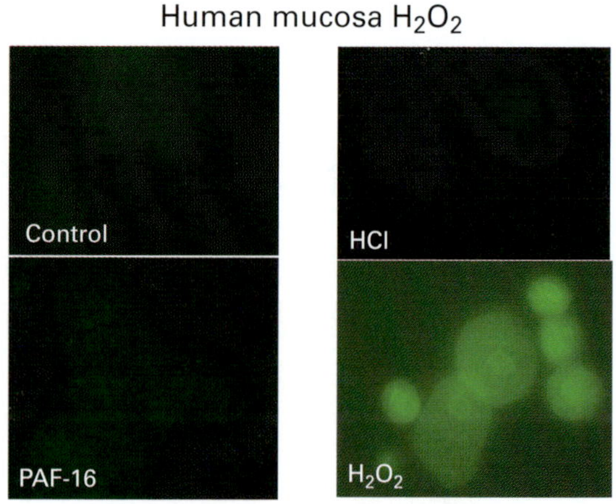

Figure 19. Rhodamine fluorescence in epithelial cells enzymatically isolated from esophageal mucosa was examined by confocal microscopy, as a probe for measurement of intracellular H_2O_2. The figure shows no ROS in epithelial cells in response to HCl or PAF-16. An H_2O_2-treated epithelial cell is shown in the right lower panel as a positive control. H_2O_2 is uncharged and penetrates the cytoplasm, demonstrating the adequacy of the technique in detecting cytoplasmic H_2O_2. (**See page 74**).

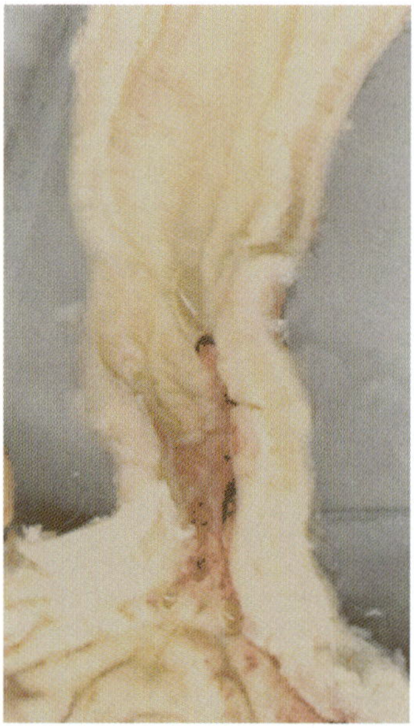

Figure 25. An esophageal specimen obtained from an organ donor exhibited hyperemia of the mucosa with scattered hemorrhagic erosions in the lower esophagus, extending across the cardia. (**See page 77**).

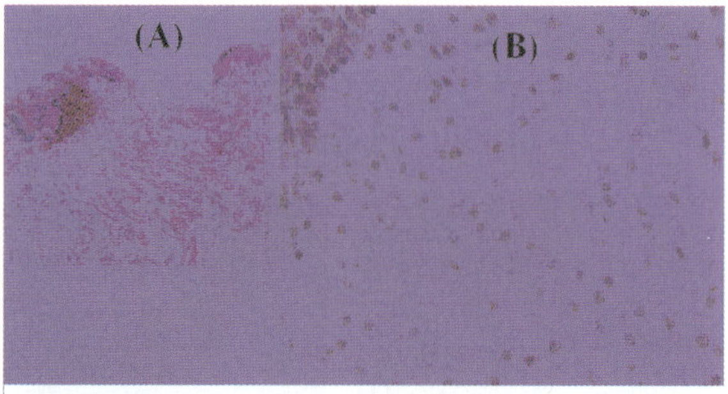

Figure 26. Panel (A) shows erosions, basal zone hyperplasia and elongation of lamina propria papillae with congestion. The enlarged area (panel B) shows inflammatory cells present in the epithelial layer. These findings are characteristic of reflux esophagitis. (**See page 77**).

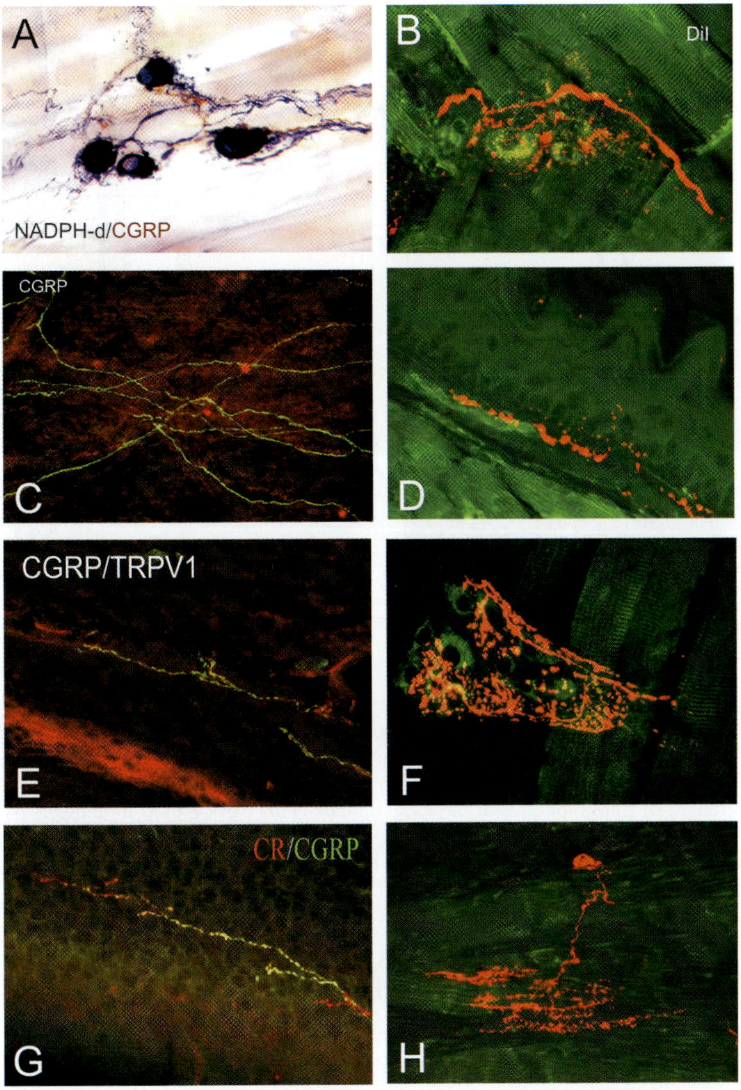

Figure 1. A. Myenteric ganglion in the rat esophagus containing four nitrergic neurons (blue NADPH diaphorase staining). CGRP positive spinal afferent fibers (brown) traverse the ganglion, forming en passant boutons on the neurons. **B.** Spinal afferent fibers (red) labelled by anterograde DiI tracing from lower thoracic spinal ganglia in the abdominal esophagus of the rat. Note numerous fine red dots indicating varicosities of the afferent axons. **C.** Meshwork of CGRP positive spinal afferent axons in a mucosal wholemount of the rat thoracic esophagus viewed en face. **D.** CGRP positive fine varicose spinal afferents (red) in the lamina propria of the rat thoracic esophagus mucosa sending delicate branches into the epithelium. **E.** Fine varicose afferent axons in the mucosa of the rat cervical esophagus co-staining for both CGRP and TRPV1 as indicated by yellow mixed color. **F.** Calretinin immunoreactive IGLEs (red) covering a myenteric ganglion (indicated by green autofluorescence of neuronal cell bodies) in the rat thoracic esophagus. **G.** Fine varicose branched vagal afferent axon beneath the epithelium of the rat cervical esophagus co-staining for both calretinin and CGRP. **H.** Intramuscular arrays (red) in the lower esophageal sphincter of the rat as stained by anterograde DiI tracing from the nodose ganglion. Note fine varicose interconnected axons coursing parallel to smooth muscle fibers displaying green autofluorescence. (**See page 90**).

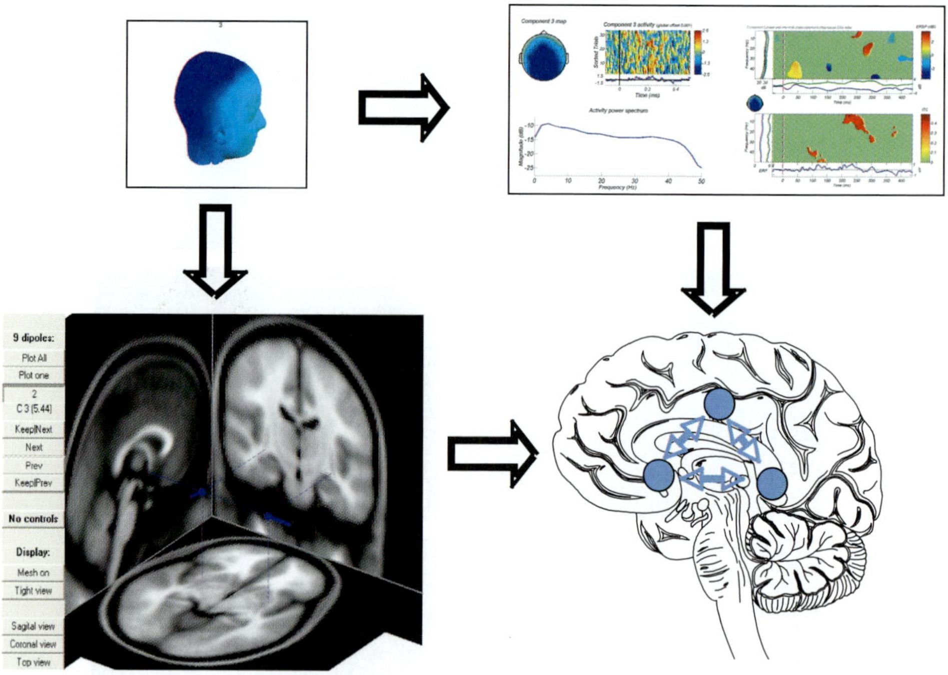

Figure 2. Independent component analysis of the surface EEG in 64 electrodes.
Top left: surface scalp map showing the interpolated projection of the component to a head model. Top right: the event related potential image consisting of 35 parallel lines representing the individual trials of the given component. The right side of this picture shows the inter-trial coherence images with the strength of phase locking of the EEG signals. This can be used in analysis of connectivity between brain centers. Bottom left: the equivalent current dipole projected into a standardized brain image. Bottom right: the connectivity analysis being an attempt to describe dynamic links between neuronal centers - "the brain web". For detailed information see [19]. (**See page 106**).

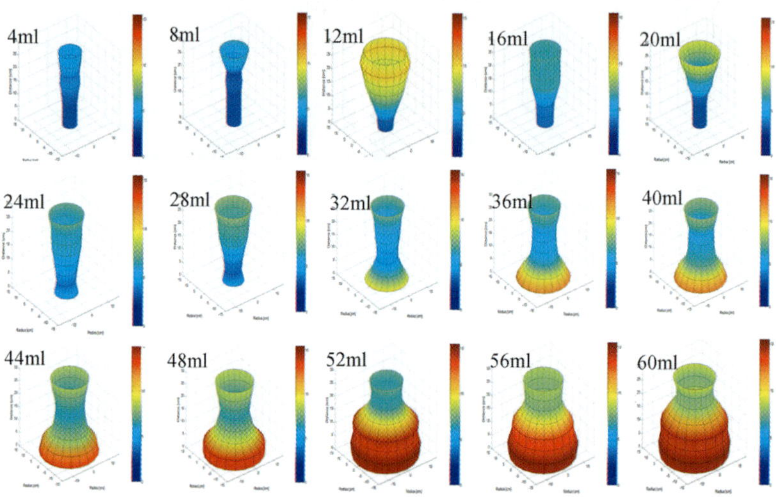

Figure 2. Reconstruction of the geometry of the esophago-gastric junction from a healthy subject shown at various bag fill volumes. The color represents radii (mm). Modified from a previous publication. (Courtesy of Dr. McMahon). (**See page 148**).

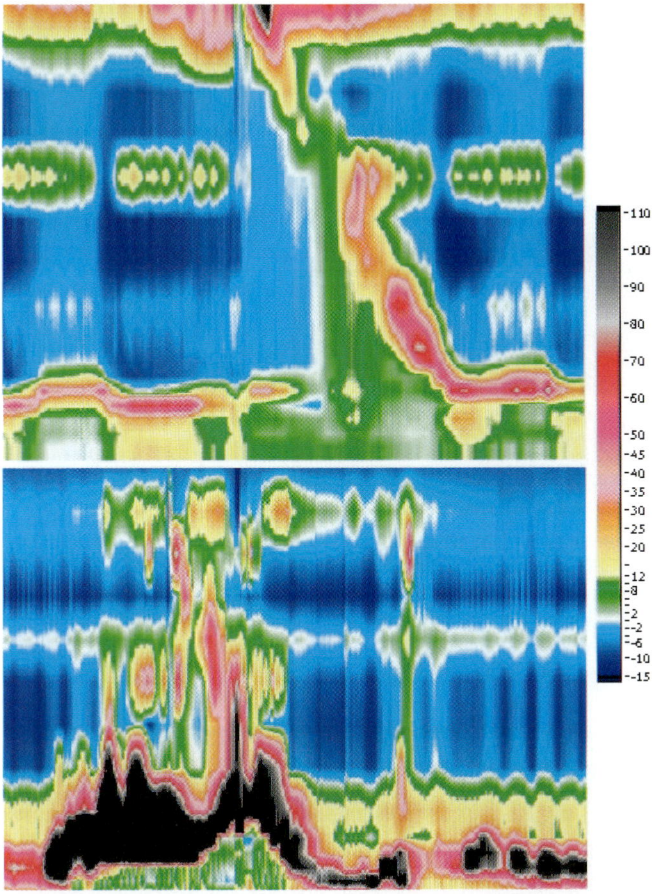

Figure 1. HRM from a patient with chest pain. The stationary study is shown in the top panel (normal). An ambulatory HRM study was done and the data in the bottom panel was collected during a period of chest discomfort. Note the increase in pressure in the LES, uncoordinated contractions in the body of the esophagus and esophageal shortening indicating longitudinal muscle contraction. (**See page 196**).

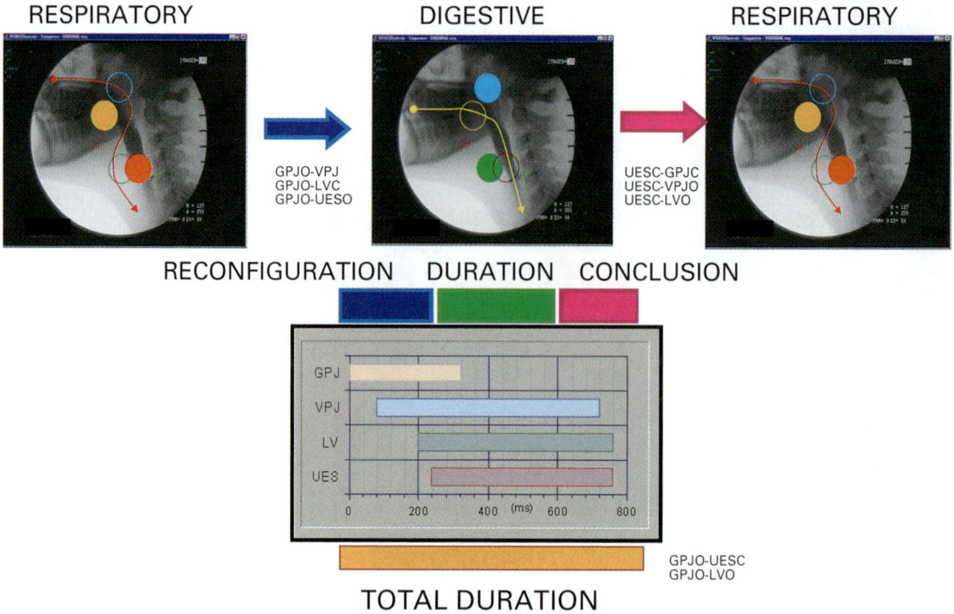

Figure 1. Configuration of the oropharynx during swallow response. Each phase of the response (reconfiguration, duration and conclusion) is defined by opening (O) or closing (C) events occurring at the glossopalatal junction (GPJ), velopharyngeal junction (VPJ), laryngeal vestibule (LV), and upper esophageal sphincter (UES). (**See page 226**).

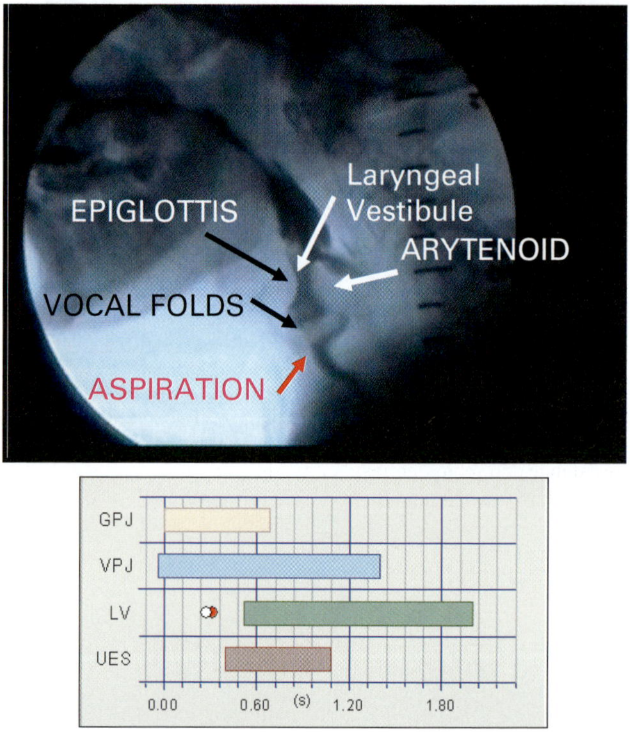

Figure 2. Swallow response in a patient with neurogenic dysphagia and aspiration during swallow. Diagram at the bottom of each tracing depicts timing of swallow response showing severe delay in LVC and UESO. White dots represent timing of laryngeal penetration and the red point, time of aspiration. (**See page 226**).

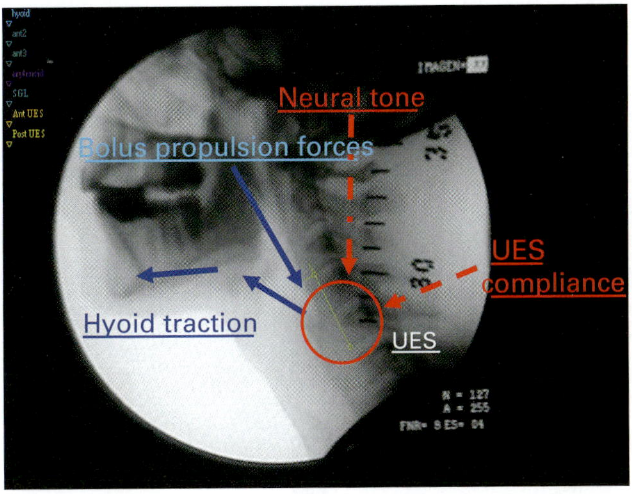

Figure 3. Mechanisms of UES opening. Timing of swallow response, the extent of hyoid motion and UES opening and bolus propulsion forces can be assessed during videofluoroscopic studies. UES relaxation and compliance is assessed by pharyngo-esophageal manometry. (**See page 227**).

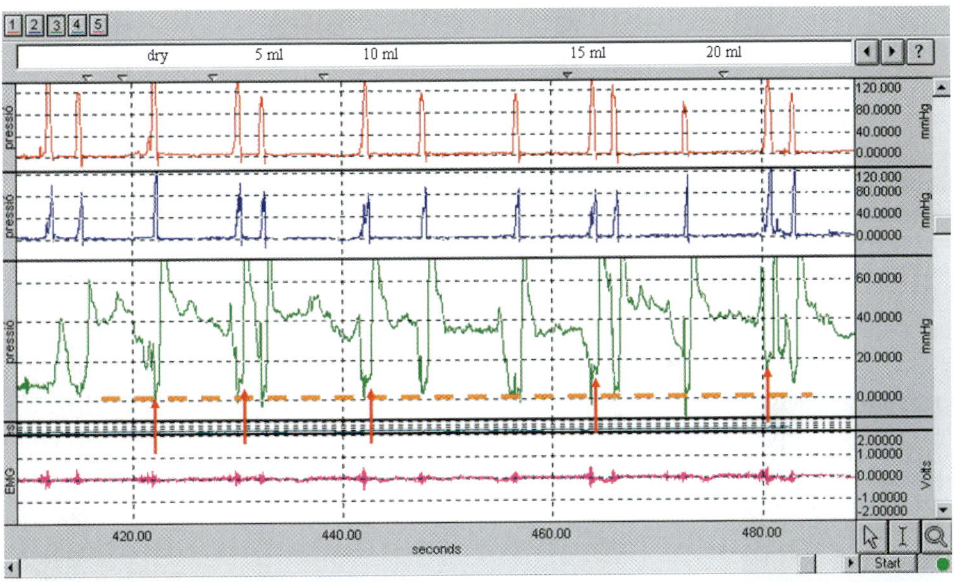

Figure 4. Pharyngeoesophageal manometry with surface EMG of hyoid muscles. Representative tracing in a patient with a Zenker diverticulum showing reduced sphincter compliance. Note that residual pressure is normal during dry swallows and that fibrosis of the sphincter causes increased resistance and increased residual (nadir) pressures with increased bolus volume. Note that nadir UES pressure is over 20 mmHg during 20 mL swallows. (**See page 228**).

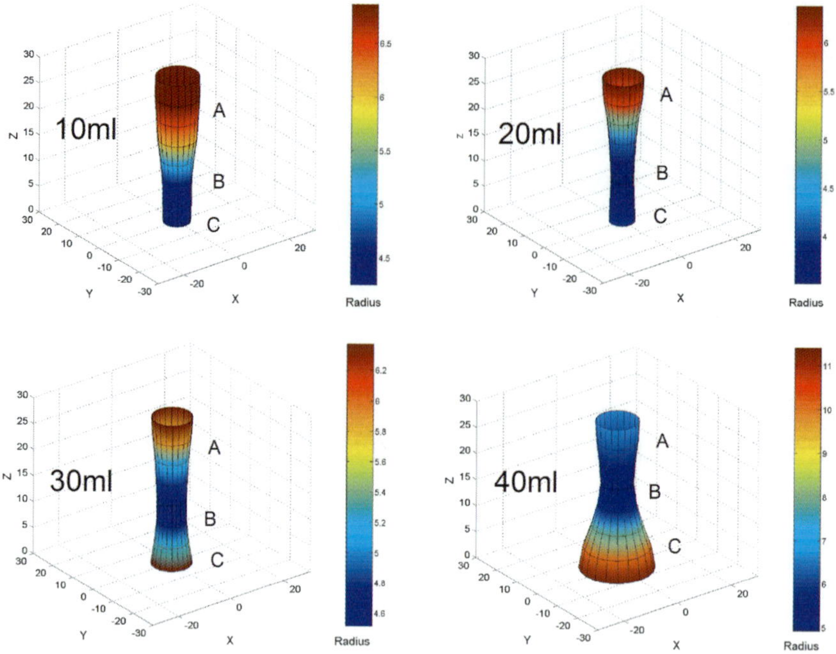

Figure 3. Three dimensional reconstruction of the geometry of the EGJ shown at bag fill volumes of 10 ml, 20 ml, 30 ml and 40 ml, respectively. The color represents radii (mm). In each case A represents the position in the luminal image of the ampulla of the esophagus, B represents the EGJ and C represents the point at which the esophagus enters the stomach. x, y and z are the three orthogonal directions (mm). (Courtesy of Dr. McMahon). (**See page 248**).

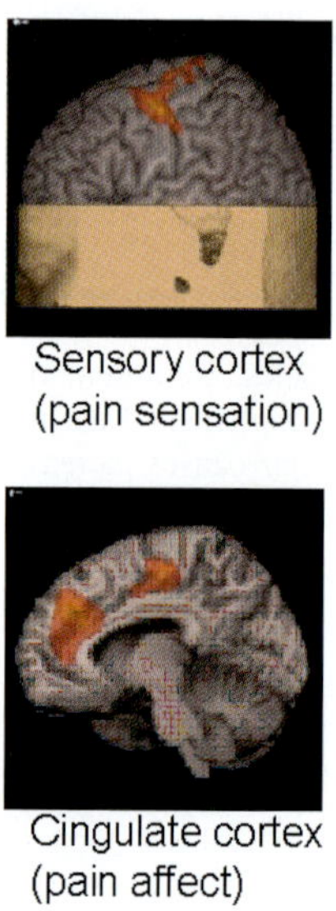

Figure 1. This figure shows the evoked field response recorded with MEG/SAM following painful and non-painful electrical stimulation of the esophagus. The top trace is recorded from a virtual electrode positioned in the lateral portion of the primary somatosensory cortex and the peak latency of this response is 90 ms. This corresponds to the P1 component of the EEP and is consistent with this regions role in the sensory discriminatory aspects of pain processing. The lower trace is recorded from a virtual electrode positioned in the perigenual cingulate cortex and the peak latency of this response is 140 ms. This later response is consistent with this regions involvement in affection/ cognitive processing of esophageal pain. (Figure reproduced with permission from [12]). (**See page 254**).

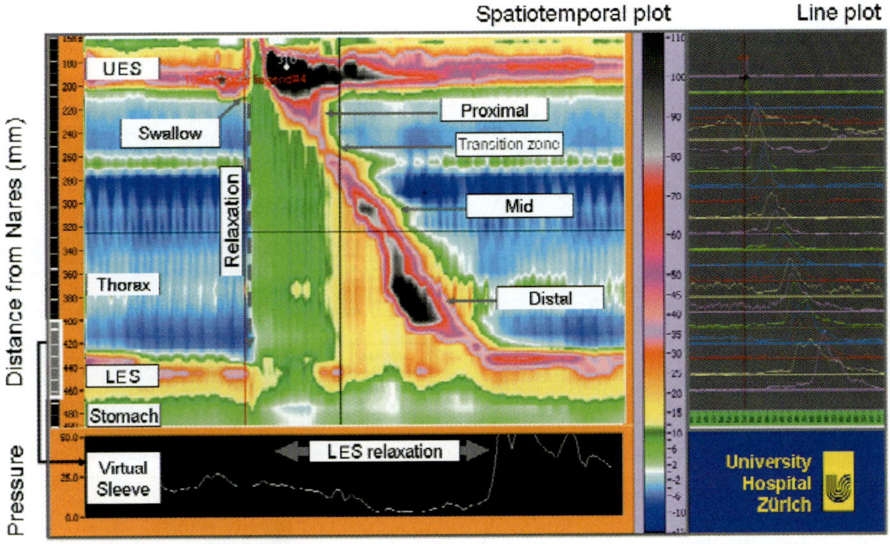

Figure 1. Normal water swallow as assessed by 32-channel, water perfused high resolution manometry (HRM). Time is on the x-axis and distance from the nares is on the y-axis. Each pressure is assigned a colour. The spatiotemporal plot presents the same information as the line plots; however the large volume of data is easier to appreciate in a single image than multiple line plots. Normal esophageal function is clearly demonstrated including the synchronous relaxation of the upper and lower esophageal sphincter on swallowing, and the increasing pressure and duration of the peristaltic wave as it passes distally. In addition subtle but functionally important pressure events are demonstrated. These include the transition zone (pressure trough) between the proximal and middle esophagus, the 'common cavity' pressure rise after the water swallow and the build up of intra-bolus pressure (the force that drives bolus transport) as peristalsis approaches the LES. (**See page 285**).

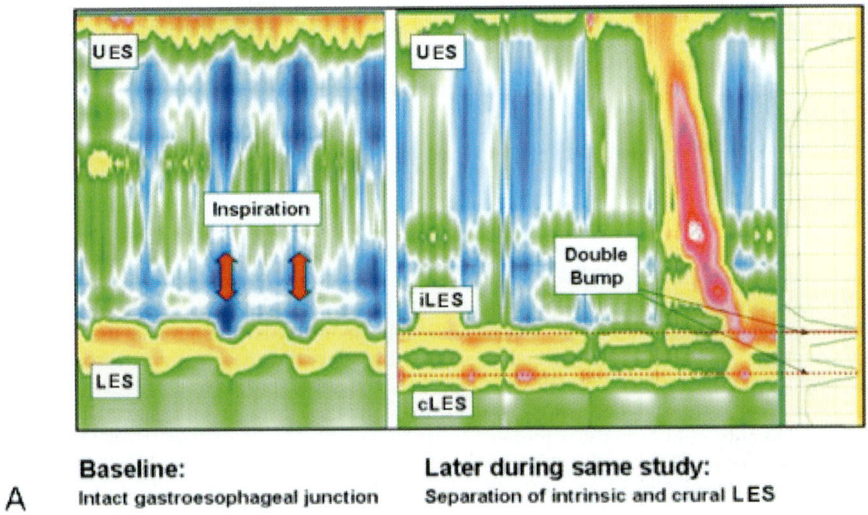

Figure 2. A. Contour plots of an individual patient at two points during a stationary HRM study. The left panel shows the gastroesophageal junction (GEJ) as a single high-pressure zone that rises and falls with respiration. The right panel shows spatial separation of the high-pressure zone into the intrinsic lower esophageal sphincter (iLES) and diaphragmatic crus (cLES) Partial relaxation of both components occurs during a dry swallow. The far right panel displays pressure measurements from the pharynx to the stomach at a single moment in time; “a virtual pull-through”. Note the typical “double bump” indicating the presence of a small hiatus hernia (~3 cm). (**See page 286**).

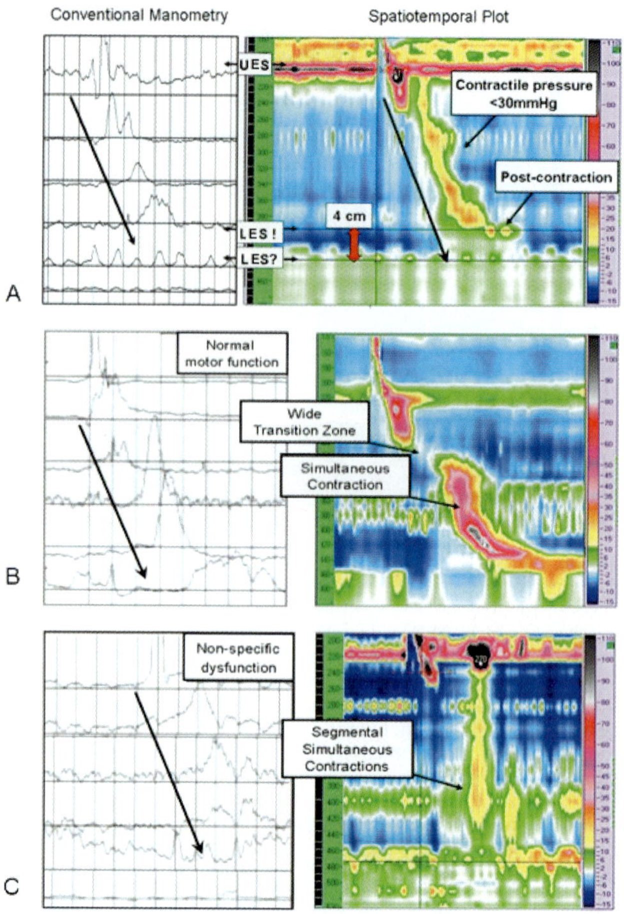

Figure 3. Three examples of conventional and high-resolution manometry in patients with reflux and/or regurgitation referred for physiological investigation. In each case conventional manometry was reported as "non-specific esophageal motor abnormality"; however HRM revealed distinct abnormalities of motor activity in each case with different effects on bolus transport. In the future HRM may guide specific management that addresses the underlying pathophysiology in such cases. **A.** This case illustrates two advantages of HRM. Firstly, the ease with which the appropriate position for pH studies can be found with HRM despite the presence of a large hiatus hernia and the absence of a high-pressure zone at the GEJ. Whereas it was not possible to locate the intrinsic LES by conventional manometry, HRM revealed the brief, weak LOS post-contraction. Secondly although this case would be labeled as "non-specific esophageal motor abnormality" or "ineffective esophageal function" on the basis of hypotensive contractile pressure, HRM reveals coordinated peristalsis from the UES to the LES indicating occlusive contraction and certainly consistent with bolus transport. **B.** Conventional manometry was essentially normal in this patient with longstanding dysphagia, chest pain and regurgitation; however HRM revealed focal abnormality of peristalsis with a wide proximal transition zone (pressure trough) and spasm in the mid-esophagus. Solid bolus escape was seen in this region on concurrent videofluoroscopy. **C.** Conventional manometry is not normal in this patient with "reflux symptoms", however the extent and nature of the motility disorder cannot be appreciated. The reason for this, clearly displayed by HRM, is that the esophageal spasm (simultaneous contraction) was not diffuse but segmental, occurring first in the mid- and then the distal-esophagus. LES function was normal and only mild reflux was present on pH studies (DeMeester score 21 (due to poor acid clearance)). Bolus escape and pendular movement of liquid barium was observed on concurrent videofluoroscopy. (Reproduced from [14]). (**See page 287**).

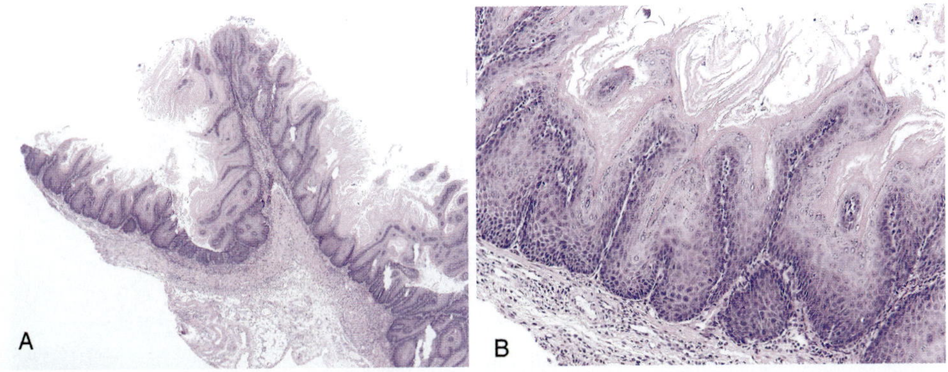

Figure 1. Squamous hyper-proliferative lesion induced by duodenal reflux displaying a papillary architecture (**A**) and prominent elongation of vascular papillae together with hyperkeratosis and parakeratosis (**B**). This epithelium was markedly acanthotic (thickened) compared to control animals. (**See page 318**).

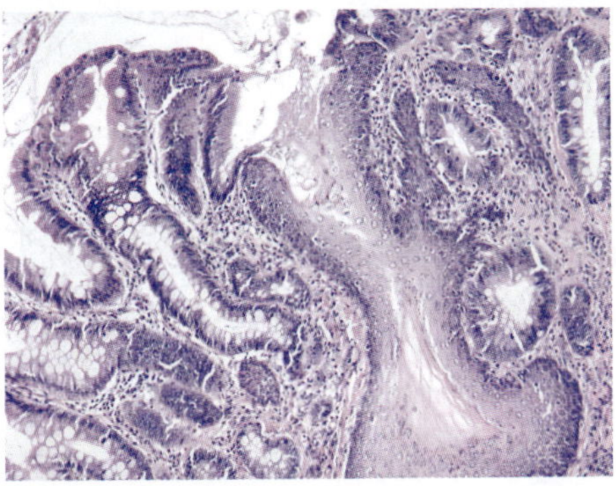

Figure 2. Lesion resembling Barrett's esophagus in duodenal reflux induced rat model. Patches of squamous mucosa are found on the right portion of this field and goblet cells are seen in the gland at the left. (**See page 318**).

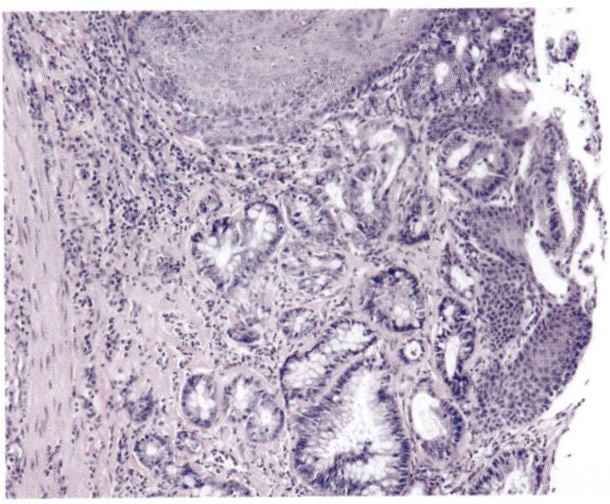

Figure 4. This lesion was found in a zone adjacent to a tumor and shows scattered glands having hyperchromatic nuclei, features similar to those found in dysplasia in Barrett's esophagus. (**See page 318**).

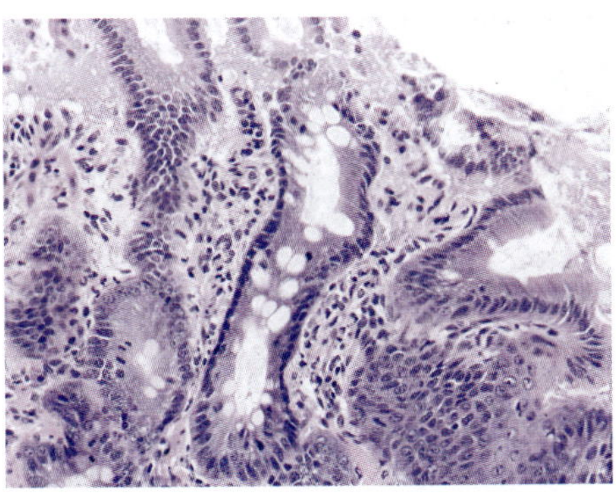

Figure 3. Higher-power view of the metaplastic focus depicted in *Figure 2*. Note the goblet cells in the gland in the center of the field. (**See page 318**).

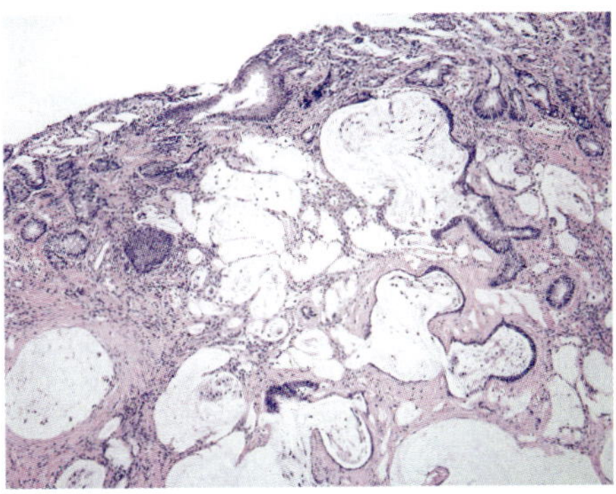

Figure 6. An adenocarcinoma-like lesion displaying an infiltrative growth pattern. (**See page 319**).

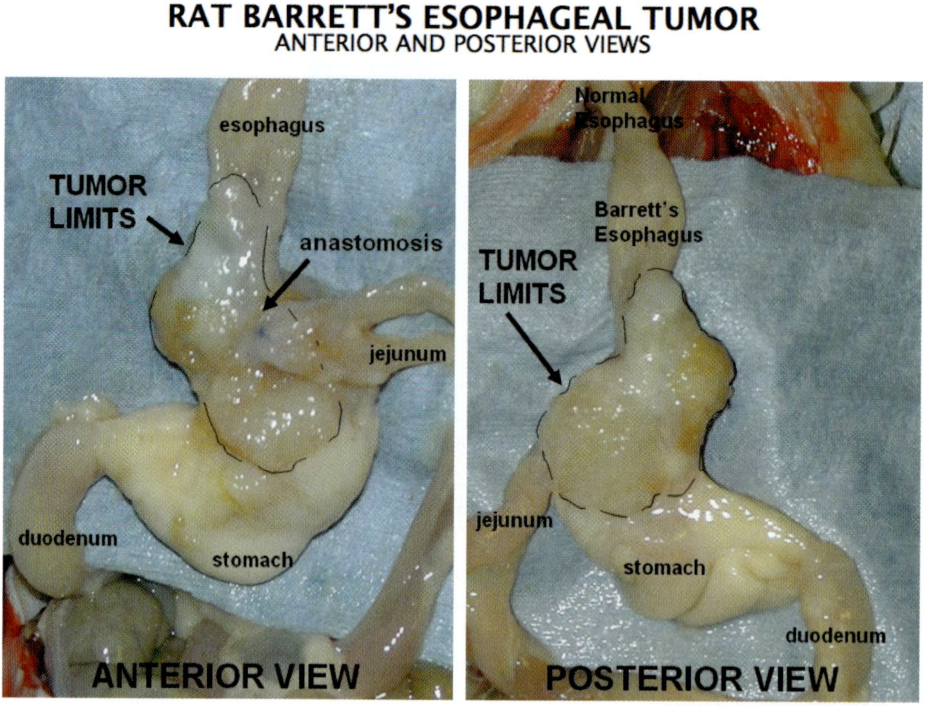

Figure 5. Gross dissections from animal models. (Courtesy of Dr, John Harmon). (**See page 319**).

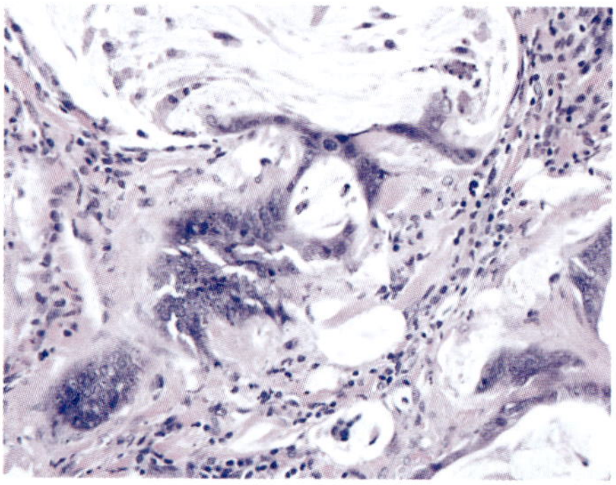

Figure 7. This adenocarcinoma-like lesion displays a dissecting growth pattern into surrounding connective tissue and an apparent tissue response. The proliferating nuclei appear enlarged and irregular. (**See page 319**).

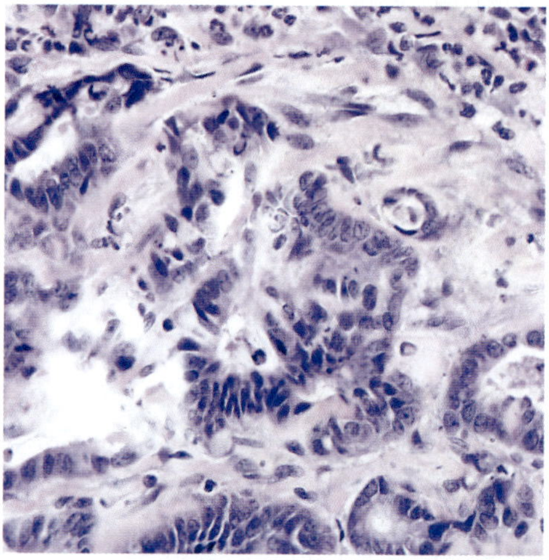

Figure 8. Another adenocarcinoma-like lesion displaying irregular nuclear contours and an apparent tissue response. (**See page 320**).

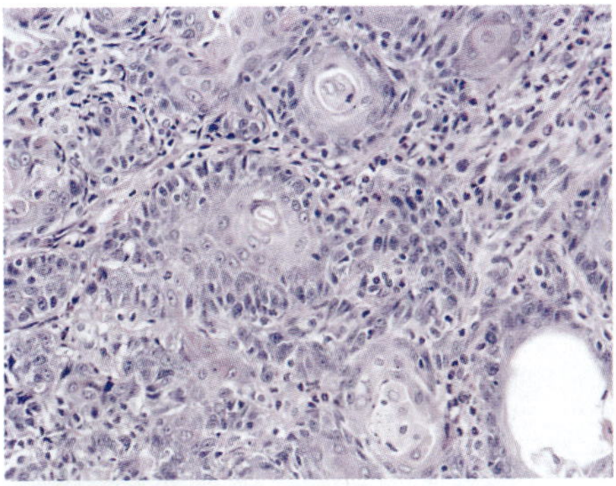

Figure 9. This tumor displays squamous differentiation, including keratinization and squamous "pearls". Some examples have adenosquamous features as well. (**See page 320**).

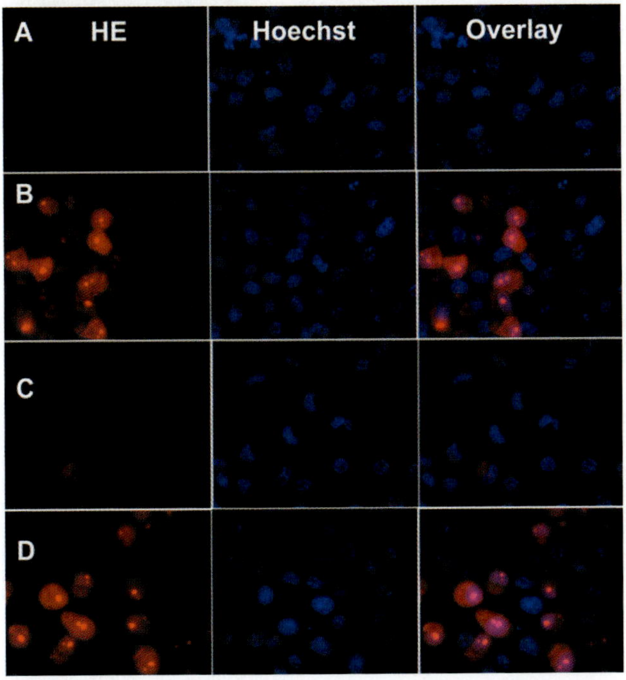

Figure 2. Oxidative stress in Seg-1 cells. Seg-1 cells were untreated (**A**) or exposed for 1 minute to pH 2 (**B**), 0.5 mM TDCA in neutral medium at pH 7.4 (**C**) or 0.5 mM TDCA in medium acidified to pH 2 (**D**), washed and stained with HE for 25 minutes and then with Hoechst 33342 for 5 minutes. The red signal represents oxidative damage (HE) while the blue signal represents nuclei (Hoechst 33342). (**See page 329**).

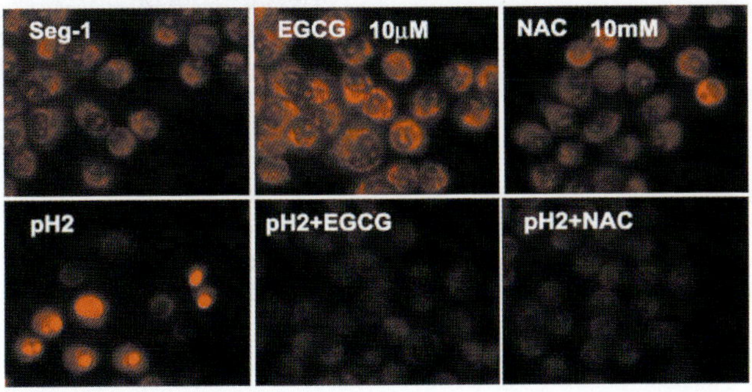

Figure 3. Oxidative stress induced in Seg-1 by pH 2 is inhibited by the pretreatment for 60 minutes with anti-oxidants such as EGCG or N-acetyl-cysteine (NAC). Red signal represents HE, a marker of oxidative stress. (**See page 330**).

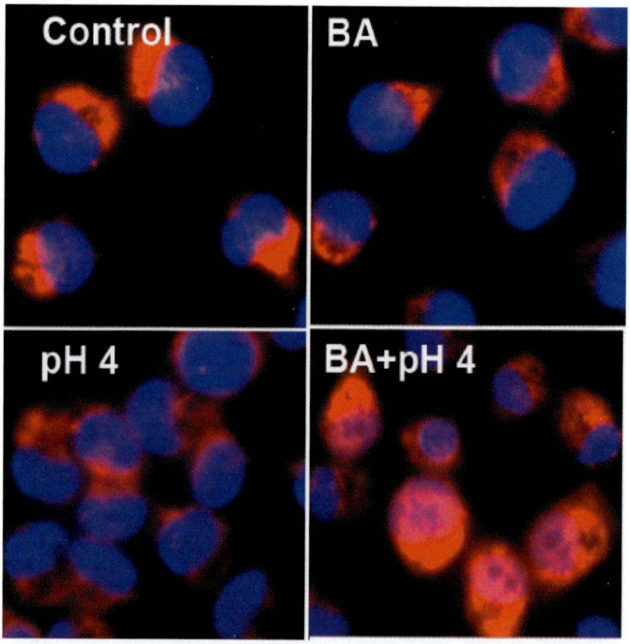

Figure 4. STAT3 translocation to the nucleus after 10 minutes treatment with 0.1 mM bile acid cocktail (BA) in acidified medium to pH4. The red signal represents STAT3, and the blue signal represents nucleus (DAPI staining). (**See page 331**).

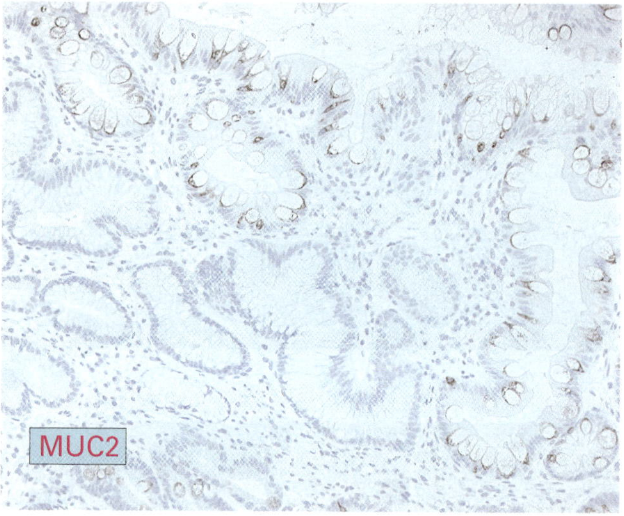

Figure 1. MUC6 which stains goblet cell mucin. (**See page 340**).

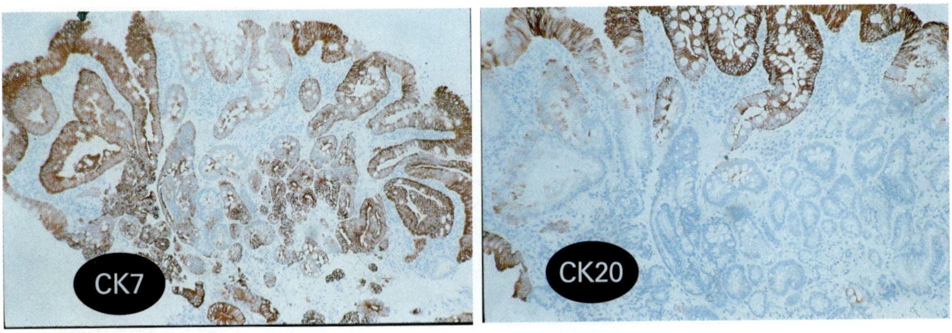

Figure 2. CK7 and CK20 in the "classical" cytokeratin pattern associated with Barrett's esophagus. a) CK7 stains both the surface and deep epithelium b) CK20 is limited to the superficial; part of the mucosa (**See page 340**).

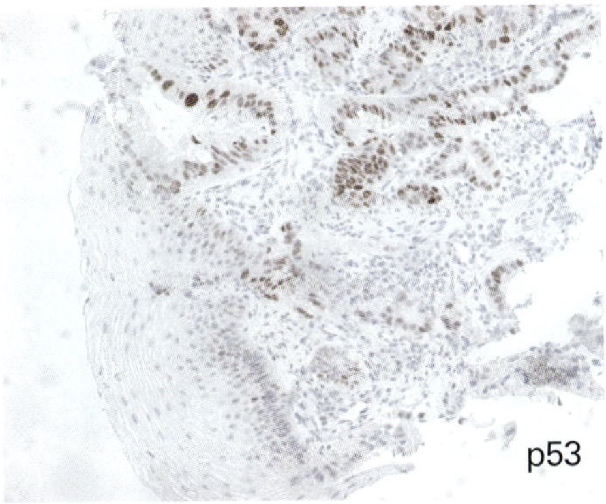

Figure 3. p53 immunostaining in a biopsy indefinite for dysplasia showing irregular immunoreactivity in the glandular mucosa extending close to the surface (left) adjacent to the squamous mucosa (left side). (**See page 341**).

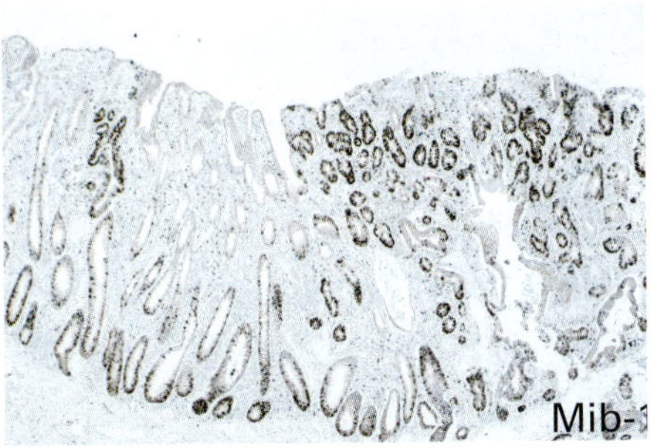

Figure 4. Mib-1 which stains the Ki-67 antigen associated with cell proliferation. On the left pits are stained primarily in the lower replicative zone except for one focus. However, on the right there is an area of dysplasia in which almost all of the cells are reactive virtually to the surface. Interestingly this virtually mirrored the p53 pattern of immunoreactivity. (**See page 342**).

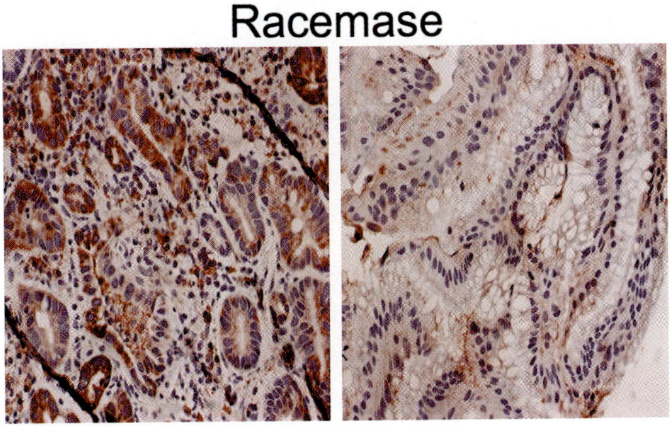

Figure 5. Racemase activity. Left shows strong staining in Barrett's esophagus with HGD and intramucosal carcinoma.) Right: non-dysplastic mucosa with minimal racemase immunoreactivity. (**See page 342**).

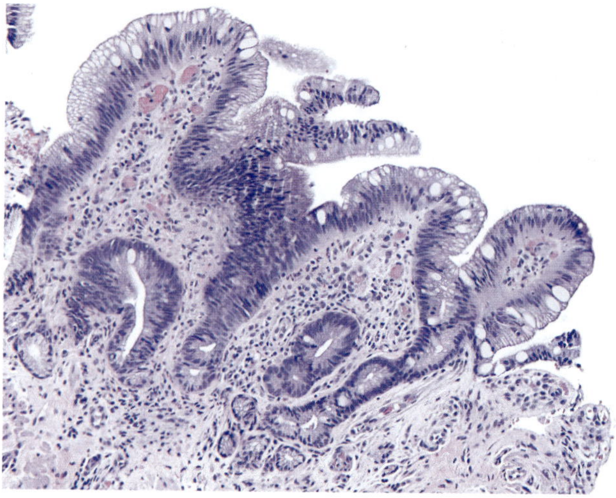

Figure 1. Indefinite for dysplasia. This focus has many intraepithelial neutrophils and merges with surrounding columnar epithelium that clearly lacks dysplasia. (**See page 347**).

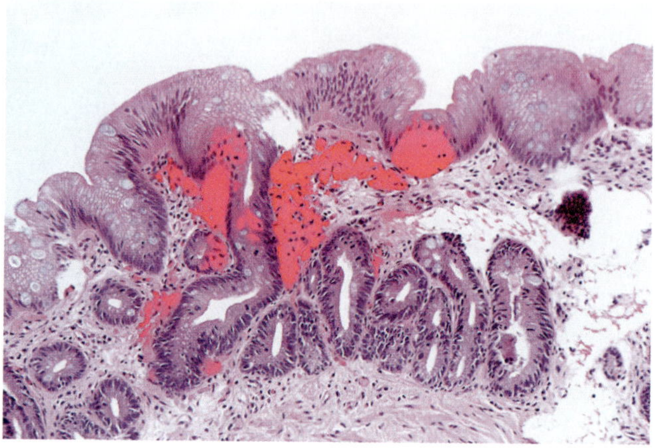

Figure 2. Indefinite for dysplasia. This focus lacks an abrupt transition with surrounding areas. (**See page 348**).

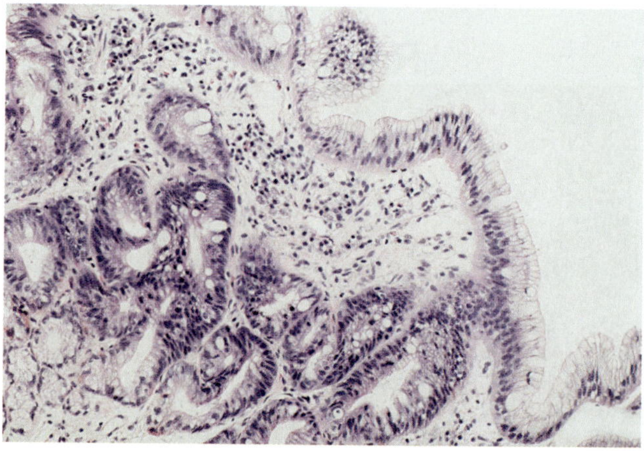

Figure 3. Indefinite for dysplasia. This lesion has too much surface maturation to be regarded as dysplastic. (**See page 348**).

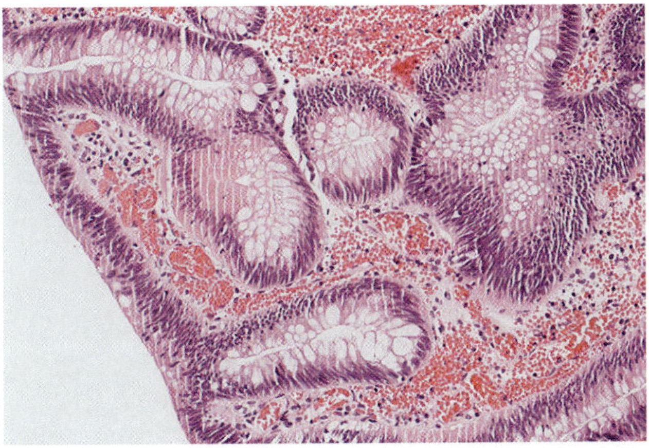

Figure 4. Occasional cases of low-grade dysplasia are indistinguishable from colon adenomas. (**See page 349**).

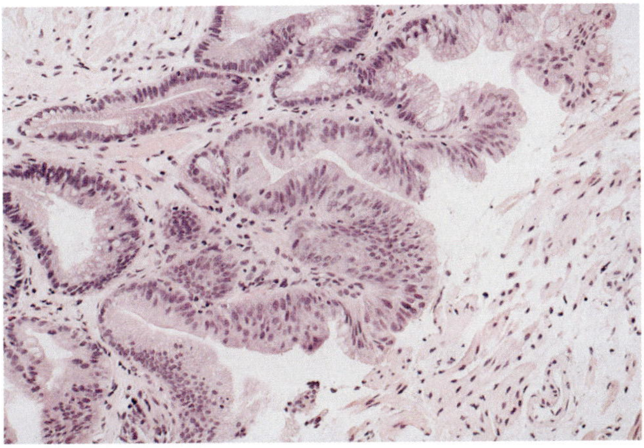

Figure 5. Another example of low-grade dysplasia. Changes extend to the epithelial surface and are homogeneous. (**See page 349**).

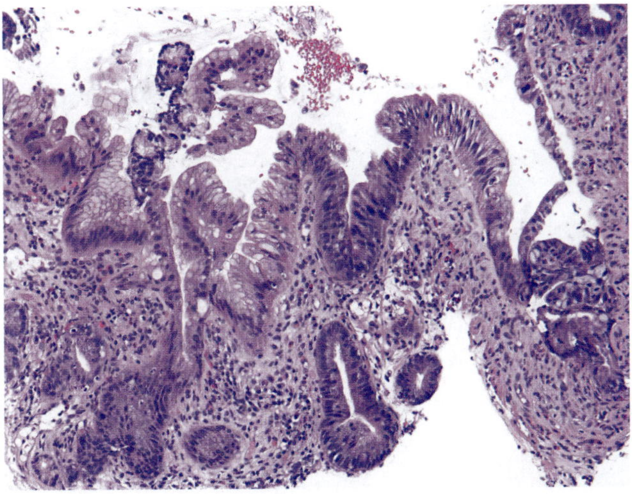

Figure 6. "Early" low-grade dysplasia. Note the abrupt transition between the dysplastic focus and the adjoining epithelium. (**See page 350**).

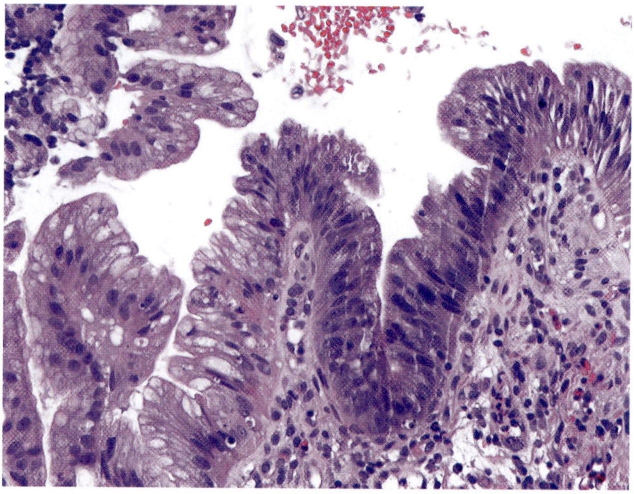

Figure 7. Higher magnification of the focus in *Figure 6*. (**See page 350**).

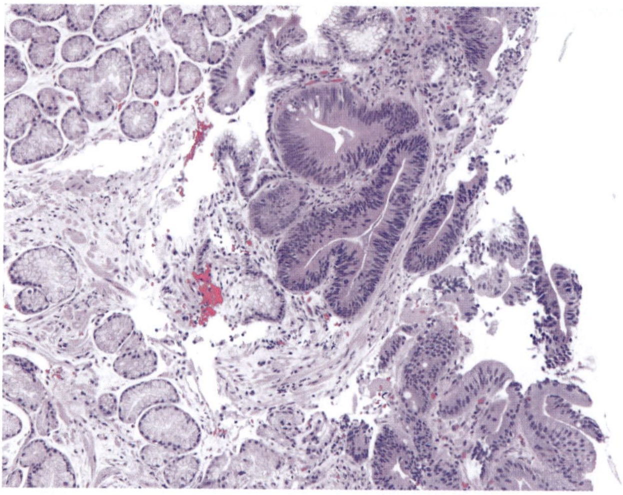

Figure 8. Another example of low-grade dysplasia in which the dysplastic focus is sharply distinct from surrounding tissue, appearing "clonal". (**See page 350**).

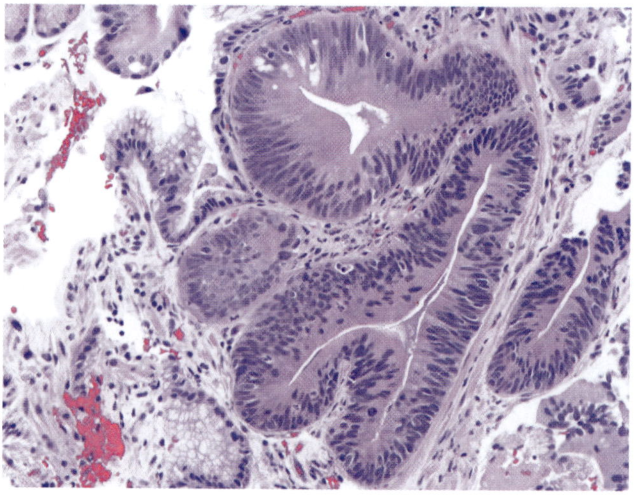

Figure 9. Higher magnification of Figure 8. (**See page 351**).

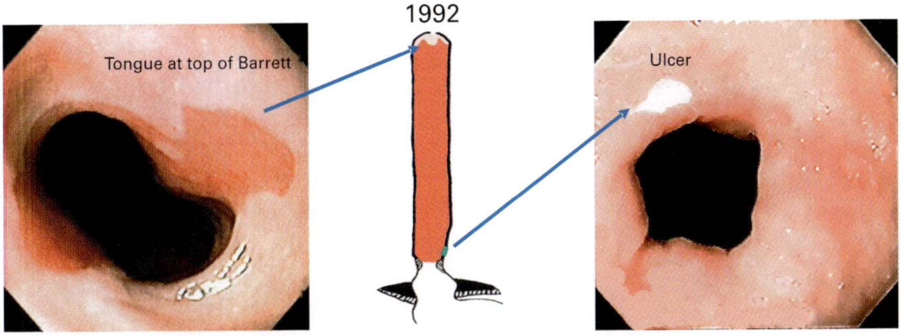

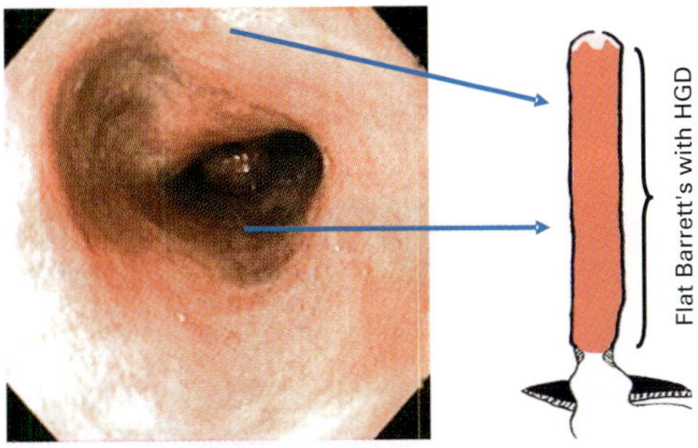

Figure 1. Perfectly flat Barrett's mucosa with HGD. (**See page 355**).

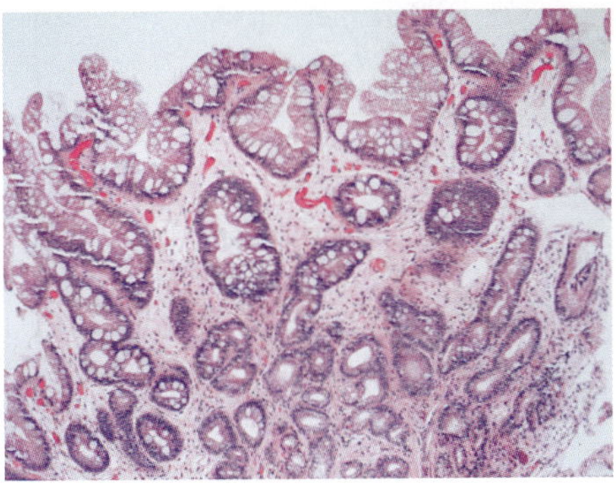

Figure 2. February 1994. (**See page 356**).

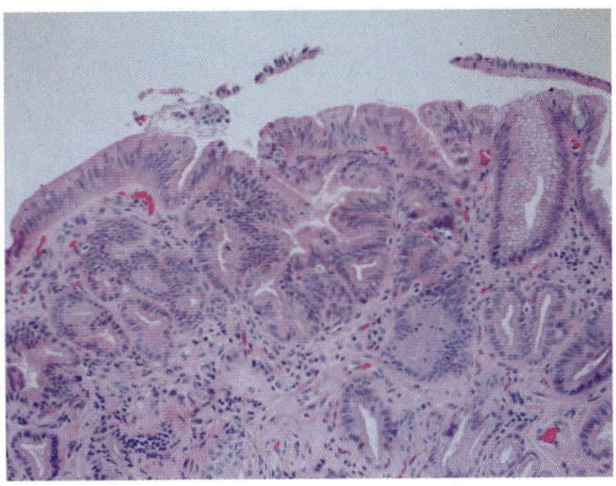

Figure 3. January 1996. (**See page 356**).

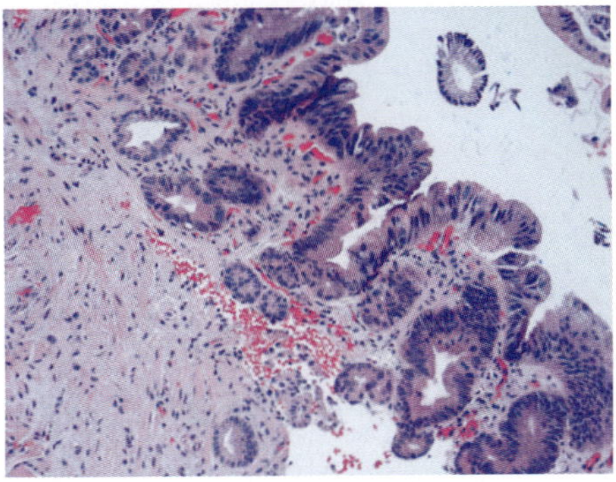

Figure 4. April 1999. (**See page 356**).

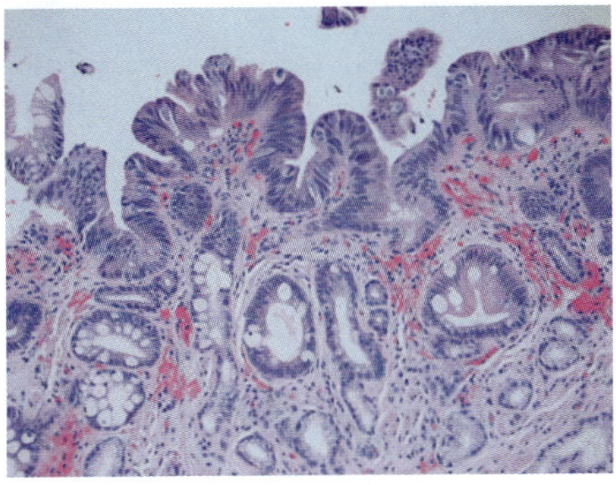

Figure 5. October 2002. (**See page 356**).

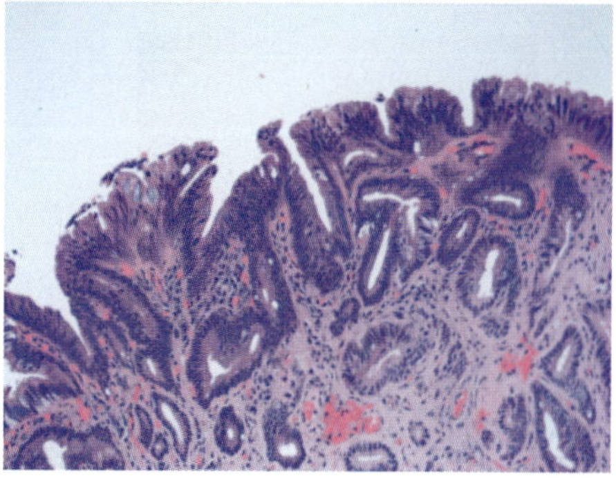

Figure 6. June 2005. (**See page 356**).

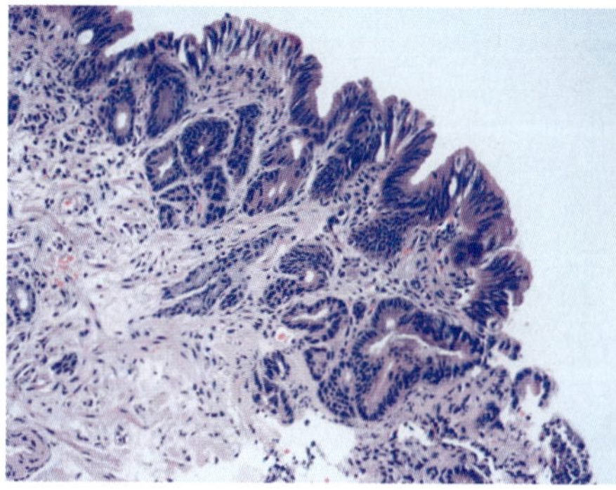

Figure 7. April 2006. (**See page 356**).

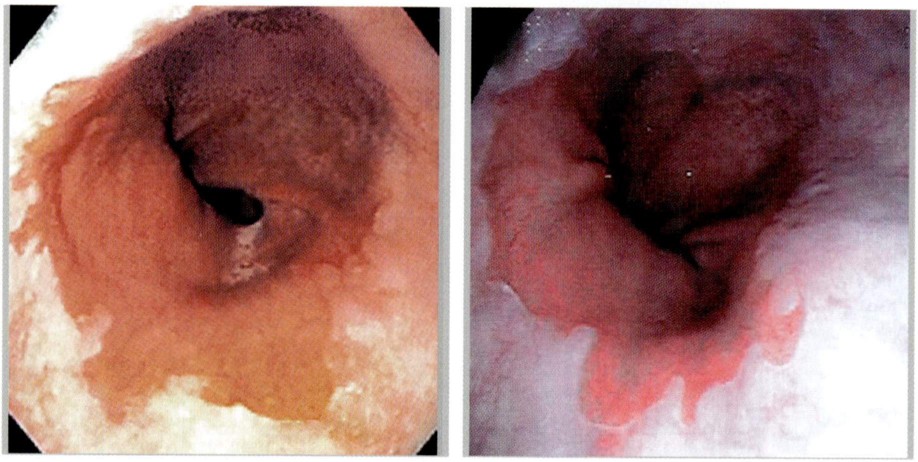

Figure 8. Perfectly flat Barrett's mucosa. (**See page 358**).

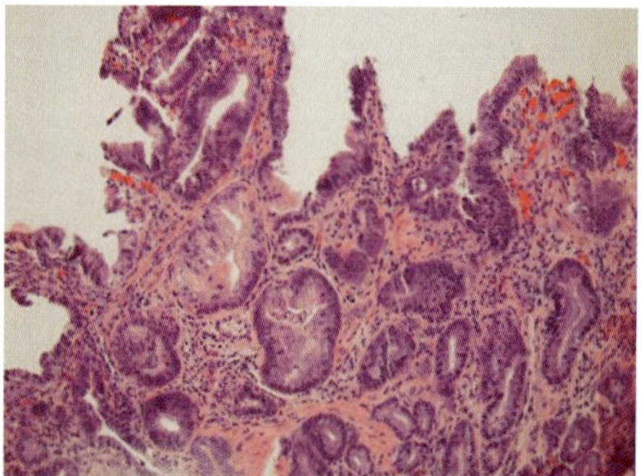

Figure 9. September 5, 2000. (**See page 358**).

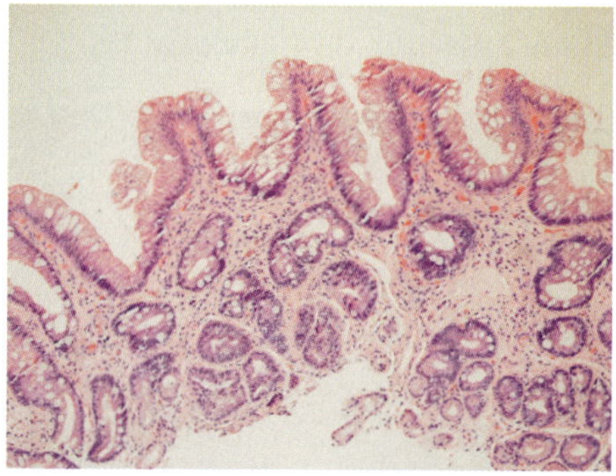

Figure 10. October 3, 2000. (**See page 358**).

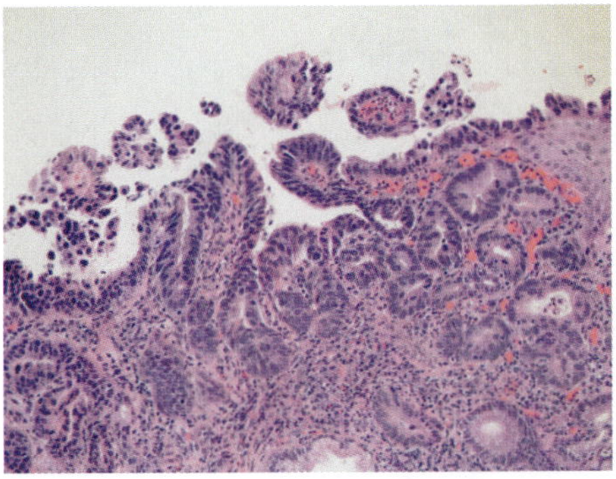

Figure 11. October 16, 2000. (**See page 358**).

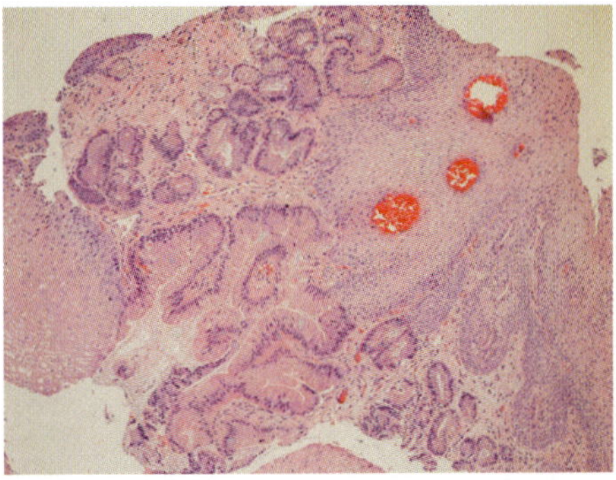

Figure 12. December 10, 2000. (**See page 358**).

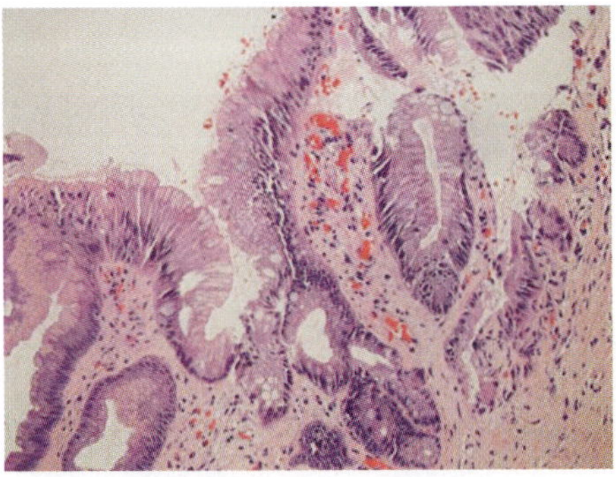

Figure 13. 2002. (**See page 359**).

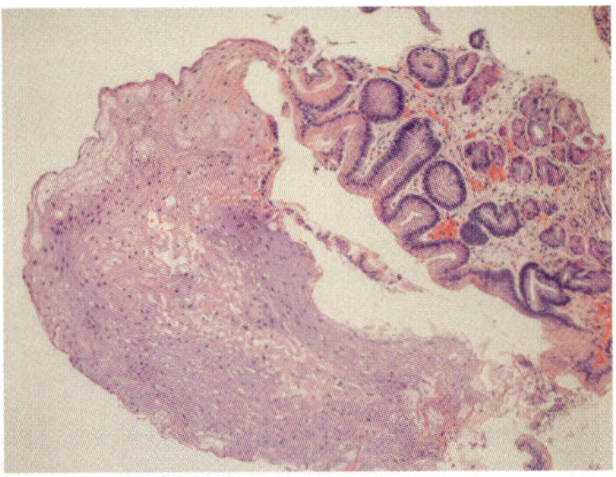

Figure 14. 2006. (**See page 359**).

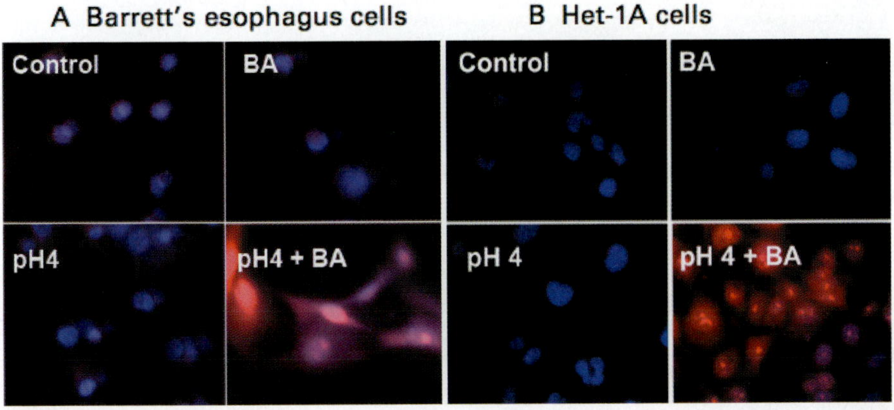

Figure 2. Detection of mitochondrial superoxide in Barrett's esophagus cells (CP-D cells) and HET-1A cells after treatment with pH 4 and/or bile acid cocktail by fluorescence microscopy. Cells were treated for 5 or 1.5 minutes, respectively, with control medium (pH 7.4), medium containing 0.1 mM bile acids cocktail (BA), medium acidified to pH 4 and medium acidified to pH 4 and containing bile acid cocktail. The cells were then washed and stained with 5 μM MitoSOX Red to measure mitochondrial superoxide (red signal). Cells were also stained with 10 μM Hoechst 3222 to visualize the nuclei (blue signal). Panel A shows Barrett's esophagus cells immortalized by hTERT transfection, panel B shows HET-1A cells. (**See page 403**).

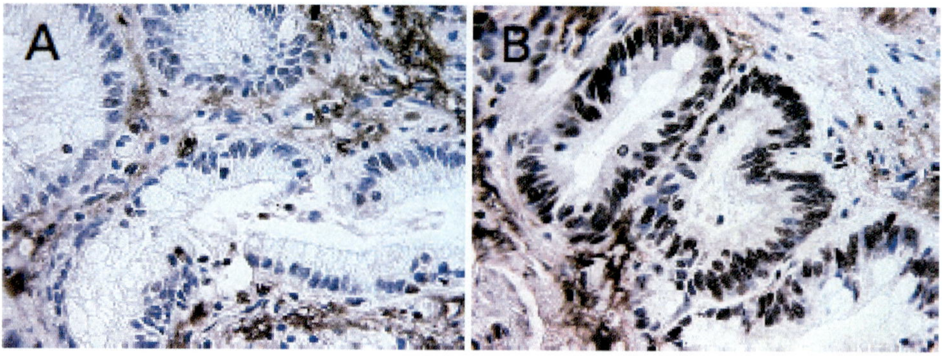

Figure 3. Immunohistochemical staining pattern of 8-OH-dG in Barrett's esophagus tissues. Barrett's esophagus biopsies were incubated in control medium **(A)** or medium acidified to pH 4 and supplemented with 0.5mM bile acid cocktail **(B)**. Note the intense nuclear staining of 8-OH-dG in epithelial cells after incubation with pH 4 and bile acid cocktail. (**See page 404**).

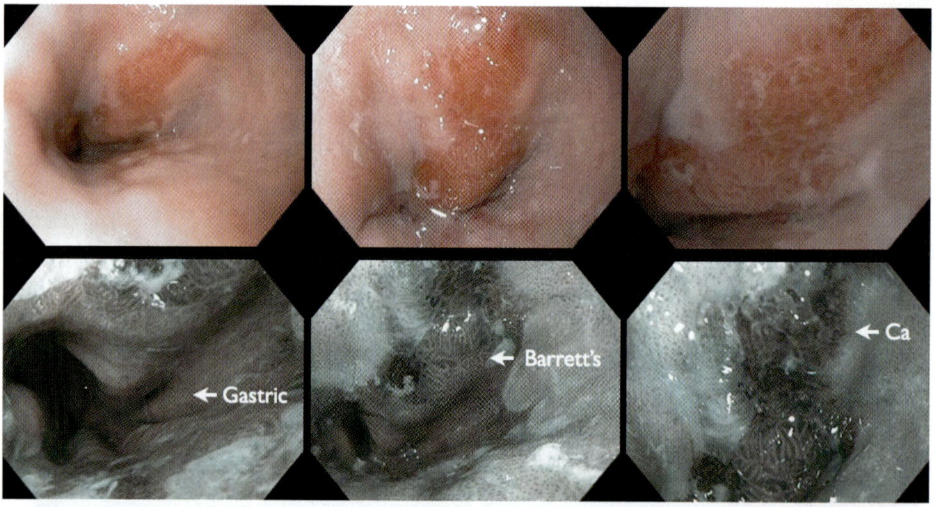

Figure 1. NBI in early esophageal adenocarcinoma (Courtesy: Roy Soetikno, MD, Stanford, CA). (**See page 400**).

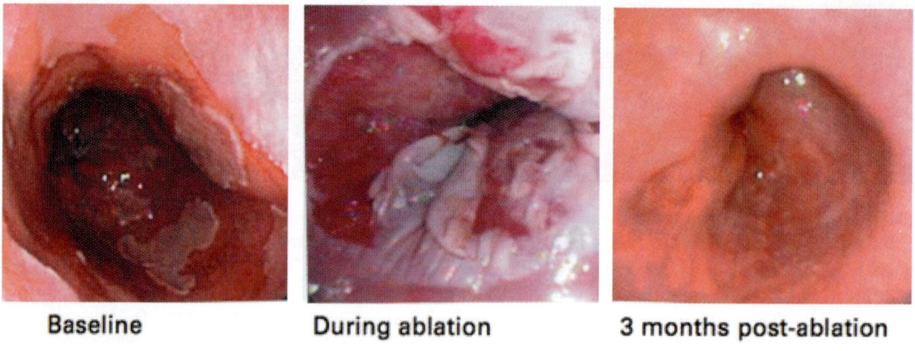

Figure 5. Long-segment Barrett's esophagus before, during and after radiofrequency ablation using Halo^{360} balloon system. (**See page 412**).

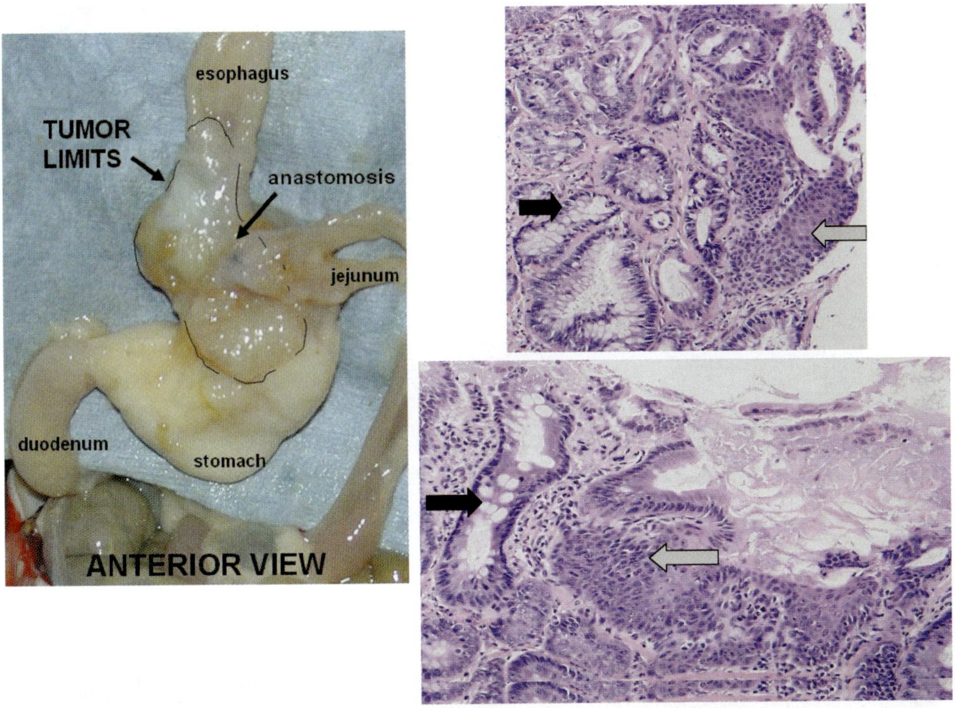

Figure 1. Surgical model of esophageal adenocarcinoma (grey arrow: normal squamous epithelium; black arrow: Barrett's columnar metaplasia with goblet cells). (**See page 426**).

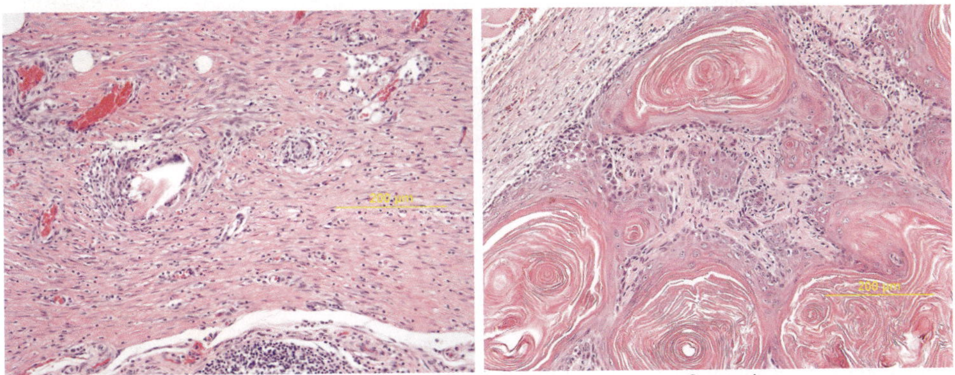

Figure 4. Histology of implantation site at day 14. (**See page 429**).

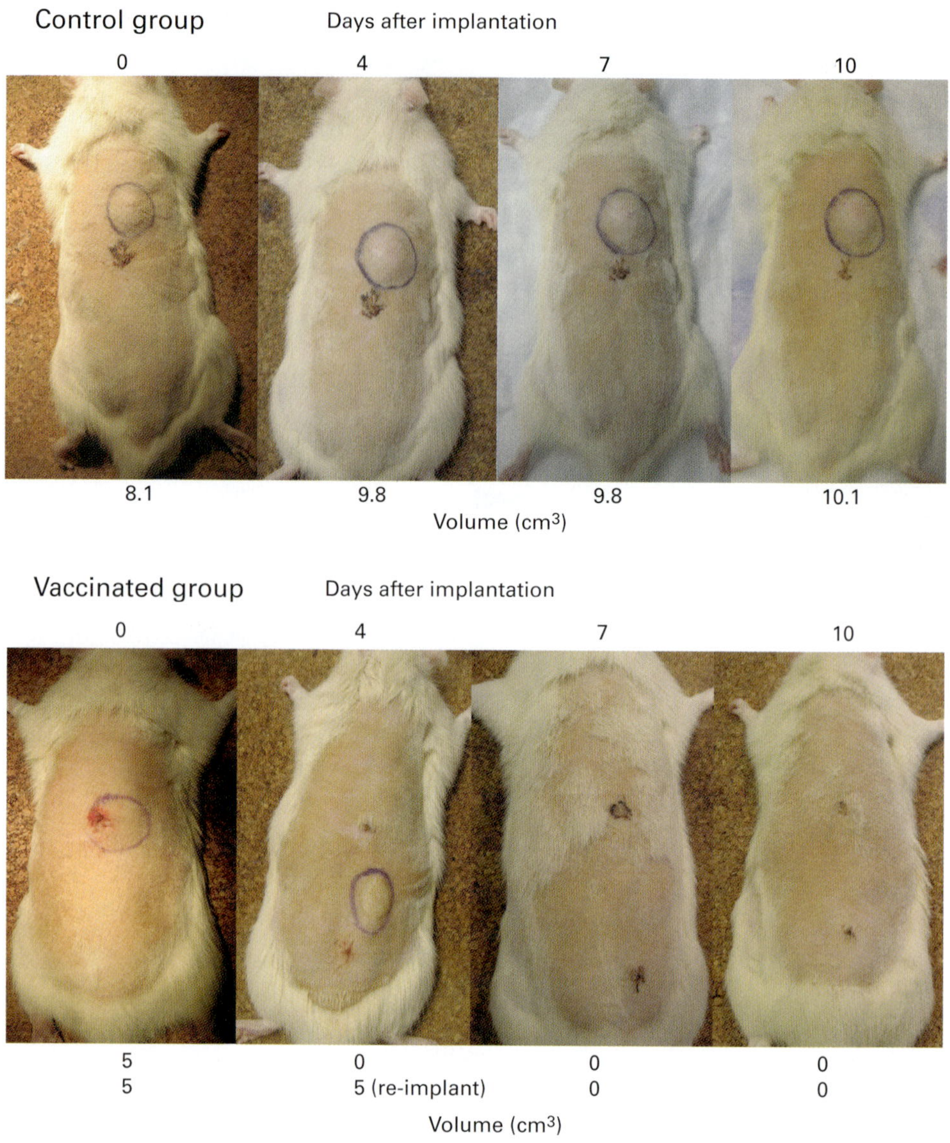

Figure 3. Tumor growth after vaccination. Note: for vaccinated group, animal #2 was re-implanted with tumor at a separate site at day 3 after initial tumor implantation (purple circle). (**See page 428**).).

Contents

Motor function of the foregut

Sensory function of the foregut

Brain - Foregut connections

Imaging techniques in the diagnosis of diseases of the foregut

Pathophysiology and controversies in gastroesophageal reflux disease

Controversies in Barrett's esophagus and Barrett's cancer

Esophageal dilation in esophageal strictures

Zenker's diverticula

Contributors

ABU-SUDOH ABADIA M., MD, Department of Gastroenterology, University Hospital Vall d'Hebron, Barcelona, Spain

APPELMAN H.D., MD, Professor of Surgical Pathology, The University of Michigan Hospitals, Ann Arbor, MI, USA

ARMENGOL MIRO J., MD, Profesor of Gastroenterology, University Hospital Vall' d'Hebron, Barcelona, Spain

AZIZ Q., MD, Professor of Gastroenterology GI Sciences, University of Manchester, Clinical Sciences Building, Hope Hospital, Salford, UK

BALDOLI D., MD, Department of Medical and Surgical Sciences, Section of General Surgery, University of Milan, IRCCS, Policlinico San Donato, Milan, Italy

BIANCANI P., PhD, Professor of Biochemistry, Rhode Island Hospital and Brown University, Providence, RI, USA

BOLLSCHWEILER E., MD, Department of Visceral and Vascular Surgery, University of Cologne, Cologne, Germany

BONA D., MD, Department of Medical and Surgical Sciences, Section of General Surgery, University of Milan, IRCCS, Policlinico San Donato, Milan, Italy

BONAVINA L., MD, Professor of Surgery, University of Milan, Department of Medical and Surgical Sciences, Policlinico San Donato, Milan, Italy

BOYCE H.W., MD, Professor of Medicine and Radiology, Joy McCann Culverhouse, University of South Florida Medical Center, Tampa, FL, USA

BRAVI I., MD, Department of Gastroenterology, University of Milan, IRCCS, Ospedale Maggiore Policlinico, Mangiagalli e Regina Elena, Milan, Italy

BROSSARD E., MD, Otolaryngology, Head and Neck Surgery, CHUV, Lausanne, Switzerland

BUTTAR N., MD, Barrett's Esophagus and GI Research Unit, Miles and Shirley Fiterman Center for Digestive Diseases, Mayo Clinic College of Medicine, Rochester, MN, USA

CANDELORO L., MD, Department of Clinical Sciences, University 'La Sapienza', Rome, Italy

CANTU P., MD, Department of Gastroenterology, University of Milan, IRCCS, Ospedale Maggiore Policlinico, Mangiagalli e Regina Elena, Milan, Italy

CAPARELLO C., MD, Department of Gastroenterology, University of Milan, IRCCS, Ospedale Maggiore Policlinico, Mangiagalli e Regina Elena, Milan, Italy

CASSIANI R.A., SLP, Department of Medicine, Faculty of Medicine of Ribeirao Preto, University of Sao Paulo, Brazil

CASSON A.G., MB, FRCSC, FACS, Professor of Surgery, University of Saskatchewan and Skaskaton Health Region, Royal University Hospital, Saskatoon, SK, Canada

CHAUDHURI D.N., MD, Department of Radiology and Nuclear Medicine, Eastern Virginia Medical School and VA Medical Center, Hampton, VA, and University of Texas Health Science Center and VA Medical Center, San Antonio, TX, USA

CHAUDHURI Tubin K., MD, FACNP, Professor of Radiology, University of Texas Health Science Center, San Antonio, TX, USA

CHAUDHURI Tapan K., MD, FACG, Professor of Radiology, Clinical Director, Nuclear Medicine, Eastern Virginia Medical School and VA Medical Center, Hampton, VA, USA

CHEJFEC G., MD, Professor of Pathology and Deputy Head Department of Pathology University of Illinois, College of Medicine, Chicago, IL, USA

CHEUNG TK, MD, Department of Medicine, University of Hong Kong, Hong Kong PR, China

CICALA M., MD, PhD, Professor of Gastroenterology, Department of Clinical Sciences, University 'La Sapienza', Rome, Italy.

CLAVE P., MD, PhD, Functional Investigations Unit, Department of Surgery, Hospital de Mataró, Consorci Sanitari del Maresme, Spain

CLEMONS N.J., PhD, Medical Research Centre Cancer Cell Unit, Hutchison-MRC Research Centre, Hills Road, Cambridge, UK

COLLARD J.-M., MD, PhD, Professor of Surgery, Unit of Upper GI Surgery, Louvain Medical School, Brussels, Belgium

CONTINI S., Department of Surgery, School of Medicine and Dentistry, University of Parma, Parma, Italy

COOK I.J.S., MD, FRACP, Professor of Medicine, Director, Department of Gastroenterology, St George Hospital, University of NSW, Sydney, Australia

DANTAS R.O., MD, Professor of Medicine, Faculty of Medicine of Ribeirão Preto, Brazil

DEMARS C., Barrett's Esophagus and GI Research Unit, Miles and Shirley Fiterman Center for Digestive Diseases, Mayo Clinic College of Medicine, Rochester, MN, USA

DEVAULT K.R., MD, Professor of Medicine, Chair, Gastroenterology and Hepatology, Mayo Clinic College of Medicine, Jacksonville, FL, USA

DOT BLACH J., MD, Department of Gastroenterology, University Hospital Vall d'Hebron, Barcelona, Spain

DREWES A.M., MD, PhD, DMSc, Center for Visceral Biomechanics and Pain, Department of Gastroenterology, Aalborg Hospital, Aalborg, Denmark

DVORAK K., MD, Ass Research Professor, Department of Cell Biology and Anatomy, College of Medicine, Arizona Cancer Center, The University of Arizona, Tucson, AZ, USA

ELIAKIM R., MD, Professor and Head Department of Gastroenterology, Rambam Health Care Center, Rappaport School of Medicine, Technion-Israel Institute of Technology, Haifa, Israel

EMERENZIANI S., MD, University 'La Sapienza', Rome, Italy

ESCHER A., MD, Department of Otolaryngology, Head and Neck Surgery, CHUV, Lausanne, Switzerland

FALK G.W., MD, MS, Professor of Medicine, Center for Swallowing and Esophageal Disorders, Department of Gastroenterology and Hepatology, Cleveland Clinic Foundation, Cleveland, OH, USA

FINK S., MD, Department of Radiology and Nuclear Medicine, Eastern Virginia Medical School and VA Medical Center, Hampton Virginia, and University of Texas Health Science Center and VA Medical Center, San Antonio, TX, USA

FITZGERALD R., MD, Medical Research Centre Cancer Cell Unit, Hutchison-MRC Research Centre, Hills Road, Cambridge, CB2 2XZ, UK

FORNARI F., MD, Centre for Gastroenterological Research, KU Leuven, Belgium

FOX M., MD, MA (Oxon), MRCP, Research Consultant, University Hospital Zurich, Zurich, Switzerland

GAREWAL H.S., MD, Professor of Medicine, Arizona Cancer Center, The University of Arizona, and Section of Hematology/Oncology, Southern Arizona Veteran's Affair Health Care System (SAVAHCS), Tucson, AZ, USA

GIBSON M., MD, Ass Professor of Medicine, Co-Leader Lung and Thoracic Malignancies Program, Department of Medicine University of Pittsburgh Cancer Institute, Pittsburgh, PA, USA

GODART B., MD, Department of Digestive Diseases and Nutrition, CHU Trousseau, Tours, France

GONCETTE R., MD, Unit of Radiology, Louvain Medical School, Brussels, Belgium

GOYAL R.K., MD, Mallinckrodt Professor of Medicine, VA Boston Healthcare System, Harvard Medical School, Boston, MA, USA

GREGERSEN H., MD, Dr m Sci, MPM, Professor of Medicine and Engineering, Center for Visceral Biomechanics and Pain, Aalborg Hospital, Aalborg, Denmark

GRIGOLON A., MD, Department of Gastroenterology, University of Milan, IRCCS, Ospedale Maggiore Policlinico, Mangiagalli e Regina Elena, Milan, Italy

GUTSCHOW C., MD, Department of Surgery, University of Cologne, Cologne, Germany

HABIB F.I., MD, Department of Clinical Sciences , University 'La Sapienza', Rome, Italy

HANNIG C., MD, Professor of Diagnostic Radiology Technical University of Munich, Klinikums rechts der Isar, Munich, Germany

HARNETT K.M., MD, Motility Research Laboratory, Rhode Island Hospital and Brown University, Providence, RI, USA

HEBBARD G.S., MD, Director of Gastroenterology, The Royal Melbourne Hospital, Melbourne, VI, Australia

HOBSON A.R., PhD, Clinical Scientist, Neurology & GI CEDD, Clinical Pharmacology and Discovery Medicine, GSK R&D Limited, New Frontiers Science Park, Harlow, Essex, UK

HOLSCHER A.H., MD, Professor of Surgery, Chairman Department of Visceral and Vascular Surgery, University of Cologne, Cologne, Germany

JADCHERLA S.R., MD, FRCPI, DCH, Associate Professor, Department of Pediatrics, Director, Neonatal and Infant Feeding Disorders Program, Columbus Children's Hospital & Research Institute, The Ohio State University College of Medicine and Public Health, Columbus, OH, USA

LAFACE L., MD, Department of Medical and Surgical Sciences, Section of General Surgery, University of Milan, IRCCS Policlinico San Donato, Milan, Italy

LAO O.B., MD, University of Washington, Department of Surgery, Seattle, WA, USA

LAO-SIRIEIX P., MD, Medical Research Centre Cancer Cell Unit, Hutchison-MRC Research Centre, Hills Road, Cambridge, UK

LEHMANN A., PhD, Associate Professor, Gastrointestinal Biology, Integrative Pharmacology, AstraZeneca R&D Mölndal, Mölndal, Sweden

LIGHTDALE C.J., MD, Professor of Clinical Medicine Columbia University, New York, NY, USA

MAJEWSKI M., MD, Gastroenterology Research Laboratory, Kansas University Medical Center, Kansas City, KS, USA

MALEKZADEH R., MD, Digestive Disease Research Center, Shariati Hospital, Tehran University of Medical Sciences, Tehran, Iran

MALFERTHEINER P., MD, Professor of Medicine, Department of Gastroenterology, Hepatology and Infectious Diseases, Otto-von-Guericke University, Magdeburg, Germany

MARTIN HARRIS B., PhD, CCC, SLP, Ass. Professor of Otolaryngology, Head and Neck Director MUSC, Trammel Institute for Voice and Swallowing, Medical University of South Carolina, Charleston, SC, USA

METMAN E.H., MD, Professor of Gastroenterology, Department of Digestive Diseases and Nutrition, CHU Trousseau, Tours, France

MILLER L.S., MD, Associate Professor of Medicine, Temple University Hospital, Philadelphia, PA, USA

MIWA K., MD, Director, Toyama Rosai Hospital, Uozu, Japan

MOKKALA V., MBBS, Barrett's Esophagus and GI Research Unit, Miles and Shirley Fiterman Center for Digestive Diseases, Mayo Clinic College of Medicine, Rochester, MN, USA

MOLTENI P., MD, Division of Gastroenterology, "L. Sacco" University Hospital, Milan, Italy

MONKEMULLER K., MD, Department of Gastroenterology, Hepatology and Infectious Diseases, Otto-von-Guericke University, Magdeburg, Germany

MONNIER P., MD, Professor and Head Department of Otolaryngology, Head and Neck Surgery, CHUV Lausanne, Switzerland

MONTGOMERY E., MD, Associate Professor of Pathology, Johns Hopkins Medical Institutions, Baltimore, MD, USA

NASSERI-MOGHADDAM S., MD, Digestive Disease Research Center, Shariati Hospital, Tehran University of Medical Sciences, Tehran, Iran

NEGREANU L., MD, Department of Digestive Diseases and Nutrition, CHU Trousseau, Tours, France

NEUHUBER W.L., MD, Professor of Anatomy Institute of Anatomy, University of Erlangen-Nürnberg, Erlangen, Germany

NEUMANN H., MD, Department of Gastroenterology, Hepatology and Infectious Diseases, Otto-von-Guericke University, Magdeburg, Germany

NILTON FELIX V., MD, Professor of Surgery, Sao Paulo University, Digestive Motility and Neurogastroenterology Lab, Sao Paulo, Brazil

OELSCHLAGER B.K., MD, Assistant Professor, Department of Surgery University of Washington School of Medicine, Seattle, WA, USA

ORLANDO R.C., MD, Professor of Medicine & Physiology, University of North Carolina at Chapel Hill, Chapel Hill, NC, USA

PACE F., MD, Professor of Gastroenterology-Hepatology, Division of Gastroenterology, "L. Sacco" University Hospital, Milan, Italy

PALLOTTA S., MD, Division of Gastroenterology, "L. Sacco" University Hospital, Milan, Italy

PANDOLFINO J.E., MD, Ass Professor of Medicine, Division Gastroenterology Hepatology, Northwestern University's Feinberg School of Medicine Chicago, IL, USA

PENAGINI R., MD, Professor of Gastroenterology, University of Milan, IRCCS, Ospedale Maggiore Policlinico, Mangiagalli e Regina Elena, Milan, Italy

PICON L., MD, Department of Digestive Diseases and Nutrition, CHU Trousseau, Tours, France

PIOTET E., MD, Department of Otolaryngology, Head and Neck Surgery, CHUV, Lausanne, Switzerland

POHL D., MD, Division of Gastroenterology and Hepatology, University Hospital Zurich, Switzerland

POKIESER P., MD, Department of Radiology, Medical University of Vienna, Austria

RIBOLSI M., MD, Division of Gastroenterology and Hepatology, University Hospital Zurich, Switzerland

RICHTER J.E., MD, FACP, FACG, Professor and Chairman Department of Medicine, Temple University, Philadelphia, PA, USA

RIDDELL R.H., MD, Professor of Laboratory Medicine and Pathobiology, University of Toronto and Mount Sinai Hospital, Toronto, ON, Canada

ROMAGNOLI R., MD, Unit of Upper GI Surgery, Louvain Medical School, Brussels, Belgium

SAINO G., MD, University of Milan, Department of Medical and Surgical Sciences, Section of General Surgery, Policlinico San Donato IRCCS, Milan, Italy

SAROSIEK I., MD, Gastroenterology Research Laboratory, Kansas University Medical Center, Kansas City, KS, USA

SAROSIEK J., MD, MD, PhD, FACG, Research Professor of Medicine, Director, Gastroenterology Research Laboratory, Kansas University Medical Center, Kansas City, KS, USA

SCARPIGNATO C., MD, DSc, PharmD, FRCP, FCP, FACG, Laboratory of Clinical Pharmacology, Department of Anatomy, Pharmacology & Forensic Sciences, School of Medicine and Dentistry, University of Parma, Parma, Italy

SCHARITZER M., MD, Department of Radiology, Medical University of Vienna, Austria

SCHINDLER A., MD, Department of Clinical Sciences "L. Sacco", University of Milan, Milan, Italy

SCHNELL T., MD, Department of Medicine, Hines Veterans Hospital, Hines, IL, USA

SHARMA A., MD, Ass Professor, Department of GI Sciences, University of Manchester, Clinical Sciences Building, Hope Hospital, Salford, UK

SIFRIM D MD, Ph.D, Centre for Gastroenterological Research KU Leuven, Belgium

SONTAG S. Department of Medicine, Hines Veterans Hospital, Hines, IL, USA

SONTAG S.J., MD Professor of Medicine Department of Medicine, Hines Veterans Hospital, Hines, IL, USA

STRAUMANN A., MD, Department of Gastroenterology, Kantonsspital Olten, Olten, Switzerland

TATUM R.P., MD, FACS, Ass Professor of Surgery, Department of Surgery, University of Washington Seattle, WA, USA

TIPNIS N.A., MD, Ass Professor, Department of Pediatrics, Medical College of Wisconsin, Milwaukee, WI, USA

TRIADAFILOPOULOS G., MD, Clinical Professor of Medicine, Division of Gastroenterology and Hepatology, Stanford University School of Medicine, Stanford, CA, USA

TUTUIAN R., MD, Head, Gastrointestinal Function Unit, Division of Gastroenterology and Hepatology, University Hospital Zurich, Switzerland

WONG B.C.Y., MD, Department of Medicine, University of Hong Kong, Hong Kong, PR China

WONG R.K.H., MD, Professor of Medicine, Chief Gastroenterology, Walter Reed Army Medical Center, Washington, DC, USA

WUTTGE HANNIG A.C., MD, Radiology Preactice, Nuclear Medicine, Munich, Germany

Motor function of the foregut

Endoscopic morphology of the esophagogastric junction

C.J. Lightdale (New York)

The Paris Workshop

The endoscopic morphology of the esophagogastric junction (EGJ) has been a surprisingly difficult and controversial area, which has increased in importance with the rising incidence of Barrett's esophagus and adenocarcinomas of the distal esophagus and EGJ [1]. On December 11-12, 2004, a remarkable Workshop on Columnar Metaplasia in the Esophagus and the Esophagogastric Junction was held in Paris, France [2]. A detailed review of the endoscopic morphology of the EGJ was carried out among the assembled international experts, and the following discussion is largely based on the insights and conclusions that emerged from the Workshop.

The esophagogastric junction at endoscopy

During upper gastrointestinal endoscopy, there has been controversy as to how to measure and detect the precise place where the esophagus ends and the stomach begins. The EGJ is the point where the tubular esophagus joins the stomach at the cardia, with an angle between the opened esophagus and the gastric greater curvature. The distal esophagus and the gastric cardia constitute the esophagogastric region, with specific anatomical landmarks. There are no conspicuous proximal and distal limits of the EGJ region. The landmarks are selected arbitrarily, with 2 cm above and below the actual junction a frequent standard. In clinical practice, the upper digestive tract is often classified into 3 sectors: esophagus, EGJ, and stomach [2].

The squamocolumnar junction (the Z-line)

The esophagus is lined by stratified squamous epithelium. The stomach is lined by secretory and absorptive columnar epithelium. The squamocolumnar junction (SCJ) is also called the Z-line (Z from Zero or the point where the squamous epithelial lining ends); its appearance is that of a serrated line. In the normal situation this conspicuous landmark is located in the distal esophagus, just above the pinch of the diaphragm and the dilated lumen of the stomach. In endoscopic vision, the normal esophagus is covered with a pale, pearl-gray-pink, epithelium with an even surface, while the stomach lining has a darker red velvety epithelium with crests and pits.

The top of the gastric folds and the esophageal palisade vessels

Important markers of the EGJ are the proximal extent of the gastric folds and the distal extent of the esophageal longitudinal palisade vessels [2] The top of the gastric folds must be measured with the lumen partially decompressed, as air distension can flatten and markedly alter the location of the top of the gastric folds. On the other hand, the palisade vessels in the distal 2 cm of the esophagus, at the level of the lower esophageal sphincter, are best seen with the lumen distended by air insufflation. The top of the gastric folds has been widely used as the endoscopic marker for the EGJ in the West, whereas in Japan the distal extent of the palisade vessels has been more commonly used to determine the EGJ.

Gastric islands in the distal esophagus

At the EGJ, the columnar epithelium of the cardia and the squamous epithelium of the esophagus frequently overlap. The length of this overlap varies in the range of 5 to 10 mm. At endoscopy, islands of gastric mucosa can often be found in the distal 1 cm segment of the esophagus. These islands correspond to more superficial areas of the epithelial overlap, and protrude slightly through the covering squamous epithelium. The islands often have a yellowish color. These islands of cardia mucosa remain unstained after endoscopic dye spraying with iodine-potassium iodide solution (e.g., Lugol's solution), and are easily discerned using narrow band imaging.

The diaphragmatic pinch

At endoscopy, another landmark of the EGJ is the passage of the distal esophagus through the diaphragmatic hiatus into the abdomen. This area can usually be discerned as a slight constriction or "pinch" of the lumen, which is normally visible just distal to the Z-line. The proximal extent of the gastric folds is normally within 1 cm of the diaphragmatic pinch. Thus, 3 markers of the normal EDJ are the diaphragmatic pinch, the top of the gastric folds, and the SCJ (Z-line). These anatomical landmarks should be routinely looked for and recorded, as measured in centimeter distances from the incisor teeth during withdrawal of the endoscope from the stomach with the lumen partially decompressed [3].

The three major endoscopic landmarks at the esophagogastric junction

In the normal situation the three landmarks are is close vicinity: The top of the gastric folds is localized in the abdomen just below the diaphragmatic pinch, and the SCJ is usually within a few millimeters of the top of the folds. A minimal sliding (a few millimeters) of the EGJ just above the diaphragmatic pinch is frequent, without formation of a hiatal hernia. Precise analyses have been conducted on anatomical specimens to assess the distance between the Z-line and the junction of the esophagus and stomach, Distances ranged on average from 11 mm in Western countries to just 3 mm in Japan [4,5]. Measuring such small distances at endoscopy in the living patient is difficult and not reliable.

The landmarks in hiatal hernia

In the presence of a hiatal hernia, the relationship of the 3 endoscopic landmarks of the EGJ has changed owing to the intrathoracic localization of the proximal stomach. The Z-line and the top of the gastric folds are now moved above or proximal to the diaphragmatic pinch. While most patients with Barrett's esophagus have a hiatal hernia, a hiatal hernia itself should never be confused with Barrett's esophagus. In patients with a hiatal hernia and no Barrett's esophagus, the Z-line is still within 1 cm of the top of the gastric folds.

The landmarks in Barrett's esophagus

In Barrett's esophagus, a segment of the esophagus is lined with metaplastic columnar epithelium, and the SCJ is displaced proximally above the top of the gastric folds. This is relatively easy to discern at endoscopy in segments greater than 1 cm, but can be difficult for small tongue-like extensions less than 1 cm. The length of the metaplastic columnar segment is the distance between the Z-line and the top of the gastric folds. The reliability of the evaluation depends on the precision of the determination of the EGJ at endoscopy. A segment of columnar metaplasia in the esophagus is classified as "long" (> 3 cm) or "short" (< 3 cm) [6-8].

The Prague C&M classification

Recently a new classification of the endoscopic extent of Barrett's esophagus has been introduced and validated, the Prague C&M classification [9] Using this classification system, the endoscopist assesses the distance between the upper end of the gastric folds and the upper margin of the segment with circumferential metaplasia (the "C" value in the classification). The maximal proximal extent of the metaplastic segment is also estimated (the "M" value in the classification) .The evaluation has proven reproducible between operators when the segment reaches at least 1 cm in length (RC = 0.72). However, for very short segments of Barrett's esophagus (less than 1 cm) the system was not reliable (RC = 0.22). Even among experts [9]. The value of chromoendoscopy, magnification endoscopy, and other new optical methods to detect very short segments of columnar lined esophagus are current areas of endoscopic research [2].

Gastric folds *versus* palisade vessels

Whether to use the distal extent of the palisade vessels (as often practiced in Japan), or the top of the gastric folds (as used in the West) to mark the EGJ has been an unresolved issue [2]. In a recent study from Japan, 84 endoscopists reviewed photographs from 30 patients with Barrett's esophagus. The initial interobserver agreement (K) for the distal end of the esophagus was only 0.14 (unacceptable). After training in the Prague C&M classification using the top of the gastric folds rather than the distal extent of the palisade vessels as the EGJ, the result significantly improved to K = 0.35 [10].

Squamous islands in Barrett's esophagus

Squamous islands are common in Barrett's esophagus, and squamous islands in the columnar mucosa at the EGJ may also serve as markers of the distal end of the esophagus. At the EGJ, in very short segments of columnar metaplasia, the presence of very small squamous islands just below the slightly displaced SCJ confirms that the zone explored corresponds to the esophagus. Reports of squamous epithelium in the cardia following ablation therapy for Barrett's esophagus more likely reflect a wrong assessment of the true location of the EGJ, as it seems unlikely that squamous epithelium truly extends into the stomach [11,12].

Conclusions

In summary, the EGJ is best identified at endoscopy using three endoscopic landmarks: the SCJ or Z-line, the top of the gastric folds with the lumen partially decompressed of air, and the diaphragmatic pinch. A hiatal hernia is seen when the top of the gastric folds is seen proximal to the diaphragmatic pinch. The columnar-lined esophagus or Barrett's esophagus is diagnosed when the Z-line is above the top of the gastric folds, with the caveat that very short segments of Barrett's esophagus, less than 1.0 cm in length, can be difficult to diagnose with certainty.

For the endoscopist, the EGJ and the Z-line have a special, challenging natural beauty (*Table I*). Endoscopic evaluation of the EGJ has become of increasing importance with the rising incidence of Barrett's esophagus and esophageal adenocarcinoma.

Table I. The line called Z by C.J. Lightdale, MD with apologies to Joyce Kilmer (1886-1918).

I think that I shall never see
A line as lovely as the Z.
A line, the proper British said,
Should be (for zero) Zed, instead.
A line that in its Zig-Zag direction,
Mimes the letter Z to perfection.
A line upon whose craggy shore,
Waves of acid pound and pour.
A line where squamous and columnar dance,
And Barrett's metaplasia may advance.
Fools can do endoscopy,
But only God can make the Z.

References

1. Pohl H, Welch HG. The role of overdiagnosis and reclassification in the marked increase of esophageal adenocarcinoma incidence. J Natl Cancer Inst 2005;97:142-6.
2. Paris Workshop on Columnar metaplasia in the esophagus and the esophagogastric junction. Paris, France, December 11-12, 2004. Endoscopy 2005;37:879-920.
3. Sharma P, McQuaid K, Dent J, et al. A critical review of the diagnosis and management of Barrett's esophagus: the AGA Chicago Workshop. Gastroenterology 2004;127:310-30.
4. Bombeck CT, Dillard DH, Nyhus LM. Muscular anatomy of the gastroesophageal junction and role of phrenoesophageal ligament; autopsy study of sphincter mechanism. Ann Surg 1966 ;164:643-54.

5. Takubo K, Arai T, Sawabe M, et al. Structures of the normal esophagus and Barrett's esophagus. Esophagus 2003;1:37-47.
6. Falk GW. Barrett's esophagus. Gastroenterology 2002;122:1569-91.
7. Shaheen NJ. .Advances in Barrett's esophagus and esophageal adenocarcinoma. Gastroenterology 2005;128:1554-66.
8. Jankowski JA, Harrison RF, Perry I, et al. Barrett's metaplasia. Lancet 2000;356:2079-85.
9. Sharma P, Dent J, Armstrong D, et al. The development and validation of an endoscopic grading system for Barrett's esophagus: the Prague C&M criteria. Gastroenterology 2006;131:1392-9.
10. Amano Y, Ishimura N, Furuta K, et al. Which landmark results in a more consistent diagnosis of Barrett's esophagus, the gastric folds or the palisade vessels? Gastrointest Endosc 2006;64:206-11.
11. Fass R, Sampliner RE. Extension of squamous epithelium into the proximal stomach: a newly recognized mucosal abnormality. Endoscopy 2000;32:27-32.
12. Wallner B, Sylvan A. Janunger KG, et al. Immunohistochemical markers for Barrett's esophagus and associations to esophageal Z-line appearance. Scand J Gastroenterol 2001;15:886-89.

Where is the gastroesophageal pH step-up under fasting conditions and following a meal?

J.E. Pandolfino (Chicago)

The acid environment at the esophagogastric junction (EGJ) has garnered considerable interest in recent years following the description of the "acid pocket" by Fletcher *et al.* in 2001 [1]. Using pH catheter pull through data from 40 dyspeptic patients, they reported that a "pocket" of acid existed at the EGJ after meals and that this "pocket" escaped the normal buffering effect of that same meal. This explained the otherwise paradoxical finding on dual probe esophageal and gastric pH monitoring of greater pH values in the stomach compared to the esophagus during post-prandial reflux. An additional finding reported by Fletcher *et al.* was that the "acid pocket" extended almost 2 cm proximal to the squamocolumnar junction (SCJ) after a meal.

Since the initial report of the "acid pocket", two studies have assessed acid exposure close to the SCJ and confirmed that it is significantly greater than when measured using conventional electrode placement. Fletcher *et al.* used endo-clips to secure a four-channel pH catheter to the esophageal mucosa and reported that acid exposure was 6 fold greater 0.5 cm proximal to the SCJ compared to a 5.5 cm proximal position [2]. Our group also reported significant increases in acid exposure 1 cm proximal to the SCJ compared to 6 cm proximal using Bravo™ pH capsules attached to the mucosa, especially in the post-prandial period [3]. However, neither of these studies explored the mechanism behind distal esophageal acid exposure; specifically, whether it was secondary to the distal sphincter splaying open secondary to gastric distention enveloping an "acid pocket" [1] or a remnant of previous brief reflux events.

To better understand the acid environment surrounding the SCJ, we performed a pH electrode pull-through with a clip placed at the SCJ that could be identified with concurrent fluoroscopy and high-resolution manometry permitting localization of the margins of the sphincteric region of the EGJ. Our results support that the pH step-up occurred uniformly at or below the SCJ in asymptomatic controls regardless of position or meal state (*Figure 1*).

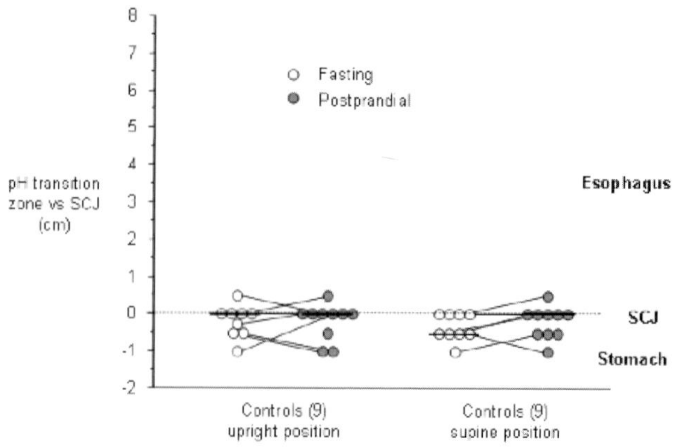

Figure 1. Position of pH step up before and after a standardized meal in controls. The position is referenced to 0 which correlates to the clip at the SCJ.

In contrast, the pH step-up extended above the SCJ in gastroesophageal reflux disease (GERD) patients and this was exaggerated in the post-prandial state and also in the supine position (*Figure 2*). However, this occurred in the context of an intact EGJ high-pressure zone. These findings suggest that in the GERD patients, although the pH transition point may extend above the SCJ it is more likely in the form of an acid film coating the mucosa rather than a "pocket" of acidic fluid. Furthermore, the observation that in some GERD patients the pH transition point was well above the EGJ high-pressure zone supports the contention that this was likely the remnant of a reflux event (*Figure 3*).

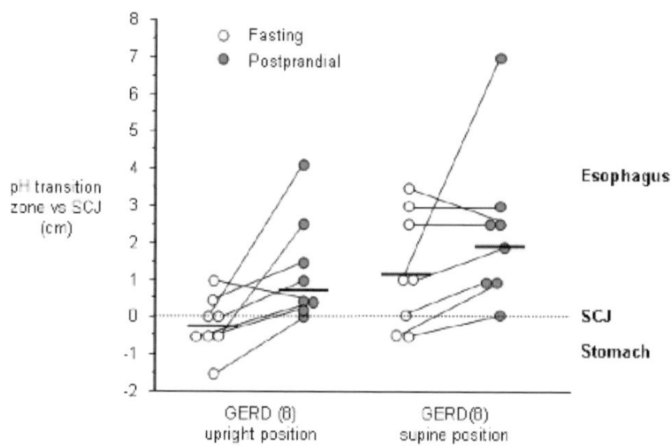

Figure 2. Position of pH step up before and after a standardized meal in GERD patients. The position is referenced to 0 which correlates to the clip at the SCJ.

In asymptomatic controls, the pH step-up occurs at or just distal to the SCJ, while in the GERD patients it extended into and even across the EGJ high-pressure zone. However, even in the case of GERD patients, this occurred in the context of a contracted sphincter suggesting to us that it is not an extension of a "pocket" of fluid sitting below the EGJ. The ultimate mechanism causing the pH step-up to occur above the SCJ and LES in GERD patients remains to be determined but the observation that it was most pronounced in patients with overt hiatal hernias suggests it may be related to mechanical distortion of the EGJ or poorly cleared reflux events.

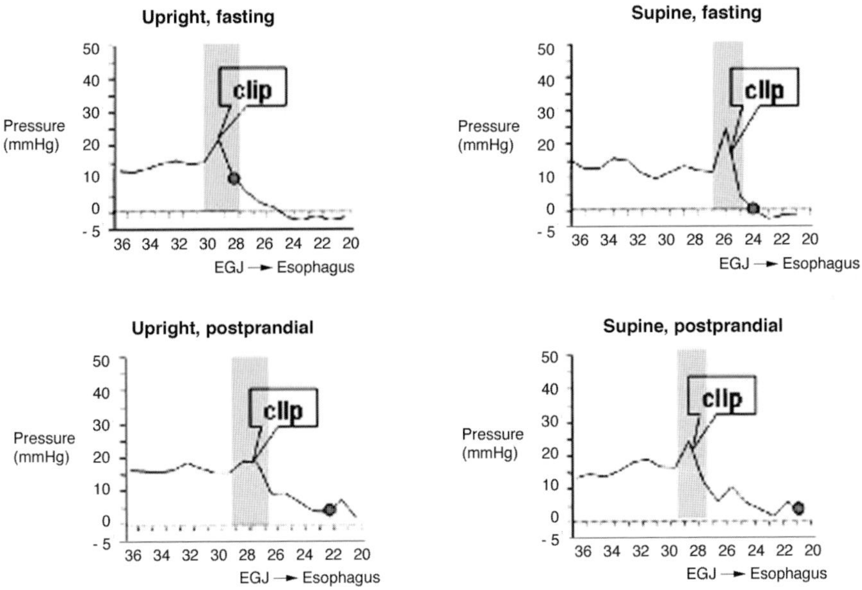

Figure 3. Representative examples of manometric data from a GERD patient illustrating the relative positions of the SCJ, proximal pH transition point (gray dot), and the EGJ high pressure zone (shaded band) during fasting and the post-prandial state in both postures. Note that the pH transition point occurs well below the upper margin of the EGJ high-pressure zone in the control subject but proximal to the SCJ in the GERD patient in every condition except fasting upright. Also note that, despite the proximal pH transition point being localized proximal to the EGJ high pressure zone in the GERD patient, the EGJ is intact and intraesophageal pressure is less than intragastric pressure suggesting no free communication between these spaces.

References

1. Fletcher J, Wirz A, Young J, Vallance R, McColl KE. Unbuffered highly acidic gastric juice exists at the gastroesophageal junction after a meal. Gastroenterology 2001;121:775-83.
2. Fletcher J, Wirz A, Henry E, McColl KE. Studies of acid exposure immediately above the gastro-oesophageal squamocolumnar junction: evidence of short segment reflux. Gut 2004;53:168-73.

Where, and what, are the three (or four) components of the distal esophageal high-pressure zone?

L. Miller (Philadelphia)

The high-pressure zone at the gastroesophageal junction (GEJ) regulates the flow of food from the esophagus into the stomach and acts as an antireflux barrier to gastric contents that are composed of acid, pepsin, food byproducts and bile. Several structures at the esophagogastric junction (EGJ) are important in maintaining an antireflux barrier. The intrinsic muscles of the distal esophagus (lower esophageal sphincter – LES) and proximal stomach (gastric sling fiber/clasp fiber complex) constitute the internal mechanism of the high-pressure zone, and the crural diaphragm constitutes the external mechanism. The phrenoesophageal ligament anchors the distal esophagus to the crural diaphragm [1,2].

Resting (baseline) intraluminal pressure at the EGJ is a measure of the strength of the antireflux barrier. Since the lower esophageal sphincter, gastric sling fiber/clasp fiber complex and the crural diaphragm are anatomically superimposed in normal individuals; intraluminal pressure is due to the combination of all of these muscles. Distinguishing the individual components of the distal esophageal high pressure zone is important because it emphasizes the individual contribution of each structure to the antireflux barrier and makes clear which components are defective in gastroesophageal reflux disease (GERD).

Until now, it has not been possible to accurately separate the GEJ high-pressure zone into its component parts and to study the mechanical properties of these components individually and as a group. The anatomic and physiologic relationships between the three components of the GEJ high-pressure zone, (the LES, the crural diaphragm and the gastric sling fiber/clasp fiber complex) were evaluated using simultaneous ultrasound and manometry (*Figure 1*) with pharmacologic manipulation during respiration in the following series of studies.

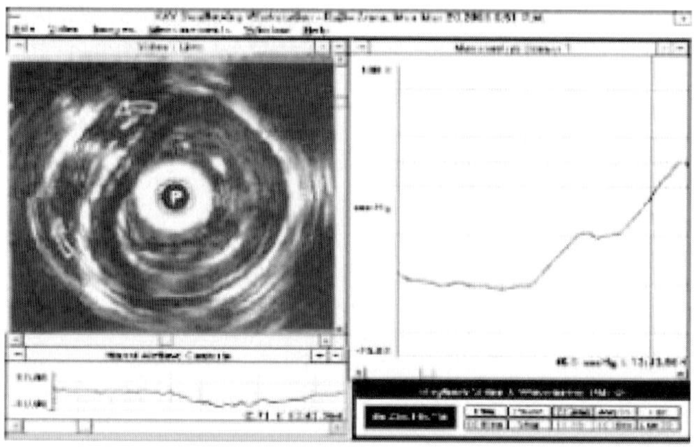

Figure 1. Picture showing the ultrasound image and the corresponding manometric pressure (46.0 mmHg). Note that the ultrasound image on the left is occurring at the time, indicated by the vertical line, as the manometry tracing on the right. This allows synchronization of the ultrasound image with the pressure generated by the muscles in that image.

Use of simultaneous ultrasound and manometry to isolate the LES, crural diaphragm and gastric sling fiber/clasp fiber complex in normal control subjects using simultaneous ultrasound and manometry during pharmacologic attenuation of the smooth muscle components (LES and gastric sling fiber/clasp fiber complex) [3].

High-frequency ultrasound was co-localized with manometric pressure in 15 healthy volunteers during breath holding in inspiration and expiration with a machine pull-through of a simultaneous ultrasound and manometry catheter assembly from the stomach into the thoracic esophagus at a constant velocity. Pullthroughs were repeated before and after intravenous administration of atropine to attenuate the pressure from intrinsic sphincter components (LES and gastric sling fiber/clasp fiber complex). The inferior margin of the right crural diaphragm and the initiation of the pull-through (pull-through start position) were used as axial spatial references. The difference between subtractions of the pre-atropine minus the post-atropine pressure profiles (the intrinsic sphincter components) displayed two distinct peaks in both inspiration and expiration, roughly 1.5-1.6 cm apart. The distal peak represents the gastric sling fiber/clasp fiber pressure profile while the proximal peak represents the intrinsic LES pressure profile (*Figure 2*). By superimposing the three pressure curves, (pre-atropine, post-atropine and the pre minus the post-atropine subtraction curve) it was possible to separate and study each of the components of the GEJ high-pressure zone individually and as an overlapping group for the first time.

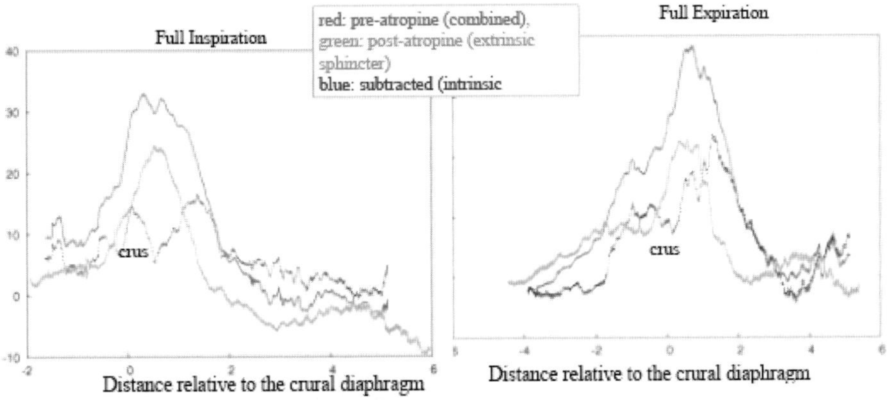

Figure 2. The combined high-pressure zone and its extrinsic and intrinsic components for both the full inspiration (FI on left) and full expiration respiratory (FE on right) states in 15 normal control subjects. The red line represents the pre-atropine pressure curve (combined external and internal sphincters). The green line represents the post-atropine pressure curve (the extrinsic sphincter). The blue line represents the pre-atropine minus the post-atropine subtraction curve (the intrinsic sphincter components). Note that in both the subtraction curves (full inspiration and full expiration) there are two peaks. The distal peak represents the gastric sling fiber/clasp fiber complex and the proximal curve represents the LES. (See page IX for colour figure).

Using this technique it was found that each component moved with respect to each of the other components during respiration. Specifically, it was found that the crus muscle moved proximally 1.95 cm between inspiration and expiration, with a 200% increase in the length of the high-pressure zone with expiration. The inferior margin of the right crus muscle was found to be at the inferior margin of the post-atropine high pressure zone in both full inspiration and full expiration and extended superiorly 1.83 cm during full inspiration and 1.73 cm during full expiration to cover the GEJ high pressure zone thus defining the external sphincter and indicating that the width of the crural diaphragm remained constant. The difference between the pre-minus the post-atropine subtraction curves (internal sphincter components) displayed two peaks in full inspiration and full expiration (*Figure 2*). In full inspiration, the proximal peak extended above the external sphincter (crural diaphragm) while the lower peak straddled the external sphincter. In full expiration, the external sphincter shifted superiorly relative to the two-peaked internal sphincter to overlap the proximal internal sphincter peak, while the lower internal sphincter peak shifted distally relative to the crus muscle. The gastric sling fiber/clasp fiber complex, crural diaphragm and intrinsic LES contributed approximately 13%, 62% and 25% to the GEJ high-pressure zone pressure profile during inspiration and 20%, 39% and 44% during expiration respectively as measured by the area under the pressure curves. In summary, this study localized each component of the GEJ high-pressure zone spatially with respect to each of the other components, determined what percent each component contributed to the antireflux barrier at the GEJ high-pressure zone, determined how each component moved with respect to each of the other components during respiration, defined the width of the crural diaphragm and the width of each of the intrinsic sphincter components both anatomically and physiologically and determined that the gastric sling fiber/clasp fiber complex and the intrinsic LES separate during expiration.

Simultaneous ultrasound and manometry during pharmacologic paralysis of the crural-diaphragm allows spatial localization of the two components of the intrinsic GEJ high-pressure zone (the LES and gastric sling fiber/clasp fiber complex) [4].
The results of the above study were confirmed and extended by pharmacologically paralyzing the crural diaphragm (the external sphincter rather than the internal sphincter as in the study above) in order to define the components of the intrinsic GEJ high-pressure zone. Seven normal control patients undergoing general anesthesia for non-esophageal surgery were evaluated by placing a simultaneous ultrasound/manometry probe into the stomach. Cis-atracurium was given to paralyze the crural diaphragm. The probe was withdrawn at a constant velocity of 5 mm/sec and ultrasound images and pressure tracings were recorded simultaneously during inspiratory and expiratory pause on the ventilator. Ensemble averaging of the pressure curves was plotted against the geographic location of the beginning of the crural diaphragm as in the study above. Tracings were compared to normal subjects who were evaluated with and without atropine ablation of the intrinsic components of the GEJ high-pressure zone. In the normal volunteers, the difference between the pre-atropine and post-atropine pressure curves (the intrinsic sphincter components) displayed the two peaks already described. The ensemble averaging of the seven patients undergoing crural diaphragm paralysis demonstrated residual pressure profiles from the intrinsic sphincter components. The same two peaks, in the same geographic location with respect to the crural diaphragm, imaged on ultrasound, were seen during crural diaphragm paralysis as were seen on the atropine subtraction curves in the 15 normal volunteers in the prior study (*Figure 3*). It was concluded that skeletal muscle paralysis of the crural diaphragm allowed spatial localization of the two intrinsic GEJ high-pressure zone sphincter components (the LES and the gastric sling fiber/clasp fiber complex). These results were consistent with localization of the individual sphincter components using smooth muscle attenuation of the intrinsic components with atropine (above). The distal intrinsic high-pressure zone component represents the gastric sling fiber/clasp fiber complex while the proximal component represents the intrinsic LES.

Pharmacologic augmentation of the intrinsic sphincter components to isolate the LES and the gastric sling fibers/clasp fiber complex [5].
In a third confirmatory study the anatomic and physiologic relationships between the components of the GEJ high-pressure zone were evaluated using pharmacologic augmentation of the intrinsic high-pressure zone components. The intrinsic and extrinsic

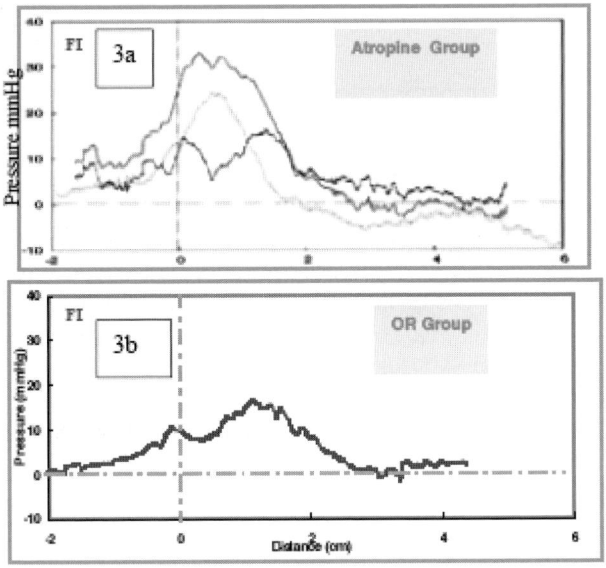

Figure 3. a. This graphs show the ensemble averaging of the normal control group who were evaluated pre- and post-atropine. **b.** This graphs show the ensemble averaging of seven patients undergoing crural diaphragm paralysis (OR group). This graph represents the residual pressure profiles only from the intrinsic sphincter components. Comparing these curves with the normal control atropine group pressure curves in blue, the same two peaks in both full inspiration) is demonstrated at the same relative geographic location with respect to the right crural diaphragm. Therefore, the results from crural diaphragm paralysis are consistent with localization of the intrinsic esophageal sphincter components using smooth muscle ablation with atropine in normal control subjects. The distal peaks represent the pressure profile from the gastric sling fiber/clasp fiber complex while the proximal peaks represent the pressure profile from the intrinsic LES. (See page IX for colour figure).

sphincters of the GEJ high-pressure zone were evaluated using simultaneous ultrasound and manometry with pharmacologic augmentation of the intrinsic (smooth muscle) high-pressure zone components in 14 healthy volunteers. Pull-throughs were repeated before and after oral administration of 100 mg of bethanechol to increase the pressure from the intrinsic (smooth muscle) high-pressure zone components. As in the prior studies, the inferior margin of the right leaf of the right crural diaphragm was used as a spatial reference. The difference between subtraction curves of the post-bethanechol minus the pre-bethanechol pressure profiles (the intrinsic sphincter components) displayed two distinct peaks in both inspiration and expiration. The distal peak once again represented the gastric sling fiber/clasp fiber pressure profile while the proximal peak represented the intrinsic LES pressure profile (*Figure 4*). By superimposing these pressure curves, it was once again possible to study each and separate out all of the individual components of the GEJ high-pressure zone. In conclusion, using simultaneous ultrasound and manometry along with pharmacologic augmentation of the intrinsic (smooth muscle) high-pressure zone components, the GEJ high-pressure zone can be divided into its three component parts, the intrinsic LES, the crural diaphragm and the gastric sling fiber/clasp fiber complex. These individual components were localized spatially within the high-pressure zone. The locations of the gastric sling fibers, crural diaphragm and LES is consistent with prior studies using atropine subtraction curves to ablate the intrinsic sphincter components and cis-atracurium pressure curves to ablate the extrinsic sphincter components.

Figure 4. This is the post-bethanechol curve minus the pre-bethanechol curve of 14 normal control subjects in full inspiration. Note the two pressure peaks, the distal pressure peak represents the gastric sling fiber/clasp fiber complex while the proximal peak represents the LES. These peaks are in the same relative position as the atropine subtraction curves and the cisatracurium curves above.

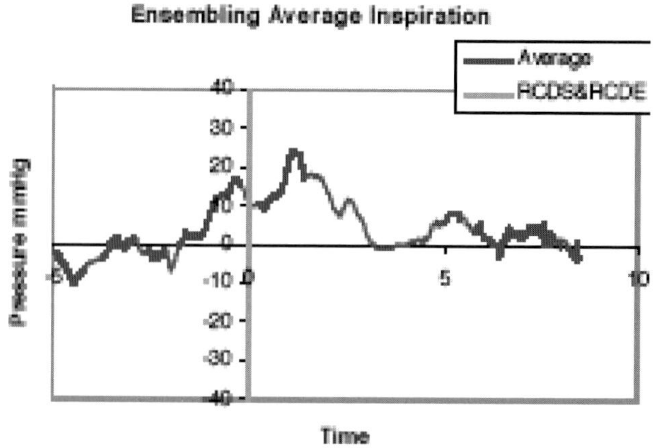

Pharmacological separation of the GEJ high-pressure zone demonstrates an absent gastric sling fiber pressure profile in patients with GERD [7].

A number of studies were performed to evaluate and compare the relative contributions of each of the components of the GEJ high-pressure zone in GERD patients and normal control subjects, in order to determine which abnormalities predispose patients to reflux. High-frequency endoluminal ultrasound and simultaneous manometry was used to evaluate 7 patients with documented GERD during inspiration and expiration as in the previous studies in normal volunteers. As described above, the difference between pre-atropine and post-atropine pressure profiles in normal volunteers (the intrinsic sphincter components) displayed two peaks in inspiration and expiration. However, in GERD patients the subtraction curve between the pre-atropine and post-atropine pressure profiles demonstrated that the distal peak pressure profile (gastric sling fiber/clasp fiber complex) was totally absent in both the inspiratory and expiratory phases of all of the GERD patients (100%) (*Figure 5*). The proximal peak representing the LES, was present in the same axial location relative to the crural diaphragm as in the normal volunteers. The intrinsic LES and crural diaphragm were found to move proximally away from the start point during expiration similar to the normal controls. It was concluded that GERD patients lack the pressure profile consistent with the gastric sling fiber/clasp fiber complex.

Endoscopic plication (EndoCinch) repairs a physiologic defect in patients with GERD: absent pressure profile due to the gastric sling fibers [8-10].

To further define this abnormality and the effects of endoscopic plication in patients with GERD a study was performed to define the mechanism of action of endoscopic plication in the treatment of GERD. High-frequency ultrasound and simultaneous manometry was used to evaluate 10 GERD patients during inspiration and expiration in a fashion similar to the previous studies. Pull-throughs were repeated before and after intravenous administration of atropine. Eight of the 10 patients (80%) had significant clinical benefit after endoscopic plication with elimination or with a marked decrease in symptoms. Pre-EndoCinch, all of the patients demonstrated the absent gastric sling fiber/clasp fiber pressure profile described above. Post-EndoCinch the distal pressure profile (gastric sling fiber/clasp fiber pressure profile) was reestablished in the GERD patients at the same location as the distal pressure peak in normal volunteers (*Figure 6*). It was concluded that that the GERD patients lack the pressure profile due to the gastric sling fibers and that endoscopic plications reestablishes this distal pressure profile. We hypothesize that endoscopic-plication works, at least in part, by replacing this missing physiologic pressure profile.

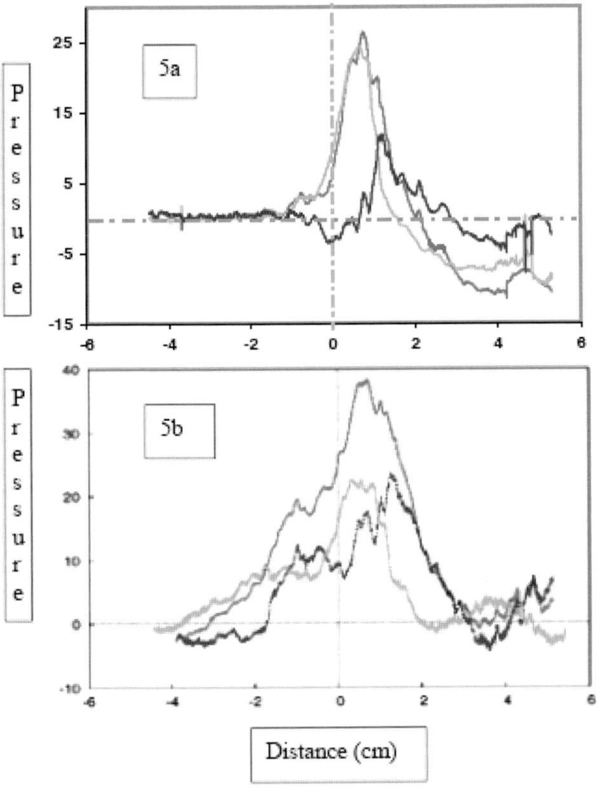

Figure 5. In GERD patients **(a)** the subtraction curves between the pre- and post-atropine pressure profiles demonstrated that the distal peak (gastric sling fiber/clasp fiber pressure profile) was totally absent in both full inspiration (FI, left graph) and full expiration (FE, right graph). The proximal peak representing the LES was present in the same axial position relative to the right crural diaphragm as in the normal volunteers **(b)**. Note: red curve represents pre-atropine pressure; green curve represents post-atropine pressure; blue curve represents post-atropine subtracted from preatropine pressures, to extract the intrinsic sphincter contribution to the GEJ high pressure zone. The vertical dashed line represents the start of the crural diaphragm, used as an axial reference mark. (See page X for colour figure).

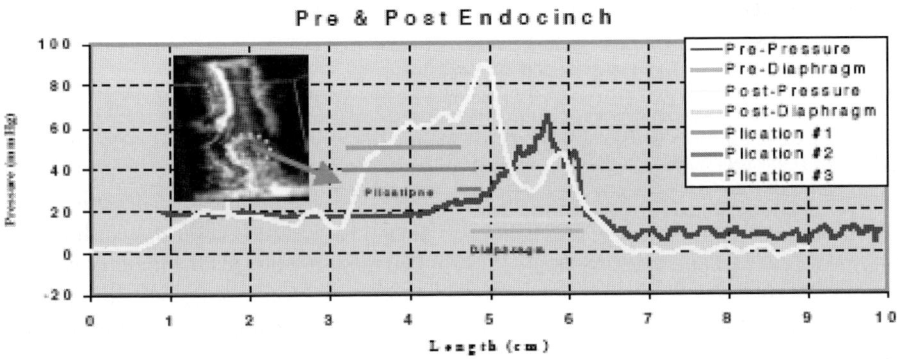

Figure 6. This picture shows the pressure profiles through the GEJ high pressure zone pre- and post-EndoCinch in a patient with GERD referenced to the right crural diaphragm. Note, the blue curve represents the pre-the EndoCinch pressure profile, while the yellow curve represents the post-EndoCinch pressure profile. The horizontal lines represent the locations of the endoscopic plications (red, pink and green lines), and the right crural diaphragm (light blue, and light green lines) located by ultrasound imaging. (See page X for colour figure).

Summary

Until now, it has not been possible to accurately separate the GEJ high-pressure zone into its component parts and to study the mechanical properties of these components individually and as a group. This was accomplish in normal volunteers and in GERD patients using a technique that employs sonography and manometry simultaneously during pharmacologic manipulation of the GEJ high-pressure zone. Three components of the GEJ high-pressure zone, the intrinsic LES, gastric sling fiber/clasp fiber complex and crural diaphragm were isolated in the normal volunteers. Each component was localized spatially with respect to each of the other components and the contribution of each component to the antireflux barrier GEJ high-pressure zone was determined. It was found that each component moved with respect to each of the other components during respiration. The width of the crural diaphragm and the intrinsic sphincter was defined, and it was determined that the intrinsic lower esophageal sphincter moved proximally during expiration due to lengthening of the esophagogastric segment.

In studies on GERD patients it was discovered that an abnormality of the gastric sling fiber/clasp fiber complex exists. The distal pressure profile due to the gastric sling fiber/clasp fiber complex, seen in normal control subjects, was lacking in all patients studied with GERD. It was further found in subsequent studies that the lack of this pressure profile decreased the stiffness of the GEJ high-pressure zone, allowing pathologic distension of this area. It was also found that mechanical plication of this area in GERD patients increased the stiffness of the area, making the mechanics of distension in the distal esophagus and proximal stomach more like the mechanics in normal volunteers. We propose a comprehensive theory of GERD based on the above findings in which a defective gastric sling fiber/clasp fiber complex leads to reduced stiffness of the GEJ making the junction easier to distend.

References

1. Ingelfinger FJ. Esophageal motility. Physiol Rev 1958;38:533-84.
2. Boyle JT, Altschuler SM, Nixon TE, Tuchman DN, Pack AI, Cohen S. Role of the diaphragm in the genesis of lower esophageal sphincter pressure in the cat. Gastroenterology 1985;88:723-30.
3. Ulerich R, Miller L, Dai Q, Brasseur JG. Pharmacologic separation of the gastroesophageal segment (GES) into extrinsic and intrinsic sphincters. Gastroenterology 2003;124:A-259.
4. Dai QS, Soliman AS, Dilipkumar P, et al. Simultaneous ultrasound and manometry during pharmacologic paralysis of the crural diaphragm allows spatial localization of the two componenets of the intrinsic gastroesophageal junction high pressure zone (GEJHPZ). Gastroenterology 2004;126:A-636-W1437.
5. Neela D, Korimilli A, Dai Q, Brasseur J, Parkman H, Miller L. Pharmacologic augmentation of the intrinsic sphincter components, isolates the gastric sling fibers, crural diaphragm and intrinsic lower esophageal sphincter at the gastroesophageal junction. Submitted to DDW 2005
6. Korimilli A, Dai Q, Schwartz B, Parkman H, Brasseur J, Miller L. Location and orientation of the gastric sling fibers and crural diaphragm at the high-pressure zone of the distal esophagus. Submitted to DDW 2005
7. Miller LS, James B, Ulerich R, Thomas B, Thomas A, Dai Q. A New Theory to explain the pathophysiology of GERD. Pharmacological separation of the gastroesophageal junction high pressure zone (GEJHPZ) demonstrates an absent gastric sling fiber pressure profile in patients with GERD. Gastroenterology 2004;126:A-503.
8. Miller LS, Dai Q, Dimitriou J, Schiffer B, Brasseur J. Endoscopic plication (Endocinch) repairs a physiologic defect in patients with gastroesophageal reflux disease (GERD): absent pressure profile due to the gastric sling fibers. Gastroenterology 2004;126:A-330.
9. Schiffner BJ, Miller L, Dai Q, Dimitriou J, Brasseur J. Opening stiffness and geometry of teh esophagogastric segment in health, with GERD, and after endoscopic surgery. Submitted to DDW 2005
10. Dai Q, Brasseur JG, Dimitriou J, et al. 2-D and 3-D endoluminal ultrasound localization of endoscopic plications with simultaneous manometry (location of plications and depth of sutures). Gastroenterology DDW 2004;126.

Intragastric micromanometry in the human being

J.-M. Collard, R. Romagnoli (Brussels)

Contraction in the distal part of the human stomach results from superimposition of two different types of electrical activity in the gastric wall [1]. A first current, named pacesetter potential or slow wave, is spontaneously generated at a rate of about 3 cycles/minute by the gastric pacemaker in the upper segment of the body of the stomach along the greater curvature [2-4]. It propagates downwards through the distal stomach from cell to cell [5], and it dictates the rhythm, velocity, and direction of contractions (*Figure 1*). A second current [6,7], named action potential, is randomly generated by the muscle cells during the depolarisation period that is induced by the slow wave. Its occurrence, amplitude, and duration are closely related to the local neurohormonal environment. During phase I of the interdigestive motor complex [7,8], action potentials are absent and no contractions occur. Action potentials are present randomly during phase II of the fasting period as well as during the fed period and give rise to random contractions of the gastric wall. They are omnipresent during phase III of the fasting period, so that a contraction occurs roughly every 20 seconds. The classic concept is that not all electrical events are followed by recordable mechanical activity [9] and comes from intraluminal recordings of the gastric contractility using large steps of pressure (from 10-20 mmHg) on the vertical axis of the tracings, so that only pressure waves of 10 or more mmHg can be seen. We aimed to challenge this concept by careful analysis of selected gastric manometric tracings that were magnified using small steps of pressure on the vertical axis, to see what happens when no pressure wave is visible on the usual scales [10].

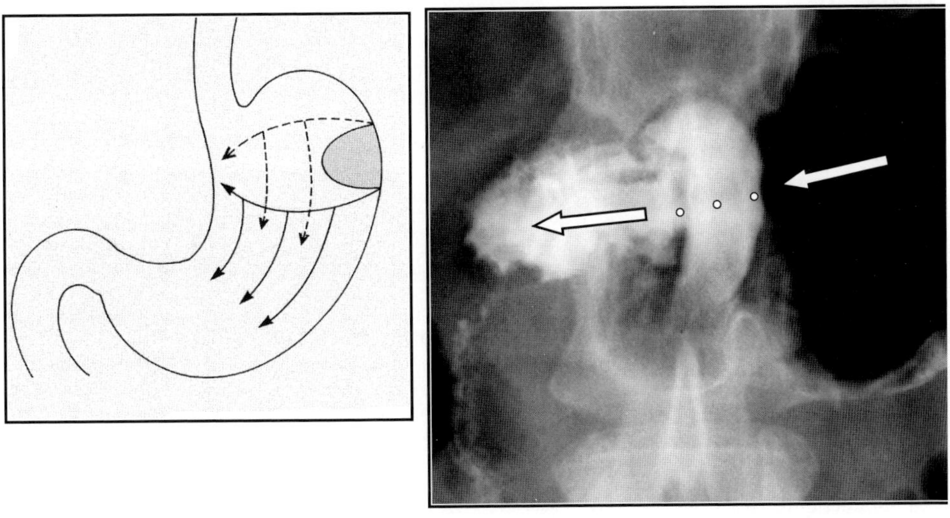

Figure 1. Gastric pacemaker and a propulsive gastric contraction sweeping over the antrum.

Study design

Gastric motility was studied manometrically in 10 healthy volunteers who had no previous foregut diseases or operations and in 31 patients with a history of subtotal esophagectomy and elevation of the denervated whole stomach up to the neck as esophageal replacement [11,12]. Thirteen of these 31 patients were given erythromycin, a motilin-receptor agonist [13] which enhances post-operative motor recovery of the denervated stomach [14]. Erythromycin chlorhydrate (Abbott, Chicago, MI) was perfused intravenously in a dose of 1 or 2 g/day until the patient started oral feeding again, and erythromycin ethylsuccinate was given orally in a dose of 1 g/day thereafter.

A 6-channel polyvinyl probe was positioned under manometric and fluoroscopic control in the gastric cavity of the patients who had had esophagectomy, so that the 6 recording side holes were located at a distance proximal to the pylorus of 2, 4, 7, 12, 17, and 22 cm, respectively [10,13,14] (*Figure 2*). The distal segment of the 6-channel probe used in control subjects was pushed into the duodenum, to prevent relative displacement of the recording holes towards the gastric wall on contraction, as there were no post-operative perigastric adhesions. The two distal holes were located in the duodenal lumen and the other four in the gastric cavity at distances proximal to the pylorus of 1, 2, 4, and 7 cm, respectively. Each channel was perfused with distilled water at a rate of 0.6 ml/minute using a pneumohydraulic pump, microcapillary catheters, and external transducers (Peter Von Berg, Kirchseson, Germany). Electrical impulses were transmitted to a polygraphic system (P.C. Polygram H.R., Synectics Medical, Stockholm, Sweden) that was connected to a personal computer through an analog-digital interface (Combi-interface 93-9506, Synectics Medical, Stockholm, Sweden). The computer was equipped with software (Polygram 6.30, Upper G-I Edition, Gastrosoft Inc., Irving, Tx) that permitted semiautomatic recognition of the best fit of intraluminal pressure waves using an auto-find threshold at 9 mmHg. Retrospectively, it was possible to modify the scale of the horizontal axis (tracing speed) in each tracing as well as that of the vertical axis (pressure steps ranging from 0.2-2.000 mmHg).

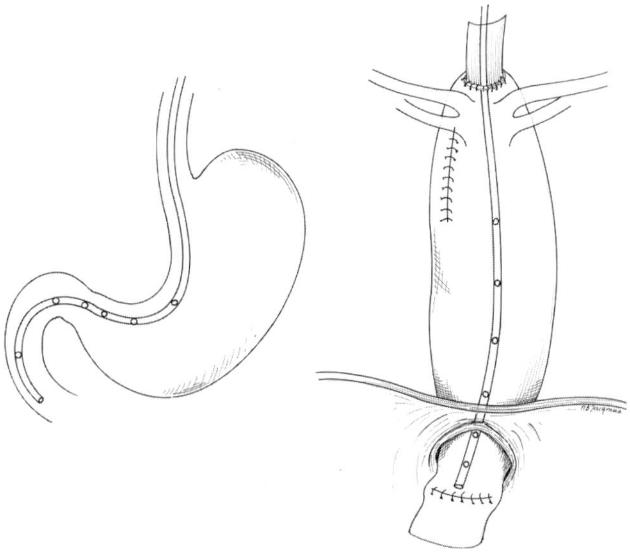

Figure 2. Position of the manometric probe in healthy volunteers (left) and in patients with a gastric transplant as o-esophageal replacement (right).

The subjects were invited to remain supine with the head and chest at a 50° angle for the whole period of recording. Fasting gastric motility was recorded for 2-3 hours until the subject was invited to take a standard solid-liquid meal of 800 kcal. Seven of the 13 patients who were taking erythromycin were studied in the fasting state only. Fed gastric motility was recorded in 34 subjects from 1-2 hours after the probe was repositioned at the same level as in the fasting period under manometric or fluoroscopic control. In addition, the investigator watched the computer screen all the time so as to reposition the probe immediately if it got displaced by high amplitude gastric contractions.

Pressure waves reflecting contractions within the gastric wall were defined as pressure elevations from baseline that occurred at a rate of about 3 cycles/minute, the rate at which the gastric pacemaker generates electrical impulses. These pressure waves could easily be differentiated from respiratory movements at about 16 cycles/minute and cannot be confused with heart beats at about 70 cycles/minute. Baseline was set using both the manual and automatic baseline calculation systems included in the manometric software.

Pressure waves were called macrowaves when they were detectable by the semiautomatic software (amplitude > 9 mmHg), and microwaves (< 9 mmHg) when they could be disclosed only by careful reading of the tracing using small steps of pressure (from 0.2-1 mmHg) on the vertical axis. Macrowaves were further classified into three subcategories according to amplitude (9-50 mmHg, 50-200 mmHg, and > 200 mmHg), and the frequency distribution of both microwaves and macrowaves (percentages of pressure wave according to amplitude) was established for each subject.

The three classic motor patterns that characterise the fasting period were identified visually before magnification of the tracings according to the following definitions : phase I = period of recording without any macrowaves detectable, lasting more than 10 minutes, and just following phase III; phase II = period with less than 3 macrowaves/ minute, and lasting more than 10 minutes; and phase III = burst of macrowaves at a rate of 3 or more than 3 cycles/minute lasting more than 2 minutes. The fed pattern was defined as a phase II-like activity that occurred just after ingestion of food and lasted at least 60 minutes. Each subject's own contraction rate in both the fasting and fed states was estimated by counting all pressure waves in selected strips of 10 minutes each, coming from three different antral channels at least, and displaying mechanical events that could be identified and differentiated from respiratory movements or artefacts (more than 6,000 pressure waves were analysed). Manometric strips that contained the most prominent microwaves were used to estimate amplitude (more than 1,700 microwaves were analysed). The nonparametric Wilcoxon rank sum, Kruskal-Wallis, and Mann-Whitney tests were used appropriately.

Manometric findings

Inspection of selected manometric strips with the vertical axis scaled up allows the observer to see microwaves of less than 9 mmHg in amplitude that are invisible on the usual scales (*Figure 3*). Microwaves are much more readily identifiable in tracings from the denervated stomach that has been pulled up to the neck as an esophageal replacement than in those from the normally innervated stomach, particularly in the fasting state (*Figure 4*). In addition, long manometric strips that are devoid of artefacts and displayed prominent microwaves are less common in healthy volunteers than after gastric transposition. This is

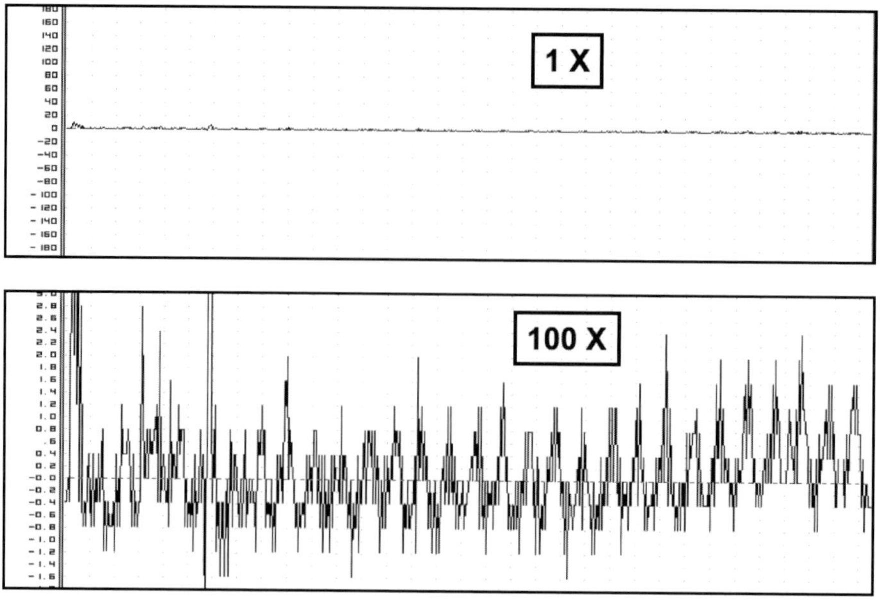

Figure 3. Disclosure of microcontractions occurring at a rate of about 3 cycles per minute after magnification of the vertical axis of the upper tracing by 100 (lower tracing) in a patient having a gastric transplant as esophageal replacement.

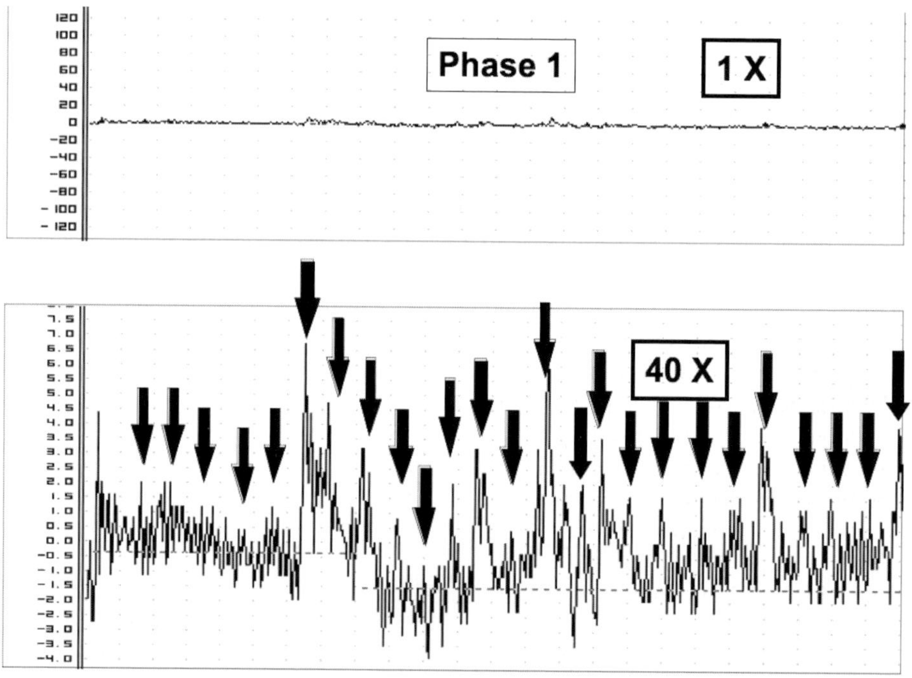

Figure 4. Disclosure of microcontractions occurring at a rate of about 3 cycles per minute after magnification of the vertical axis of the upper tracing by 40 (lower tracing) in a healthy subject. Note that identification of the microcontractions is more difficult than in *Figure 3*.

likely related to the anatomical modifications of the gastric pouch after elevation of the stomach up to the neck. Indeed, perfused catheters placed in the gastric lumen record variations in intraluminal pressure induced by contractions of the gastric wall as a resistance to fluid outflow through side holes [15]. So, detection of a gastric contraction depends on the relationship between side holes of the probe and the gastric wall. This relationship is much closer in a stomach that has been elongated into a narrow tubular structure for esophageal replacement than in the rather globular stomach *in situ*, and it may vary from one moment to another in the same subject as a result of slight displacement of the probe in the gastric lumen on contraction. A study of human and canine antral motility [16] in which 25 mmHg pressure steps were used on the vertical axis of the tracings showed that intraluminal catheters failed to detect more than half the mechanical events recorded by serosal strain gauges.

Microwaves are recorded as either peristaltic or synchronous variations in intraluminal pressure. In this respect, the fact that the perfused-catheter manometric method was designed initially for the virtual esophageal lumen [15] before it became the classic method for assessment of gastric contractility, explains why weak mechanical events may be recorded as synchronous rather than as peristaltic mechanical phenomena in a lumen like the stomach. Disappearance of a similar common – cavity effect may explain the apparent return of peristalsis in the achalasic esophagus after treatment [17].

Counting of all intraluminal pressure waves regardless of amplitude allows estimation of the contraction rate of individual stomachs, which ranged in the present study from 2.43 to 3.60 cycles/minute. It seems that the human stomach shows a mechanical activity at a rate of about 3 cycles/minute, which is the rate at which the gastric pacemaker generates electrical slow waves [3,4,8]. This phenomenon can be observed at all levels of the contractile part of the stomach, irrespective of gastric connections with the extrinsic nervous pathways [18,19]. As shown by *Figure 5*, during phase I, microwaves are the only pressure waves detectable in the gastric lumen. During phase II and after feeding, they come between macrowaves, so that the stomach shows mechanical activity that is recorded as a mixture of microwaves and macrowaves. During phase III, all pressure waves are of high amplitude and are visible on the usual scales. It thus appears that analysis of manometric strips in which microwaves are identified confirms the relevance but redefines the contents of the classic phases of the gastric motor activity. These do not differ from each other by the frequency at which a variation in intraluminal pressure is detected, but by their respective frequency distribution of pressure waves according to amplitude. On the basis of the range of amplitude of contractions, phase I of the interdigestive motor complex should not be considered as a resting period during which the stomach does not contract at all [9], but as a phase containing low-amplitude variations in intraluminal pressure ($\leq$ 9 mmHg) during which the gastric machinery is idling, just like the engine of a car when the lights are at red. As for phase II of the interdigestive motor complex and the fed motor pattern, they consist of a mixture of macrowaves (> 9 mm Hg) that are identifiable irrespective of the scale used on the vertical axis of the tracings, and of microwaves (< 9 mm Hg) that become visible only when the vertical axis has been scaled up.

Food ingestion speeds up the contraction rate as an adaptive response of the gastric wall to the arrival of nutrients (*Figure 6*). Post-prandial acceleration of the mechanical activity correlates with the increase in the frequency of electrical slow waves that has been noted in the gastric wall of anaesthetised subjects who have had oleic acid put into the stomach [20]. This acceleration has also been shown by cutaneous electrogastrography [21]. Both the

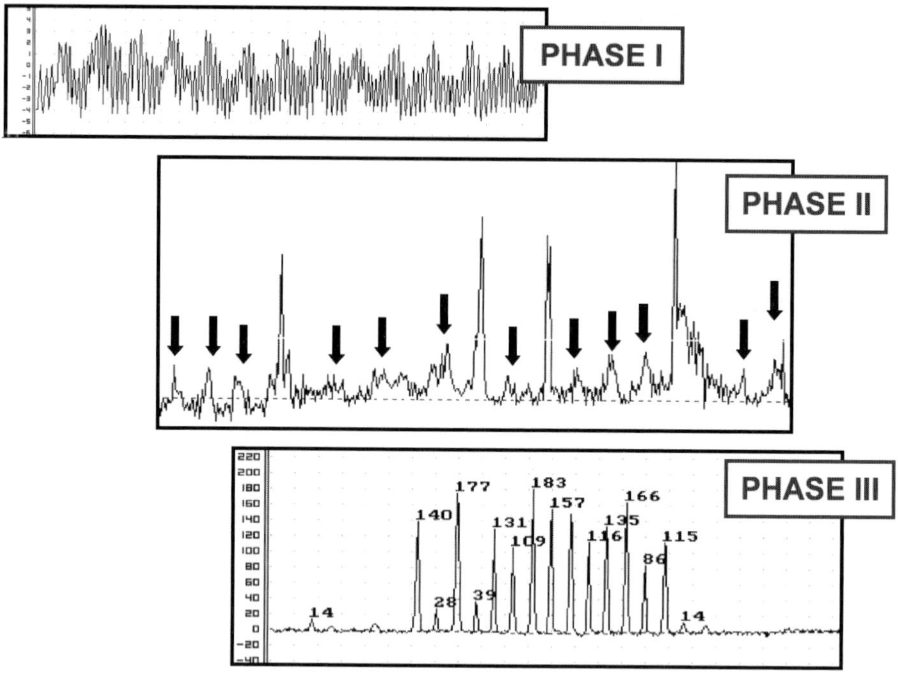

Figure 5. Phases of the fasting gastric contractility differ from each other by their respective frequency distribution of contractions according to amplitude rather than by the rate at which a contraction occurs.

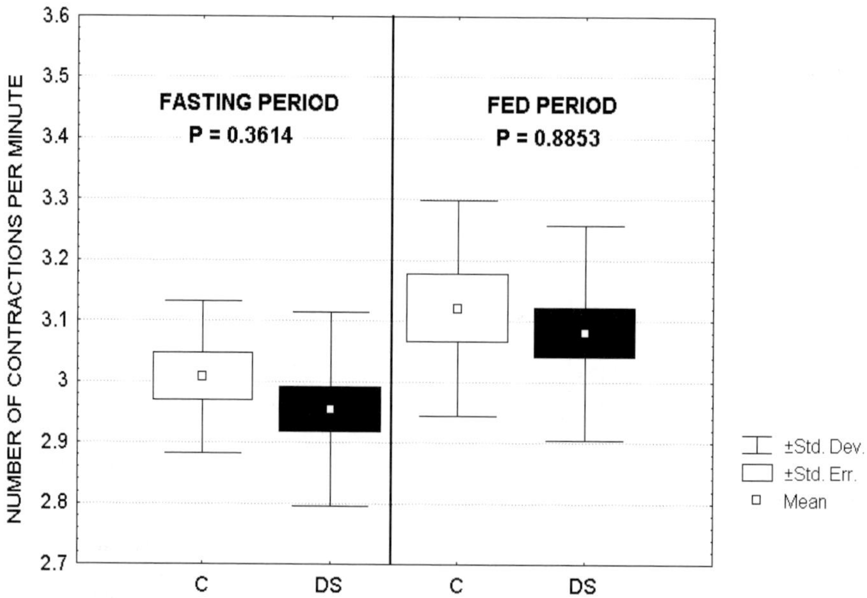

Figure 6. Contraction rate in control subjects (C, blank boxes) and in patients with a denervated stomach pulled-up to the neck (DS, black boxes) during the fasting (left) and fed (right) periods of recording.

parallelism between the basal rhythm of contractions and the rate at which electrical slow waves are generated by the pacemaker, and their respective acceleration following food ingestion, therefore, support the concept that each electrical slow wave triggers mechanical activity in the human stomach. This one-to-one electrical-mechanical relationship has previously been shown *in vivo* in dogs [16,18] and in isolated human antral muscle segments [22]. Although the same authors [16,18,22] have shown that low amplitude contractions can be triggered by an electrical slow wave in the absence of any action potential, further electrophysiological studies should establish the actual role of each current throughout the range of amplitudes of intraluminal microwaves.

Calculation of the rate at which an individual stomach contracts together with the estimation of the frequency distribution of intraluminal pressure waves according to amplitude is a relevant method for assessment of gastric motility and its disorders. In this respect, *Figure 7* shows the variations in this frequency distribution secondary to food ingestion in healthy volunteers. Likewise, *Figure 8* shows the way the gastric antrum spontaneously recovers more and more contractility over time following bilateral truncal vagotomy. As shown with erythromycin therapy after vagotomy (*Figure 9*), this assessment method of gastric contractility also allows quantification of the effect of any prokinetic treatment, as well as comparison of two different treatments.

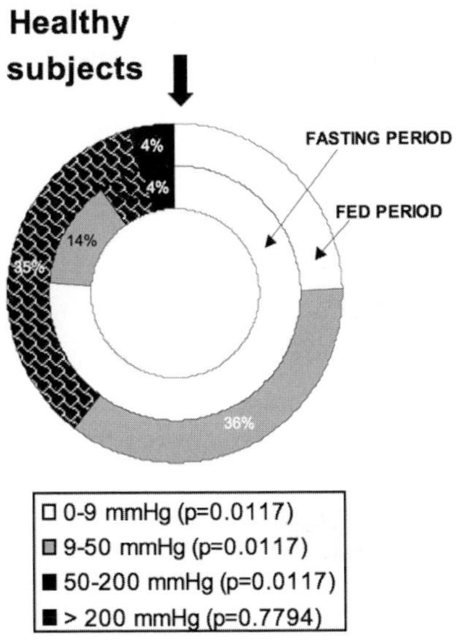

Figure 7. Frequency distribution of intraluminal pressure waves classified according to amplitude in the fasting (internal ring) and fed (external ring) periods of recording in heathy volunteers. The 360° of each circumference correspond to 100 % of intraluminal pressure waves (counterclockwise reading from the vertical black arrow).

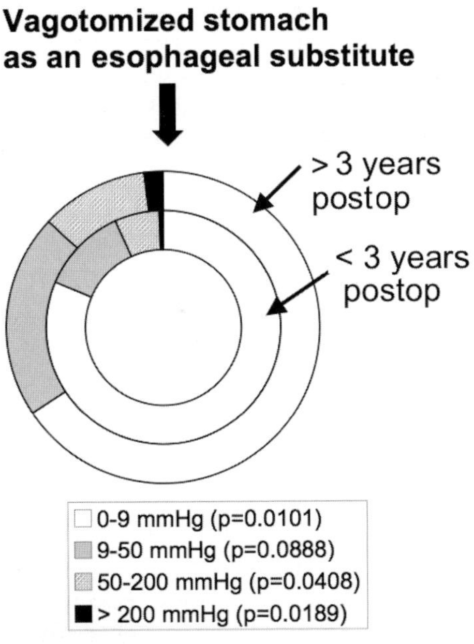

Figure 8. Frequency distribution of intraluminal pressure waves classified according to amplitude < 3 years (internal ring) and > 3 years (external ring) after truncal vagotomy, subtotal esophagectomy, and gastric pull-up. The 360° of each circumference correspond to 100 % of intraluminal pressure waves (counterclockwise reading from the vertical black arrow).

Figure 9. Frequency distribution of intraluminal pressure waves classified according to amplitude after truncal vagotomy, subtotal esophagectomy and gastric pull-up (internal ring), and after truncal vagotomy, subtotal esophagectomy and gastric pull-up plus continuous intravenous administration of erythromycin (1g: medial ring; 2 g: external ring). The 360° of each circumference correspond to 10 % of intraluminal pressure waves (counterclockwise reading from the vertical black arrow).

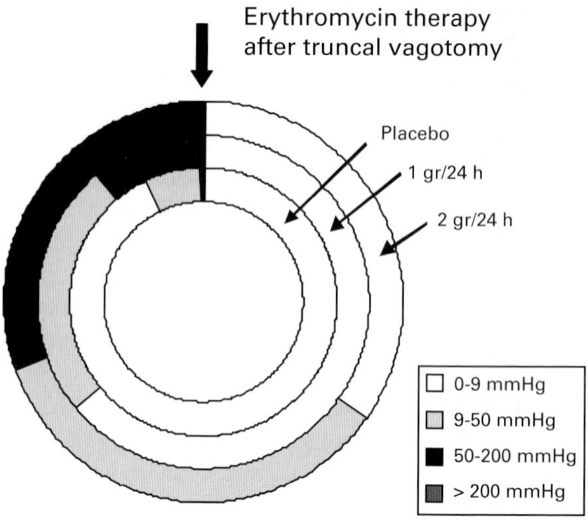

Conclusions

Human stomach exhibits a recordable mechanical activity at a rate of about 3 cycles per minute, i.e. the rate at which the gastric pacemaker generates pacesetter electrical potentials so that the classic phases of the gastric motor activity differ from each other by their respective frequency distribution of pressure waves according to amplitude rather than by the frequency at which a variation in intraluminal pressure is detected.

Proper identification of microwaves requires rigorous selection of typical manometric strips and some habituation to the reading of magnified tracings. It also depends on the closeness of the relationship between the intraluminal recording probe and the gastric wall.

References

1. Richter HM. In: Read NW, ed. Gastro-intestinal motility. Which test? Petersfield: Wrightson Biomedical Publishing, 1989:163-174.
2. Christensen J, Rick GA, Lowe LS. Distribution of interstitial cells of cajal in stomach and colon of cat, dog, ferret, opossum, rat, guinea pig, and rabbit. J Auton Nerv Syst 1992;37:47-56.
3. Hinder RA, Kelly KA. Human gastric pacesetter potential: site of origin, spread, and response to gastric transection and proximal gastric vagotomy. Am J Surg 1977;133:29-33.
4. Kwong NK, Brown BH, Whittaker GE, Duthie HL. Electrical activity of the gastric antrum in man. Br J Surg 1970;57:913-6.
5. Larson DM, Gilbert RJ, Beyer EC. Two-dimentional coupling by gap junctions in cultured gastric smooth muscle monolayers. Am J Physiol 1992;263:G261-8.
6. Kelly KA, Code CF. Effect of transthoracic vagotomy on canine gastric electrical activity. Gastroenterology 1969;57:51-8.
7. Kelly KA, La Force RC. Role of the gastric pacesetter potential defined by electrical pacing. Can J Physiol Pharmacol 1972;50:1017-9.
8. Code CF, Marlett JA. The interdigestive myo-electric complex of the stomach and small bowel of dogs. J. Physiol 1975;246:289-309.
9. Rao SSC, Schulze-Delrieu K. In: Kumar D, Wingate D, eds. An illustrated guide to gastrointestinal motility. Edinburgh, Churchill Livingstone, 1993:373-92.
10. Collard JM, Romagnoli R. Human stomach has a recordable mechanical activity at a rate of about 3 cycles per minute. Eur J Surg 2001;167:188-94.
11. Collard JM, Tinton N, Malaise J, Romagnoli R, Otte JB, Kestens PJ. Esophageal replacement. Gastric tube or whole stomach? Ann Thorac Surg 1995;60:261-7.

12. Collard JM, Romagnoli R, Otte JB, Kestens PJ. The denervated stomach as an esophageal substitute is a contractile organ. Ann Surg 1998;227:33-9.
13. Peeters T, Matthijs G, Depoortere I, Cachet T, Hoogmartens J, Van Trappen G. Erythomycin is a motilin receptor agonist. Am J Physiol 1989;257:G470-4.
14. Collard JM, Romagnoli R, Otte JB, Kestens PJ. Erythromycin enhances early postoperative contractility of the denervated whole stomach as an esophageal substitute. Ann Surg 1999;229:337-43.
15. Arndorfer RC, Stef JJ, Dodds WJ, Linehan JH, Hogan WJ. Improved infusion system for intraluminal esophageal manometry. Gastroenterology 1977;73:23-7.
16. You CH, Chey WY. Study of electromechanical activity of the stomach in humans and in dogs with particular attention to tachygastria. Gastroenterology 1984;86:1460-8.
17. Van Trappen G, Janssens J, Hellemans J, Coremans G. Achalasia, diffuse esophageal spasm, and related motility disorders. Gastroenterology 1979;76:450-7.
18. Nelsen TH, Eigenbrodt EH, Keoshian LA, Bunker C, Johnson L. Alterations in muscular and electrical activity of the stomach following vagotomy. Arch Surg 1967;94:821-35.
19. Stoddard CJ, Smallwood R, Brown BH, Duthie HL. The immediate and delayed effects of different types of vagotomy on human gastric myoelectrical activity. Gut 1975;16:165-70.
20. Duthie HL, Kwong NK, Brown BH, Whittaker GE. Pacesetter potential of the human gastroduodenal junction. Gut 1971;12:250-6.
21. Parkman HP, Harris AD, Miller MA, Fisher RS. Influence of age, gender, and menstrual cycle on the normal electrogastrogram. Am J Gastroenterol 1996;91:127-33.
22. You CH, Lee KY, Chey WY, Menguy R. In vitro myoelectric study of antral muscle from the patients of tachygastria. Dig Dis Sci 1980;25:A17.

How should "ineffective esophageal motility" be defined?

M. Ribolsi, R. Tutuian (Zurich)

After revisiting the manometric characteristics in patients with non-specific motor disorders (NEMD) in 1997 Leite *et al.* noticed that these patients had in common an increased proportion of esophageal contractions with amplitudes less than 30 mmHg. Based on this observation the authors proposed the term "ineffective esophageal motility" (IEM) to be used instead of NEMD as these patients had specific findings [1]. They defined IEM as the presence of 30% or more contractions with an amplitude less than 30 mmHg in the distal esophagus. The rationales for these criteria were provided normal manometry values from 95 healthy volunteers [2] and data from combined video-fluoroscopic and manometry examinations documenting complete bolus transit when the contraction amplitude in the distal esophagus exceeded 30 mmHg [3]. This definition of IEM is used by Spechler and Castell in the most recent classification of esophageal motility abnormalities [4].

The term and concept of IEM have been challenged over the years, some investigators arguing that the current definition of manometric ineffective swallows does not distinguish between:

- contractions with distal esophageal peristaltic wave amplitude < 30 mmHg;
- simultaneous contractions with amplitudes < 30 mmHg in the distal esophagus;
- failed peristalsis in which the peristaltic wave does not traverse the entire length of the distal esophagus;
- absent peristalsis.

One point of controversy is the clinical importance of finding IEM in patients with gastroesophageal reflux disease (GERD). Approximately 20-50% of GERD patients are found to have IEM during esophageal manometry [5,6]. Although patients with IEM were found to have a higher number of reflux episodes and a delayed esophageal acid clearance time (defined as the period that the esophageal mucosa remains at a pH < 4 after gastroesophageal reflux) than those without IEM [1] the percentage of patients with IEM is similar in erosive and in nonerosive GERD patients, and there is also no difference between the severity of IEM in erosive and in nonerosive GERD patients. Therefore while some authors have suggested that IEM could be a marker for GERD, and possibly contribution to the pathophysiologic mechanism of disease, other authors have challenged this association [5,7-9]. Most recently Simren *et al.* evaluated the relationship between the number of manometric ineffective contractions, chemical clearance and volume clearance in a group of healthy volunteers in whom low amplitude contractions were induced using sildenafil. In these healthy volunteers who underwent combined manometry, pH and impedance monitoring the authors noted that in upright position volume clearance was slightly prolonged only in presence of severe IEM (abnormal peristaltic waves > 80% of the times) while in supine position, severe IEM significantly delayed chemical and volume clearance. On the other hand moderate IEM (30-80% abnormal peristalsis) had no impact on esophageal acid and bolus clearance times neither in upright nor in recumbent position. Based on these findings the authors concluded that only the presence of 80% or more manometric ineffective swallows are clinically relevant in the pathogenesis of GERD.

Another point of controversy is the clinical importance of identifying IEM in patients scheduled to undergo fundoplication. The presence of manometric ineffective contractions was thought to increase the risk of developing post-operative dysphagia and identifying IEM in the pre-operative setting might require adjusting the fundoplication (i.e. would be an argument to perform only a partial fundoplication). Fibbe *et al.* evaluated 200 patients scheduled to undergo laparoscopic fundoplication that were stratified based on the presence of IEM (100 patients with IEM and 100 patients with normal motility) prior to being randomized to either 360° (Nissen) or 270° (Toupet) fundoplication [10]. Although patients with IEM had more severe reflux symptoms and lower esophageal sphincter resting pressures compared to those with normal manometry, IEM was more frequently found in patients complaining of dysphagia pre-operatively the presence of IEM did not predict the development of post-operative dysphagia. Based on these findings the authors concluded that esophageal dysmotility reflects more severe disease, does not affect post-operative clinical outcome, is not corrected by fundoplication, is independent of the surgical procedure performed, may occur as a result of fundoplication and it's presence doesn't require a tailoring of surgical management.

We have analyzed the relationship between manometric ineffective contractions and bolus transit in both healthy volunteers and patients with manometric IEM. The study in healthy volunteers revealed that during liquid swallows almost half (47.6%) of manometric ineffective swallows had complete bolus transit and during viscous swallows little over one third (34.7%) of manometric ineffective swallows had complete bolus transit [11]. In patients with IEM we found during the per-swallow analysis that no manometric cut-off value of the distal esophageal amplitude can be both highly sensitive and highly specific of predicting complete bolus transit and that the likelihood of an abnormal bolus transit increases parallel to the number of distal esophageal sites with low amplitude. In the per-patient analysis we noticed that the majority of patients with 30-40% manometric ineffective swallows had normal bolus transit while the majority of patients with 50% or more manometric ineffective swallows had abnormal bolus transit [12]. We interpreted these findings as suggestive of using a cut-off value of 50% ineffective swallows to define ineffective esophageal manometry. In a subsequent study including 120 patients with traditional IEM and 192 patients with normal manometry we noticed that the new IEM criterion would have a positive predictive value of 72% and a negative predictive value of 89% to anticipate abnormal bolus transit.

In summary, the currently used criterion of 30% or more manometric contractions with an amplitude < 30 mmHg in the distal esophagus is sensitive but not specific in identifying abnormal bolus transit. Evaluating bolus transit at the same time with esophageal contractions, ideally with combined impedance-manometry as this method is free of ionizing radiation, allows determining which patients with IEM have abnormal bolus transit. Therefore during combined MII-EM testing IEM can be defined as 30% or more manometric ineffective contractions and abnormal bolus transit. During conventional esophageal manometry defining IEM as the presence of 50% or more manometric ineffective contractions will increase the specificity of this diagnosis to be associated with abnormal esophageal bolus transit.

References

1. Leite LP, Johnston BT, Barrett J, et al. Ineffective esophageal motility (IEM): the primary finding in patients with non-specific esophageal motility disorder. Dig Dis Sci 1997;42:1859-65.
2. Richter JE, Wu WC, Johns DN, et al. Esophageal manometry in 95 healthy adult volunteers. Dig Dis Sci 1987;32:583-92.
3. Kahrilas PJ, Doods WJ, Hogan WJ. Effect of peristaltic dysfunction on esophageal volume clearance. Gastroenterology 1988;94:73-80.
4. Spechler SJ, Castell DO. Classification of oesophageal motility abnormalities. Gut 2001;49:145-51.
5. Ho SC, Chang CS, Wu CY, et al. Ineffective esophageal motility is a primary motility disorder in gastroesophageal reflux disease. Dig Dis Sci 2002;47:652-6.
6. Fouad YM, Katz PO, Hatlebakk JG, et al. Ineffective esophageal motility: the most common motility abnormality in patients with GERD-associated respiratory symptoms. Am J Gastroenterol 1999;94:1464-7
7. Diener U, Patti MG, Molena D, et al. Esophageal dysmotility and gastroesophageal reflux disease. J Gastrointest Surg 2001; 5:260-5.
8. Mittal RK, Lange RC, McCallum RW. Identification and mechanism of delayed esophageal acid clearance in subjects with hiatus hernia. Gastroenterology 1987;92:130-5.
9. Lin S, Ke M, Xu J, et al. Impaired esophageal emptying in reflux disease. Am J Gastroenterol 1994;89:1003-6.
10. Fibbe C, Layer P, Keller J, Strate U, Emmermann A, Zornig C. Esophageal motility in reflux disease before and after fundoplication: a prospective, randomized, clinical, and manometric study. Gastroenterology 2001;121:5-14.
11. Tutuian R, Vela MF, Balaji N, et al. Esophageal function testing using combined multichannel intraluminal impedance and manometry. Multicenter study of healthy volunteers. Clin Gastroenterol Hepatol 2003;1:174-82.
12. Tutuian R, Castell DO. Clarification of the esophageal function defect in patients with manometric ineffective esophageal motility: studies using combined impedance-manometry. Clin Gastroenterol Hepatol 2004;2:230-6.

Is there a relationship between the proportion of longitudinal or circular muscle and the motility of the esophageal body?

I. Sarosiek, M. Majewski, J. Sarosiek (Kansas City)

The role of esophagus in the physiology of the upper alimentary tract is to act as pathway for ingested food to be delivered into the gastric lumen. The unique role of the esophagus is closely related to the fact that this is the only segment of the alimentary tract where solid food bolus is destined to be propelled strongly enough to rich its destination – the gastric lumen. This requirement must be reflected in its anatomy and structure-related physiology.

The muscularis propria of the esophagus is composed of an inner circular smooth muscle (CSM) layer and an outer longitudinal smooth muscle (LSM) layer. Only highly synchronized contractile activities of circular and longitudinal muscles would make solid food bolus propulsion mechanically efficient and clinically comfortable to the patients. In this process, the CSM of the esophageal wall was originally thought to be primarily responsible for generating intraluminal pressure followed by its closure giving the ingested bolus propelling force necessary to deliver its content into the stomach [1]. However, neither the propagation velocity nor the strength of circular muscle contraction correlates with the esophageal propulsive giving an impression that perhaps longitudinal muscle may have a significant role in bolus aborad propulsion [2]. The LSM contraction is recognized for local longitudinal shortening of the esophagus during peristaltic waves and providing some rigidity to the esophageal conduit during bolus propulsion [2-4]. Since LSM contraction-related local longitudinal shortening is overlapping CSM contraction and circular shortening, the methodology employed to measure both phenomena at the same moment is pivotal for the qualitative and quantitative changes recorded during peristaltic waves to recognize contribution of both muscle layers.

The mucosal clips methodology employed during the earlier studies required optimalization in selection of number of clips and their distribution along the segment of musculature in experimental protocol [1,2]. This has resulted in a search for novel solutions and high resolution intraluminal ultrasound probe with simultaneous manometry recordings seemed to significantly improve our capability in addressing the contemporary issue of interrelationship between the CSM and LSM in setting the most energy efficient way in developing the propulsive power of peristaltic waves for delivering the liquid and/or solid food bolus from the oral cavity to the gastric lumen.

Review of methodology employed in assessment of the thickness of longitudinal *versus* circular muscle at baseline and during contraction

Although the placement of mucosal metal clips with preset spacing allowed to trace their axial movement during longitudinal muscle contraction and shortening there were a number of issue that require to be addressed before correct selection of their spatial distribution:

- the larger the space between mucosal metal clips, more global phenomenon was going to be recorded;
- the shorter the space between metal clips, greater was the impact of local longitudinal muscle contraction on clips displacement and calculation of minimum shortening (Lengthcontr/Lengthres);
- movement of mucosal clips was also influenced by contractions of the muscularis mucosa that not always was synchronized with LSM contractions, affecting its precision;
- slippage of the mucosa relative to submucosa resulting from the connective tissue elasticity also influenced its accuracy [2].

Coupling endoscopic ultrasonography and intraluminal manometry with basic principle of mechanics (the law of mass conservation) made possible direct measurements of local shortening of the esophagus concurrently with intraluminal pressure during normal bolus transport [3].

In the next step in mastering the technique of the measurement of muscle shortening along the normal esophagus during swallowing, the high-resolution endoluminal ultrasound (HREUS) transducer and manometry probe were combined [1].

Catheter-based high-frequency intraluminal ultrasound imaging, especially when combined with manometry, pH and impedance measurements techniques became a powerful tool to study esophageal motor function and dysfunction *in vivo* in humans [5].

Evaluation of the structure/function relationship of the longitudinal muscle *versus* circular muscle in esophageal health

Using metal clips spaced 4.5cm proximally from the squamocolumnar junction it was demonstrated that that esophageal shortening was coordinated with circular muscle contraction such that each propagated distally as overlapping segments of contraction at a velocity of about 2.5 cm/sec [2]. Propulsive force within the proximal segment occurred after shortening, during the circular muscle contraction, with the magnitude of propulsive force correlated with the degree of shortening with the LSM contraction leading the CSM [2]. Propulsive force occurred during both proximal CSM and distal LSM contractions.

Propulsive force within a defined esophageal segment occurred after passage of the contracting segment of longitudinal muscle, at which time circular muscle contraction within the segment under study was coupled with LSM contraction downstream. Furthermore, the magnitude of propulsive force generated within the studied segment correlated less with the magnitude of the CSM but more with the magnitude of LSM contraction [2]. The length of the LSM segment that was contracting concurrently was at least 4.5 cm and perhaps even as long as 12 cm segment [2]. There are a few mechanistic hypotheses that try to explain this phenomenon:
- LSM contraction works to slip the esophagus over the bolus;
- to increase the rigidity of the esophageal wall;
- to increase the density of circular muscle fibers orad to the bolus, thereby increasing the mechanical advantage of circular muscle contraction.

Thus LSM contraction may be important in promoting esophageal transit of solids, as once the CSM contraction hold the solid food bolus, aborad motion of this bolus and the force magnitude seem to be directly proportional to the magnitude and duration of distal LSM contraction rather than the CSM contraction [2].

Therefore, based on metal clip methodology, both CSM and LSM contractions occur at propagating segment during peristalsis, with the LSM contraction leading the contracting complex. Furthermore, propulsive force within the peristaltic wave is mainly determined by the amplitude and duration of the esophageal shortening in the distal segment driven by LSM contraction [2].

On the other hand, using novel methodology employing endoscopic ultrasonography with intraluminal manometry, two clear phases of local longitudinal shortening were observed during bolus transport [2]. During luminal filling by bolus fluid, the muscle layer distended and the muscle thickness decreased in the absence of CSM or LSM contraction. This was followed by local contraction, first in longitudinal muscle, then in circular muscle. Maximal longitudinal shortening occurred nearly coincidentally with peak intraluminal pressure. LSM contraction begun before and ended after CSM contraction. Larger longitudinal shortening was correlated with higher pressure amplitude suggesting that CSM contractile forces were enhanced by LSM shortening [2]. This indicated that a peristaltic wave of LSM contraction envelops the wave of CSM contraction as it passes through the middle esophagus with peak longitudinal contraction aligned with peak CSM contraction. Thus coordination of the two waves may be a physiological response to the mechanical influence of longitudinal shortening, which increases contractile force while reducing average muscle fiber tension by increasing CSM fiber density locally near the bolus tail [2].

Using the HREUS transducer and manometry probe it was demonstrated that both CSM and LSM shortened longitudinally more at distal then proximal esophagus during swallowing of the bolus of liquids [1]. Peak intraluminal pressure strongly correlates with peak muscle thickness of both layers at all esophageal levels.

This increase in local longitudinal shortening in the distal esophagus increases the efficiency of peristaltic contraction and likely contributes to the axial displacement of the LES preceding hiatal opening and esophageal emptying [1].

Using catheter-based high-frequency intraluminal ultrasound imaging, combined with manometry, revealed that there is synchrony in the timing and the amplitude of contraction between the circular and longitudinal muscle layers [5]. Contractile synchrony between the two muscle layers is important and provides biomechanical advantage to the contraction process; the increase in the muscle thickness (caused by LSM contraction) at the site of peak pressure (caused by CSM contraction) reduced the esophageal wall stress (in accordance with the Laplace law) [5].

How this phenomenon takes shape during swallowing solid food bolus remains to be determined. This is of special clinical importance as esophagus is the only gastrointestinal (GI) tract organ that has to be well equipped to propel solid food in aborad direction and patients with swallowing disorders develop first solid food dysphagia before going into more generalized phenomenon of both solids and liquids dysphagia.

Exploration of the structure/function relationship of the longitudinal muscle *versus* circular muscle in esophageal disease

Disturbances of esophageal clearance in some individuals with normal manometric examination may be explained by disordered LSM contractions [2]. Thus the diminished propulsive force like that observed in patients with reflux esophagitis that improves after endoscopic healing could be related to attenuated LSM contraction as a result of persistent inflammation-related shortening [2,6,7].

Catheter-based high-frequency intraluminal ultrasound imaging, combined with manometry, has demonstrated that a sustained contraction of the longitudinal muscle layer is temporarily related to esophageal chest pain and even heartburn [5].
Achalasia, diffuse esophageal spasm and nutcracker esophagus are associated with hypertrophy of circular and longitudinal muscle layers [5]. In patients with high amplitude esophageal contractions (nutcracker esophagus), however, asynchrony in the contraction of two muscle layers can be demonstrated: peak LSM contraction occur earlier than the peak of CSM contraction during peristalsis leading to higher stress within the esophageal wall [8].

One has to recognize, however, that lubrication of the solid food bolus with adequate flow of saliva and subsequently lubrication within the esophageal lumen by continuous secretion from esophageal submucosal mucous glands helps significantly in propulsion of solid food bolus making the esophageal motility event highly efficient and comfortable for the patients in health and disease [9-18]. This is schematically outlined in *Figure 1.*

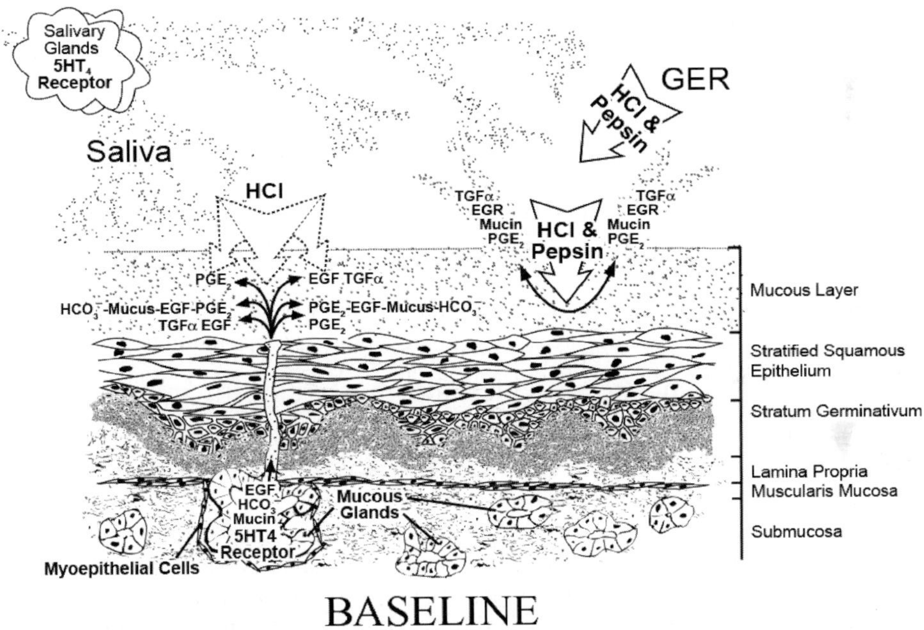

Figure 1. Schematic outline of the lubricating role of salivary and esophageal submucosal mucous glands always exhibiting significant rate of secretion at baseline that remains greatly influenced by cholinergic, adrenergic and serotonergic pathways [12,16-18].

References

1. Dai Q, Korimilli A, Thangada VK, Chung CY, Parkman H, Brasseur J, Miller LS. Muscle shortening along the normal esophagus during swallowing. Dig Dis Sci 2006;51(1):105-9.
2. Pouderoux P, Lin S, Kahrilas PJ. Timing, propagation, coordination, and effect of esophageal shortening during peristalsis. Gastroenterology 1997;112(4):1147-54.

3. Nicosia MA, Brasseur JG, Liu JB, Miller LS. Local longitudinal muscle shortening of the human esophagus from high-frequency ultrasonography. Am J Physiol Gastrointest Liver Physiol 2001;281(4):G1022-33.
4. Crist JR, He XD, Goyal RK. Chloride-mediated inhibitory junction potentials in opossum esophageal circular smooth muscle. Am J Physiol 1991;261:G752-62.
5. Mittal RK, Liu J, Puckett JL, et al. Sensory and motor function of the esophagus: lessons from ultrasound imaging. Gastroenterology 2005;128(2):487-97.
6. Christensen J, Lund GF. Esophageal responses to distension and electrical stimulation. J Clin Invest 1969;48(2):408-19.
7. Williams D, Thompson DG, Heggie L, O'Hanrahan T, Bancewicz J. Esophageal clearance function following treatment of esophagitis. Gastroenterology 1994;106(1):108-16.
8. Dogan I, Mittal RK. Esophageal motor disorders: recent advances. Curr Opin Gastroenterol 2006;22(4):417-22.
9. Sarosiek J, McCallum RW. Mechanisms of oesophageal mucosal defence. Best Pract Res Clin Gastroenterol 2000;14(5):701-17.
10. Goldin GF, Marcinkiewicz M, Zbroch T, Bityutskiy LP, McCallum RW, Sarosiek J. Esophagoprotective potential of cisapride. An additional benefit for gastroesophageal reflux disease. Dig Dis Sci 1997;42(7):1362-9.
11. Namiot Z, Yu ZJ, Piascik R, Hetzel DP, McCallum RW, Sarosiek J. Modulatory effect of esophageal intraluminal mechanical and chemical stressors on salivary prostaglandin E2 in humans. Am J Med Sci 1997;313(2):90-8.
12. Sarosiek J, Scheurich CJ, Marcinkiewicz M, McCallum RW. Enhancement of salivary esophagoprotection: rationale for a physiological approach to gastroesophageal reflux disease. Gastroenterology 1996;110(3):675-81.
13. Sarosiek J, McCallum RW. Do salivary organic components play a protective role in health and disease of the esophageal mucosa? Digestion 199556:32-7;.
14. Sarosiek J, McCallum RW. What role do salivary inorganic components play in health and disease of the esophageal mucosa? Digestion 1995;56:24-31.
15. Sarosiek J, McCallum RW. What is the secretory potential of submucosal mucous glands within the human gullet in health and disease? Digestion 1995;56:15-23.
16. Namiot Z, Sarosiek J, Marcinkiewicz M, Edmunds MC, McCallum RW. Declined human esophageal mucin secretion in patients with severe reflux esophagitis. Dig Dis Sci 1994;39(12):2523-9.
17. Namiot Z, Sarosiek J, Rourk RM, Hetzel DP, McCallum RW. Human esophageal secretion: mucosal response to luminal acid and pepsin. Gastroenterology 1994;106(4):973-81.
18. Majewski M, Jaworski T, Sarosiek I, et al. Significant enhancement of esophageal pre-epithelial defense by tegaserod: implications for an esophagoprotective effect. Clin Gastroenterol Hepatol 2007;5(4):430-8.

Among the available gastrointestinal function tests, which one provides the most relevant information on motility of the esophagus?

G.W. Falk (Cleveland)

There are a variety of studies that provide information on esophageal motility. These include barium radiography, standard manometry, high resolution manometry, combined impedance manometry testing and endoscopic ultrasonography. This chapter will review the information provided by standard manometry, high resolution manometry and combined impedance manometry testing.

Standard manometry

Standard manometry can be performed with either water perfused or solid state catheters with sensors placed at 3 to 5 cm intervals. This technique is widely available and has been in use for many years. The technique is well standardized normal values have been established and the equipment is relatively inexpensive, especially if water perfused catheters are used. Standardized classification systems for esophageal motility disorders are widely disseminated [1]. The key disadvantage of conventional manometry is that the pressure sensors are relatively widely spaced apart, and thus there is no information available on the activity between these pressure recording sites. This technique is not optimal for predicting bolus transport, and most importantly, there is considerable interobserver variability in assessment of the tracings. Dayar *et al.* found that manometric diagnosis for conditions other than achalasia and normal are highly variable with poor interobserver variability among both experienced and less experienced interpreters [2]

High resolution manometry

High resolution manometry is a relatively new technique which involves the placement of multiple sensors at closely spaced intervals < 2 cm instead of the standard 5 cm. This can be accomplished by either solid state or water perfused catheters. The results can be displayed as conventional pressure waves or by color, two dimensional contour plots whereby contraction amplitude is represented by different colors. This allows for a more complete definition of the intraluminal pressure environment and minimizes spatial gaps inherent with conventional manometry. It has the advantages of ease and efficiency of recording, as the catheter is never moved during the study and there is no need for a sleeve sensor at the lower esophageal sphincter. The close spacing of sensors allows for a better dynamic visualization of the esophagus and hence better ability to detect esophageal motor abnormalities. The key disadvantage of the technique is cost. The solid state catheters, which are typically used, are expensive to purchase and replace. Furthermore, it is unclear if this technique is superior to conventional manometry in clinical practice [3]. However, one study has compared high resolution to conventional manometry in patients with endoscopy-negative dysphagia [4]. High resolution manometry was more accurate than conventional manometry at predicting mild to moderate bolus transport abnormalities seen on videofluoroscopy and could detect subtle abnormalities in patients with endoscopy negative dysphagia not seen with conventional manometry. However, both techniques were comparable at predicting normal bolus transport as well as severe bolus transport abnormalities.

Combined impedance manometry testing

Esophageal impedance allows for the simultaneous assessment of esophageal motility and bolus transit. This is accomplished by measuring the impedance between pairs of rings placed 2 cm apart along a combined impedance manometry catheter. It is the only test that allows one to determine if motility abnormalities are accompanied by abnormalities in bolus transit. Normally, there is complete bolus transit of > 80% of liquid swallows and > 70% of viscous swallows [5]. The key advantage of this technique is that it is the only method that provides direct information on bolus transit and motility simultaneously. Impedance testing has shown that about approximately 50% of patients with manometric ineffective esophageal motility in fact have normal bolus transit [6]. Impedance recordings can also identify bolus transit abnormalities in patients with nonobstructive dysphagia and normal conventional esophageal manometry [7].

The key disadvantages are that the study is relatively difficult and time intensive to interpret, involves a learning curve, and the observation that in normal individuals, swallows with dysmotility often have complete bolus transit. It is anticipated that combined impedance high resolution catheters will be forthcoming shortly.

Conclusions

The ideal test to provide complete information on esophageal motor function and bolus transit would be combined high resolution manometry and impedance. Such probes are currently under development and should soon be available. There are no direct comparisons between high resolution manometry and combined impedance manometry. High resolution manometry is more intuitive with simpler analysis and interpretation than combined impedance manometry. Furthermore, information regarding bolus transit may be inferred with high resolution manometry. In contrast, only combined impedance manometry provides information on bolus transit in patients with esophageal motility disorders and individuals with symptoms of dysphagia in the absence of motility abnormalities. It remains to be seen whether meticulous definition of motor function, bolus function or both will influence the care of patients with esophageal symptoms.

References

1. Spechler SJ, Castell DO. Classification of oesophageal motility abnormalities. Gut 2001;49:145-51.
2. Nayar DS, Khandwala F, Achkar E, et al. Esophageal manometry: assessment of interpreter consistency. Clin Gastroenterol Hepatol 2005;3:218-24.
3. Pandolfino JE, Kahrilas PJ. AGA technical review on the clinical use of esophageal manometry. Gastroenterology 2005;128:209-24.
4. Fox M, Hebbard G, Janiak P, et al. High-resolution manometry predicts the success of oesophageal bolus transport and identifies clinically important abnormalities not detected by conventional manometry. Neurogastroenterol Motil 2004;16:533-42.
5. Tutuian R, Vela MF, Balaji NS, et al. Esophageal function testing with combined multichannel intraluminal impedance and manometry: multicenter study in healthy volunteers. Clin Gastroenterol Hepatol 2003;1:174-82.
6. Tutuian R, Castell DO. Combined multichannel intraluminal impedance and manometry clarifies esophageal function abnormalities: study in 350 patients. Am J Gastroenterol 2004;99:1011-9.
7. Conchillo JM, Nguyen NQ, Samsom M, Holloway RH, Smout AJ. Multichannel intraluminal impedance monitoring in the evaluation of patients with non-obstructive dysphagia. Am J Gastroenterol 2005;100:2624-32.

How can complete relaxation of the lower esophageal sphincter in patients with typical achalasia be explained?

J.E. Richter (Philadelphia)

The traditional manometric criteria for achalasia require the demonstration of the absence of peristalsis in the esophageal body and incomplete lower esophageal sphincter (LES) relaxation. However, we and others [1,2] have described patients with clinical symptoms (dysphagia for solids/liquids and bland regurgitation) and radiologic findings suggestive of achalasia in whom esophageal manometry demonstrates aperistalsis but with apparent complete LES relaxation, raising doubt as to the diagnosis of achalasia. How can this be explained?

To study this issue, we retrospectively identified from manometric records between January 1, 1983 and December 31, 1984, 23 patients with achalasia, of whom 7 (30%) had mean LES relaxation > 90%; i.e., "complete relaxation" [1]. These latter patients were younger, their duration of dysphagia shorter, they had less weight loss and their esophagram showed minimal dilation compared to the patients with more classical achalasia with aperistalsis and incomplete LES relaxation. Mean LES pressure and mean distal esophageal amplitude was similar in both groups. However, the duration of LES relaxation was significantly shorter (3.2 + 0.4 seconds) when compared to healthy controls with normal LES relaxation (6.6 + 0.4 seconds). The clinical course of these atypical achalasia patients resembles classic achalasia.

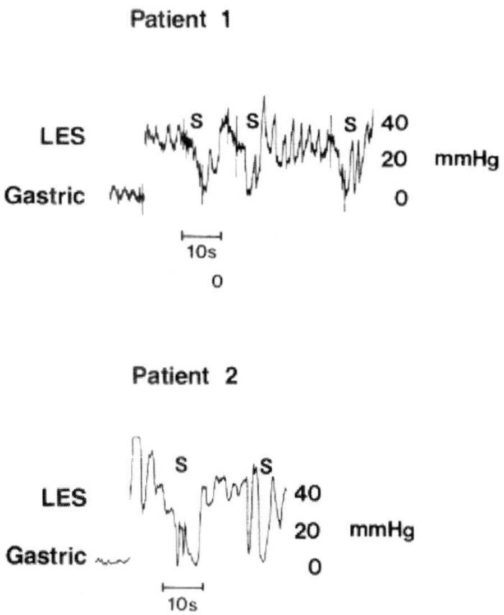

Figure 1. Representative manometry tracings showing complete but shortened lower esophageal sphincter (LES) relaxation to gastric baseline in two patients using a Dent sleeve (S = swallow).

How can we account for this apparently complete albeit shortened LES relaxation in achalasia? This could be an artifact due to the catheter orifice moving out of the LES due to esophageal shortening by the longitudinal muscle during swallowing. However, the demonstration of complete LES relaxation in two patients with the Dent sleeve, which should eliminate longitudinal catheter movement seen with the standard side hole catheters by remaining in contact with the LES during swallowing, seems to confirm that this is a true finding (*Figure 1*).

Rather, the LES relaxation in these patients is to gastric baseline, but not functionally adequate for normal esophageal emptying. The normal LES should open to a luminal diameter of > 20 mm. In contrast to LES opening, the relaxation of the LES to gastric baseline only requires the sphincter to partially open off the manometry catheter, which traditionally has a diameter of 4-5 mm. Thus, "complete" LES relaxation does not equate to normal LES opening required for functional esophageal emptying. This concept is supported by three findings from our study:

- the shortened LES relaxation in the atypical achalasia patients compared to normals. This short relaxation represents the sphincter "winking" at the catheter, rather than the 6 to 10 seconds seen with normal LES opening and closing;
- the degree of impaired esophageal emptying of a radionuclide solid meal in these atypical patients *versus* those with classic achalasia (*Figure 2*). The former group is significantly

delayed compared to normal controls, but not to the degree seen in achalasia patients with incomplete LES relaxation;

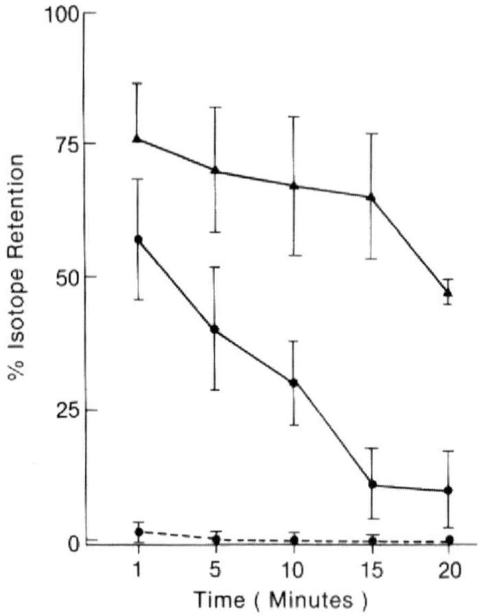

Figure 2. Comparison of radionuclide esophageal solid emptying (expresses as a percent isotope retention) in 7 study patients (solid line), 7 normal volunteers (dotted line) and 4 patients with traditional achalasia (solid line with triangles).

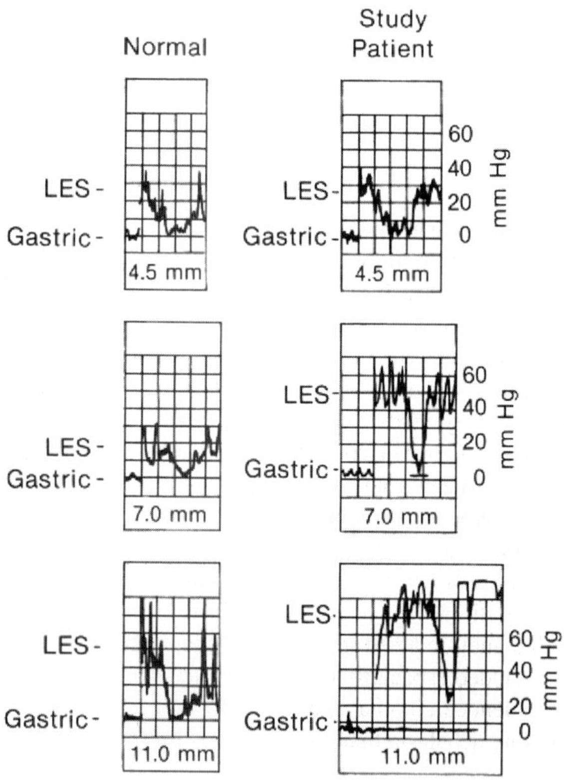

Figure 3. Effect of catheter diameter on LES relaxation in 2 normal subjects and 1 study patient using three different sized manometry catheters; 4.5, 7.0 and 11.0 mm in diameter.

- as shown in *Figure 3*, this complete relaxation is an artifact of the luminal diameter of the catheter. To address this possible factor, we constructed catheters with different diameters: 4.5, 7.0 and 11.0 mm. Complete LES relaxation with all three catheters was observed in two normal subjects. In contrast, the one atypical achalasia patient showed complete LES relaxation with the two smaller catheters, but only 70% relaxation with the 11.0 mm catheter.

Therefore, there is a subset of achalasia patients with apparent complete LES relaxation by manometry. However, the duration of LES relaxation is shorter than seen in healthy subjects and they have evidence of impaired esophageal emptying. In my experience in four academic medical centers, these patients can account for 10%-15% of patients with achalasia.

References

1. Katz PO, Richter JE, Cowan R, Castell DO. Apparent complete LES relaxation in achalasia. Gastroenterology 1986;90;978-83.
2. Hirano I, Tatum RP, Shi G, Sang Q, Joehl RJ, Kahrilas PJ. Manometric heterogeneity in patients with idiopathic achalasia. Gastroenterology 2001;120:789-98.

Comparison of medical, endoscopic, and surgical therapy for esophageal achalasia

L. Bonavina, D. Baldoli, L. Laface (Milan)

Achalasia is the most commonly diagnosed primary esophageal motor disorder and the second most common functional esophageal disease. The motor disorder in achalasia is characterized by incomplete relaxation of the lower esophageal sphincter (LES) and aperistalsis of the esophageal body secondary to loss of inhibitory ganglion cells in the myenteric plexus. The etiology of the disease is unknown, with genetic, autoimmune, infectious, and environmental factors being implicated. Defective esophageal emptying progressively leads to dilatation and tortuosity of the esophagus. The disease is usually diagnosed between 20 and 40 years or after 60 years of age. Achalasia has an insidious onset. Dysphagia and food regurgitation are the two major presenting symptoms of the disease. Nocturnal regurgitation often leads to recurrent episodes of aspiration pneumonia. In about one third of patients the diagnosis of achalasia is delayed by the reported symptoms of chest pain and heartburn simulating gastroesophageal reflux (GER) disease. As the disease progresses, inability to swallow causes malnutrition and weight loss. Malignancy-induced secondary achalasia, often referred as pseudoachalasia, should always be excluded especially in elderly patients. Both squamous-cell carcinoma of the esophagus and adenocarcinoma appear to develop with greater frequency in patients with long-standing achalasia than in the normal population [1,2].

Current therapy of achalasia is palliative and is directed toward elimination of the outflow resistance caused by failure of the LES to relax completely upon swallowing. The first successfully treated case of achalasia was reported in 1674 by Thomas Willis who used a whale bone to forcibly dilate the cardia. The first surgical myotomy was performed in 1913 by Ernst Heller.

Pharmacological therapy

Sublingual nitrates (isosorbide dinitrate) and calcium channel blockers (nifedipine) have been used with various degrees of success in achalasia [3]. Symptom relief is transient and limited to patients with early stage disease, and side effects include peripheral edema, dizziness, and headache. A prospective, placebo-controlled, randomised trial has found a significant reduction in LES pressure and symptoms with nifedipine, but dysphagia was still reported in the treated group. Moreover, the reduction of LES pressure was about one half the typical response from endoscopic dilatation or surgical myotomy, and there was no improvement in esophageal emptying [4]. Sildenafil, a phosphodiesterase-5-inhibitor, has been shown more recently to induce LES relaxation by increasing the availability of nitric oxide [5]. However, the effect is transient and side effects are significant. Therefore, oral pharmacotherapy is reserved for patients who are unwilling or unable to tolerate more invasive forms of treatment. Occasionally, oral pharmacotherapy can be prescribed for short-term relief of symptoms in patients awaiting endoscopic or surgical therapy.

Endoscopic therapy

Endoscopic treatment of achalasia consists of injective treatment with botulinum toxin or pneumatic dilation. Direct injection of botulinum toxin at the level of LES is expected to decrease resting tone by blocking the release of acetylcoline from presynaptic nerve endings. A placebo-controlled randomised trial has proven the effectiveness of this treatment [6]. However, only about two-thirds of patients continue to demonstrate symptomatic benefit at 6 months, and average duration of response is estimated at 0.7 to 1.6 years. When repeat injections are used, success rates up to 75% have been reported at a mean follow-up of 2 years [7]. For this reason, injection therapy with botulinum toxin should be reserved to patients who are uneligible for a more definitive treatment such as pneumatic dilation or surgical myotomy.

It appears that sustained symptomatic relief of dysphagia can only be achieved by endoscopic pneumatic dilation or by surgical myotomy [8]. Pneumatic dilation performed with polyethylene ballons under conscious sedation has the advantage of being an outpatient procedure, but a 1-5% risk of esophageal perforation exists, and most authors have reported success rates not exceeding 70% at one year, even with repeat treatments. Retrospective studies have shown better results with myotomy performed by an experienced surgeon, and in the only prospective randomised trial myotomy gave better long-term results compared with pneumatic dilatation [9]. In addition, it has been estimated that the cumulative risk of any subsequent intervention for achalasia at 10 years is 63.5% for individuals treated initially with pneumatic dilation, and 37.5% for individuals treated initially with surgical myotomy [10]. Young patients and those not responding to a single pneumatic dilatation should be offered surgery [11]. Over the past two decades, the advent of minimally invasive technology has made surgery a more attractive option as a first-line therapy to both patients and referring physicians. It has been shown that pneumatic dilation is 72% effective *versus* 92% for the laparoscopic Heller myotomy (*Table I*). In addition, laparoscopic techniques have sharply reduced surgical morbidity [12].

Table I. Pooled response rate of achalasia treatments (from [12]).

Therapy		n	Weighted response rate	Weighted follow-up
Botulinum toxin		149	32%	1.1 years
Pneumatic dilation		1,276	72%	4.9 years
Heller myotomy	Thoracotomy	1,221	84%	5 years
	Laparotomy	732	85%	7.6 years
	Laparoscopy	171	92%	1.2 years

Surgical therapy

The goal of surgical therapy in the treatment of achalasia is extramucosal division of both layers of the esophageal muscolaris propria and of the oblique gastric fibers, the so-called Heller myotomy. For many years this operation has been performed through a laparotomy, often with the addition of a fundoplication, or through a left thoracotomy. The extent of the myotomy in the stomach, which in part depends on the type of surgical access, has long been a matter of controversy [13]. Ellis, the pioneer of the transthoracic approach, advocated a limited (< 1 cm) gastric myotomy without an antireflux procedure. However, at a very late follow-up the level of symptomatic improvement markedly deteriorated over time with this approach, and the rate of excellent results (i.e., asymptomatic patients) progressively decreased from 54% at 10 years to 32% at 20 years [14]. The majority of European surgeons have instead favored the transabdominal approach which includes a longer gastric myotomy (1 to 2 cm) and a fundoplication to protect the esophagus from iatrogenic GER. Another debated issue has been the direction of the myotomy over the stomach, which may be closer to the lesser curve or to the greater curve, and, as a consequence, can divide the semicircular (clasp) fibers and the oblique (sling) fibers in distinct proportions [15].

A third major issue is the opportunity to add an antireflux repair to the myotomy. The rationale for considering a concomitant fundoplication is the assumption that a well performed surgical myotomy renders the LES incompetent. Furthermore, gastric contents propelled retrograde into an aperistaltic esophagus are not effectively cleared, thus magnifying the damage caused by post-operative reflux. The majority of surgeons worldwide presently favor a transabdominal approach and add to the myotomy a partial fundoplication, either a 180 degree anterior (Dor) or a 270 degree posterior fundoplication (Toupet). The partial fundoplication, as opposed to the 360 degree Nissen repair, does not cause significant resistance to esophageal emptying, therefore reducing the risk of post-operative dysphagia. The main advantage of an anterior Dor fundoplication is that this technique does not require mobilization of the distal esophagus and cardia, and provides a natural patch over the denuded esophageal mucosa. Overall, there has been a greater than

90% symptomatic relief and a less than 10% incidence of pH proven GER with this approach [16]. This operation should be proposed as the first therapeutic option also in patients with sigmoid-shaped esophagus, although the chances of symptomatic relief are reduced in such circumstances, and in some of these individuals an esophagectomy can eventually be required [17].

During the early times of the minimally invasive surgical approach, both laparoscopy and thoracoscopy have been used to perform a Heller myotomy. However, it soon became clear that laparoscopy offers several inherent advantages, including superior visualization of the gastroesophageal junction (GEJ), a single lumen endotracheal intubation, the ability to add an antireflux procedure, and a shorter hospital stay. In addition, laparoscopy showed a better symptomatic outcome and a lesser incidence of post-operative GER [18].

The first laparoscopic Heller procedures were performed in England and in Italy during the early 1990s [19,20]. Compared to the open abdominal approach, a technical innovation introduced in the laparoscopic era has been the use of intraoperative endoscopy as a means of precisely identifying the GEJ, checking for the completeness of the myotomy, and testing for the presence of occult perforations. During the early phase of the learning curve, a Rigiflex balloon dilator was also used to distend the cardia in order to facilitate division of all residual muscle fibers [21]. Subsequently, transillumination and air inflation provided by the endoscope were considered appropriate to assist the myotomy [22]. Further demonstration of the effectiveness of intraoperative endoscopy came from a study showing that endoscopic and laparoscopic criteria were discordant in the identification of the esophagogastric junction (EGJ) in 58% of the cases, the cardia being in all these cases at a more distal site with endoscopic criteria. As a consequence, based on the laparoscopic appearance, the surgeon may err by underestimating the caudal extent of the myotomy and can perform a too short myotomy on the gastric side [23]. Although we are still convinced of the effectiveness of intraoperative endoscopy during the learning curve of this operation and during reoperative surgery, we have now discontinued this practice in our high-volume referral center where between 15 and 20 patients per year undergo Heller myotomy as a primary treatment for achalasia.

A common reason for an incomplete myotomy on the gastric side is the fear of producing a mucosal injury, which typically occurs just at the EGJ. The mean reported rate of mucosal perforation is about 5%, but the frequency is largerly dependent on surgeon's experience. There are no consequences if the mucosal injury is detected intraoperatively and repaired with interrupted stitches [22].

The principle of limited surgical dissection of the cardia, already advocated by some surgeons in the open era [16], has been successfully reproduced in many centers with the minimally invasive laparoscopic approach. Dissection is limited to the anterior and lateral attachments of the phrenoesophageal membrane as this allows enough space to perform the myotomy and helps to prevent the occurrence of post-operative GER. Only in patients with an associated hiatal hernia or epiphrenic diverticulum the distal esophagus is encircled and a posterior crural repair is performed. The myotomy is carried out for about 6 cm on the esophagus, toward the left of the anterior vagus nerve, and up to 2 cm on the gastric side to include the oblique fibers.

Despite the minimal surgical dissection herein described, an antireflux repair added to the Heller myotomy appears to be beneficial. The anterior Dor fundoplication is a technically simple procedure, quick and safe to perform laparoscopically. It does not require mobilization of the cardia, and places a gastric fundic patch over the myotomy site to protect the mucosa and prevent re-healing of the myotomy. The Heller-Dor operation is carried out in about one hour by an expert surgeon, and post-operative length of stay averages 2 days.

Studies including large number of patients have shown that an extramucosal myotomy of the esophagus and cardia combined with an anterior fundoplication can be performed safely and effectively through laparoscopy, with clinical and functional results similar to that obtained with the open transabdominal approach and relief of dysphagia in more than 90% of patients [24-29]. Although previous endoscopic treatments, such as balloon dilatation or intrasphincteric botulinum toxin injection, may cause submucosal scarring at the EGJ resulting in a more difficult surgical procedure and an increased operative morbility, no statistically significant differences as far as concern the clinical outcome have been reported [22].

In a recent report, at a minimum follow-up of 6 years after the operation, about 82% of patients were satisfied with the treatment and were able to eat normally; more than a half of the symptomatic recurrences occurred during the first year of follow-up and were effectively treated with pneumatic dilations. Nine (12.7%) patients either had abnormal acid exposure on post-operative 24-hour pH study or were on treatment with proton pump inhibitors for reflux symptoms; however, in none of these individuals did endoscopy reveal more than grade A esophagitis [30].

The issue of whether an antireflux procedure should be added to the Heller myotomy has long been controversial. Recently, a randomised double-blind clinical trial comparing the outcome of laparoscopic myotomy plus Dor fundoplication *versus* myotomy alone has shown that the former operation is superior in terms of reflux control. The addition of a Dor fundoplication reduces the risk of pathologic GER by 9-fold as tested by 24-hour esophageal pH monitoring. Even the median esophageal acid exposure was lower in the Heller-Dor group, indicating that the few unfortunate individuals in whom reflux might occur are easily managed with medical therapy [31].

References

1. Streitz J, Ellis F, Gibb P, Heatley G. Achalasia and squamous cell carcinoma of the esophagus: analysis of 241 patients. Ann Thorac Surg 1995;59:1604-9.
2. Zendehdel K, Nyren O, Edberg A, Ye W. Risk of esophageal adenocarcinoma in achalasia patients, a retrospective cohort study from Sweden. A J Gastroenterol 2007;102:1-5.
3. Bortolotti M, Labò G. Clinical and manometric effects of nifedipine in patients with esophageal achalasia. Gastroenterology 1981;80:39-44.
4. Bortolotti M, Mari C, Lopilato C, et al. Effects of sildenafil on esophageal motility of patients with idiopathic achalasia. Gastroenterology 2000;118:253-7.
5. Traube M, Dubovik S, Lange R, et al. The role of nifedipine therapy in achalasia:results of a randomised,double-blind,placebo-controlled study. Am J Gastroenterol 1989;84:1259-62.
6. Pasricha P, Ravich W, Hendrix T, et al. Botulinum toxin for the treatment of achalasia. N Engl J Med 1995;332:774-8.
7. Annese V, Basciani M, Borrelli O, et al. Intrasphincteric injection of botulinum toxin is effective in the long-term treatment of esophageal achalasia. Muscle Nerve 1998;21:1540-42.
8. Peracchia A, Bonavina L. Achalasia: dilation, injection or surgery? Can J Gastroenterol 2000;14:441-3.
9. Csendes A, Braghetto I, Henriquez A, Cortes C. Late results of a prospective randomised study comparing forceful dilatation and oesophagomyotomy in patients with achalasia. Gut 1989;30:299-304.
10. Lopushinsky S, Urbach D. Pneumatic dilatation and surgical myotomy for achalasia. JAMA 2006;296:2227-33.
11. Eckardt V, Gockel I, Berhard G. Pneumatic dilation for achalasia: late results of a prospective follow up investigation. Gut 2004;53:629-33.
12. Spiess A, Kahrilas P. Treating achalasia. From whalebone to laparoscope. JAMA 1998;280:638-42.
13. Bonavina L. Minimally invasive surgery for esophageal achalasia. World J Gastroenterol 2006;12:5921-5.
14. Ellis F. Oesophagomyotomy for achalasia. A 22-year experience. Br J Surg 1993:80:882-5.

15. Korn O, Braghetto I, Burdiles P, Csendes A. Cardiomyotomy in achalasia: which fibers do we cut? Dis Esoph 2000;13:104-7.
16. Bonavina L, Nosadini A, Bardini, et al. Primary treatment of esophageal achalasia. Long-term results of myotomy and Dor fundoplication. Arch Surg 1992;127:222-6.
17. Orringer M, Stirling M. Esophageal resection for achalasia: indications and results. Ann Thorac Surg 1989;47:340-5.
18. Stewart K, Finley R, Clifton J, et al. Thoracoscopic versus laparoscopic modified Heller myotomy for achalasia: efficacy and safety in 87 patients. J Am Coll Surg 1999;189:164-70.
19. Shimi S, Nathanson L, Cuschieri A. Laparoscopic cardiomyotomy for achalasia. J R Coll Surg Edinb 1991:36:152-4.
20. Peracchia A, Ancona E, Ruol A, et al. Use of mini-invasive procedures in esophageal surgery. Chirurgie 1992;118:305-9.
21. Ancona E, Peracchia A, Zaninotto G, et al. Heller laparoscopic cardiomyotomy with anterior antireflux fundoplication (Dor) in the treatment of esophageal achalasia. Surg Endosc 1993;7:459-61.
22. Bonavina L, Incarbone R, Antoniazzi L, et al. Previous endoscopic treatment does not affect complication rate and outcome of laparoscopic Heller myotomy and anterior fundoplication for oesophageal achalasia. Ital J Gastroenterol Hepatol 1999;31:827-30.
23. Alves A, Perniceni T, Godeberge P, et al. Laparoscopic Heller's cardiomyotomy in achalasia. Is intraoperative endoscopy useful, and why? Surg Endosc 1999;13:600-3.
24. Rosati R, Fumagalli U, Bona S, et al. Evaluating results of laparoscopic surgery for esophageal achalasia. Surg Endosc 1998;12:270-3.
25. Patti M, Pellegrini C, Horgan S, et al. Minimally invasive surgery for achalasia. An eight-year experience with with 168 patients. Ann Surg 1999;230:587-94.
26. Zaninotto G, Costantini M, Molena D, et al. Treatment of esophageal achalasia with laparoscopic Heller myotomy and Dor partial fundoplication: prospective evaluation of 100 consecutive patients. J Gastrointest Surg 2000;4:282-9.
27. Ackroyd R, Watson D, Devitt P, Jamieson G. Laparoscopic cardiomyotomy and anterior partial fundoplication for achalasia. Surg Endosc 2001;15:683-6.
28. Finley R, Clifton J, Stewart K, et al. Laparoscopic Heller myotomy improves esophageal emptying and the symptoms of achalasia. Arch Surg 2001;136:892-6.
29. Donahue P, Horgan S, Liu K, et al. Floppy Dor fundoplication after esophagocardiomyotomy for achalasia. Surgery 2002;132:716-23.
30. Costantini M, Zaninotto G, Guirroli E, et al. The laparoscopic Heller-Dor operation remains an effective treatment for esophageal achalasia at a minimum of 6-year follow-up. Surg Endosc 2005;19:345-51.
31. Richards W, Torquati A, Holzman M, et al. Heller myotomy versus Heller myotomy with Dor fundoplication for achalasia. A prospective randomised double-blind clinical trial. Ann Surg 2004;240:405-15.

Esophageal function testing in achalasia patients

O.B. Lao, B.K. Oelschlager (Seattle)

Pre-operative and diagnostic studies

Dysphagia for both liquids and solids is usually the presenting symptom that elicits further studies into esophageal motility that eventually lead to a diagnosis of achalasia. While that is the most common complaint, other symptoms such as swallowing difficulty, weight loss, regurgitation, chest pain, heart-burn, choking and/or frequent cough can also be described. There are a variety of studies that can be undertaken to evaluate these symptoms.

Achalasia results from the degeneration of neurons within the myenteric plexus of the esophageal wall. The loss of these nitrogen-oxide producing, inhibitory neurons allows unopposed cholinergic stimulation and prevents effective relaxation of the lower esophageal sphincter (LES)

An upper-gastrointestinal (GI) fluoroscopy study or barium swallow may show the characteristic signs of absent peristalsis and a dilated esophagus. Classically, a "bird's beak" esophagus is demonstrated as the tapered distal esophagus narrows at the esophageal sphincter. Full evaluation of LES mechanism relies on real-time evaluation and will commonly show a failure of the LES to relax.

Despite the above mentioned characteristic findings on fluoroscopy, the diagnosis of achalasia is confirmed by esophageal manometry and, therefore, should always be undertaken to fully evaluate the esophagus when achalasia is suspected. This study should demonstrate an aperistaltic esophagus with an associated non-relaxing LES. The specific pressures obtained in the LES are not characteristic and should not be used to define achalasia as a spectrum of pressures can be found; fewer than half of patients have a hypertensive LES [1]. Still, as Gorodner *et al.* point out in their paper, one must always include connective tissue disorders, such as scleroderma, in the differential for patients with hypotensive LES in the setting of an aperistaltic esophagus. Usually other findings can differentiate the two, for example fluoroscopy will demonstrate a wide open gastroesophageal junction (GEJ) in scleroderma as oppose to the typical "bird's beak" of achalasia.

Multichannel intraluminal impedance (MII), in addition to manometry, offers the advantage of providing evaluation of bolus transit along with the evaluation of esophageal contraction. The combination of MII with manometry may provide for greater specificity in identifying those manometric abnormalities that are associated with altered esophageal function. Achalasia, along with scleroderma, diffuse esophageal spasm and ineffective esophageal motility all are associated with disorders in bolus transit that can be measured by MII. Moreover, MII is able to separate these disorders of esophageal motility from those with pressure defects such as nutcracker esophagus, hypertensive LES and hypotensive LES along with poorly relaxing LES [2]. Some studies have attempted to describe the impedance characteristics of achalasia as low esophageal baseline impedance, failed bolus transport, regurgitation of luminal contents during swallowing and air trapping during deglutition [3]; while other studies have called into question the ability of MII to accurately help diagnose achalasia [4]. There is no question that esophageal transit is very abnormal in achalasia, but this may be the case in other esophageal disorders, thus MII is inferior to standard manometry for diagnosis.

Upper endoscopy can also be used to differentiate achalasia from connective tissue disorders in that achalasia will have evidence of a dilated esophagus with retained food while scleroderma may show distal esophagitis and strictures resulting from reflux and a very patent GEJ. Endoscopy is also helpful to evaluate for esophagitis separate from connective tissue disorders along with other structural abnormalities such as strictures and/or tumors like squamous or adenocarcinoma of the distal esophagus that may be leading to the patient's symptoms. Lastly, esophageal endoscopy is critical to rule-out pseudo-achalasia that is diagnosed when a tumor or carcinoma is found within the cardia of the stomach that then extends towards the esophagus leading to mechanical obstruction.

Esophageal scintigraphy is yet another option to study the function of the esophagus [5]. Dynamic scintigraphy utilizes a radioactive liquid or semisolid bolus and has the advantage of being well-tolerated by patients while closely reflecting the underlying physiology under study. This test is less invasive than those mentioned above and requires relatively minimum cooperation by patients. Achalasia is seen as a delay in transit times through the esophagus just as with fluoroscopy. There is evidence of distal esophageal retention that does not clear with the upright position or swallowing liquid; in contrast to scleroderma.

Despite all of these studies to evaluate the esophagus and diagnose achalasia, there is still debate as to the prognostic significance of the results. Some authors have endorsed the idea that a higher preoperative resting LES pressure is a predictor for the resolution of the symptoms of dysphagia post-operatively [6]. The average LES resting pressure of those that had resolution of dysphagia was 35.9 mmHg whereas those that had persistent dysphagia had initial resting pressures in the LES of only 24.5 mmHg. Others suggest that the finding of a hypertensive LES does not have prognostic value in the treatment of achalasia [1]. These studies may appear to be in disagreement, however the second study stratified patients according to their LES pressure ranging from less than 14 mmHg, between 14-24 mmHg and greater than 24 mmHg finding no difference in relief of dysphagia after myotomy. It may be that those patients with extremely high LES pressures benefit from achalasia treatment more than those with normal or even slightly elevated pressures, but it is still not clear.

Intra-operative studies

There are two main studies that can be performed intra-operatively during a myotomy: endoscopy and manometry. Endoscopy is usually performed to assess for structural changes or abnormalities along with evidence of perforation during an operation. During the operation, many surgeons use manometry to guide the extent and length of their myotomy. In a study of 139 patients that underwent 136 myotomies, 34% of those patients had evidence of residual high pressure of the LES after initial myotomy, resulting in the lengthening of the myotomy [7]. The myotomy was continued until completion that was noted by a dimunition in pressure to 3 mmHg or less, the implication being that the manometry changed therapy (and potentially outcomes). A retrospective review of the data shows that the majority of those requiring revision occurred in the first half of those treated demonstrating an obvious learning curve with myotomy for achalasia. The authors conclude their study by noting that the addition of manometry to endoscopy would be helpful especially during the initial experience of the laparoscopic surgeon. More experienced surgeons may simply choose to perform a more complete, extended myotomy without concurrent manometry.

At the University of Washington, we have published on our experience with the extended gastric myotomy [8]. Our study compared 52 patients with a standard esophagogastric myotomy, 1-1.5 cm below the GEJ, to 58 patients that had an extended myotomy to 3 cm below the GEJ. We found that there was less recurrent, severe dysphagia, less requirement for re-intervention and no indication for re-operations in the extended myotomy group. Our long-term results have reinforced our initial findings of the durability of the extended gastric myotomy in preventing the symptoms of recurrent dysphagia and also the need for re-intervention for those symptoms [9]. One can either do an extended myotomy or perhaps get similar results by tailoring the extent of myotomy to the findings on intra-operative manometry.

Post-operative studies

In the post-operative period, patients usually have resolution of their initial achalasia symptoms; however in a few patients symptoms may persist or recur and require work-up. The most common post-operative complaint is persistence of dysphagia that was the presenting complaint. In this case, one should be concerned about incomplete myotomy. Further testing would be warranted in this setting including barium swallow and/or fluoroscopy to rule out a physical or obstructive cause that may have arisen due to the intervention. The timed barium swallow has been advocated as a simple and reproducible test to assess esophageal emptying in patients with achalasia both prior to and after treatment [10]. The height and width of the barium column and thus the esophagus is measured along with a measurement of the open LES. These values can be used to quantitatively gauge effectiveness of an intervention. Qualitatively, the progression of barium through the swallow can be judged to assess effectiveness of an intervention with good intra- and inter-observer reliability. The authors recommend waiting one month before assessing esophageal emptying to avoid post-procedural changes that may confound interpretation of findings such as edema and spasm. In another study, the post-operative width of the esophagus in the short-term was a useful gauge for predicting clinical outcome [11]. They found that patients with an esophageal diameter 4 cm or less had complete resolution of symptoms at one year after the operation. For patients with intractable esophageal symptoms despite surgical intervention, all of them had esophageal diameters greater than 4 cm.

An esophagogram is not enough to evaluate persistent symptoms after intervention. Manometry is necessary to evaluate for residual high-pressure zones within the LES and also evaluate the total and abdominal length of the LES. In a study by Zaninotto *et al.*, 10 of 113 patients that underwent laparoscopic Heller myotomy were symptomatic at a median of five months after their operation [12]. When comparing their post-operative tests to 74 asymptomatic patients, the factors that differentiated them were a longer overall LES length, a longer abdominal LES length. LES pressure was similar in the two groups despite the difference in symptoms. This study reveals the importance of completely obliterating the LES in an effort to perform a successful operation for achalasia.

If the post-operative symptoms are different than those that the patient presented with, other studies should be undertaken to evaluate for reflux disease, that frequently found as a long-term outcome of achalasia treatment. In fact, at 20 years of follow-up approximately 20% of patients will suffer from pathologic acid reflux disease [13]. Endoscopy, manometry and pH testing would be crucial to evaluate for reflux physiology and esophagitis. New heartburn, chest pain and regurgitation should be investigated with the understanding that these symptoms may not be related to achalasia, but rather a result of treatment. When recurrent or new symptoms arise in patients with achalasia, one should always be weary of the possibility of the late occurrence of carcinoma, gastroesophageal reflux, a tight fundoplication if one was used, and an inadequate myotomy [14].

The use of MII in the post-operative setting has not been studied very well. In an unpublished study from the University of Washington, we studied patients with MII and manometry and compared 38 patients that had no therapy, and were called "untreated achalasia", with 26 patients that either had endoscopic therapy or underwent Heller myotomy. The results of impedance testing demonstrated significantly better clearance of both liquid and viscous boluses in the endoscopic and myotomy groups compared to untreated achalasia patients. Though promising, further studies, with larger sample sizes, are necessary to confirm the benefit in documenting outcomes of intervention for achalasia.

Those patients that are found to have persistence of their achalasia symptoms and documentation of persistence of their LES on manometry and esophagogram have several options for treatment. Pneumatic dilations have been shown to be effective in treating incomplete myotomies in the post-operative achalasia patient [13]. Important in their description of dilation is the delay of four months after the initial operation before undertaking pneumatic dilation. Other options include repeated myotomy and if this is undertaken, an extended gastric myotomy, as described above, is recommended to ensure adequate clearance of the LES [9]. Lastly, for patients that are still symptomatic and have failed less invasive methods, one can consider esophagectomy and reconstruction to relieve severe, debilitating symptoms.

Summary

The pre-operative evaluation of achalasia must include manometry and endoscopy. The addition of fluoroscopy and MII may support specific diagnoses, but they are not critical. Intra-operative performance of endoscopy and manometry have been shown to aid in the successful performance of myotomy for achalasia. Post-operative studies should be targeted to symptomatology. Manometry is key to evaluate for residual high-pressure zones and an incomplete myotomy.

References

1. Gorodner M, Galvani C, Fisichella PM, Patti MG. Preoperative lower esophageal sphincter pressure has little influence on the outcome of laparoscopic Heller myotomy for achalasia. Surg Endosc 2004;18:774-8.
2. Tutuian R, Castell D. Combined multichannel intraluminal impedance and manometry clarifies esophageal function abnormalities: study in 350 patients. Am J Gastroenterol 2004;99(6):1011-9.
3. Nguyen HN, Domingues GR, Winograd R, Lammert F, Silny J, Matern S. Impedance characteristics of esophageal motor function in achalasia. Dis Esophagus. 2004;17:44-50.
4. Conchillo JM, Nguyen NQ, Samsom M, Holloway RH, Smout A. Multichannel intraluminal impedance monitoring in the evaluation of patients with non-obstructive dysphagia. Am J Gastroenterol 2005;100(12):2624-32.
5. Mariana G, Boni G, Barreca M, et al. Radionuclide gastroesophageal motor studies. J Nucl Med 2004;45(6):1004-28.
6. Arain MA, Peters JH, Tamhankar AP. Preoperative lower esophageal sphincter pressure affects outcome of laparoscopic esophageal myotomy for achalasia. J Gastrointest Surg 2004;8(3): 328-34.
7. Chapman JR, Joehl RJ, Murayama KM, et al. Achalasia treatment Improved outcome of laparoscopic myotomy with operative manometry. Arch Surg 2004;139:508-13.
8. Oelschlager BK, Chang L, Pellegrini CA. Improved outcome after extended gastric myotomy for achalasia. Arch Surg 2003;138(5):490-5.
9. Wright AS, Williams CW, Pellegrini CA, Oelschlager BK. Long-term outcomes confirm the superior efficacy of extended Heller myotomy with Toupet fundoplication for achalasia. Surg Endosc 2007;21(5):713-8.
10. De Oliveira JMA, Birgisson S, Doinoff C, et al. Timed barium swallow: a simple technique for evaluating esophageal emptying in patients with achalasia. Am J Roentgenol 1997;169(2):473-9.
11. Pechlivanides G, Chrysos E, Athanasakis E, et al. Laparoscopic Heller cardiomyotomy and Dor fundoplication for achalasia: possible factors predicting outcome. Arch Surg 2001;136:1240-3.
12. Zaninotto G, Costantini M, Portale G, et al. Etiology, diagnosis, and treatment of failures after laparoscopic Heller myotomy for achalasia. Ann Surg 2002;235(2):186-92.
13. Csendes A, Braghetto I, Burdiles P, Korn O, Csendes P, Henriquez A. Very late results with esophagomyotomy for patients with achalasia. Ann Surg 2006;243(2):196-203.
14. Ellis HF. Failure after esophagomyotomy for esophageal motor disorders. Causes, prevention, and management. Chest Surg Clin N Am 1997;7:476-88.

What are the absolute manometric criteria for making the diagnosis of diffuse esophageal spasm?

E.-H. Metman, L. Negreanu, B. Godart (Tours)

Diffuse esophageal spasm (DES) has no well defined pathophysiology and its natural history is still poorly understood. It could represent a range of motility changes associated with subtle neural dysfunctions, gastroesophageal reflux (GER), or anxiety states.

Despite the recent technical advances in manometry, its diagnosis remains a challenge because of the variability of manometric findings and an obvious lack of general agreement on its definition.

The term "diffuse spasm of the lower part of the esophagus" was used for the first time by Moersch and Camp in 1934 [1] on radiologic examination. In this first description it was "distal" and "diffuse" [2]

The first manometric description was made in 1958 by Creamer *et al.* [3] and then by Fleschler and Kramer [4].

In 1974 Vantrappen and Hellemans [5] described in a comprehensive report a syndrome with multiple causes characterized by:
- frequent radiological abnormalities;
- simultaneous pressure peaks of repetitive and multiphasic waves and of giant waves, occasional spontaneous activity and some peristaltic contractions;
- normal or high pressure of the lower esophageal sphincter (LES) and decreased deglutitive relaxation.

The associated conditions were idiopathic muscular hypertrophy of the lower esophagus and the hypertensive LES.

In 1979 Vantrappen *et al.* [6] realized a classification of the esophageal motility disorders following three criteria: esophageal peristalsis, relaxation of the LES and the character of the esophageal contractions (vigorous or not). In a reappraisal in 1982, Vantrappen proposed the value of 30% non peristaltic contractions for diagnosing DES [7]. LES was often found normal in accord with Di Marino and Cohen [8].

In a rather disturbing definition in 1984 Richter *et al.* used as principal criteria for diagnosing DES the presence of simultaneous contractions after at least 10% (but less than 100%) of wet swallows irrespective of other features [9].

Allen and DiMarino [10] offered with timidity their results separating DES with high pressures waves from DES with low pressure waves based on the amplitude of distal esophageal contractions and its relation with the clinical presentation. From the 60 patients diagnosed manometrically with diffuse esophageal spasm, those with chest pain had high pressures and those with dysphagia had lower pressures. The authors suggested that a diagnosis of DES might be inadequate in patients with low contraction amplitudes.

Controversies upon reflux associated DES and idiopathic DES appeared appeared in the eighties before the recognition of the ineffective esophageal motility (IEM) in 1997 by Leite *et al.* They defined IEM by the presence of either low amplitude (< 30 mmHg) peristaltic or simultaneous contractions in the distal esophagus, or failed peristalsis in which the wave does not traverse the entire length of the distal esophagus [11].

The presence of high amplitude non peristaltic contractions was considered necessary for diagnosis of DES by Vantrappen [5]. In the Spechler and Castell [12] and Richter's [13] new classifications published in 2001, only an amplitude greater than 30 mmHg of the simultaneous contractions was proposed for the diagnosis of diffuse esophageal spasm. In the same paper, Richter redefined the DES by the presence of simultaneous contractions after 20% or more of wet swallows [13].

For Spechler and Castell the features that can be commonly found but are not required for manometric diagnosis of DES include: spontaneous contractions, repetitive contractions, multiple peaked contractions, and intermittent normal peristalsis [12]. The presence of long-duration contractions, repetitive waves (three peaks or more), and spontaneous non-swallow induced contractions were manometric findings less consistently found in DES and considered secondary criteria by Richter [13].

As for the LES anormalities in diffuse esophageal spasm there is also controversy.

Vantrappen *et al.* excluded the possibility of associated LES abnormalities [4]. Spechler and Castell also considered that the association of LES relaxation abnormalities with simultaneous esophageal contractions should be better characterized as an atypical disorder of LES relaxation and not as diffuse esophageal spasm [12]. On the other hand Richter accepted the possibility of LES abnormalities as secondary findings that can be seen in DES [13]. However, one must remain prudent as a low basal pressure in the LES is more commonly seen in patients with GER, suggesting that the motility abnormalities might be secondary to GER disease (GERD) [11]. For a better classification of these patients it would be interesting to know their future evolution: was it really DES, non specific motor disorder, early achalasia or GERD related motility abnormalities?

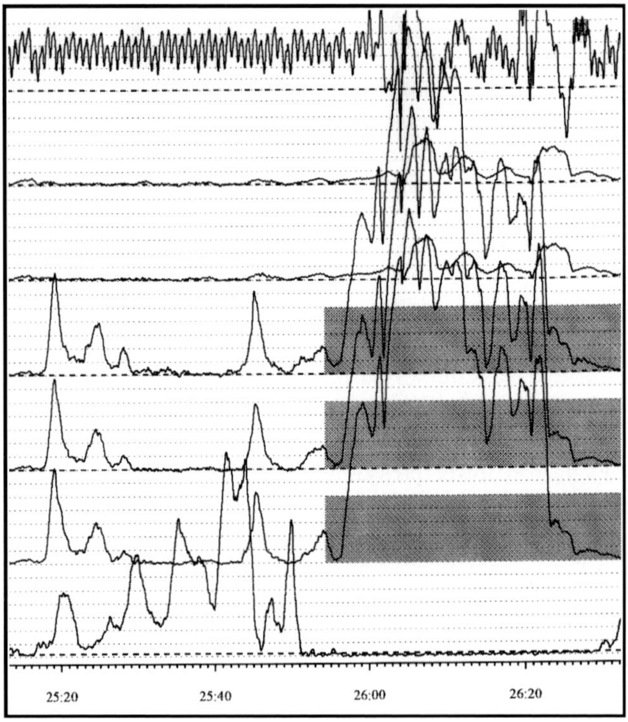

Figure 1.

There are no gold standards to establish the specificity of the manometric criteria: radiology, provocation tests, echoendoscopy and even histology being neither specific nor reliable. Important features of DES as the sustained esophageal contractions and the esophageal shortening were evidenced by echoendoscopy [14]. Sustained contractions and shortening could be observed on standard manometry [15] (*Figure 1*). But these modifications can also be observed in achalasia in our experience.

The 24-hour manometry showed poor concordance with standard manometry and no clear cut off in the percentage of simultaneous waves between different disorders. The importance of spasm waves occurring with pain was evidenced by Barham [16]. In his patients DES diagnosis upon standard manometric examination – on more than 10% of simultaneous waves- was rarely confirmed by 24-hour manometry.

In a recent paper a very poor concordance between observers was shown for the manometric diagnoses using classic criteria except for achalasia and normal. The authors challenged the classic dogma in their conclusion that manometric diagnoses other than achalasia and normal must be redefined or eliminated from practice [17]. Impedance-manometry could perhaps in the future but not yet help to distinguish muscular spasm from other syndromes [18].

In conclusion, clinically and manometrically DES remains an elusive entity because of its rarity and lack of consensus on its definition. It is and should remain a rare disease.

We suggest these criteria for the diagnosis upon standard manometry:

- more than 20% of simultaneous waves (and some peristalsis) with two of the following:
  - high pressure or prolonged duration waves,
  - repetitive waves,
  - spontaneous activity,
  - LES relaxation disorders,
  - or with sustained esophageal contraction (at best accompanied by pain on 24-hour manometry),
  - and absence of hypotensive sphincter;
- the presence of an associated esophageal muscular hypertrophy is of clinical and therapeutic importance.

References

1. Moersch HJ, Camp JD. Diffuse spasm of the lower part of the esophagus. Ann Otol Rhinol Laryngol 1934;43:1165-73.
2. Sperandio M, Tutuian R, Gideon M, Katz PO, Castell DO. Diffuse esophageal spasm: not diffuse but distal esophageal spasm (DES). Dig Dis Sci 2003;48:1380-4.
3. Creamer B, Donoghue FE, Code CF. Pattern of esophageal motility in diffuse spasm. Gastroenterology 1958;34:782-6.
4. Kramer P, Fleshler B, McNally E, Harris LD. Oesophageal sensitivity to Mecholyl in symptomatic diffuse spasm. Gut 1967;8(2):120-7.
5. Vantrappen G, Hellemans J. Diffuse esophageal spasm. In: Vantrappen G, Hellemans J, eds. Diseases of the esophagus. Berlin: Springer Verlag, 1974: 355-66.
6. Vantrappen G, Janssens J, Hellemans J, Coremans G. Achalasia, diffuse esophageal spasm, and related motility disorders. Gastroenterology 1979;76:450-7.
7. Vantrappen G, Hellemans J. Oesophageal spasm and other muscular dysfunction. Clin Gastroenterol 1982;11:453-77.
8. DiMarino AJ, Cohen S. Characteristics of lower esophageal sphincter function in symptomatic diffuse esophageal spasm. Gastroenterology 1974; 66:1-6.
9. Richter JE, Castell DO. Diffuse esophageal spasm: a reappraisal. Ann Intern Med 1984;100:242-5.
10. Allen M, DiMarino A. Manometric diagnosis of diffuse esophageal spasm. Dig Dis Sci 1996;41:1346-9.
11. Leite LP, Jhonston BT, Barrett J, Castell JA, Castell DO. Ineffective esophageal motility (IEM). The primary finding in patients with non-specific esophageal motility disorder. Dig Dis Sci 1997;42:1859-65.

12. Spechler SJ, Castell DO. Classification of oesophageal motility abnormalities. Gut 2001;49:145-51.
13. Richter JE. Oesophageal motility disorders. Lancet 2001;358:823-8.
14. Mittal RK, Kassab G, Puckett JL, Liu J. Hypertrophy of the muscularis propria of the lower esophageal sphincter and the body of the esophagus in patients with primary motility disorders of the esophagus.Am J Gastroenterol 2003;98:1705-12.
15. Metman EH, Picon L, d'Alteroche L, Lagasse JP, Addra B. Oesophageal shortening associated with non cardiac chest pain (NCCP). A new manometric pattern. Neurogastroenterol Motil 1998;10: 471.
16. Barham CP, Gotley DC, Fowler A, Mills A, Alderson D. Diffuse oesophageal spasm: diagnosis by ambulatory 24 hour manometry. Gut 1997; 41:151-5.
17. Nayar DS, Khandwala F, Achkar E, et al. Esophageal manometry; assessment of interpreter consistency. Clin Gastroenterol Hepatol 2005;3:218-24.
18. Tutuian R, Mainie I, Agrawal A, Gideon RM, Katz PO, Castell DO. Symptom and function heterogenicity among patients with distal esophageal spasm: studies using combined impedance-manometry. Am J Gastroenterol 2006;101:464-9.

What criteria differentiate diffuse esophageal spasm from nutcracker esophagus?

V. Nilton Felix (São Paulo)

The primary and secondary esophageal motor disorders are progressively better described and better known, but controversies are always present and justify continuous discussion about them.

Diffuse esophageal spasm (DES) and nutcracker esophagus, characterised by dysphagia and chest pain, are two functional diseases that exemplify those controversies beginning in diagnostic criteria and arriving to treatment basis.

DES is mainly a primary disorder and nutcracker esophagus, in most times, a secondary one, and differences between them can be found basically, but not exclusively, on manometric study of the esophagus (*Table I*).

Symptomatic DES is an uncommon motility disorder in which wet swallows are followed by non-propulsive contractions, without evidences of its evolution to achalasia.

DES is manifested clinically by episodes of dysphagia and chest pain and is found in less than 5% of patients undergoing esophageal motility testing for dysphagia.

Spastic contractions of the esophagus eventually can be seen radiographically, and manometrically DES is characterised by signals of uncoordinated activity in the smooth muscle portion of the esophagus [1], more frequent on its distal portion [2].

There is disagreement on how spastic activity manifests itself manometrically, compromising an universally accepted diagnostic criteria for the condition: different investigators have used different manometric criteria for DES regarding the requirement for the presence of spontaneous and repetitive contractions and the need to demonstrate esophageal contractions that are of high amplitude and prolonged duration.

DES is defined manometrically when more than 10% (but < 100%) of wet swallows are followed by simultaneous esophageal contractions, with mean amplitude > 30 mmHg [1].

Table I. Differences between diffuse esophageal spasm and nutcracker esophagus.

	Diffuse esophageal spasm	Nutcraker esophagus
Etiology (mostly)	Primary	Secondary
Peristalsis	Absent in > 10% and < 100% of the wet deglutition waves	Normal
Spastic contractions on the distal esophagus	Frequent	Absent
Contraction amplitude on the distal esophagus	Occasionally abnormal	> 180 mmHg
Duration of contractions	Occasionally abnormal	Frequently > 6 sec
Radiographic signals (when present)	Esophageal spasm	Marked progressive esophageal contractions
Esophageal diverticula	Can occur	Absent
Usual clinical treatment	Calcium channel blocking agents	PPI
Eventual surgical treatment	LES myotomy	Fundoplicature

Features that can be found commonly but are not required for manometric diagnosis include spontaneous contractions, repetitive contractions, multiple peaked contractions, and intermittent normal peristalsis, almost always without any lower esophageal sphincter (LES) disorder.

Ten dysphagic patients, clinically suspected to have DES, complaining chest pain during meals (mean age: 46 ± 15.9 years; 8 women and 2 men), were submitted to endoscopic and manometric studies in the last years [3]. The Synectics® perfusion computerized system was used to perform the manometric exam.

Eight patients had normal esophageal endoscopic exam and light esophagitis (Savary I) was present in two, but with normal esophageal prolonged pHmetry.

Manometric study data confirmed the clinical diagnosis (mean ± SE):

- LES pressure (mmHg) = 16.21 ± 6.36;
- LES relaxing pressure (mmHg) = 0.21 ± 0.56;
- LES extension (cm) = 3.45 ± 0.79;
- contraction amplitude on distal esophagus = 103.66 ± 31.07;
- normal peristalsis (10 wet deglutition's percentile) = 25.16 ± 11.05 (*versus* spastic and simultaneous contractions).

LES was absolutely normal in the series, as well as the amplitude of the deglutition waves on distal esophagus; there was a significant low normal peristaltic contractions percentile in these DES patients, probably causing dysphagia.

The low amplitude simultaneous contractions seen in scleroderma differ substantially from those normal or high amplitude simultaneous contractions of the idiopathic DES and LES is clearly compromised in achalasia. There is no reason to have misunderstanding among these motor disturbances.

Treatment is mostly clinical, with nitrates and calcium channel blocking agents used in order to decrease smooth muscle activity. Tranquilizers and antidepressant may be used and psychological assessment may be useful.

Intractable symptoms may be surgically treated by LES myotomy [4] or botulinum toxin [5] in selected patients.

When a diverticulum of the esophageal body is present, associated myotomy and fundoplicature are essential procedures to prevent recurrences after diverticulectomy [6]. Motor abnormalities remain unchanged, after myotomy, but there is a marked reduction of the amplitude of the multi-peaked contractions on the distal esophagus [7].

"Nutcracker esophagus" is a term coined by Castell *et al.* for the condition in which patients with non-cardiac chest pain and/or dysphagia exhibit peristaltic waves in the distal esophagus with mean amplitudes exceeding normal values by more than 2 SD [8].

Patients with nutcracker esophagus demonstrate a hypersensitive esophagus. Intraesophageal balloon distensions often reproduce their chest pain, and so visceral hyperalgesia of the esophagus may be relevant to the pathogenesis of their chest pain [9].

Areas of disparity among published reports regarding the manometric criteria for nutcracker esophagus have included the precise amplitude of the peristaltic waves required for the diagnosis.

Whereas the nutcracker esophagus has been defined by the presence of peristaltic waves with mean amplitudes > 2 SD above normal, the precise amplitude required for the diagnosis can vary depending on the data used to establish normal values, and a number of subsequent reports on nutcracker esophagus have used 180 mmHg as the diagnostic criterion [10].

Peristaltic wave amplitude varies considerably throughout the esophagus, both in normal individuals and in patients with nutcracker esophagus [11,12] and some studies have shown that high amplitude contractions may involve the esophagus in a segmental fashion, with high amplitude peristaltic waves found only in the distal esophagus [13,14].

Summarizing, the manometric feature proposed for a diagnosis of nutcracker esophagus is a mean distal esophageal peristaltic wave amplitude > 180 mmHg measured as the average amplitude of 10 swallows at two recording sites positioned 3 and 8 cm above the LES.

Peristaltic contractions of long duration (> 6 sec) are commonly viewed, but are not required for manometric diagnosis of nutcracker esophagus and resting pressure of the LES is usually normal.

Regular progressive and marked contractions on the esophageal body, typical radiographic images of nutcracker esophagus, are uncommonly found.

Associated gastroesophageal reflux have been observed in 80% of our cases of nutcracker esophagus and the use of proton pump inhibitors has obtained excellent chest pain control (more than 90%).

Twelve patients submitted to fundoplicature, operated on for erosive reflux esophagitis associated to symptomatic nutcracker esophagus, had presented normal esophageal endoscopy after one year, and 66.66% of them became completely asymptomatic and converted motility pattern to normal.

References

1. Richter JE, Castell DO. Diffuse esophageal spasm: a reappraisal. Ann Intern Med 1984;100:242-5.
2. Sperandio M, Tutuian R, Gideon RM, Katz PO, Castell DO. Diffuse esophageal spasm: not diffuse but distal esophageal spasm (DES). Dig Dis Sci 2003;48:1380-4.
3. Felix VN, Viebig RG. Diffuse esophageal spasm. Manometric data exclude some principles of treatment. Dis Esophagus 2003;17(S1):A87.

4. Stein HJ, DeMeester TR, Hinder RA. Outpatient physiological testing and surgical management of foregut motility disorders. Curr Prac Surg 1992;418-545.
5. Storr M, Linke R, Nicolaus M, Göke B, Schirra J. Injection of botulinum toxin for diffuse esophageal spasm. Dtsch Med Wochenschr 2005;130:266-9.
6. Duranceau A, Pera M. Motor disorders of the esophagus. Dis Esophagus 1995;8:159-66.
7. Felix VN. Divertículos do esôfago distal. In: Pinotti HW, ed. Acesso ao esôfago torácico por transecção mediana do diafragma. São Paulo: Atheneu, 1999:105-10.
8. Dalton CB, Castell DO, Richter JE. The changing faces of the nutcracker esophagus. Am J Gastroenterol 1988;83:623-8.
9. Mujica VR, Mudipalli RS, Rao SS. Pathophysiology of chest pain in patients with nutcracker esophagus. Am J Gastroenterol. 2001;96:1371-7.
10. Achem SR, Benjamin SB. Esophageal dysmotility (spastic dysmotility). In: Castell DO, ed. The esophagus, 2nd ed. Boston: Little, Brown and Company, 1995;247-68.
11. Richter JE, Wu WC, Hohns DN. Esophageal manometry in 95 healthy adult volunteers. Variability of pressures with age and frequency of "abnormal" contractions. Dig Dis Sci 1987;32:583-92.
12. Clouse RE, Staiano A. Topography of normal and high-amplitude esophageal peristalsis. Am J Physiol 1993;265:1098-107.
13. Achem SR, Kolts BE, Burton L. Segmental versus diffuse nutcracker esophagus: an intermittent motility pattern. Am J Gastroenterol 1993;88:847-51.
14. Freidin N, Mittal RK, Traube M. Segmental high amplitude peristaltic contractions in the distal esophagus. Am J Gastroenterol 1989;84:619-23.

Can sensory function of the esophageal body be predicted by motility pattern?

R.P. Tatum (Seattle)

A link between esophageal motility events and esophageal sensation has been postulated for over 100 years, since the time of Osler [1]. This issue most frequently arises in the evaluation of patients with non-cardiac or unexplained chest pain, particularly in the situation in which evidence for pathologic acid reflux cannot be demonstrated. Esophageal dysmotility is found on manometry in 25-30% of patients undergoing workup for unexplained chest pain. Unfortunately, however, pain episodes rarely occur during standard manometric studies, making the establishment of an association between motility events and sensory function elusive [2]. Further, this is difficult to demonstrate on prolonged motility studies as well: for example in a study using 24-hour ambulatory manometry, Lacima *et al.* found that only 16% of non-cardiac chest pain patients had motility-associated pain episodes. The most common motility disorder in these patients was nutcracker esophagus, and less frequently diffuse esophageal spasm [3].

Provocative testing

Over the last several decades, multiple provocative tests have been developed to investigate the sensory properties of the esophageal body, including the acid perfusion test, the edrophonium test, intraesophageal balloon distension (IEBD), and others. All of these have been performed in conjunction with esophageal manometry in attempt to discover and explain a relationship between the motor and sensory function of the esophagus.

The acid perfusion test, in which acid is instilled into the distal esophagus and the patient reports the subsequent development of painful stimuli, was first described by Bernstein in 1958 [4]. While it is among the most simple of the provocative tests to perform, there is considerable variability in response rates [5], and less than 50% of patients reporting non-cardiac chest pain test positive [6]. Allen *et al.* found that "feeble" peristalsis was associated with a positive acid perfusion test in 78% of patients. They speculated that this may be because this finding frequently occurs in conjunction with a hypotensive LES, or alternatively because weak peristalsis may be a result of chronic acid exposure [7]. Hewson *et al.,* using the acid perfusion test and subsequent 24-hour ambulatory manometry, described a correlation between a positive test and a variety of abnormal pressure episodes. However, no one specific motility pattern was associated with increased sensitivity [8].

Intravenous edrophonium can be used as a provocative test in which peristaltic amplitudes are increased pharmacologically. The test is considered positive when this produces a pain episode, and suggests an esophageal origin for non-cardiac chest pain. Ultimately, this test seems less useful in linking sensitivity to motility pattern. In the study by Hewson *et al.*, a positive edrophonium test was significantly associated with acid-induced chest pain events on 24-hour pH monitoring but not motility-induced pain events on ambulatory manometry [8]. A 2003 study by Lacima *et al.* reported poor correlation between pain provoked by edrophonium administration and esophageal motility abnormalities [3].

IEBD has been used in a number of investigations to characterize esophageal sensitivity. The technique was described in the early 20th century, prior to the introduction of the acid perfusion test. It has been performed using a variety of techniques, but with little true standardization, and like the acid perfusion test, typically relies upon the subjective report of the patient regarding the onset of sensation and onset of pain [5]. Further, as the balloon distension test alone does not examine the biomechanical properties of esophageal muscle, its interpretation is not purely objective [1]. Nonetheless, a number of studies using this technique have demonstrated some association between motility and esophageal sensitivity. Using combined IEBD and standard esophageal manometry, Clouse *et al.* found that patients who had high rates of multipeaked peristaltic contractions were more likely to have increased sensitivity to balloon distension: 52% of patients with positive IEBD had multipeaked contractions *versus* only 25% of patients with negative IEBD [9]. Börjesson *et al.,* using simultaneous manometry and IEBD, were able to positively correlate both baseline peristaltic amplitude and velocity with esophageal pain sensitivity to balloon distension in patients referred for non-cardiac chest pain. They suggested that this relationship between sensitivity and motor function may be related to an increase in cholinergic activity in these patients [10]. Bohn *et al.* evaluated 19 patients complaining of non-obstructive dysphagia using IEBD and manometry. A high number of these patients were shown to be hypersensitive (defined by sensation at less than 6 cc of balloon inflation), and 42% had both hypersensitivity and motor abnormalities on manometry. However, there was no correlation between any one particular motor abnormality and the presence or degree of hypersensitivity to balloon distension [11].

Patients with achalasia, though they often report symptoms of chest pain, have been shown to have diminished sensitivity to IEBD [12,13]. Brackbill *et al.*, performing balloon distension with a barostat on 9 post-myotomy achalasia patients as well as 9 healthy volunteers found that though both groups were comparable with respect to threshold of initial sensation, the achalasia patients had a significantly higher pain threshold. Further, using the acid perfusion test, they demonstrated significantly reduced chemosensitivity in these patients compared to controls [13]. This is consistent with the observation that achalasia patients frequently experience silent acid reflux after Heller myotomy. However, the answer to the question of why chest pain is often seen in achalasia patients despite these findings remains elusive.

Esophageal sensitivity and longitudinal muscle contraction

Recently, high-frequency intraluminal ultrasound (HFIUS) has been used to better define the biomechanical properties of the esophageal wall. HFIUS permits examination of longitudinal muscle activity, complementing manometry which essentially evaluates only circular muscle contraction. Using this technique, it has been demonstrated that sustained longitudinal muscle contractions produce pain in the absence of circular muscle contraction, and are not observed on standard manometry [14]. Combining HFIUS with manometry and balloon distension, Takeda *et al.* determined that distension-induced sensation, most often perceived as heartburn, is related to esophageal circumference and esophageal strain (the ratio of change in esophageal circumference during distension to the baseline circumference). Further, strain and therefore sensitivity is greater in subjects of smaller stature and weight, as the baseline esophageal circumference is lower in these than in larger subjects [15].

Motility patterns of greatest interest in esophageal hypersensitivity

The most common manometric abnormalities found in patients presenting with non-cardiac chest pain are nutcracker esophagus (30-50%), and diffuse esophageal spasm (DES) (15%) [1]. In both of these motility disorders, HFIUS has demonstrated an increased baseline thickness of the esophageal muscular wall and muscular cross-sectional area compared to normal subjects. The reason for this is postulated to be the result of muscular hypertrophy in these patients, rather than increased muscular tone [16].

Nutcracker esophagus, being one of the more common motility disorders seen during routine manometric investigations, has been more widely investigated. Interestingly, pain episodes in patients with nutcracker esophagus are typically not concurrent with high-amplitude contractions seen during manometric studies [17,18]. Using impedance planimetry in 10 patients with an established diagnosis of nutcracker esophagus and comparing these to 12 healthy volunteers, Mujica *et al.* discovered that the nutcracker patients experienced sensation, discomfort, and pain at significantly lower thresholds during graded balloon distension than controls. Nine out of 10 patients reported reproducibility of their chest pain with balloon distension. They suggested that nutcracker esophagus was associated with esophageal hypersensitivity, and that the sensory abnormality may be an epiphenomenon not directly related to abnormal peristaltic contractions themselves [18]. The reason for this is unclear, but it may be related to an abnormality in the interaction between the longitudinal and circular muscle layers of the esophageal wall. Using manometry as a measure of circular muscle contraction and HFIUS to measure longitudinal contraction, Jung *et al.* demonstrated significant asynchrony between the peaks of longitudinal and circular muscle contraction during peristaltic waves in 10 nutcracker esophagus patients. In healthy controls, the contractions were seen to peak nearly simultaneously. This phenomenon was observed during both hypertensive and normotensive contraction sequences. They suggested that such asynchrony leads to an increase in esophageal wall tension (since the maximal increase in esophageal pressure occurs at a different time than the maximum wall thickness), which may in turn explain the sensitivity abnormalities observed in these patients [19].

Diffuse esophageal spasm, being a relatively uncommon motility disorder, has been less well-characterized. Tutuian *et al.,* using combined impedance-manometry, demonstrated that patients with DES who present for workup of chest pain were more likely to have higher distal esophageal amplitudes but normal bolus transit compared to those presenting with dysphagia, linking contraction amplitude to particular sensory complaints [20].

Conclusion

The combined work of the last two decades, using a wide array of techniques, has yielded a somewhat complex answer to the question of the relationship between esophageal sensitivity and motility. Some associations have been established, such as a connection between the presence of multipeaked contractions and hypersensitivity, and a positive correlation of baseline peristaltic amplitude and velocity with the degree of mechanosensitivity. Further, both mechanosensory and chemosensory functions are diminished in achalasia. The evidence linking specific motility abnormalities with hypersensitivity is most compelling in patients with nutcracker esophagus. Contrary to what one might expect, this does not appear to be directly related to the abnormal esophageal contractions themselves. HFIUS is able to demonstrate abnormalities in the biomechanical properties of the esophageal wall in these patients. Thus, newer techniques such as HFIUS have the potential to shed more light on the causes that may be underlying these associations between motility patterns and esophageal sensitivity.

References

1. Chahal PS, Rao SSC. Functional chest pain: nocioception and visceral hyperalgesia. J Clin Gastroenterol 2005;39:S204-9.
2. Katz PO, Castell DO. Approach to the patient with unexplained chest pain. Am J Gastroenterol 2000;95:S4-8.
3. Lacima G, Grande L, Pera M, Francino A, Ros E. Utility of ambulatory 24-hour esophageal pH and motiliy monitoring in noncardiac chest pain. Dig Dis Sci 2003;48(5):952-61.
4. Bernstein LM, Baker LA. A clinical test for esophagitis. Gastroenterology 1958;34:760-81.
5. Shi G, Tatum RP, Joehl RJ, Kahrilas PJ. Esophageal sensitivity and symptom perception in gastroesophageal reflux disease. Curr Gastroenterol Rep 1999;1:214-19.
6. Bruley des Varannes S, Galmiche JP. Evaluation of esophageal sensitivity. In: Scarpignato C, Galmiche JP, eds. Functional evaluation of esophageal disease, frontiers in gastrointestinal research, vol. 22. Basel: Karger, 1994:344-65.
7. Allen ML, Robinson MG, Orr WC. Lower esophageal sphincter pressure, esophageal body motor functioning, and esophageal acid sensitivity. Scand J Gastroenterol 1989;24:1129-34.
8. Hewson EG, Dalton CB, Richter JE. Comparison of esophageal manometry, provocative testing, and ambulatory monitoring in patients with unexplained chest pain. Dig Dis Sci 1990;35(3):302-9.
9. Clouse RE, McCord GS, Lustman PJ, Edmundowicz SA. Clinical correlates of abnormal sensitivity to intraesophageal balloon distension. Dig Dis Sci 1991;36(8):1040-5.
10. Börjesson M, Pilhall M, Eliasson T, Norssell H, Mannheimer C, Rolny P. Esophageal visceral pain sensitivity: effects of TENS and correlation with manometric findings. Dig Dis Sci 1998;43(8):1621-8.

11. Bohn B, B onaz B, Gueddah N, et al. Oesophageal motor and sensitivity abnormalities in non-obstructive dysphagia. Eur J Gastroenterol Hepatol 2002;14:271-7.
12. Rate AJ, Hobson AR, Barlow J, Bancewicz J. Abnormal neurophysiology in patients with oesophageal motility disorders. Br J Surg 1999;86:1202-16.
13. Brackbill S, Shi G, Hirano I. Diminished mechanosensitivity and chemosensitivity in patients with achalasia. Am J Physiol Gastrointest Liver Physiol 2003;285:G1198-203.
14. Balaban, DH, Yamamoto Y, Liu J, et al. Sustained esophageal contraction: a marker of esophageal chest pain identified by Intraluminal ultrasonography. Gastroenterology 1999;116(1):29-37.
15. Takeda T, Nabae T, Kassab G, Liu J, Mittal RK. Oesophageal wall stretch: the stimulus for distension induced oesophageal sensation. Neurogastroenterol Motil 2004;16:721-8.
16. Mittal RK, Kassab G, Puckett JL, Liu J. Hypertrophy of the muscularis propria of the lower esophageal sphincter and the body of the esophagus in patients with primary motility disorders of the esophagus. Am J Gastroenterol 2003; 98(8):1705-12.
17. Mittal RK, Liu J, Puckett JL, et al. Sensory and motor function of the esophagus: lessons from ultrasound imaging. Gastroenterology 2005;128:487-97.
18. Mujica VR, Mudipalli RS, Rao SSC. Pathophysiology of chest pain in patients with nutcracker esophagus. Am J Gastroenterol 2001;96:1371-7.
19. Jung HY, Puckett JL, Bhalla V, et al. Asynchrony between the circular and the longitudinal muscle contraction in patients with nutcracker esophagus. Gastroenterology 2005;128:1179-86.
20. Tutuian R, Mainie I, Agrawal A, Gideon M, Katz PO, Castell DO. Symptom and function heterogeneity among patients with distal esophageal spasm: studies using combined impedance-manometry. Am J Gastroenterol 2006;101:464-9.

What is the role of drug treatment in the management of esophageal pain?

C. Scarpignato, S. Contini (Parma)

Noncardiac chest pain (NCCP) is a common medical problem; it accounts for 2-5% of all presentations to emergency departments [1] and is likely to constitute an even higher percentage of presentations to primary care physicians (PCPs) although one population-based study found that 77% of individuals who suffered chest pain did not consult a physician [2].

The majority of patients who present to hospital emergency departments with acute chest pain undergo a diagnostic work-up. Patients with pain that is considered to be noncardiac in nature are allowed to go home, sometimes without any treatment or diagnosis. Indeed, following the completion of cardiac investigations, it is often difficult to determine to whom the patient should be referred next. The clinical attitudes of PCPs towards NCCP patients were evaluated by Wong *et al.* [3]. It was found that the majority of NCCP patients (i.e. 79.5%) are diagnosed and treated by PCPs without referring them to a gastroenterologist. The most preferred subspecialty for the initial diagnostic evaluation of a patient presenting with chest pain however was cardiology (62%), followed by gastroenterology (17%) [3].

There are many causes of chest pain (cardiac, gastroenterological, musculoskeletal, psychiatric, pulmonary and soft tissue ones) although the relative importance of each category has not as yet been adequately defined. There is also no doubt that coronary arterial disease and esophageal disease can co-exist [4]. Strong evidence is available to show that esophageal events can modify cardiac function and *vice versa* [5,6]. Along the same lines, drugs targeting cardiovascular smooth muscle also affect gastrointestinal (GI) smooth muscle [7].

The hemodynamic response to esophageal pain can produce cardiac ischemia [8]. A subset of patients with documented coronary artery disease also have concomitant chest pain of esophageal origin; such pain is as common in this group as in patients with normal coronary arteries [9]. Indeed, patients who respond poorly to treatment for their documented ischemic heart disease can respond well to treatment of gastroesophageal reflux disease (GERD) [10]. Studies among patients with coronary heart disease and simultaneous esophageal chest pain have found that GERD was the most common cause of the latter [11,12].

Pathophysiology of noncardiac chest pain

GERD is by far the most common cause for NCCP. Typical reflux symptoms were found to be significantly and independently associated with the presence of NCCP [13,14]. NCCP was reported by 37% of the patients who experienced frequent heartburn symptoms (at least once a week) when compared with 30.7% of those with infrequent heartburn symptoms (less than once a week) and 7.9% of individuals reporting no symptoms [14]. An abnormal esophageal pH-recording can be documented in up to 50% of the subjects with NCCP [15-17], although only half of them experience chest pain during the test.

Esophageal erosions during upper GI endoscopy are present in 10-70% of the patients with NCCP, half of whom also display an abnormal esophageal exposure to acid. The wide range is likely due to the different patient populations assessed in these studies. The presence of abnormal pH test or a GERD-related esophageal mucosal injury suggests association, but not necessarily causality. However, studies have showed that up to 80% of NCCP patients with either erosive esophagitis or abnormal pH testing responded to potent antireflux treatment, suggesting that, if one of these diagnostic tests is positive, then GERD is likely the underlying cause of patient's symptoms [15-17]. An alternative method for evaluating individuals with non cardiac chest pain is an empirical trial with a proton pump inhibitor (PPI) [18]. This method involves using a short course of high-dose PPI (usually full dose twice daily) to diagnose patients with GERD-related non cardiac chest pain. The usefulness of the PPI test is basically dependent on the frequency of chest pain symptoms. If symptom frequency is low, the PPI test can be lengthened to 2 weeks, or even longer. The PPI empirical trial (e.g. PPI test) is a simple non-invasive, accurate and cost-saving test for evaluating patients with GERD-related NCCP [19].

In patients with non GERD-related NCCP, **esophageal dysmotility** is relatively uncommon, being present in only 30% of 160 NCCP patients evaluated by esophageal manometry [20]. The most common esophageal motor disorders encountered in these patients are nutcracker esophagus, hypertensive lower esophageal sphincter (LES) and non specific esophageal motor disorders (ns-EMDs) [20,21]. In a thoughtful study [22], 10 subjects with NCCP were studied with simultaneous measurement of intraluminal pressure, pH and ultrasound images of the esophagus for 24 hours. Muscle thickness was assessed by ultrasonography and compared during chest pain and asymptomatic baseline as well as control periods. Sustained esophageal contractions (never seen in healthy subjects or patients without NCCP) were detected in 18 of 24 spontaneous chest pain episodes.

Despite these exciting results, the relationship between non GERD-related NCCP and esophageal dysmotility remains an area of controversy. This is primarily due to the common documentation of esophageal dysmotility in NCCP patients undergoing stationary esophageal manometry without concomitant reports of chest pain symptoms.

Visceral hypersensitivity is a phenomenon in which the conscious perception of visceral stimulus is enhanced independent of the intensity of the stimulus. Peripheral and central mechanisms have been proposed to be responsible for visceral hypersensitivity in patients with NCCP. It has been hypothesized that peripheral sensitization of esophageal sensory afferents leads to subsequently heightened responses to physiological or pathological stimuli of the esophageal mucosa [23]. Additionally, central sensitization at the brain level or the dorsal horn of the spinal cord may modulate afferent neural function and thus enhance perception of intraluminal stimuli [23]. What causes peripheral or central sensitization remains to be determined.

Several studies [*for review see* 24] using balloon distension or electrical stimulation protocols have demonstrated that patients with non GERD-related NCCP have lower perception thresholds for pain. In addition, Tougas at McMaster University (Hamilton, Canada) [24] did suggest that a subset of patients with NCCP demonstrate autonomic dysregulation (increased vagal cardiac outflow). He further hypothesized that increased perception of esophageal stimulation may also reflect an exaggerated brainstem response. However, in most cases in which both central and autonomic factors are involved, central factors will likely lead to autonomic dysregulation.

Finally, **psychological co-morbidity** has been shown to be common in patients with NCCP. Between 17% and 43% of the patients with NCCP are estimated to suffer from some type of psychological abnormality [25]. Panic disorder, anxiety and major depression were highly prevalent in the population studied. Overall, it was found that central factors, such as stress and psychological disorders play an important role in enhancing perception of intra-esophageal stimuli [25].

Drugs for the treatment of esophageal pain

Different classes of drugs have been employed to manage NCCP sometimes empirically and sometimes based on its supposed pathophysiology. These include PPIs, smooth muscle relaxants, botulinum toxin (BoTox®), antidepressants and visceral analgesics. The very fact that so many different drugs have been tried is evidence that no single treatment serves to provide the symptom relief that clinicians and patients do require.

Proton pump inhibitors

There is little or no evidence to suggest that lifestyle changes, antacids or H_2-receptor antagonists are efficacious in the treatment of NCCP [54]. However, acid suppression with PPIs has become the cornerstone for any therapeutic intervention in GERD-related NCCP [26]. Patients are likely to benefit more from at least a double dose of PPI until symptom subside, followed by dose tapering to determine the lowest dose that can control patient's symptoms. As with other atypical manifestations of GERD, NCCP patients may require more than 2 months of therapy for optimal symptom control [27].

Seven randomized, placebo-controlled studies on PPI efficacy in NCCP were recently included in a meta-analysis [27], which confirmed that these drugs are highly effective for symptom improvement (*Figure 1*) with a pooled risk ratio for continued chest pain of 0.54 (95% C.I. 041-0.71) and number needed to treat (NNT) of only 3 (95% C.I. 2-4).

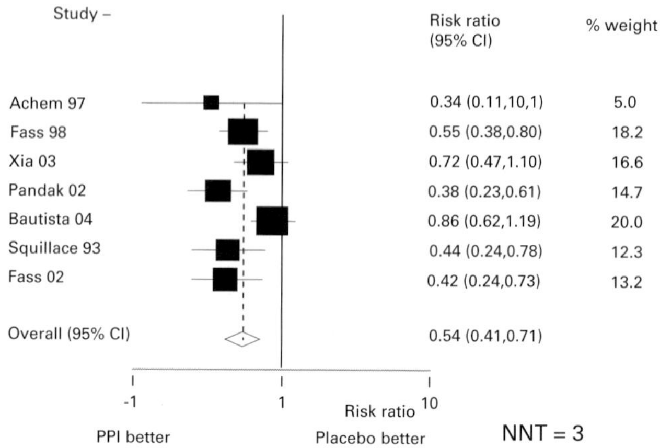

Figure 1. Forest plot showing the effect of PPI treatment on symptom improvement in NCCP. Estimates of relative risk for continued chest pain after treatment are presented with their 95% confidence intervals (from [27]).

Although data regarding the long-term efficacy of PPIs in NCCP are available only with omeprazole, it is likely that all the other members of the class will show a similar efficacy [26].

Along the same lines, antireflux surgery proved to be highly effective, thus giving further rationale to the use of acid suppression in patients with GERD-related NCCP. In carefully selected patient populations, Nissen fundoplication was able to achieve symptom relief in more than 90% of subjects [28,29].

Smooth muscle relaxants

The treatment for the majority of patients with an esophageal motor disorder, except achalasia, has been disappointing. To date, there have not been sufficient randomized controlled trials of smooth-muscle relaxants for treatment of NCCP, most of the trials carried out being small in size and inconclusive [*for review see* 30].

Despite their presence, it is unclear whether the manometric abnormalities in patients with NCCP have pathophysiologic consequences. Indeed, during manometry, patients who display simultaneous contractions consistent with diffuse esophageal spasm (DES) or the high-amplitude peristalsis observed in nutcracker esophagus are rarely symptomatic [31]. Furthermore, most of them have shown that – despite significant amelioration of the abnormal motility – there is a lack of symptomatic improvement [32]. Disturbed esophageal sensory processing is more likely to correlate with symptoms than abnormal esophageal motility [33,34]. And indeed, NCCP patients respond better to pain modulators than to smooth muscle relaxants.

Botulinum toxin

BoTox® injection into the LES represents a promising therapeutic option for NCCP, currently under evaluation. The rationale for BoTox® use in patients with NCCP relies on the following assumptions:

- clinical and manometric parameters of DES, hypertensive LES, ineffective esophageal motility (IEM) disorders may overlap those of achalasia; in addition, some patients have been shown to progress from DES to achalasia and from IEM to DES or achalasia, suggesting that these disorders likely represent a spectrum of diseases [31]. Therefore, treatments that are effective for achalasia may also be effective for other EMDs;
- several studies have shown that BoTox® injection into the LES of patients with achalasia not only improved dysphagia and regurgitation but also decreased chest pain significantly [35].

A total of 100 units of toxin are usually injected circumferentially, using five injections at the gastroesophageal junction of 20 units each. Usually, there are no procedure-related complications except for slight, short-lived chest pain in few patients. By using this technique, Miller *et al.* [36] conducted an open-label trial to ascertain the effectiveness of this approach in treating NCCP patients (*Figure 2*). The study found that BoTox® injection at LES provided significant chest pain improvement among patients with spastic EMDs. The symptomatic improvement remained stable for at least 6 months after injection (*Table I*) [37], after which some patients required re-treatment [37], as in the case of patients with non achalasia EMDs [38].

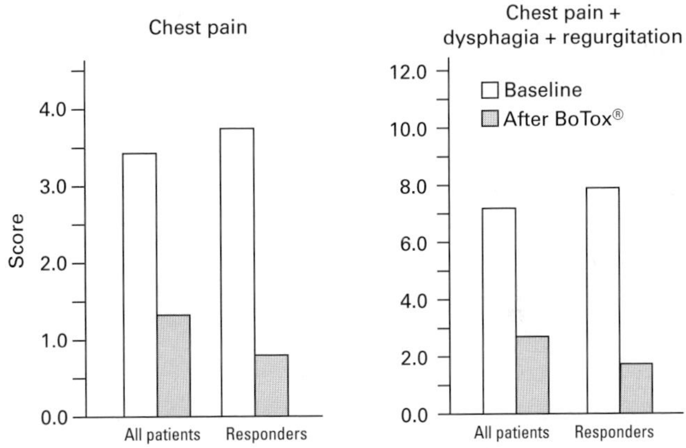

Figure 2. Symptom improvement after BoTox® injection into the LES of NCCP patients. In all the patients studied there was a significant ($p < 0.0001$) reduction of pre-treatment score (from [36]).

Table I. Duration of symptomatic improvement over time in patients with DES treated with BoTox® (from [38]).

	Median symptom score			
Baseline	Baseline	Day 1	Month 1	Month 6
Dysphagia	3.0	1.0*	1.0*	1.0*
Regurgitation	3.0	0.0*	0.0*	0.0*
NCCP	3.0	1.0*	1.0*	0.0*
Total	8.0	2.0*	2.0*	2.0*
* $p < 0.01$ compared with baseline values				

Overall, it appears that botulinum toxin injection may lead to a short-term symptomatic improvement in NCCP patients with spastic EMDs but controlled trials are needed. Similarly, the role of pneumatic dilation or long esophageal myotomy (Heller myotomy) with or without antireflux surgery in patients with NCCP and non-achalasic dysmotility remains controversial and is best avoided [26].

Antidepressants

The mechanism by which tricyclic antidepressants (TCAs) reduce visceral pain remains poorly understood. Some authors suggested a central effect, while others a peripheral one. Imipramine has been shown to increase esophageal perception thresholds for pain in normal subjects, without affecting esophageal tone, thus suggesting a visceral analgesic effect [39]. A similar effect that was independent of cardiac, esophageal or psychiatric testing results at baseline was noted in NCCP patients [26]. In a study [40] of chest pain patients with normal coronary angiography subjects were randomized to the α_2 agonist clonidine hydrochloride (0.1 mg twice daily), imipramine (50 mg) nightly with a morning placebo, or placebo twice daily for 3 weeks. As later confirmed by Cox *et al.* [41] in a placebo-controlled trial, only the patients who received imipramine showed a significant reduction in chest pain events (*Figure 3*).

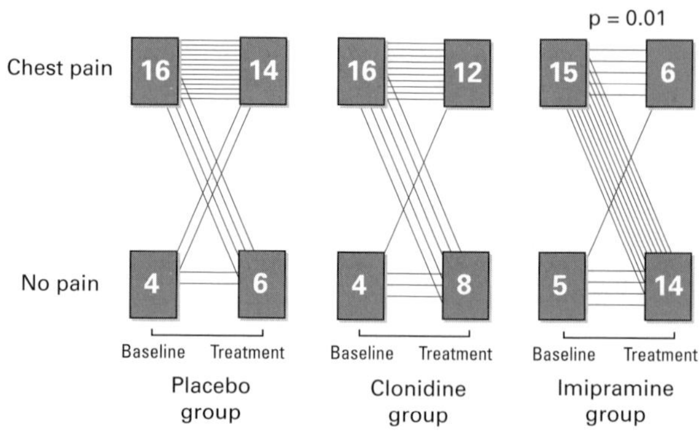

Figure 3. Patients with chest pain during right ventricular stimulation at baseline and during the treatment phase, according to treatment group. The lines between the boxes indicate whether the cardiac-pain response of individual patients changed or stayed the same from base line to the treatment phase (from [40]).

TCAs also provide a long-term effect in NCCP patients, although drop-out rate due to side effects may reach 30% [26,42]. Treatment with TCAs should start at a low dose (10-25 mg) that is administered at bedtime and then increased by 10-25 mg increments per week to a non-mood altering goal of 50-75 mg per day [42].

Compared to TCAs, selective serotonin reuptake inhibitors (SSRIs) have been less studied. Varia *et al.* [43] conducted a randomized, double-blind, placebo-controlled trial that assessed the efficacy, tolerability and safety of sertraline in patients with NCCP. Patients were randomly selected to receive sertraline or placebo in doses starting at 50 mg daily and adjusted (based on patient's clinical response) to a maximum of 200 mg. On intention-to-treat analysis, patients receiving sertraline reported a significant reduction in their chest pain scores when compared with those receiving placebo, despite lack of significant improvement in the depression score. Symptomatic improvement was accompanied by significant improvement of quality of life, which continued to deteriorate under placebo treatment (*Table II*).

Table II. Symptomatic improvement in NCCP patients after sertraline treatment (from [43]).

Parameter evaluated	Placebo		Sertraline		Difference drug-placebo	p value
	Week 0	Week 9	Week 0	Week 9		
Pain	3.50	2.96	3.94	1.47	- 1.92	0.02
BDI	9.87	7.80	9.20	6.07	- 1.07	0.58
SF-36	62.13	57.33	64.60	66.93	7.13	0.02
BDI: Beck Depression Inventory						

Low-dose trazodone (100-150 mg day), an atypical antidepressant with additional anxiolytic effects, has been shown to improve symptoms of non GERD-related NCCP patients with esophageal dysmotility, without affecting esophageal amplitude contractions. In a small double-blind, placebo-controlled trial Clouse *et al.* [44] treated patients with NCCP and esophageal dysmotility with trazodone for 6 weeks and compared their response with those receiving placebo. The treatment group demonstrated a significantly greater global improvement compared with the placebo group suggesting that trazodone may be of therapeutic value in patients with NCCP and spastic EMDs.

Antidepressants are typically reserved for NCCP patients with severe symptoms or symptoms resistant to common, first-line approaches. Such reservations relate primarily to tolerability profile rather than suspected lack of efficacy in patients with mild disease. Because of the varied effects of antidepressants at the receptor and/or mediator level [45], failure of one compound to improve symptoms is not indicative of future failure of other members of the same or different class of drugs, which may exert a synergic action and could therefore used together (*Table III*).

Table III. Antidepressants for management of patients with NCCP: tryciclic antidepressants *versus* selective serotonin reuptake inhibitors.

	TCAs	SSRIs
Primary effect	Brain-gut axis	Cognitive environment
Effective dosages	**Low**	**Conventional**
Onset of action	**Rapid**	**Delayed**
Synergism with SSRIs	Yes	–

A subset of patients with NCCP may report psychological or psychiatric abnormalities, as either the cause or an effect of their chest pain [25]. Reassurance about the benign nature of the disorder has been emphasized as an important mode of early therapeutic intervention in patients with NCCP. However, patients symptoms are seldom relieved by reassurance only, resulting in the need for additional therapeutic modalities [26], including behavioural therapy [46,47]. Patients with more severe symptoms may have abnormality at the CNS level, which are more responsive to antidepressant therapy. Indeed, increasing severity of "functional" GI symptoms is associated with greater likelihood of psychiatric abnormalities and less association of gut physiologic abnormalities to symptoms [42].

In patients who suffer from panic disorder, treatment with benzodiazepines (such as alprazolam and clonazepam) has been demonstrated to reduce panic attack frequency, chest pain episodes and anxiety score [48]. These drugs may relieve chest pain caused by esophageal disorders by reducing not only anxiety but also muscle spasm. Since emotional stress can exacerbate esophageal hypermotility [49], medications with anxiolytic properties may well be useful in the treatment of EMDs. The risk of dependance is minimal when benzodiazepines are prescribed on a short-term basis but these drugs should be used cautiously on the long-term.

Drugs affecting visceral sensitivity

Amongst the five classes (i.e. opioid agonists, serotoninergic drugs, antidepressants, somatostatin analogs and α_2-adrenergic agonists) of drugs affecting visceral sensitivity [50], only antidepressants (discussed above) have been used in the short-term treatment of patients with NCCP.

A single investigation [51] showed that octreotide significantly increases esophageal perception thresholds to balloon distension in healthy volunteers, without affecting pain thresholds or altering cortical evoked potentials to painful stimulation. Unfortunately, no study has been performed in patients with NCCP, as yet. However, the need for subcutenous administration would make octreotide an unpractical drug for the long-term treatment.

In a more recent investigation [52] tegaserod (6 mg twice daily for 2 weeks) was found capable of improving esophageal pain threshold to mechanical distension in patients with functional hearburn, some of whom complained also of chest pain. This drug may then be of value in patients with related NCCP. Unfortunately, however, tegaserod is not available in Europe and is presently under restricted use in United States [53]. New serotoninergic agents with improved safety profile are currently under development [54] and may eventually play a therapeutic role in non GERD-related NCCP.

Future research in NCCP will continue to focus on mechanisms for pain and will attempt to identify new therapeutic modalities aimed to reduce visceral pain. Research will likely concentrate primarily on the role of central and peripheral sensitization in enhancing perception of intraesophageal stimuli. Furthermore, currently available treatments for other functional gastrointestinal disorders [50,55], such as irritable bowel syndrome and functional dyspepsia, may be tested in NCCP and found useful, as well.

Conclusions

NCCP is a heterogeneous condition for which diagnosis and treatment are challenging.

GERD is probably the most important cause of NCCP and a trial with high-dose PPIs is often effective and represents a useful diagnostic test. Esophageal dysmotility is relatively uncommon and smooth muscle relaxants are almost invariably ineffective. Pain modulators offer a significant symptom improvement in patients with non GERD-related NCCP. Reassurance represents a useful therapeutic adjunct in all patients while behavioral therapy should be reserved to selected cases.

References

1. Eslick GD, Coulshed DS, Talley NJ. The burden of illness of noncardiac chest pain. Aliment Pharmacol Ther 2000;16:1217-23.
2. Eslick GD, Jones MP, Talley NJ. Non-cardiac chest pain: prevalence, risk factors, impact and consulting - a population-based study. Aliment Pharmacol Ther 2003;17:1115-24.
3. Wong WM, Beeler J, Risner-Adler S, Habib S, Bautista J, Fass R. Attitudes and referral patterns of primary care physicians when evaluating subjects with noncardiac chest pain – a national survey. Dig Dis Sci 2005;50:656-61.
4. Mellow MH, Simpson AG, Watt L, Schoolmeester L, Haye OL. Esophageal acid perfusion in coronary artery disease. Induction of myocardial ischemia. Gastroenterology 1983;85:306-12.
5. Chauhan A, Mullins PA, Taylor G, Petch MC, Schofield PM. Cardio-oesophageal reflex in humans as a mechanism for "linked angina". Eur Heart J 1996;17:407-13.
6. Makk LJ, Leesar M, Joseph A, Prince CP, Wright RA. Cardioesophageal reflexes: an invasive human study. Dig Dis Sci 2000;45:2451-4.
7. Scarpignato C, Franzé A. What is the role of smooth muscle relaxants in the treatment of diffuse esophageal spasm? In: Giuli R, McCallum RW, Skinner DB, eds. Primary motility disorders of the esophagus. Paris: John Libbey Eurotext, 1991:701-6.
8. Lux G, Van Els J, The GS, Bozkurt T, Orth KH, Behrenbeck D. Ambulatory oesophageal pressure, pH and ECG recording in patients with normal and pathological coronary angiography and intermittent chest pain. Neurogastroenterol Motil 1995;7:23-30.
9. Ghillebert G, Janssens J. Oesophageal pain in coronary artery disease. Gut 1998;42:312-9.
10. Garcia-Pulido J, Patel PH, Hunter WC, Douglas JE, Thomas E. Esophageal contribution to chest pain in patients with coronary artery disease. Chest 1990;98:806-10.
11. Bortolotti M, Marzocchi A, Bacchelli S, et al. The esophagus as a possibile cause of chest pain in patients with and without angina pectoris. Hepatogastroenterology 1990;37:316-8.
12. Schofield PM, Whorwell PJ, Brooks NH, Bennett DH, Jones PE. Oesophageal function in patients with angina pectoris: a comparison of patients with normal coronary angiograms and patients with coronary artery disease. Digestion 1989;42:70-8.
13. Locke GR 3rd, Talley NJ, Fett SL, Zinsmeister AR, Melton LJ 3rd. Prevalence and clinical spectrum of gastroesophageal reflux: a populationbased study in Olmsted County, Minnesota. Gastroenterology 1997;112:1448-56.
14. Chiocca JC, Olmos JA, Salis GB, Soifer LO, Higa R, Marcolongo M, the Argentinean Gastro-esophageal Reflux Study Group. Prevalence, clinical spectrum and atypical symptoms of gastro-oesophageal reflux in Argentina: a nationwide population-based study. Aliment Pharmacol Ther 2005;22:331-42.
15. Fass R, Naliboff B, Higa L, et al. Differential effect of long-term esophageal acid exposure on mechanosensitivity and chemosensitivity in humans. Gastroenterology 1998;115:1363-73.
16. Beedassy A, Katz PO, Gruber A, Peghini PL, Castell DO. Prior sensitization of esophageal mucosa by acid reflux predisposes to reflux-induced chest pain. J Clin Gastroenterol 2000;31:121-4.
17. Fass R, Fennerty MB, Ofman JJ, et al. The clinical and economic value of a short course of omeprazole patients with noncardiac chest pain. Gastroenterology 1998;115:42-9.
18. Wong WM. Use of proton pump inhibitor as a diagnostic test in NCCP. J Gastroenterol Hepatol 2005;20:S14-7.
19. Wang WH, Huang JQ, Zheng GF, et al. Is proton pump inhibitor testing an effective approach to diagnose gastroesophageal reflux disease in patients with noncardiac chest pain?: a meta-analysis. Arch Intern Med 2005;165:1222-8.
20. Dekel R, Pearson T, Wendel C, De Garmo P, Fennerty MB, Fass R. Assessment of oesophageal motor function in patients with dysphagia or chest pain – the Clinical Outcomes Research Initiative experience. Aliment Pharmacol Ther 2003;18:1083-9.
21. Katz PO, Dalton CB, Richter JE, Wu WC, Castell DO. Esophageal testing of patients with noncardiac chest pain or dysphagia. Results of three years experience with 1,161 patients. Ann Intern Med 1987;106:593-7.
22. Balaban DH, Yamamoto Y, Liu J, et al. Sustained esophageal contraction: a marker of esophageal chest pain identified by intraluminal ultrasonography. Gastroenterology 1999;116:29-37.
23. Hollerbach S, Bulat R, May A, et al. Abnormal cerebral processing of oesophageal stimuli in patients with non-cardiac chest pain (NCCP). Neurogastroenterol Motil 2000;12:555–65.
24. Chahal PS, Rao SS. Functional chest pain: nociception and visceral hyperalgesia. J Clin Gastroenterol 2005;39:S204-49.
25. Clouse RE, Carney RM. The psychological profile of non cardiac chest pain patients. Eur J Gastroenterol Hepatol 1995;7:1160-5.
26. Fass R, Dickman R. Non-cardiac chest pain: an update. Neurogastroenterol Motil 2006;18:408-17.
27. Cremonini F, Wise J, Moayyedi P, Talley NJ. Diagnostic and therapeutic use of proton pump inhibitors in non-cardiac chest pain: a metaanalysis. Am J Gastroenterol 2005;100:1226-32.
28. Patti MG, Molena D, Fisichella PM, Perretta S, Way LW. Gastroesophagealreflux disease (GERD) and chest pain. Results oflaparoscopic antireflux surgery. Surg Endosc 2002;16:563-6.

29. Farrell TM, Richardson WS, Trus TL, Smith CD, Hunter JG. Response of atypical symptoms of gastro-oesophageal reflux to antire-flux surgery. Br J Surg 2001;88:1649-52.
30. Eslick GD. Noncardiac chest pain: epidemiology, natural history, health care seeking, and quality of life. Gastroenterol Clin North Am 2004;33:1-23.
31. Richter JE. Oesophageal motility disorders. Lancet 2001;358:823-8.
32. Achem SR. Treatment of spastic esophageal motility disorders. Gastroenterol Clin North Am 2004;33:1071-1024.
33. Hollerbach S, Bulat R, May A, et al. Abnormal cerebral processing of oesophageal stimuli in patients with noncardiac chest pain (NCCP). Neurogastroenterol Motil 2000;12:555-65.
34. Rao SS, Hayek B, Summers RW. Functional chest pain of esophageal origin: hyperalgesia or motor dysfunction. Am J Gastroenterol 2001;96:2584-9.
35. Zhao X, Pasricha PJ. Botulinum toxin for spastic GI disorders: a systematic review. Gastrointest Endosc 2003;57:219-35.
36. Miller LS, Pullela SV, Parkman HP, et al. Treatment of chest pain in patients with noncardiac, nonreflux, nonachalasia spastic esophageal motor disorders using botulinum toxin injection into the gastroesophageal junction. Am J Gastroenterol 2002;97:1640-6.
37. Storr M, Allescher HD, Rösch T, Born P, Weigert N, Classen M. Treatment of symptomatic diffuse esophageal spasm by endoscopic injections of botulinum toxin: a prospective study with long-term follow-up. Gastrointest Endosc 2001;54:754-9.
38. Miller LS, Parkman HP, Schiano TD, et al. Treatment of symptomatic nonachalasia esophageal motor disorders with botulinum toxin injection at the lower esophageal sphincter. Dig Dis Sci 1996;41:2025-31.
39. Peghini PL, Katz PO, Castell DO. Imipramine decreases oesophageal pain perception in human male volunteers. Gut 1998;42:807-13.
40. Cannon RO 3rd, Quyyumi AA, Mincemoyer R, et al . Imipramine in patients with chest pain despite normal coronary angiograms. N Engl J Med 1994;330:1411-7.
41. Cox ID, Hann CM, Kaski JC. Low dose imipramine improves chest pain but not quality of life in patients with angina and normal coronary angiograms. Eur Heart J 1998;19:250-24.
42. Clouse RE, Lustman PJ. Use of psychopharmacological agents for functional gastrointestinal disorders. Gut 2005;54:1332-41.
43. Varia I, Logue E, O'connor C, et al. Randomized trial of sertraline in patients with unexplained chest pain of noncardiac origin. Am Heart J 2000;140:367-72.
44. Clouse RE, Lustman PJ, Eckert TC, Ferney DM, Griffith LS. Low-dose trazodone for symptomatic patients with esophageal contraction abnormalities. A double-blind, placebo-controlled trial. Gastroenterology 1987;92:1027-36.
45. Feighner JP. Mechanism of action of antidepressant medications. J Clin Psychiatry 1999;60(Suppl 4):4-11.
46. Klimes I, Mayou RA, Pearce MJ, Coles L, Fagg JR. Psychologicalc treatment for atypical non-cardiac chest pain: a controlled evaluation. Psychol Med 1990;20:605-11.
47. van Peski-Oosterbaan AS, Spinhoven P, van Rood Y, et al. Cognitive-behavioral therapy for noncardiac chest pain: a randomized trial. Am J Med 1999;106:424-9.
48. Huffman JC, Stern TA. The use of benzodiazepines in the treatment of chest pain: a review of the literature. J Emerg Med 2003;25:427-37.
49. Anderson KO, Dalton CB, Bradley LA, Richter JE. Stress induces alteration of esophageal pressures in healthy volunteers and non-cardiac chest pain patients. Dig Dis Sci 1989;34:83-91.
50. Kuiken SD, Tytgat GN, Boeckxstaens GE. Review article: drugs interfering with visceral sensitivity for the treatment of functional gastrointestinal disorders - the clinical evidence. Aliment Pharmacol Ther 2005;21:633-51.
51. Johnston BT, Shils J, Leite LP, Castell DO. Effects of octreotide on esophageal visceral perception and cerebral evoked potentials induced by balloon distension. Am J Gastroenterol 1999;94:65-70.
52. Effect of tegaserod on esophageal pain threshold, regurgitation, and symptom relief in patients with functional heartburn and mechanical sensitivity. Clin Gastroenterol Hepatol 2006;4:442-50.
53. FDA. FDA permits restricted use of Zelnorm for qualifying patients [http://www.fda.gov/bbs/topics/NEWS/2007/NEW01673.html].
54. Gershon MD, Tack J. The serotonin signaling system: from basic understanding to drug development for functional GI disorders. Gastroenterology 2007;132:397-414.
55. Camilleri M, Bueno L, de Ponti F, Fioramonti J, Lydiard RB, Tack J. Pharmacological and pharmacokinetic aspects of functional gastrointestinal disorders. Gastroenterology 2006;130:1421-34.

Onset and development of acid induced esophageal inflammation

P. Biancani, K.M. Harnett (Providence)

Acid-induced esophageal inflammation begins with refluxed acid activating proton-sensitive vanilloid type 1 receptors known as transient receptor potential vanilloid type 1 (TRPV1, also known as VR1), present in the esophageal mucosa.

These receptors are present in sensory neural fibers in lamina propria and submucosa, where they activate substance P – and CGRP – containing neurons, inducing release of substance P and CGRP from the mucosal layer. In addition TRPV1 receptors are present in mucosal epithelial cells, where they induce production of platelet activating factor (PAF). PAF is a chemotactic factor for leukocytes and stimulates them to produce hydrogen peroxide (H_2O_2).

In addition PAF diffuses to the circular muscle layer, where it induces production of interleukin-6 (IL-6) that, in turn activates a non phagocytic reduced nicotinamide adenine dinucleotide phosphate (NADPH) oxidase, that produces H_2O_2. H_2O_2 induces production of interleukin-1β (IL-1β), that causes the muscle to produce PAF, thus completing a self sustaining inflammatory cycle.

H_2O_2, produced by leukocytes and circular muscle, is uncharged and free to diffuse across plasma and nuclear membranes. H_2O_2 has high affinity for lipids, inducing lipid peroxidation, and upregulating NADPH oxidase, and it may bind to DNA bases, possibly altering cell phenotype.

Acid induced inflammatory mediators in esophageal mucosa

The transient receptor potential channel, TRPV1, was originally described in primary sensory neurons as a receptor for capsaicin and related natural irritants (collectively referred to as vanilloids) [32]. TRPV1 is a non-selective cation channel expressed by sensory nerves. It is activated by heat or by the pungent ingredient of chili peppers, capsaicin, or by endogenous hydrogen ions released in tissues during inflammation [32] or present in gastric reflux. TRPV1 is now believed to function as a molecular integrator of noxious stimuli, including acids, heat, pollutants with negative electric charge, and endogenous pro-inflammatory substances [10]. TRPV1 activation in primary afferent neurons evokes the sensation of burning pain and induces neurogenic inflammation by the release of substance P and calcitonin-gene-related peptide (CGRP) [33,34]. Upregulated TRPV1 expression has been demonstrated in disease states such as inflammatory bowel disease [34], irritable bowel syndrome [4] and, more recently, esophagitis [22].

TRPV1-associated "neurogenic inflammation" has been examined in several systems, particularly in the airways, and to a lesser extent in the digestive tract. In the digestive tract most publications have focused on the role of vanilloid receptor in inflammation, with emphasis on stimulation of substance P release [17-21,23-27], or on a role of endopeptidases in degradation of substance P, with a resulting decrease in inflammation [1,16,31]. In the ileum and colon, TRPV1 is thought to be a mediator of inflammation because, in experimental models of colitis induced by dextran sulphate sodium (DSS) [14,15], or of ileitis induced by *Clostridium difficile* toxin A [24] or anandamide [23], attenuation of colitis occurs in response to TRPV1 channel blockers [14,15] or after genetic deletion of TRPV1 [12].

To test whether this acid-sensitive receptor may be the initial mediator of acid-induced inflammation in the cat esophagus, a tubular segment of normal esophageal mucosa was removed and tied at both ends to form a mucosal sac (*Figure 1*) [8]. The sac was filled with 0.01N HCl (or normal Krebs' solution for control) and kept in oxygenated Krebs' solution at 37°C. The medium around the HCl-filled sac (supernatant) was collected after 3 hour incubation and examined for content of inflammatory mediators.

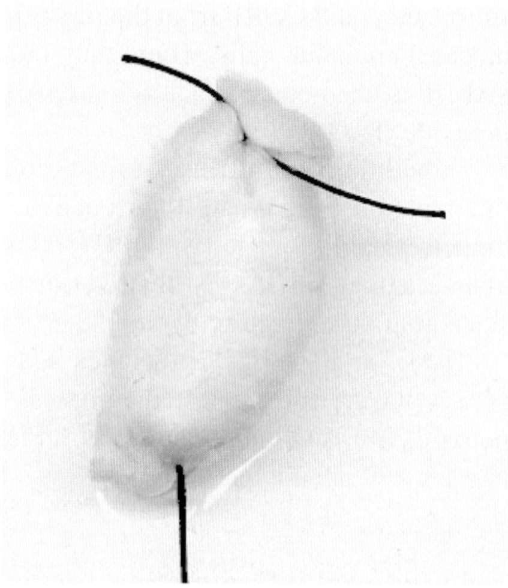

Figure 1. We produced an *in vitro* model of esophageal inflammation using an esophageal mucosa tube tied at both ends. The tube was created by removing the muscle layers from the esophagus by sharp dissection at the level of the submucosa. It had the squamous epithelium on the inside and the submucosa on the outside. HCl or Kreb's buffer was injected inside the tube, which was then kept in oxygenated Kreb's buffer at 36°C for 3 hours. (1 ml Kreb's buffer/100 mg mucosa). After 3 hours the supernatant outside the tube was collected and analyzed or used to incubate circular muscle strips. (See page XI for colour figure).

Substance P levels increased six-fold in mucosal tissue and in supernatant in response to HCl (*Figure 2*), while CGRP levels increased 200 times in the mucosa and 10 times in the supernatant (*Figure 3*). The HCl-induced increases in substance P and CGRP in mucosa and in supernatant were abolished when the TRPV1 receptor antagonist 5'-iodoresiniferatoxin (IRTX) was added inside the mucosal sac, or when tetrodotoxin (TTX) was added inside the sac and to the supernatant, suggesting that TRPV1-induced production of substance P and CGRP was neurally mediated.

TRPV1, however, has also been demonstrated in non-neural cells, for instance in keratinocytes of the epidermis [29,30], in the human keratinocyte cell line HaCat [29], in the human bronchial epithelial cell line BEAS-2B [33], in bladder urothelium and smooth muscle [2,3], liver [28], polymorphonuclear granulocytes [13] and macrophages [5].

To examine a role of non neural TRPV1 receptor we induced contraction esophageal circular muscle strips in response to electric field stimulation (EFS), that is neurally mediated. EFS-induced contraction was almost abolished by incubation in the supernatant of HCl-filled (*Figure 4*) or of capsaicin filled (*Figure 5*) mucosal sac. This supernatant-induced inhibition was reversed by application of the TRPV1 antagonist IRTX inside the mucosal sac, confirming presence of capsaicin-sensitive TRPV1 receptors in the mucosal wall.

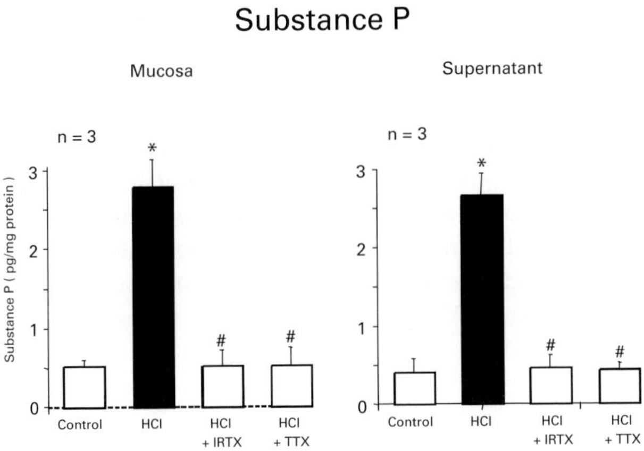

Figure 2. When *in vitro* mucosa is exposed to HCl for 3 hours, substance P levels increase 6 times in the mucosa and in the supernatant when compared to control (pH 7.4) (* p < 0.5 ANOVA). The HCl-induced increase in substance P is abolished by the TRPV1 receptor antagonist IRTX and by the neural blocker TTX both in the mucosa and in the supernatant (# p < 0.5 ANOVA). Bars represent mean ± SEM of 3 experiments.

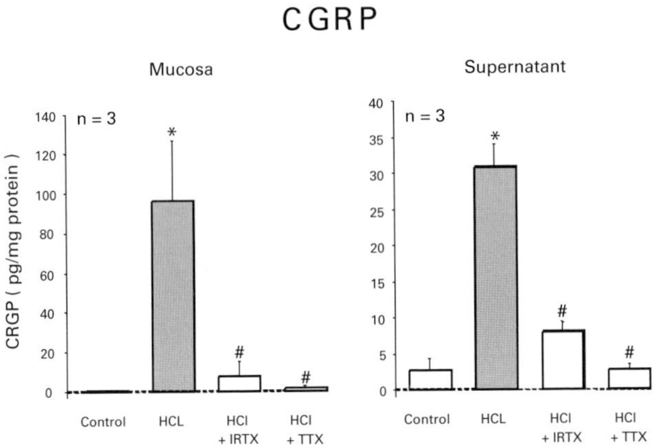

Figure 3. When *in vitro* mucosa is exposed to HCl for 3 hours, CGRP levels increase 200 times in the mucosa and 10 times in the supernatant when compared to control (pH 7.4) (* p < 0.5 ANOVA). The HCl-induced increase in CGRP is abolished by the TRPV1 receptor antagonist IRTX and by the neural blocker TTX both in the mucosa and in the supernatant (# p < 0.5 ANOVA). Bars represent mean ± SEM of 3 experiments.

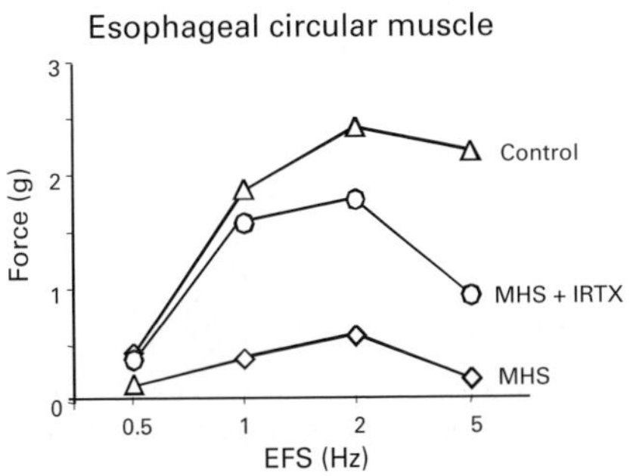

Figure 4. Contraction of esophageal circular muscle (Control) in response to electrical field stimulation (EFS) is almost abolished by supernatant of HCl-filled mucosal sac (MHS). The reduction is reversed by application of the TRPV1 antagonist IRTX (10^{-5}M) inside the mucosal sac (MHS + IRTX), confirming presence of TRPV1 vanilloid receptors in the mucosal wall.

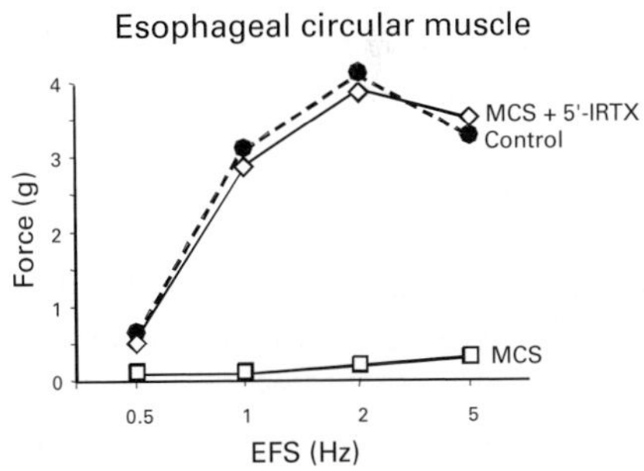

Figure 5. Contraction of esophageal circular muscle (Control) in response to electrical field stimulation (EFS) is almost abolished by supernatant of capsaicin-filled mucosal sac (MCS). The reduction is reversed by application of the TRPV1 antagonist IRTX (10^{-5}M) inside the mucosal sac (MCS + 5'IRTX), confirming presence of TRPV1 vanilloid receptors in the mucosal wall.

The reduction in contraction caused by supernatant of capsaicin-filled sac was almost abolished by pre-exposure of the muscle to the PAF receptor antagonist CV9388 (*Figure 6*). This is consistent with release of PAF by mucosa in response to activation of TRPV1 by capsaicin and indicates that PAF is the major inflammatory mediator affecting circular muscle contraction. Measurements of PAF in mucosa tissue and in mucosa supernatant confirmed that PAF levels increased 4-5 times in the HCl-filled mucosal sac and in its supernatant when compared to control (Kreb's filled mucosal sac at pH 7.4) (*Figure 7*). The HCl-induced increase in PAF was abolished by the TRPV1 receptor antagonist IRTX. The increase in PAF levels in mucosa and supernatant, however, were not affected by neural block with TTX, indicating that production of PAF may arise from non neural pathways, and most likely from the esophageal epithelium.

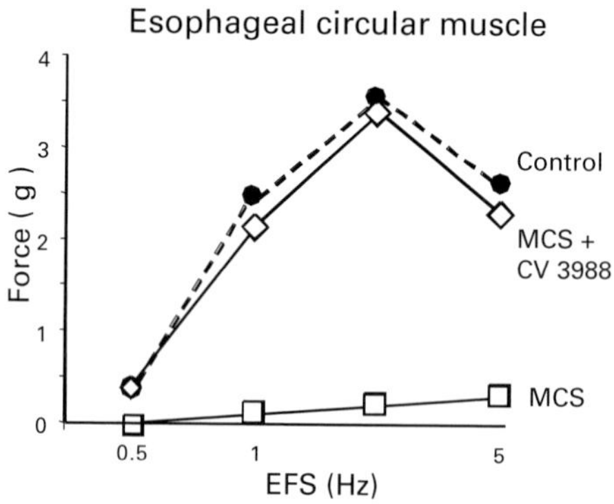

Figure 6. EFS-induced contraction of esophageal circular muscle (control) is almost abolished by supernatant of capsaicin (10^{-6} M) - filled mucosal sac (MCS). The reduction is reversed by pre-exposure of the muscle to the PAF receptor antagonist CV3988 (MCS + CV3988-10^{-6}M). This is consistent with release of PAF by mucosa in response to activation of TRPV1 by capsaicin, and suggests that PAF may be the inflammatory mediator most responsible for impairment of EFS-induced (i.e. neurally induced) contraction of circular muscle.

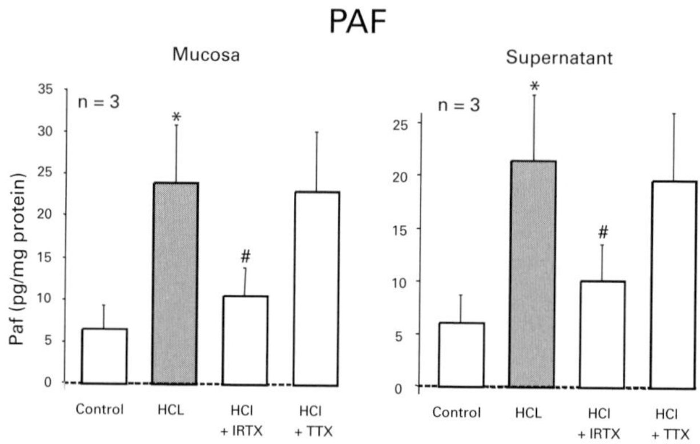

Figure 7. When *in vitro* mucosa is exposed to HCl for 3 hours, PAF levels increase 4-5 times in the mucosa and in the supernatant when compared to control (pH 7.4) (* $p < 0.5$ ANOVA). The HCl-induced increase in PAF is abolished by the TRPV1 receptor antagonist IRTX (# $p < 0.5$ ANOVA) and not affected by the neural blocker TTX both in the mucosa and in the supernatant indicating that production of PAF arises from non neural tissues. Bars represent mean ± SEM of 3 experiments.

The presence of TRPV1 receptor mRNA in esophageal mucosa was examined by RT-PCR (*Figure 8*). Primers were derived from conserved regions of mRNA sequences of humans, rat, dog, mouse guinea pig and rabbit. The BLAST database confirmed that the primers were specific for TRPV1. The band produced using these primers was sequenced,

TRPV1 in whole mucosa

Primers:
Sense: GACTTCAAGGCTGTCTTCATCATCC
Antisense : CAGGGAGAAGCTCAGGGTGCGC

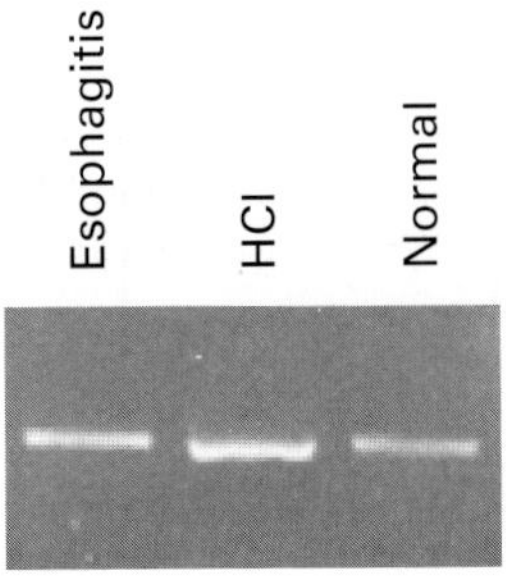

Figure 8. RT-PCR was performed in cat esophageal mucosa with primers selected from conserved regions of published sequences for humans, rat, dog, mouse, guinea pig and rabbit. Expression of TRPV1 mRNA increased after 3 hours exposure to HCl and after induction of experimental esophagitis by repeated perfusion of 0.1 N HCl for 1 hour on three succesive days.

obtaining the sequence of cat TRPV1 with 95% homology to human TRPV1. RT-PCR of mucosa exposed to HCl for 3 hours showed upregulation of TRPV1 cat receptor mRNA

To demonstrate the expression of TRPV1 receptor mRNA in non-neural cells, esophageal epithelial cells were enzymatically isolated, sorted by flow cytometry, and a 90-95% pure cell preparation was obtained. RT-PCR confirmed the presence of TRPV1 receptor mRNA in these cat esophageal epithelial cells (*Figure 9*). These isolated epithelial cells produced PAF in response to HCl, and the response was abolished by IRTX, supporting the presence of HCl-sensitive TRPV1 receptors in these cells (*Figure 10*).
We conclude that HCl-induced activation of TRPV1 receptors in esophageal mucosa results in upregulation of TRPV1 receptor mRNA, neurally mediated release of substance P and CGRP, and non-neurally mediated release of PAF from epithelial cells (*Figure 11*).

TRPV1 in mucosa and epithelial cells

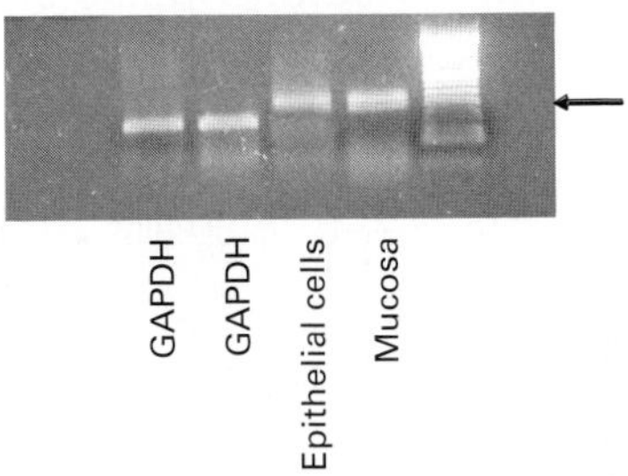

Figure 9. To demonstrate the presence of TRPV1 receptor mRNA in non-neural cells, esophageal epithelial cells were enzymatically isolated and sorted by flow cytometry. Primers were derived from conserved regions of mRNA sequences of humans, rat, dog, mouse, guinea pig and rabbit. RT-PCR confirmed the presence of TRPV1 receptor mRNA in these cat esophageal epithelial cells.

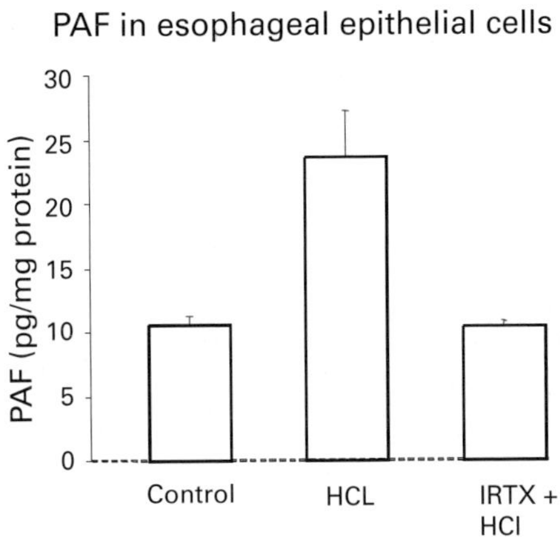

Figure 10. In enzymatically isolated epithelial cells, sorted to 95% purity by flow cytometry, 3 hour exposure to HCl more than doubled PAF levels ($p < 0.5$ ANOVA) The increase in PAF was abolished by the TRPV1 receptor antagonist IRTX (10^{-5}M).

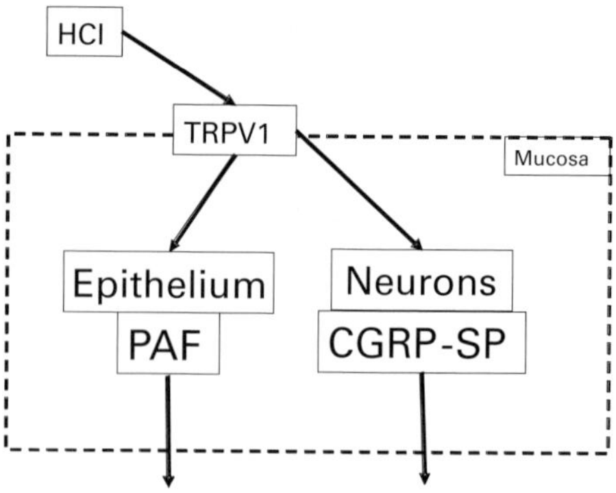

Figure 11. HCl-induced activation of TRPV1 receptors in esophageal mucosa results in neurally mediated release of substance P and CGRP, and non-neurally mediated release of PAF from epithelial cells

Inflammatory mediators and circular muscle contraction

The data presented to this point were obtained in cat. The following data have been obtained in cat [7] and in human esophagi from organ donors. Because the data are quite similar in both species, only the human data will be shown.

Contraction of human esophageal circular muscle is affected by the inflammatory mediators release by the mucosa, rather than by diffusion of HCl through the mucosal barrier, because when esophageal circular muscle is directly exposed to HCl (pH 4, 2-3 hours) no change in EFS-induced contraction occurs (*Figure 12*). When the mucosal sac is filled with HCl at the same pH, however, IL-1β, and PAF are formed in the mucosa, and PAF is released into the surrounding medium, to affect circular muscle function, whereas IL-1β is not released and remains in the mucosa, (*Figures 13 and 14*). In the circular muscle layer PAF inhibits neurally mediated contraction (*Figure 15*) as it inhibits release of acetylcholine from cholinergic neurons (*Figure 16*).

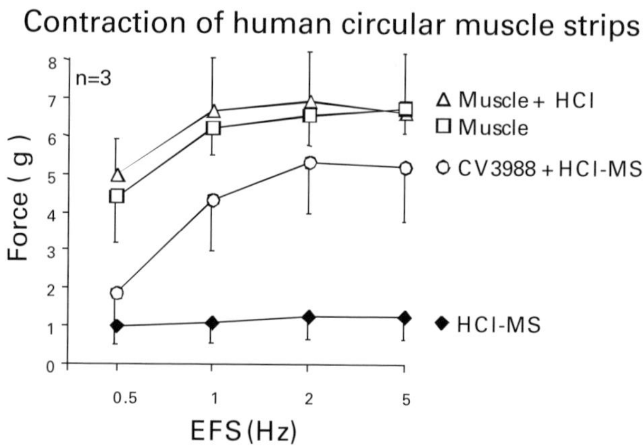

Figure 12. Direct application of HCl (pH 4.0, 3 hour) to circular muscle strips (Muscle + HCl) did not change contraction in response to electrical field stimulation (supramaximal voltage, 02 ms), when compared to untreated muscle (Muscle). Supernatant of HCl-filled mucosa (HCL-MS, pH 4, 3 hours), however, almost abolished the contraction ($p < 0.05$ ANOVA for comparison of HCL-MS to Muscle + HCl) The supernatant-induced inhibition was reversed when the competitive PAF antagonist CV3988 (10^{-6} M) was added to the supernatant of the HCl-filled mucosal sac (CV3988 + HCl-MS) ($p < 0.05$ ANOVA for comparison of CV3988+HCl-MS to HCL-MS . Means ± SEM are shown for 3 esophagus samples

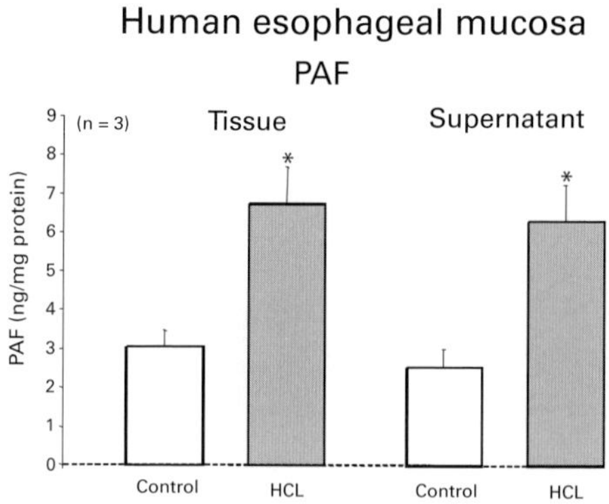

Figure 13. In the mucosa sac preparation, exposure to HCl (pH 4.0, 3 hours) caused a significant ($p < 0.05$) increase in the mucosa tissue content of PAF when compared to normal Krebs'-treated mucosa (control) ($p < 0.05$, paired t-test). HCl similarly increased PAF in the supernatant surrounding the mucosal sac ($p < 0.05$, t-test). The PAF concentration was quantified by using a platelet activating factor [^{3}H] (PAF) scintillation proximity assay system (Amersham Pharmacia Biotech Inc). Means ± SEM are shown for 3 esophageal samples.

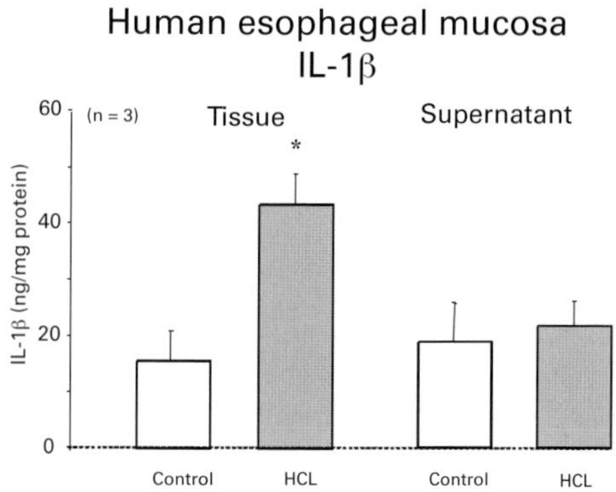

Figure 14. When mucosa was exposed to HCl, IL-1β increased significantly in the mucosa (paired t-test, $p < 0.05$) but not in the supernatant surrounding the mucosal sac. IL-1β levels were measured by enzyme immunoassay (R&D Systems, Minneapolis, MN). Means ± SEM are shown for 3 esophagus samples.

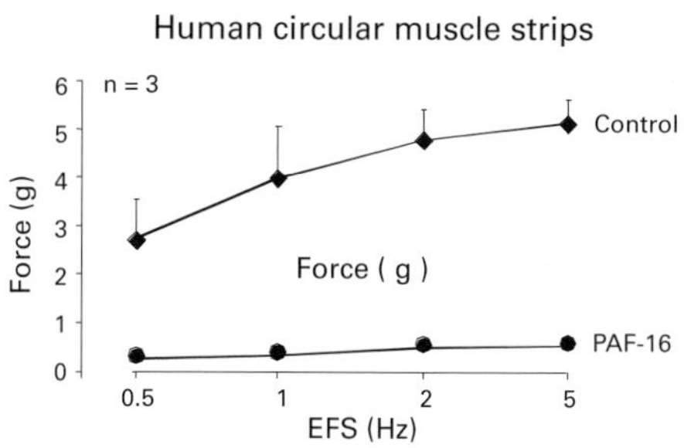

Figure 15. Incubation of normal esophageal smooth muscle strips in the PAF analog PAF-16 (10^{-5} M, 1-2 hours) almost abolished contraction in response to electrical field stimulation (EFS) ($p < 0.05$ ANOVA). Means ± SEM are shown for 3 esophagus samples.

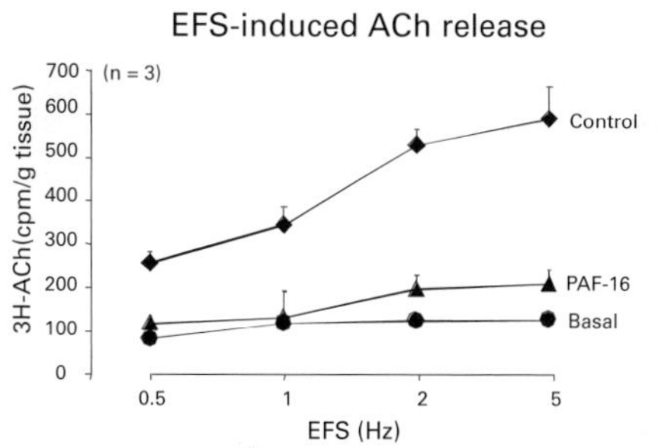

Figure 16. Electrical field stimulation (EFS)-induced release of ACh from esophageal circular muscle strips is shown as control. Incubation of normal muscle strips in PAF-16 (10^{-5} M, 1-2 hours) reduced ACh release to basal levels ($p < 0.05$ ANOVA for comparison of PAF-16 to control), suggesting that PAF inhibits EFS-induced contraction by inhibiting release of ACh. Means ± SEM are shown for 3 esophagus samples

In addition PAF induces formation of H_2O_2 in the circular muscle (*Figures 17 and 18*). It is noteworthy that the initial production of H_2O_2 occurs only in the circular muscle and not in the mucosa (*Figure 19*). These data therefore indicate that involvement of the circular muscle is an important step in the onset of the inflammatory process.

Figure 17. When esophageal circular muscle was exposed to PAF-16 (10^{-5} M) H_2O_2 levels in the muscle increased significantly (* $p < 0.05$ ANOVA compared to control). The increase was significantly reduced by the NADPH inhibitor apocynin (10^{-5} M) (# $p < 0.05$ ANOVA) The data indicate that PAF-induced production of H_2O_2 depends on activation of NADPH oxidase. Bars represent mean ± SEM of 3 experiments. The cartoon on the upper right side represents a possible pathway consistent with these results. The pathway will be modified in subsequent figures, so as to remain consistent with this and the following figures.

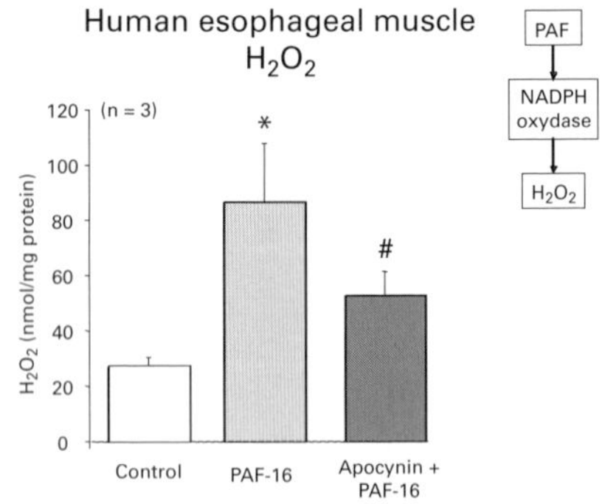

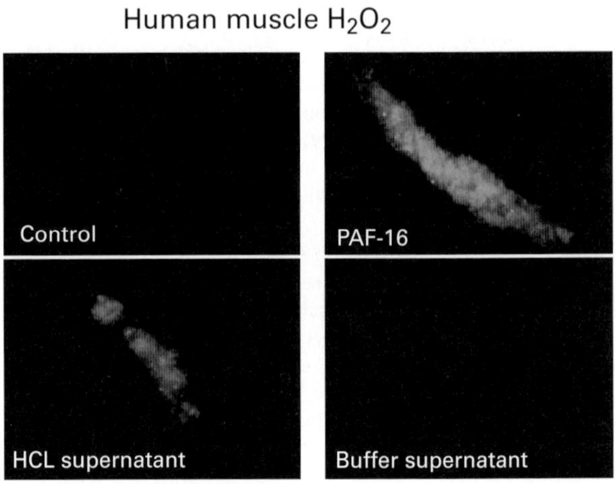

Figure 18. Rhodamine fluorescence in muscle cells enzymatically isolated from esophageal circular muscle layer as a probe for measurement of intracellular ROS. Dihydro-rhodamine (DHR 123) enters the cells as a freely permeable dye which, when oxidized, is converted to rhodamine 123, which is not membrane permeable. Rhodamine 123 is a common laser dye, which is excitable at 488 detectable at 515 nm, under confocal microscopy. Rhodamine 123 fluoresces when exposed to reactive oxygen species (ROS), including H_2O_2. ROS levels were low in normal esophageal smooth muscle cells (Control) and were not affected by supernatant of normal Krebs' treated mucosa (Buffer supernatant). In contrast incubating normal smooth muscle cells with supernatant of HCl (pH 5.8)-filled mucosa (HCl supernatant), or with PAF-16, visibly increased cytoplasmic ROS, confirming the data in *Figure 17*, and indicating that PAF induced-fluorescence is most likely a reflection of NADPH-dependent production of H_2O_2. (See page XI for colour figure).

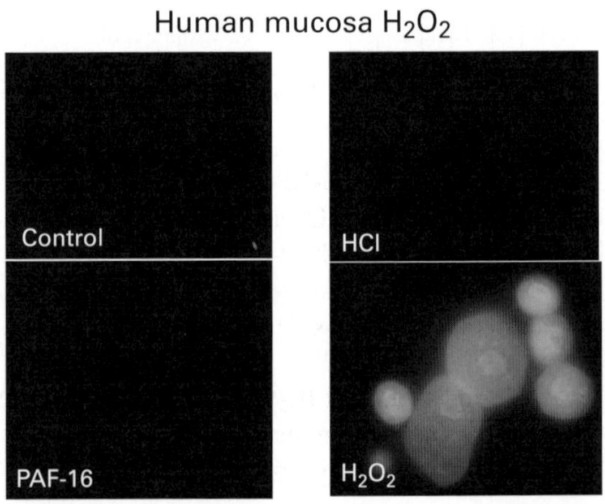

Figure 19. Rhodamine fluorescence in epithelial cells enzymatically isolated from esophageal mucosa was examined by confocal microscopy, as a probe for measurement of intracellular H_2O_2. The figure shows no ROS in epithelial cells in response to HCl or PAF-16. An H_2O_2-treated epithelial cell is shown in the right lower panel as a positive control. H_2O_2 is uncharged and penetrates the cytoplasm, demonstrating the adequacy of the technique in detecting cytoplasmic H_2O_2. (See page XII for colour figure).

In addition PAF induces formation of the pro-inflammatory cytokine IL-6 in the circular muscle (*Figure 20*), without involving production of H_2O_2 as the H_2O_2 scavenger catalase does not significantly inhibit PAF induced formation of IL-6.

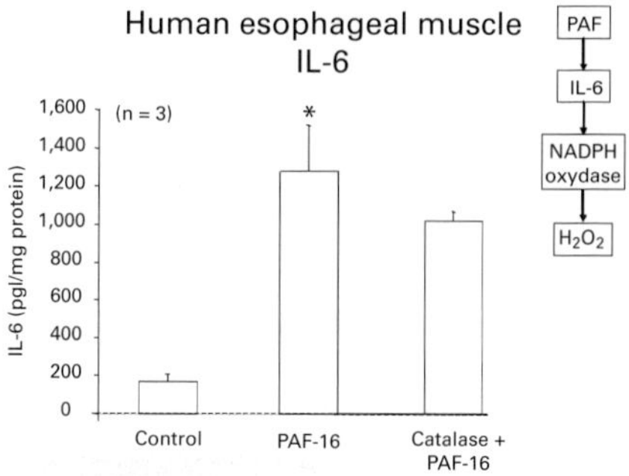

Figure 20. When esophageal circular muscle was exposed to PAF-16 (10^{-5} M) IL-6 levels in the muscle increased significantly (* $p < 0.05$ ANOVA) when compared to control. The increase was not affected by the H_2O_2 scavenger catalase (1,000 u/ml) when compared to PAF alone. The data indicate that PAF-induced production of IL-6 is direct and not mediated by H_2O_2. Bars represent mean ± SEM of 3 experiments.

Figure 21 indicates that IL-6 induces production of H_2O_2 by activating NADPH oxidase, as H_2O_2 production is significantly reduced by the NADPH oxidase inhibitor apocynin. This IL-6-induced production of H_2O_2 is PAF independent, as it is not affected by the PAF receptor antagonist CV3988. These data support the sequence of events indicated in the panel in the upper right hand of the figure: PAF induces formation of IL-6 that, in turn, induces activation of NADPH oxidase and formation of H_2O_2.

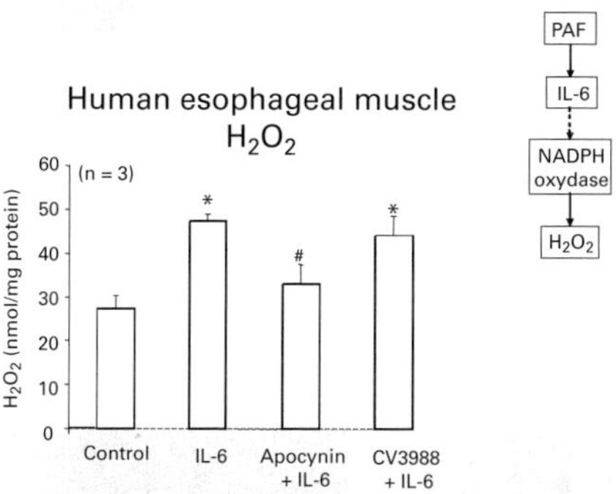

Figure 21. When esophageal circular muscle was exposed to IL-6 (2 u/ml) H_2O_2 levels in the muscle increased significantly (* $p < 0.05$ ANOVA compared to control). The increase was abolished by the NADPH inhibitor apocynin (10^{-5} M) (# $p < 0.05$ ANOVA when compared to IL-6-treated muscle), indicating IL-6-induced activation of NADPH oxidase. The IL-6-induced increase in H_2O_2 was not affected by the PAF receptor antagonist CV3988 (10^{-6} M) and remained different from control (* $p < 0.05$ ANOVA). These data indicate that IL-6-dependent production of H_2O_2 does not involve PAF. Bars represent mean ± SEM of 3 experiments.

Similarly to IL-6, IL-1β increased in the muscle after exposure to PAF (*Figure 22*). The figure indicates that H_2O_2 and PAF caused an increase in IL-1β levels. The PAF-induced increase was equally reduced by apocynin and by IL-6 antibodies. These data are consistent with a sequential pathway, involving PAF-induced production of IL-6, followed by activation of NADPH oxidase and production of H_2O_2 that finally, results in production of IL-1β.

Figure 23 indicates that IL-6 may induce production of PAF, through production of H_2O_2, because IL-6 induced production of PAF was abolished by the NADPH inhibitor apocynin. H_2O_2, in turn induced production of PAF, in part through IL-1b, because H_2O_2-induced production of PAF was partly reduced by immuno-neutralization of IL-1β. The partial reduction in formation of PAF by immuno-neutralization of IL-1β, suggests the presence of an IL-1β-independent pathway, possibly mediating direct formation of PAF in response to H_2O_2.

Figure 24 summarizes possible pathways that are consistent with these data.

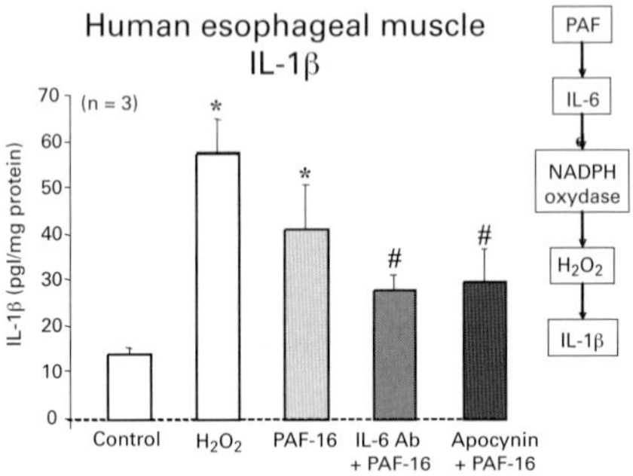

Figure 22. When esophageal circular muscle was exposed to H_2O_2 (70 μM), IL-1β in the muscle increased significantly (* $p < 0.05$ ANOVA compared to control). PAF-16 also increased IL-1β. The increase induced by PAF-16 was abolished by immuno-neutralization of IL-6 (# $p < 0.05$ ANOVA, when compared to PAF-16 alone). and by the NADPH inhibitor apocynin (10^{-5} M) (# $p < 0.05$ ANOVA, when compared to PAF-16 alone). The data indicate PAF may induce production of IL-1β by sequential formation of IL-6, causing production of H_2O_2 that, finally, induces production of IL-1β. Bars represent mean — SEM of 3 experiments.

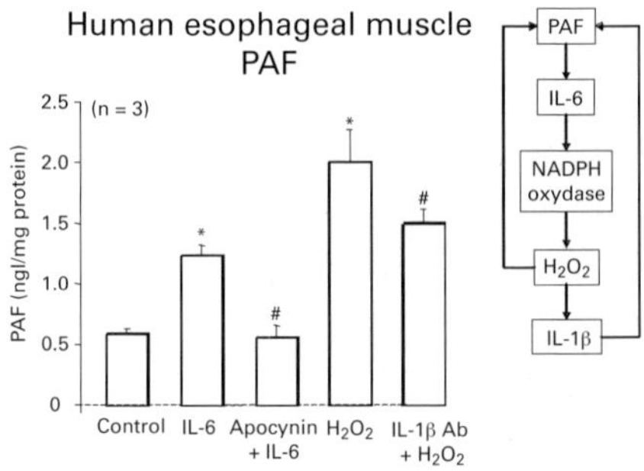

Figure 23. When esophageal circular muscle was exposed to IL-6 (2 u/ml), PAF in the muscle increased significantly (* $p < 0.05$ ANOVA compared to control). H_2O_2 (70 μM) also increased PAF. The increase induced by IL-6 was abolished by the NADPH inhibitor apocynin (10^{-5} M) (# $p < 0.05$ ANOVA, when compared to IL-6 alone). The increase induced by H_2O_2 was partly reduced by immuno-neutralization of IL-1β (# $p < 0.05$ ANOVA, when compared to H_2O_2 alone). The data indicate IL-6 may induce production of PAF by activation of NADPH oxidase, causing production of H_2O_2. H_2O_2, in turn, causes production of PAF, either directly or, in part, by inducing production of IL-1β. Bars represent mean ± SEM of 3 experiments.

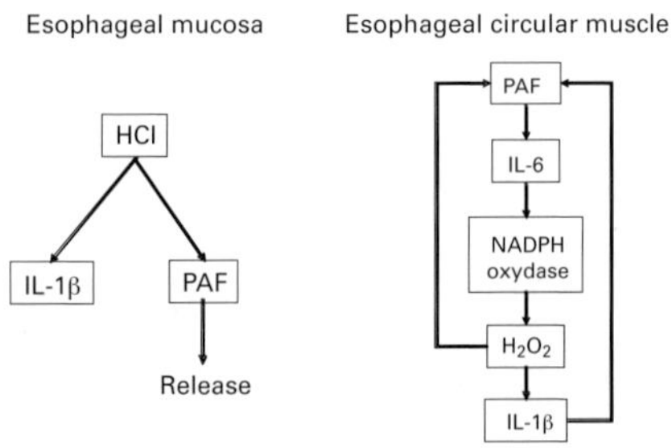

Figure 24. In mucosa HCL causes formation of IL-1β and PAF (left panel). PAF is then released to affect the circular muscle. IL-1β remains in the mucosa. In the circular muscle (right panel) PAF, released by the mucosa causes the sequential production of IL-6, H_2O_2 and IL-1β that, in turn, induce production of PAF by the circular muscle. PAF is only partly produced by IL-1β, because the IL-1β antibody partly reduced PAF formation. The data suggest that H_2O_2 may induce formation of PAF directly, and in part through formation of IL-1β.

Inflammatory mediators in chronic esophagitis

The previous data were obtained in normal human esophageal specimens after short (3-hour) exposure of esophageal mucosa to acid, and short (3-hour) exposure of circular muscle to mucosa supernatant. To examine whether the data may also be applicable to chronic esophagitis we refer to a human organ donor specimen with histologically demonstrated erosive esophagitis [9] (*Figures 25 and 26*). In this specimen the circular muscle was taken from the lower esophageal sphincter (LES). Essentially the same inflammatory processes are present in the body of the esophagus and in the LES. This is not surprising as the inflammation begins with damage to the epithelial cells in the mucosa. When mounted in a warm (37°C) oygenated muscle chamber, normal-LES circular muscle strips gradually develop tone and reach a steady state tone (3.25 ± 0.2 grams) after 3-4 hours. In contrast, circular muscle strips from esophagitis LES developed little tone (0.7 grams), a value falling outside of the normal tone minus 2 standard deviations. When circular muscle strips from the esophagitis LES were exposed to catalase (800 U/ml), tone increased within 15-30 min and reached a value of 2.7 g, a value similar to that of strips from normal LES (*Figure 27*). These findings suggest that H_2O_2 may be present in circular muscle of esophagitis LES, and responsible for reduced tone when inflammation is present. Upregulation of NADPH oxidases is a possible mechanism for overproduction of H_2O_2. We therefore examined by RT-PCR whether any NADPH oxidases are present in human esophageal circular muscle, and upregulated by esophagitis. We designed primers for NOX1, NOX2, NOX3, NOX4, NOX5, and found that these membrane-bound catalytic components of the NADPH oxidase enzyme are all present in esophageal circular muscle, but only NOX5 mRNA was increased in the human specimen with esophagitis, as shown in *Figure 28A*. Increased NOX5 cDNA in the esophagitis specimen was confirmed by real-time RT-PCR, when compared to normal human esophageal

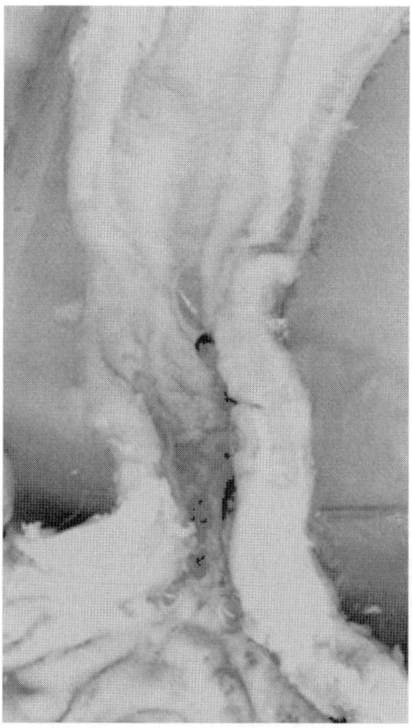

Figure 25. An esophageal specimen obtained from an organ donor exhibited hyperemia of the mucosa with scattered hemorrhagic erosions in the lower esophagus, extending across the cardia. (See page XII for colour figure).

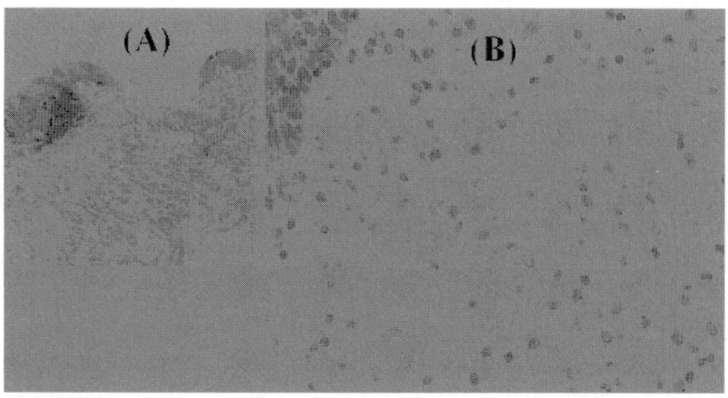

Figure 26. Panel (A) shows erosions, basal zone hyperplasia and elongation of lamina propria papillae with congestion. The enlarged area (panel B) shows inflammatory cells present in the epithelial layer. These findings are characteristic of reflux esophagitis. (See page XII for colour figure).

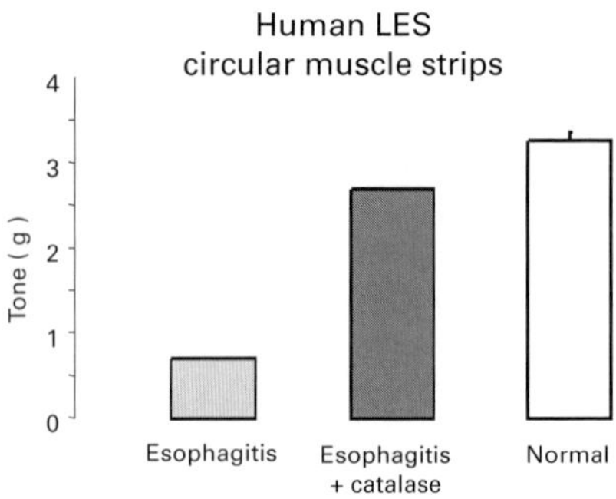

Figure 27. Circular muscle strips were mounted in muscle chambers, stretched to 2.5 grams to bring them near conditions of optimum force development, and equilibrated for 4-6 hour while perfused continuously with oxygenated physiologic salt solution at 37°C. During this time the tension in LES strips increased, attaining a steady level at 3-4 hour. In LES circular muscle strips from the esophagitis specimen obtained from an organ donor tone was lower than in normal strips almost to a normal level. These data indicate that H_2O_2 may be responsible for the reduced tone in esophagitis. Means ± SE are shown for 3 normal LES samples.

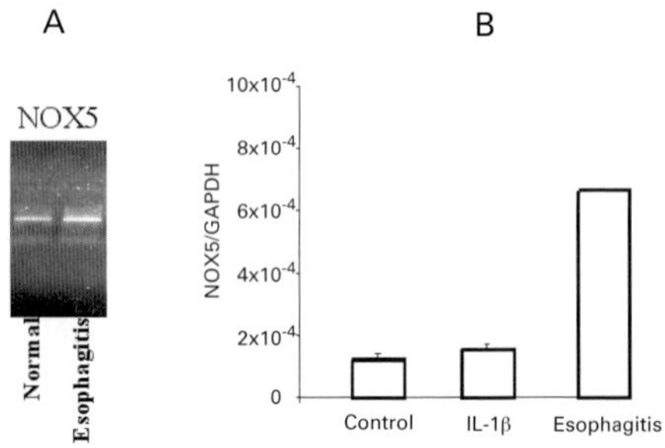

Figure 28. LES circular muscle was examined by RT-PCR for the presence of NADPH oxidases. We used published primers for NOX1, NOX2, NOX3, NOX4, NOX5, and found that these components of the NADPH oxidase enzyme are all present in esophageal circular muscle, but only NOX5 mRNA was increased in the human specimen with esophagitis, as shown in panel A. Increased NOX5 cDNA in the esophagitis specimen was confirmed by real-time RT-PCR, when compared to normal human esophageal circular muscle, as shown in panel B.
Means ± SE are shown for 3 normal (control) and for 3 IL-1β-treated LES samples.

circular muscle, as shown in *Figure 28B*. The figure shows increased levels of NOX5 cDNA in the esophagitis specimen when compared to normals. Three-hour exposure to IL-1β did not increase NOX5 cDNA, even though IL-1β increases H_2O_2 levels in normal circular muscle as shown in *Figure 29*. This is not surprising as NADPH oxidase-mediated production of H_2O_2 may be regulated at multiple levels, even when its expression is not upregulated.

Figure 29 shows H_2O_2 levels in normal and esophagitis circular muscle tissue. Basal H_2O_2 levels were elevated in circular muscle of esophagitis LES, exceeding normal levels by more than two standard deviations. We have previously shown that, in cat LES, IL-1β [6] and other cytokines, presumably released by inflammatory cells or the damaged esophageal epithelium, may contribute to production of H_2O_2. This possibility was tested in circular muscle from normal LES. Exposure of normal LES circular muscle to IL-1β increased production of H_2O_2 to a level approaching that of esophagitis muscle (*Figure 29*).

Finally we tested for the presence of PAF in circular muscle in this chronic esophagitis specimen. *Figure 30* shows that PAF levels were elevated in the human esophagitis sample and exceeded those of the normal sample by more than two standard deviations. Incubation of normal LES circular muscle in H_2O_2 (70 mM, 2 hour) significantly increased PAF levels ($p < 0.01$).

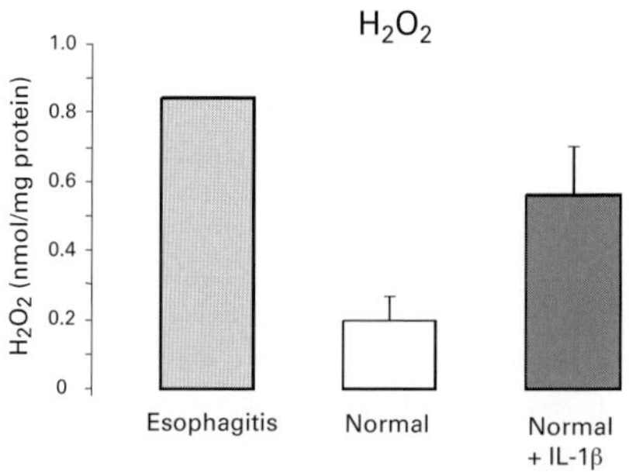

Figure 29. IL-1β and esophagitis increase H_2O_2 levels in LES circular smooth muscle. H_2O_2 levels of LES circular smooth muscle were measured by colorimetric assay. H_2O_2 levels were four-fold higher in LES muscle from the esophagitis specimen compared with normal muscle. Treatment of normal LES circular smooth muscle with IL-1≤ (200 U/ml, 2 hr) increased H_2O_2 levels compared with untreated muscle. Means — SE are shown for 3 normal and for 3 IL-

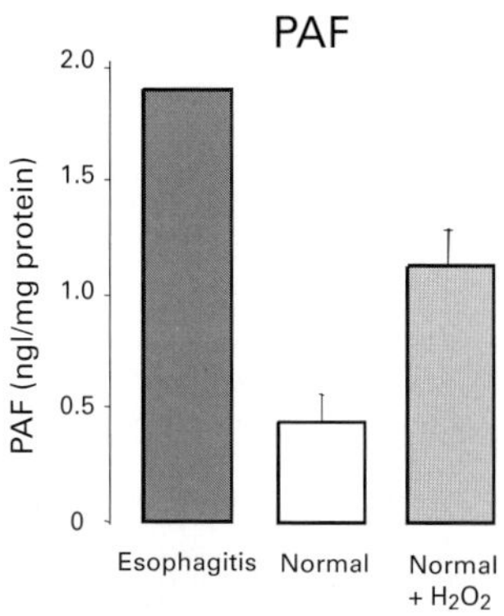

Figure 30. Esophagitis and H_2O_2 increase PAF production in LES. The PAF concentration was quantified by using a platelet activating factor [^{3}H] (PAF) scintillation proximity assay system (Amersham Pharmacia Biotech Inc). In esophagitis circular muscle PAF levels were four times higher than in normal LES. In normal LES muscle, PAF levels were significantly increased ($p < 0.01$, unpaired t-test) by H_2O_2 (70 mM, 2 hour).

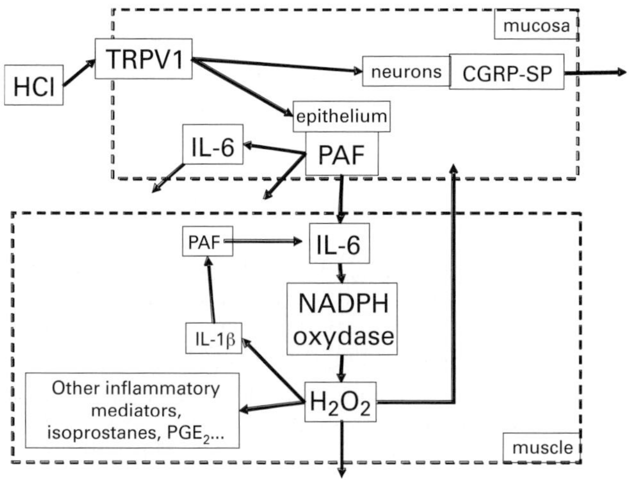

Figure 31. The data suggest that exposure of esophageal mucosa to acid activates TRPV1 receptors, inducing neurally mediated formation of substance P and CGRP, and production of PAF by the epithelium. These inflammatory mediators are released by the mucosa to activate leukocytes and to affect circular muscle contraction. PAF alone is sufficient to almost completely inhibit release of ACh from cholinergic neurons, thus inhibiting esophageal circular muscle contraction. In addition PAF induces sequential production of IL-6, H_2O_2, IL-1β, and PAF in the circular muscle. In LES circular muscle IL-6, H_2O_2, IL-1β, and PAF all contribute to reducing LES tone. Once these inflammatory mediators are present, any one of them may contribute to sequential formation of the others, possibly initiating a self-sustaining cycle.

These data are consistent with the model illustrated in *Figure 31*. Taken together the data suggest that PAF, released by the mucosa, induces sequential production of IL-6, H_2O_2, IL-1β, and PAF in the circular muscle. Once these inflammatory mediators are present, any one of them may contribute to sequential formation of the others, possibly initiating a self-sustaining cycle.

From the data we conclude that PAF and H_2O_2 may be two major inflammatory mediators in esophagitis. PAF, initially released by the mucosa affects circular muscle contraction and induces production of H_2O_2. H_2O_2 is uncharged, freely diffusible through cellular membranes, and likely to interact with membrane lipids, causing lipid peroxidation and peroxidation-induced inflammatory mediators. H_2O_2 may contribute to further production of PAF and cause upregulation of NADPH oxidase in the mucosa and muscle. H_2O_2 may also interact with DNA bases (more than 20 different oxidatively altered purines and pyrimidines have been detected and characterized [11]), perhaps inducing alterations of cell phenotype and possibly resulting in permanent mutations.

References

1. Barbara G, De Giorgio R, Stanghellini V, et al. Neutral endopeptidase (EC 3.4.24.11) downregulates the onset of intestinal inflammation in the nematode infected mouse. Gut 2003;52:1457-64.
2. Birder LA, Kanai AJ, de Groat WC, et al. Vanilloid receptor expression suggests a sensory role for urinary bladder epithelial cells. Proc Natl Acad Sci USA 2001;98:13396-401.
3. Birder LA, Nakamura Y, Kiss S, et al. Altered urinary bladder function in mice lacking the vanilloid receptor TRPV1. Nat Neurosci 2002;5:856-60.
4. Chan CL, Facer P, Davis JB, et al. Sensory fibres expressing capsaicin receptor TRPV1 in patients with rectal hypersensitivity and faecal urgency. Lancet 2003;361:385-91.
5. Chen CW, Lee ST, Wu WT, Fu WM, Ho FM, Lin WW. Signal transduction for inhibition of inducible nitric oxide synthase and cyclooxygenase-2 induction by capsaicin and related analogs in macrophages. Br J Pharmacol 2003140:1077-87.
6. Cheng L, Cao W, Behar J, Biancani P, Harnett KM. Inflammation induced changes in arachidonic acid metabolism in cat LES circular muscle. Am J Physiol Gastrointest Liver Physiol 2005;288:G787-97.
7. Cheng L, Cao W, Fiocchi C, Behar J, Biancani P, Harnett KM. HCl-induced inflammatory mediators in cat esophageal mucosa and inflammatory mediators in esophageal circular muscle in an in vitro model of esophagitis. Am J Physiol Gastrointest Liver Physiol 2006; 290(6):G1307-17.
8. Cheng L, Cao W, Fiocchi C, Behar J, Biancani P, Harnett KM. In vitro model of acute esophagitis in the cat. Am J Physiol Gastrointest Liver Physiol 2005;289:G860-9.
9. Cheng L, Harnett KM, Cao W, et al . Hydrogen peroxide reduces lower esophageal sphincter tone in human esophagitis. Gastroenterology 2005;129:1675-85.
10. Cortright DN, Szallasi A. Biochemical pharmacology of the vanilloid receptor TRPV1. An update. Eur J Biochem 2004;271:1814-9.
11. Dizdaroglu M. Oxidative damage to DNA in mammalian chromatin. Mutat Res 1992;275:331-42.
12. Fujino K, de la Fuente SG, Takami Y, Takahashi T, Mantyh CR. Attenuation of acid induced oesophagitis in VR-1 deficient mice. Gut 2006;55:34-40.
13. Heiner I, Eisfeld J, Halaszovich CR, et al. Expression profile of the transient receptor potential (TRP) family in neutrophil granulocytes: evidence for currents through long TRP channel 2 induced by ADP-ribose and NAD. Biochem J 2003;371:1045-53.
14. Kihara N, de la Fuente SG, Fujino K, Takahashi T, Pappas TN, Mantyh CR. Vanilloid receptor-1 containing primary sensory neurones mediate dextran sulphate sodium induced colitis in rats. Gut 2003;52:713-9.
15. Kimball ES, Wallace NH, Schneider CR, D'Andrea MR, Hornby PJ. Vanilloid receptor 1 antagonists attenuate disease severity in dextran sulphate sodium-induced colitis in mice. Neurogastroenterol Motil 2004;16:811-8.
16. Kirkwood KS, Bunnett NW, Maa J, et al. Deletion of neutral endopeptidase exacerbates intestinal inflammation induced by Clostridium difficile toxin A. Am J Physiol Gastrointest Liver Physiol 2001;281:G544-51.
17. Mantyh CR, Maggio JE, Mantyh PW, Vigna SR, Pappas TN. Increased substance P receptor expression by blood vessels and lymphoid aggregates in Clostridium difficile-induced pseudomembranous colitis. Dig Dis Sci 1996;41:614-20.
18. Mantyh CR, McVey DC, Vigna SR. Extrinsic surgical denervation inhibits Clostridium difficile toxin A-induced enteritis in rats. Neurosci Lett 2000;292:95-8.

19. Mantyh CR, Pappas TN, Lapp JA, et al. Substance P activation of enteric neurons in response to intraluminal Clostridium difficile toxin A in the rat ileum. Gastroenterology 1996;111:1272-80.
20. Mantyh CR, Vigna SR, Bollinger RR, Mantyh PW, Maggio JE, Pappas TN. Differential expression of substance P receptors in patients with Crohn's disease and ulcerative colitis. Gastroenterology 1995;109:850-60.
21. Mantyh PW, DeMaster E, Malhotra A, et al. Receptor endocytosis and dendrite reshaping in spinal neurons after somatosensory stimulation. Science 1995;268:1629-32.
22. Matthews PJ, Aziz Q, Facer P, Davis JB, Thompson DG, Anand P. Increased capsaicin receptor TRPV1 nerve fibres in the inflamed human oesophagus. Eur J Gastroenterol Hepatol 2004;16:897-902.
23. McVey DC, Schmid PC, Schmid HH, Vigna SR. Endocannabinoids induce ileitis in rats via the capsaicin receptor (VR1). J Pharmacol Exp Ther 2003;304:713-22.
24. McVey DC, Vigna SR. The capsaicin VR1 receptor mediates substance P release in toxin A-induced enteritis in rats. Peptides 2001;22:1439-46.
25. McVey DC, Vigna SR. The role of leukotriene B4 in Clostridium difficile toxin A-induced ileitis in rats. Gastroenterology 2005;128:1306-16.
26. Nathan JD, Patel AA, McVey DC, et al. Capsaicin vanilloid receptor-1 mediates substance P release in experimental pancreatitis. Am J Physiol Gastrointest Liver Physiol 2001;281:G1322-8.
27. Nathan JD, Peng RY, Wang Y, McVey DC, Vigna SR, Liddle RA. Primary sensory neurons: a common final pathway for inflammation in experimental pancreatitis in rats. Am J Physiol Gastrointest Liver Physiol 2002;283:G938-46.
28. Reilly CA, Taylor JL, Lanza DL, Carr BA, Crouch DJ, Yost GS. Capsaicinoids cause inflammation and epithelial cell death through activation of vanilloid receptors. Toxicol Sci 2003;73:170-81.
29. Southall MD, Li T, Gharibova LS, Pei Y, Nicol GD, Travers JB. Activation of epidermal vanilloid receptor-1 induces release of proinflammatory mediators in human keratinocytes. J Pharmacol Exp Ther 2003;304:217-22.
30. Stander S, Moormann C, Schumacher M, et al. Expression of vanilloid receptor subtype 1 in cutaneous sensory nerve fibers, mast cells, and epithelial cells of appendage structures. Exp Dermatol 2004;13:129-39.
31. Sturiale S, Barbara G, Qiu B, et al. Neutral endopeptidase (EC 3.4.24.11) terminates colitis by degrading substance P. Proc Natl Acad Sci USA 1999;96:11653-8.
32. Szallasi A,Blumberg PM. Vanilloid (Capsaicin) receptors and mechanisms. Pharmacol Rev 1999;51:159-212.
33. Veronesi B, Carter JD, Devlin RB, Simon SA, Oortgiesen M. Neuropeptides and capsaicin stimulate the release of inflammatory cytokines in a human bronchial epithelial cell line. Neuropeptides 1999;33:447-56.
34. Yiangou Y, Facer P, Dyer NH, et al. Vanilloid receptor 1 immunoreactivity in inflamed human bowel. Lancet 2001;357:1338-9.

Esophageal motility disorders after esophageal banding

O.B. Lao, B.K. Oelschlager (Seattle)

Surgery and obesity

Obesity is a major health problem for the western world because of its association with an increased rate of mortality. In patients where diet, exercise and medication fail to provide for adequate weight control, surgery has become a main option. Surgery has proven to have the most predictable and lasting effect on morbid obesity [1]. There are a variety of surgical options for weight control including the gastric band, vertical banded gastroplasty and gastric bypass.

The laparoscopic adjustable band continues to gain popularity for the treatment of obesity because of its ease of placement and low surgical risk compared to the other surgical alternatives. The theory behind the procedure is the creation of a small pouch in the upper portion of the stomach with a controlled and adjustable stoma to limit food intake and promote early satiety. This is done by placing a hollow, flexible silicone ring around the upper portion of the stomach that can be filled and adjusted to various degrees with saline. Despite the prevalence of the gastric band, there is still a great deal that is not known about its long term effects.

Obesity and esophageal motility

Gastroesophageal reflux (GER) is present in approximately 25% of the adult population and has a strong relationship with obesity. Weight loss is commonly recommended as part of the first-line management of reflux symptoms. The etiology behind this relationship is not clearly defined, but is believed to be related to the increase in intraabdominal pressure and increased likelihood of hiatal hernia in obese patients. Obese patients have been shown to have an incidence of reflux symptoms anywhere between 30-60% [2,3].

Morbid obesity itself is also associated with esophageal motility disorders. One study demonstrated motility disorders in 40-60% of obese patients considering weight loss surgery including the presence of achalasia, diffuse esophageal spasm, hypotensive lower esophageal sphincter mechanism (LESM) and nutcracker esophagus [3]. At the University of Washington, we have found that not only do many patients have abnormal manometry (23%), when using impedance technology up to 60% of morbidly obese patients have delayed or incomplete bolus clearance through the esophagus. Notable among these findings is a lack of symptoms among the obese patients who were found to have motility disorders. This may be due to impaired parasympathetic and sympathetic responsiveness to stomach distention.

Altering esophageal motility

The location of the gastric band relative to the normal LESM is paramount to its effects on the esophagus and stomach. The band is intended to be placed at a location that facilitates the creation of a pouch or "neo stomach" with a volume of approximately 10-30 cc. The distal end of that pouch is controlled by the band and its inflation with saline. The volume of this pouch and the outlet to the larger stomach is controlled by the amount of saline that is used to inflate the band.

Since the band is placed at or very near the LESM, implantation of the gastric band in that location and its subsequent inflation can result in relative obstruction of the esophagus. Studies done in the 1960s demonstrated that the esophagus will respond to an acute obstruction by initiating a sustained force to the obstruction oriented to drive a presumed bolus toward the stomach. These researchers termed this the "esophageal propulsive force" (EPF) [4]. This EPF persists until resolution of the obstruction and during this time, normal peristalsis is delayed and interrupted. This condition mimics the symptoms of achalasia for the patient with dysphagia and the sensation of regurgitation. Aperistalsis and impaired relaxation of the LESM is the hallmark if achalasia that is thought to result from the inflammation around and loss of the ganglion cells in the myenteric plexus of the distal esophagus. Similar physiology can be created by placing the band near and around the LESM.

There is experience with a prosthesis near or around the gastroesophageal junction and LESM. Such a device is the Angelchik prosthesis that was introduced in 1979 as a treatment for GER disease (GERD). Initially intended to recreate the dysfunctional LES, the Angelchik prosthesis has encountered numerous complications such as esophagitis, esophageal stricture and obstruction, transient and persistent dysphagia, migration or slippage, breakage and also erosion into the gastric lumen. These complications have required endoscopic and laproscopic treatment along with laparotomy for removal of the prosthesis as well as reconstruction [5]. Because of the frequency of serious complications that have arisen with the use of the Angelchik prosthesis, surgeons soon abandoned this method for the treatment of reflux disease.

The other commonly performed restrictive gastric banding procedure is the vertical banded gastroplasty. In this procedure, initially described in 1981, a pouch is created and isolated from the lesser curve of the stomach and restricted by the use of a prosthesis. This combination effectively limits the size of the pouch to a volume that is created by the staple line and the "new pylorus" created by the prosthesis. Complications that have arisen with the use of this procedure include inadequate weight loss, persistent GER and persistent emesis. Migration or slippage of the prosthesis has also been reported. The lack of effective weight loss using vertical banded gastroplasty has led a large number of patients to undergo reoperation for converstion to Roux-en-Y gastric bypass for durable results [6,7].

Experience with adjustable bands

Proponents of the adjustable bands suggest that they are much less likely to cause the above mentioned problems because of their adjustable nature. There have been very few studies done to study their effect on esophageal physiology, and none have studied the long-term effects of the band on the esophagus. What has been done provides a little insight into the possible effects.

Effect on gastroesophageal reflux disease

Whether adjustable bands improve or exacerbate GERD is still an un answered question, but important to consider as it may have implications on its effect on esophageal motility. An Italian study [8] published in 2002 demonstrated an improvement in GERD after the placement of the band. Their study included 43 obese patients and followed 16 of them for 18 months. At baseline, they found that esophageal symptoms such as heartburn, regurgitation, dysphagia and chest pain were higher in obese patients than non-obese controls. Of the banded patients followed up at 18 months, it appeared that their regurgitation and heartburn had decreased. Dysphagia, on the other hand, appeared to increase. The authors concluded that band placement did indeed reduce the amount of acid exposure for obese patients with abnormal acid exposure pre-operatively. Despite this conclusion, the authors note that pouch dilation, which can occur after banding, can lead to retention of gastric contents and subsequent reflux of those contents into the distal esophagus.

Another study [9] published in 1998 that reviewed morbidly obese patients treated with banding or vertical-banded gastroplasty demonstrated worsening of GERD after the placement of the band. Measurements of acid exposure pre-operatively and post-operatively in band patients at three to four years of follow-up demonstrated a statistically significant difference in the percentage of acid exposure in the distal esophagus, with banding patients having a higher incidence of acid exposure after placement of the band.

While these two studies would appear to be contradictory, the difference in length of follow-up may be significant. It is perhaps possible that reflux symptoms in obese patients initially improve in the short-run after the placement of the band with subsequent worsening of those symptoms in the long-run. Similarly, it may be that patients that receive the band benefit from reduction in their esophageal symptoms from reduced acid exposure and those that suffer worsening of their reflux are those that develop pouch dilatation and subsequently reflux of the pouch into the distal esophagus.

Given the seemingly disparate information regarding GERD symptoms after the placement of the band, how should one counsel patients with regard to this subject during pre-operative counseling?

Studies done in the past two years [10,11] have suggested the need for a complete esophageal evaluation prior to the initiation of gastric banding as poor pre-operative testing may indicate the need for alternative bariatric procedures.

The first study [10] demonstrated an alteration in esophageal motility after gastric banding, specifically a weakening in the lower esophageal musculature. They also found fewer peristaltic contractions after banding and more nonspecific motility disorders following placement of the band. These poor post-operative outcomes tended to occur in patients with abnormal pre-operative acid exposure based on pH monitoring and DeMeester score. This study followed 43 patients for between 6 and 18 months after banding. Based on their results, they have suggested that patients with abnormal pH monitoring and esophageal manometry may be poor candidates for gastric banding because of the subsequent deleterious effects on the lower esophagus.

The second study [11] followed patients from 12-49 months, with a mean of 33 months and found mixed results with respect to GERD symptoms after the placement of the band. Approximately 70% of patients improved and 30% of patients remained symptomatic after banding. Of those that remained symptomatic after banding, the majority of them had pre-operative studies that demonstrated poor esophageal motility. Esophageal dilatation was noted in 35% of symptomatic patients that were banded. While the dilatation may not completely explain the presence of GERD symptoms after banding, the presence of dilatation or other motility disorders pre-operatively may be a signal to consider thorough testing and alternative bariatric procedures in that patient population.

None of these studies were able to retrospectively review their patients and find a specific test or group of findings pre-operatively that would accurately predict poor function after placement of the band. The combination of pH studies, esophageal motility studies and manometry along with endoscopy may provide more information, but cannot elucidate which gastric band patients will respond negatively to banding. Those that begin to have or continue to have GERD symptoms and poor esophageal motility after banding may subsequently need band adjustment, deflation or even removal. The long-term effect of these adjustable bands on the esophagus needs to be followed and studied closely, to make sure they do not have similar effects as their non-adjustable counterparts.

References

1. Gastrointestinal Surgery for severe obesity: NIH Consensus Development Conference Statement. Am J Clin Nutr 1992;55:615-9.
2. O'Brien TF, Stroop EM. Lower esophageal sphincter pressure (LESP) and esophageal function in obese human. J Clin Gastroenterol 1980;2:145-8.

3. Jaffin BW, Knoepflmacher P, Greenstein R. High prevalence of asymptomatic esophageal motility disorders among morbidly obese patients. Obes Surg 1999;9:390-5.
4. Winship DH, Zboralske FF. The esophageal propulsive force: esophageal response to acute obstruction. J Clin Invest 1967;9:1391-401.
5. Kauten JR, Mansour KA. Complications of the Angelchik prosthesis in the management of gastroesophageal reflux. Am Surg 1986;52(4):208-13.
6. Balsiger BM, Poggio JL, Mai J, Kelly KA, Sarr MG. Ten and more years after vertical banded gastroplasty as primary operation for morbid obesity. J Gastrointest Surg 2000;4(6):598-605.
7. Cordera F, Mai JL, Thompson GB, Sarr MG. Unsatisfactory weight loss after vertical banded gastroplasty: is conversion to Roux-en-Y gastric bypass successful? Surgery 2004;136(4):731-7.
8. Iovino P, Angrisani L, Tremolaterra F, et al. Abnormal esophageal acid exposure is common in morbidly obese patients and improves after a successful lap-band system implantation. Surg Endosc 2002;16:1631-5.
9. Ovrebo KK, Hatlebakk JG, Viste A, Bassoe HH, Svanes K. Gastro-oesophageal reflux in morbidly obese patients treated with gastric banding or vertical banded gastroplasty. Ann Surg 1998;228:51-8.
10. Suter M, Dorta, G, Giusti V, Calmes J. Gastric banding interferes with esophageal motility and gastroesophageal reflux. Arch Surg 2005;140 639-43.
11. Klaus A, Gruber I, Wetscher G, et al. Prevalent esophageal body motility disorders underlie aggravation of GERD symptoms in morbidly obese patients following adjustable gastric banding. Arch Surg 2006;141:247-51.

Sensory function of the foregut

Sensory structure responsible for sensing pain in the esophagus: do we know what it looks like?

W.L. Neuhuber (Erlangen)

Esophageal pain, often categorized less apodictically as non cardiac chest pain (NCCP), is triggered by afferent signals to the brain from nociceptors detecting potentially tissue damaging mechanical, chemical and thermal stimuli. It is important to note that thresholds of nociceptive neurons and for pain sensations are not unchangeable but can be lowered (or raised) by local factors in the esophagus or by the psychological state of the individual, respectively. Nocicceptors are conventionally related to dorsal root ganglionic afferents projecting to thoracic and cervical levels of the spinal cord where they are relayed to spinothalamic and spinoreticular second order neurons located in laminae I, V, VII and X. Convergence of input from various levels of the esophagus with afferents from other chest and abdominal organs as well as skin areas is likely to be responsible for widespread referral of esophageal pain. However, recent evidence indicated involvement also of vagal afferents in esophageal nociception [1]. Thus, sensory nerve terminals mediating esophageal pain may be connected to both spinal and vagal afferent neurons.

Spinal afferents

Knowledge about the structure of spinal afferent fibers in the esophagus derives from calcitonin gene related peptide (CGRP) immunocytochemistry and anterograde neuronal tracing from thoracic dorsal root ganglia. It has been demonstrated that more than 90% of dorsal root ganglion neurons retrogradely labeled from the esophagus contain CGRP, often colocalized with substance P [2,3]. Thus, in the absence of CGRP positive enteric neurons in the esophagus, this peptide is a convenient marker for spinal afferents in this organ. Thin calibre CGRP positive axons enter the esophagus through delicate branches from the sympathetic chain which distributes not only post-ganglionic efferents but also spinal afferents to this organ. CGRP positive spinal afferent axons assume a varicose appearance at the level of the myenteric plexus (*Figure 1A*). By virtue of this morphology, they can be

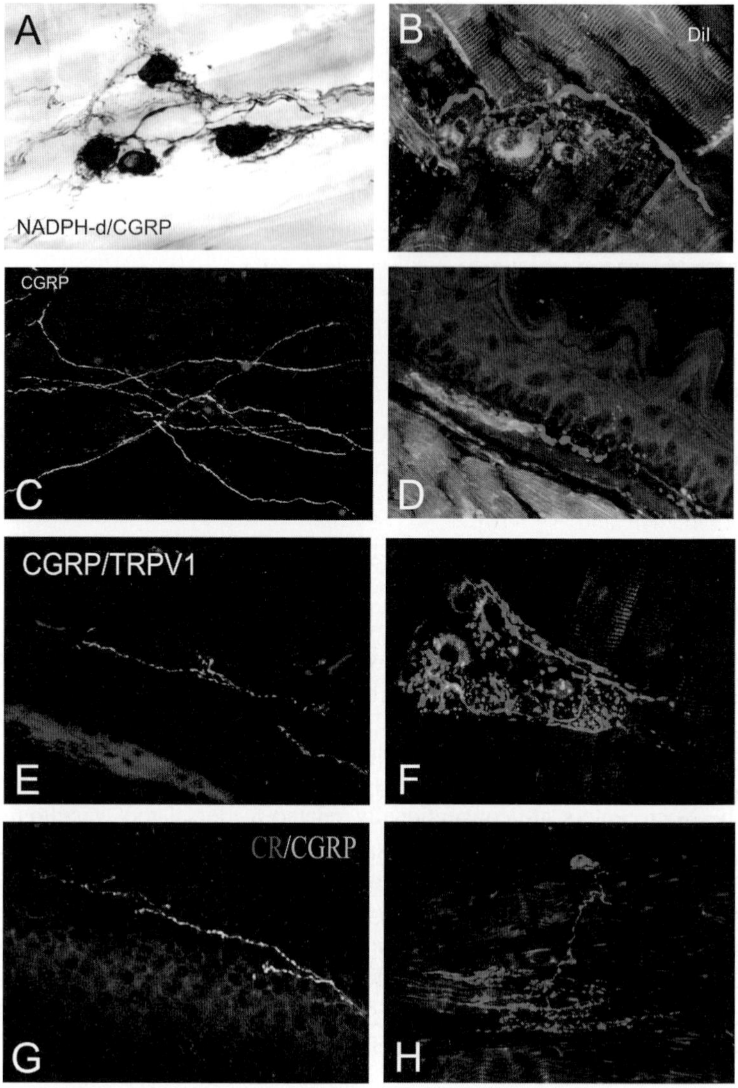

Figure 1. A. Myenteric ganglion in the rat esophagus containing four nitrergic neurons (blue NADPH diaphorase staining). CGRP positive spinal afferent fibers (brown) traverse the ganglion, forming en passant boutons on the neurons. **B.** Spinal afferent fibers (red) labelled by anterograde DiI tracing from lower thoracic spinal ganglia in the abdominal esophagus of the rat. Note numerous fine red dots indicating varicosities of the afferent axons. **C.** Meshwork of CGRP positive spinal afferent axons in a mucosal wholemount of the rat thoracic esophagus viewed en face. **D.** CGRP positive fine varicose spinal afferents (red) in the lamina propria of the rat thoracic esophagus mucosa sending delicate branches into the epithelium. **E.** Fine varicose afferent axons in the mucosa of the rat cervical esophagus co-staining for both CGRP and TRPV1 as indicated by yellow mixed color. **F.** Calretinin immunoreactive IGLEs (red) covering a myenteric ganglion (indicated by green autofluorescence of neuronal cell bodies) in the rat thoracic esophagus. **G.** Fine varicose branched vagal afferent axon beneath the epithelium of the rat cervical esophagus co-staining for both calretinin and CGRP. **H.** Intramuscular arrays (red) in the lower esophageal sphincter of the rat as stained by anterograde DiI tracing from the nodose ganglion. Note fine varicose interconnected axons coursing parallel to smooth muscle fibers displaying green autofluorescence. (See page XIII for colour figure).

readily distinguished from vagal motor axons originating in the nucleus ambiguus leading to motor endplates in the striated muscle portion of the esophagus which also stain for CGRP but are thicker and smooth contoured. Spinal afferents traverse myenteric ganglia giving off a few branches (*Figure 1B*) and directly contact myenteric neurons with their varicosities [1,4]. These findings, together with results of neurokinin-1 receptor location on myenteric neurons in the esophagus [5,6] provide a reasonable basis for local reflexes involving spinal afferents and enteric neurons. Spinal afferents continue their course through the inner layer of the muscularis propria, eventually coming in close contact to muscle fibers [6] and distribute to the submucosa where they form a rather regular meshwork (*Figure 1C*). Close relationships to blood vessels provide the structural basis for vasodilatory local effector function. In the mucosa, spinal afferent fibers course beneath the epithelium, sending delicate branches into it (*Figure 1D*). Of particular interest is the equipment of spinal afferents with the heat and proton sensitive transient receptor potential vanilloid 1 (TRPV1) (*Figure 1E*). Thus, spinal afferents display morphological and neurochemical traits compatible with a mechano-, chemo- and thermonociceptive function detecting stimuli to both mucosa and muscularis. This concurs well with results from numerous functional studies [7-10].

Vagal afferents

For quite a while, vagal afferent fibers in inner organs could be identified by anterograde tracing from the nodose ganglion only, and to some extent also by their disappearance upon nodose ganglionectomy [11-13]. By virtue of these techniques, intraganglionic laminar endings (IGLEs) [14] could be established as the most prominent vagal afferent structures throughout the rodent and cat esophagus (*Figure 1F*) [11,13,15,16]. They are intricately interwoven with the neuropil of myenteric ganglia and tightly related to teh periganglionic connective tissue [1,17]. They have been functionally identified as low threshold mechanosensors responding to both pressure and tension [18,19]. Under normal conditions, they unlikely detect noxious stimuli. However, their sensitivity can be enhanced by substances that may signal noxious events, e.g., ATP [19]. Immunohistochemical demonstration of P2X2/3 purinergic receptors in IGLEs is in line with this functional data [20,21]. It also remains to be studied whether IGLEs express TRPV1 under inflammatory conditions. Normally, they are immunonegative for TRPV1 and resistant to capsaicin [22,23].

In more recent years, vagal afferents have become amenable to immunocytochemical visualization. In rat esophagus, calretinin proved to be a rather specific marker for both IGLEs and various mucosal vagal afferent fibers [2]. This study showed a cranio-caudal gradient in density of vagal mucosal innervation. The mucosa of the upper esophagus, corresponding to the cranialmost 10 mm in rat, is densely innervated by thin calibre vagal afferents, either simple varicose fibers or axons with periodoc finger-like extensions to the epithelium along their course (*Figure 1G*). Many of these vagal afferent fibers contained CGRP, which corresponds to the frequent CGRP staining of retrogradely labeled jugular ganglion neurons innervating the esophagus [24]. There is also significant costaing for CGRP and TRPV1 in the jugular ganglion. This indicates that many of the vagal mucosal afferents innervating the upper esophagus share chemical and supposedly also functional similarities with spinal afferents. Data from a single fibe recording study in a rat *in vitro* esophagus-superior laryngeal nerve (SLN) preparation and from similar experiments in guinea-pig indicated a considerable number of high threshold mechanical, heath and chemosensitive Adelta and C fibers [25,26] the SLN carries most of the mucosal afferents from the upper esophagus).

Vagal afferent mucosal innervation declines caudally and CGRP expressing vagal afferents become rare [2].

At the level of the lower esophageal sphincter (LES), both muscular and mucosal vagal afferents are present [12]. In the LES of rodents, a particular type of muscular afferents has been identified with anterograde tracing, i.e., intramuscular arrays (IMAs) (*Figure 1H*) [16,27]. They form long trails of thin rectangular branching axons coursing parallel to the circular smooth muscle. Although originally considered as the anatomical equivalent to muscular tension or stretch receptors in the fundic stomach [28], IMAs could not yet be identified as sites of mechanosensory transduction as could IGLEs [29]. However, there remains the possibility that they represent high-threshold vagal mechanosensors probably activated under special conditions (J. Sengupta, pers. communication).

Conclusions

Considering the anatomical repertoire of afferent nerve fibers in the esophagus, spinal afferents are the most likely candidates for pain sensors. However, a particular class of vagal afferents, abundant in the upper esophagus mucosa, may represent vagal nociceptors. In the LES area, IMAs may function as high-threshold muscular sensors.

References

1. Neuhuber WL, Raab M, Berthoud HR, Worl J. Innervation of the mammalian esophagus. Adv Anat Embryol Cell Biol 2006;185:1-73.
2. Dütsch M, Eichhorn U, Wörl J, Wank M, Berthoud HR, Neuhuber WL. Vagal and spinal afferent innervation of the rat esophagus: a combined retrograde tracing and immunocytochemical study with special emphasis on calcium-binding proteins. J Comp Neurol 1998;398:289-307.
3. Uddman R, Grunditz T, Luts A, Desai H, Fernstrom G, Sundler F. Distribution and origin of the peripheral innervation of rat cervical esophagus. Dysphagia 1995;10:203-12.
4. Mazzia C, Clerc N. Ultrastructural relationships of spinal primary afferent fibres with neuronal and non-neuronal cells in the myenteric plexus of the cat oesophago-gastric junction. Neuroscience 1997;80:925-37.
5. Kuramoto H, Oomori Y, Murabayashi H, Kadowaki M, Karaki S, Kuwahara A. Localization of neurokinin 1 receptor (NK1R) immunoreactivity in rat esophagus. J Comp Neurol 2004;478:11-21.
6. Mazzia C, Clerc N. Ultrastructural analysis of spinal primary afferent fibers within the circular muscle of the cat lower esophageal sphincter. Histochem Cell Biol 2000;113:235-9.
7. Clerc N, Mei N. Thoracic esophageal mechanoreceptors connected with fibers following sympathetic pathways. Brain Res Bull 1983;10:1-7.
8. Clerc N. Afferent innervation of the lower esophageal sphincter of the cat. Pathways and functional characteristics. J Auton Nerv Syst 1984;10:213-6.
9. Sengupta JN, Saha JK, Goyal RK. Stimulus-response function studies of esophageal mechanosensitive nociceptors in sympathetic afferents of opossum. J Neurophysiol 1990;64:796-812.
10. Sengupta JN, Saha JK, Goyal RK. Differential sensitivity to bradykinin of esophageal distension-sensitive mechanoreceptors in vagal and sympathetic afferents of the opossum. J Neurophysiol 1992;68:1053-67.
11. Rodrigo J, de Felipe J, Robles-Chillida EM, Perez Anton JA, Mayo I, Gomez A. Sensory vagal nature and anatomical access paths to esophagus laminar nerve endings in myenteric ganglia. Determination by surgical degeneration methods. Acta Anat (Basel) 1982;112:47-57.
12. Clerc N, Condamin M. Selective labeling of vagal sensory nerve fibers in the lower esophageal sphincter with anterogradely transported WGA-HRP. Brain Res 1987;424:216-24.
13. Neuhuber WL. Sensory vagal innervation of the rat esophagus and cardia: a light and electron microscopic anterograde tracing study. J Auton Nerv Syst 1987;20:243-55.

14. Rodrigo J, Hernandez J, Vidal MA, Pedrosa JA. Vegetative innervation of the esophagus. II. Intraganglionic laminar endings. Acta Anatomica 1975;92:79-100.
15. Berthoud HR, Patterson LM, Neumann F, Neuhuber WL. Distribution and structure of vagal afferent intraganglionic laminar endings (IGLEs) in the rat gastrointestinal tract. Anat Embryol (Berl) 1997;195:183-91.
16. Wang FB, Powley TL. Topographic inventories of vagal afferents in gastrointestinal muscle. J Comp Neurol 2000;421:302-24.
17. Powley TL, Wang XY, Fox EA, Phillips RJ, Liu LW, Huizinga JD. Ultrastructural evidence for communication between intramuscular vagal mechanoreceptors and interstitial cells of Cajal in the rat fundus. Neurogastroenterol Motil 2008;20:69-79.
20. Castelucci P, Robbins HL, Furness JB. P2X(2) purine receptor immunoreactivity of intraganglionic laminar endings in the mouse gastrointestinal tract. Cell Tissue Res 2003;312:167-74.
18. Zagorodnyuk VP, Brookes SJ. Transduction sites of vagal mechanoreceptors in the guinea pig esophagus. J Neurosci 2000;20:6249-55.
19. Zagorodnyuk VP, Chen BN, Costa M, Brookes SJ. Mechanotransduction by intraganglionic laminar endings of vagal tension receptors in the guinea-pig oesophagus. J Physiol 2003;553:575-87.
21. Wang ZJ, Neuhuber WL. Intraganglionic laminar endings in the rat esophagus contain purinergic P2X2 and P2X3 receptor immunoreactivity. Anat Embryol (Berl) 2003;207:363-71.
22. Berthoud HR, Patterson LM, Willing AE, Mueller K, Neuhuber WL. Capsaicin-resistant vagal afferent fibers in the rat gastrointestinal tract: anatomical identification and functional integrity. Brain Res 1997;746:195-206.
23. Patterson LM, Zheng H, Ward SM, Berthoud HR. Vanilloid receptor (VR1) expression in vagal afferent neurons innervating the gastrointestinal tract. Cell Tissue Res 2003;311:277-87.
24. Wank M, Neuhuber WL. Local differences in vagal afferent innervation of the rat esophagus are reflected by neurochemical differences at the level of the sensory ganglia and by different brainstem projections. J Comp Neurol 2001;435:41-59.
25. Yu S, Undem BJ, Kollarik M. Vagal afferent nerves with nociceptive properties in guinea-pig oesophagus. J Physiol 2005;563:831-42.
26. Lennerz JK, Dentsch C, Bernardini N, Hummel T, Neuhuber WL, Reeh PW. Electrophysiological characterization of vagal afferents relevant to mucosal nociception in the rat upper oesophagus. J Physiol 2007;582:229-42.
27. Neuhuber WL, Kressel M, Stark A, Berthoud HR. Vagal efferent and afferent innervation of the rat esophagus as demonstrated by anterograde DiI and DiA tracing: focus on myenteric ganglia. J Auton Nerv Syst 1998;70:92-102.
28. Berthoud HR, Powley TL. Vagal afferent innervation of the rat fundic stomach: morphological characterization of the gastric tension receptor. J Comp Neurol 1992;319:261-76.
29. Zagorodnyuk VP, Chen BN, Brookes SJ. Intraganglionic laminar endings are mechano-transduction sites of vagal tension receptors in the guinea-pig stomach. J Physiol 2001;534:255-68.

What are the functional characteristics of esophageal sensory nociceptors?

K.M. Harnett, P. Biancani (Providence)

Pain is initiated when the peripheral terminals of a subgroup of sensory neurons are activated by noxious chemical, mechanical or thermal stimuli. These neurons, called nociceptors, transmit information regarding tissue damage to pain-processing centers in the spinal cord and brain. Nociceptors are characterized, in part, by their sensitivity to capsaicin, a natural product of capsicum peppers that is the active ingredient of many "hot" and spicy foods, that contains a 3-methoxy-4-hydroxy-benzylamine (or "vanillamine") moiety, previously shown to be a key determinant to observe potent activity in typical assays of vanilloid receptors [1]. The term vanilloid receptor was originally coined to describe the shared membrane recognition site for capsaicin and its ultrapotent analog, resiniferatoxin. Responsiveness to vanilloids is a functional signature of nociceptive neurons, although there is compelling evidence that vanilloid receptor expression is not restricted to nociceptive neurons [2]. In mammals, exposure of nociceptor terminals to capsaicin leads initially to excitation of the neuron and the consequent perception of pain and local release of inflammatory mediators.

A more detailed understanding of the molecular nature of capsaicin action and its relationship to endogenous pain signaling mechanisms was obtained through the cloning of a gene encoding a capsaicin receptor [3]. The deduced amino-acid sequence of this clone demonstrated that the capsaicin receptor is an integral membrane protein with homology to a family of putative store-operated calcium channels expressed exclusively by small-diameter neurons within sensory ganglia, providing a definitive molecular explanation for the remarkable selectivity of capsaicin action. This receptor is also a thermal sensor that is strongly activated when ambient temperatures are elevated to a range known to elicit pain in humans or pain associated behaviors in animals. Thus capsaicin elicits burning sensations through the activation of a heat-gated ion channel that is likely to contribute to the detection of painful thermal stimuli [3].

The vanilloid receptor VR1 is structurally related to the transient receptor potential (TRP) family of ion channels that have been proposed to mediate the influx of extracellular calcium in response to depletion of intracellular calcium stores [1]. One of the major functions of this channel is to act as one of several molecular transducers of painful physico-chemical stimuli, such as high temperatures (> 43°C) and acidity (the half-maximal effect occurs at pH 5.0) [4], and to intervene in inflammatory and thermal pain [1]. The detection of VR1 (now known as TRPV1) first in central neurons and more recently in epithelial cells, keratinocytes and endothelial and glial cells, is likely to expand its participation to important (physio)pathological functions other than nociception.

In the esophagus refluxate from the stomach may be present at very low pH (< 4) and may sufficient by itself to induce activation ot TRPV1 receptors.

Because TRPV1 was initially found in neurons, the role of TRPV1 in "neurogenic inflammation" of the gut has been examined to a limited extent. TRPV1-immunoreactive nerves have been demonstrated in lamina propria of esophageal biopsies from healthy subjects and esophagitis patients. In esophagitis patients the percentage of esophageal papillae positive for TRPV1 was elevated, when compared with controls [5].

TRPV1, however, has also been demonstrated in non-neural cells, for instance in keratinocytes of the epidermis [6,7], in the human keratinocyte cell line HaCat [6], in the human bronchial epithelial cell line BEAS-2B [8], in bladder urothelium and smooth muscle [9,10], liver [11], polymorphonuclear granulocytes [12] and macrophages [13].

To test whether this acid-sensitive receptor may be the initial mediator of acid-induced inflammation in the cat esophagus, a tubular segment of normal esophageal mucosa was removed and tied at both ends to form a mucosal sac [14]. The sac was filled with 0.01 N HCl (or normal Krebs' solution for control) and kept in oxygenated Krebs' solution at 37°C. The medium around the HCl-filled sac (supernatant) was collected after 3 hours incubation and examined for content of inflammatory mediators.

Substance P levels increased six-fold in mucosal tissue and in supernatant in response to HCl, while CGRP levels increased 200 times in the mucosa and 10 times in the supernatant. The HCl-induced increases in substance P and CGRP in mucosa and in supernatant were abolished when the TRPV1 receptor antagonist 5'-iodoresiniferatoxin (IRTX) was added inside the mucosal sac, or when tetrodotoxin (TTX) was added inside the sac and to the supernatant, suggesting that TRPV1-induced production of substance P and CGRP was neurally mediated.

Measurements of PAF in mucosa tissue and in mucosa supernatant (*Figure 1*) indicated that PAF levels increased 4-5 times in the HCl-filled mucosal sac and in its supernatant when compared to control (Kreb's filled mucosal sac at pH 7.4). The HCl-induced increase in PAF was abolished by the TRPV1 receptor antagonist IRTX. The increase in PAF levels in mucosa and supernatant, however, were not affected by neural block with TTX, indicating that production of PAF may arise from non neural pathways, and most likely from the esophageal epithelium.

The presence of TRPV1 receptor mRNA in esophageal mucosa was examined by RT-PCR (*Figure 2*). Primers were derived from conserved regions of mRNA sequences of humans, rat, dog, mouse guinea pig and rabbit. The BLAST database confirmed that the primers were specific for TRPV1. The band produced using these primers was sequenced,

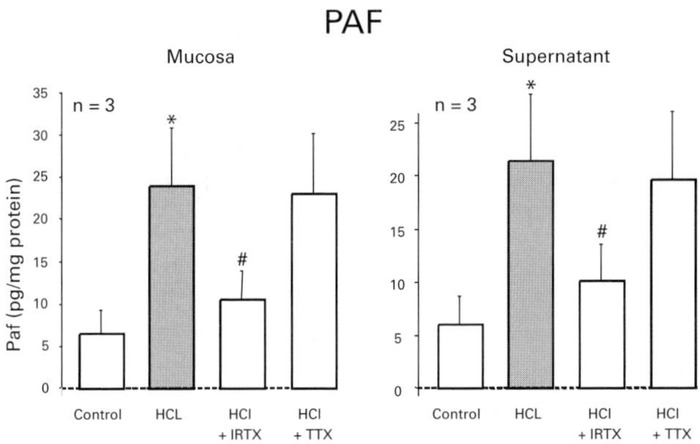

Figure 1. When in vitro mucosa is exposed to HCl for 3 hours, PAF levels increase 4-5 times in the mucosa and in the supernatant when compared to control (pH 7.4) (* $p < 0.5$ ANOVA). The HCl-induced increase in PAF is abolished by the TRPV1 receptor antagonist IRTX (# $p < 0.5$ ANOVA) and not affected by the neural blocker TTX both in the mucosa and in the supernatant indicating that production of PAF arises from non neural tissues. Bars represent mean ± SEM of 3 experiments.

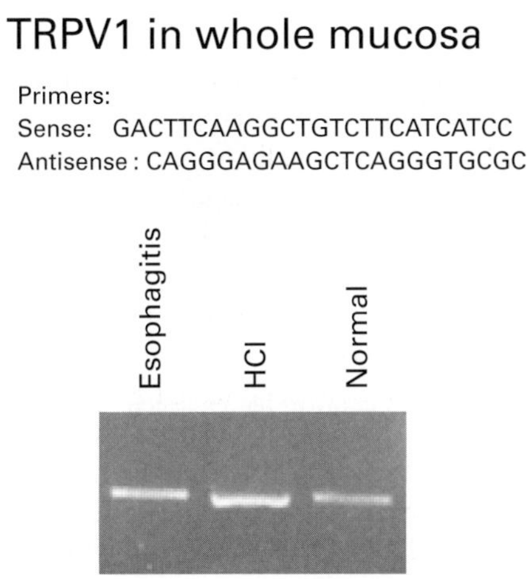

Figure 2. RT-PCR was performed in cat esophageal mucosa with primers selected from conserved regions of published sequences for humans, rat, dog, mouse, guinea pig and rabbit. Expression of TRPV1 mRNA increased after 3 hours exposure to HCl and after induction of experimental esophagitis by repeated perfusion of 0.1 N HCl for 1 hour on three successive days.

obtaining the sequence of cat TRPV1 with 95% homology to human TRPV1. RT-PCR of mucosa exposed to HCl for 3 hours showed upregulation of TRPV1 cat receptor mRNA.

To demonstrate the expression of TRPV1 receptor mRNA in non-neural cells, esophageal epithelial cells were enzymatically isolated, sorted by flow cytometry, and a 90-95% pure cell preparation was obtained. RT-PCR confirmed the presence of TRPV1 receptor mRNA in these cat esophageal epithelial cells (*Figure 3*). These isolated epithelial cells produced PAF in response to HCl, and the response was abolished by IRTX, supporting the presence of HCl-sensitive TRPV1 receptors in these cells (*Figure 4*).

To confirm the presence of TRPV1 receptor mRNA in a pure esophageal epithelial cell preparation TRPV1 mRNA was obtained in the human esophageal epithelial cell line HET-1A, using primers for the human mRNA sequence (*Figure 5*).

In fura 2-loaded HET-1A cells, capsaicin (10^{-5} M), caused a gradual increase in cytosolic Ca^{2+} levels confirming the presence of functional TRPV1 receptors in these epithelial cells (*Figure 6*).

In addition, preliminary work indicates that capsaicin-induced PAF production in these cells (*Figure 7*). PAF production was reduced by prior 30 minutes exposure to the p38 MAPK inhibitor SB203589 (10^{-5} M), and was abolished by the cytosolic

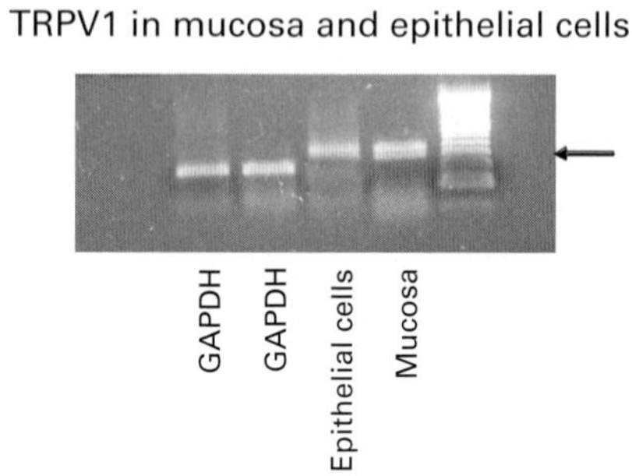

Figure 3. To demonstrate the presence of TRPV1 receptor mRNA in non-neural cells, esophageal epithelial cells were enzymatically isolated and sorted by flow cytometry. Primers were derived from conserved regions of mRNA sequences of humans, rat, dog, mouse, guinea pig and rabbit. RT-PCR confirmed the presence of TRPV1 receptor mRNA in these cat esophageal epithelial cells.

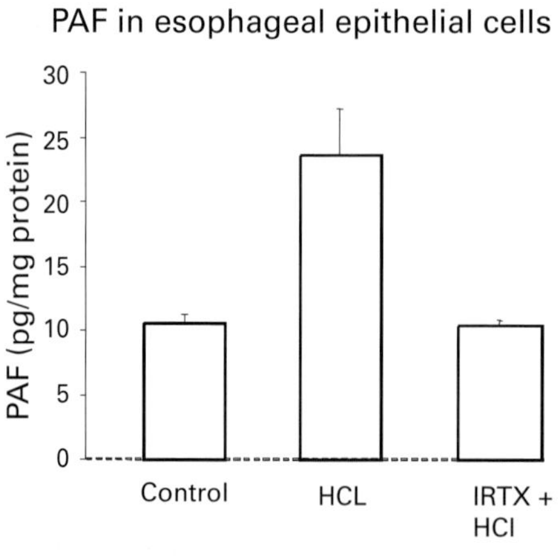

Figure 4. In enzymatically isolated epithelial cells, sorted to 95% purity by flow cytometry, 3 hour exposure to HCl more than doubled PAF levels ($p < 0.5$ ANOVA) The increase in PAF was abolished by the TRPV1 receptor antagonist IRTX (10^{-5} M).

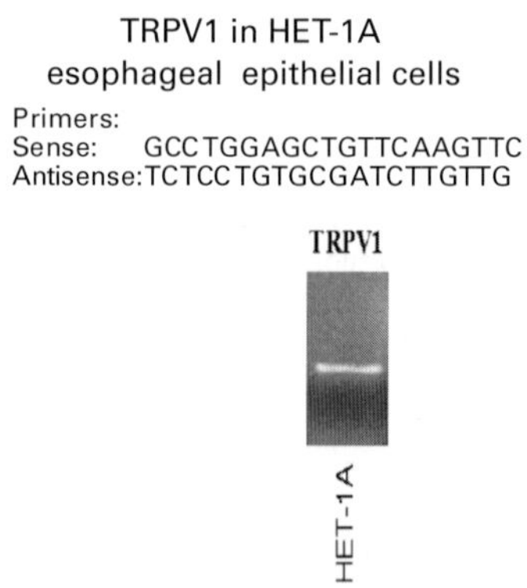

Figure 5. To confirm the presence of TRPV1 receptors in esophageal epithelial cells TRPV1 mRNA was obtained in the human esophageal epithelial cell line HET-1A, using primers designed for the human TRPV1.

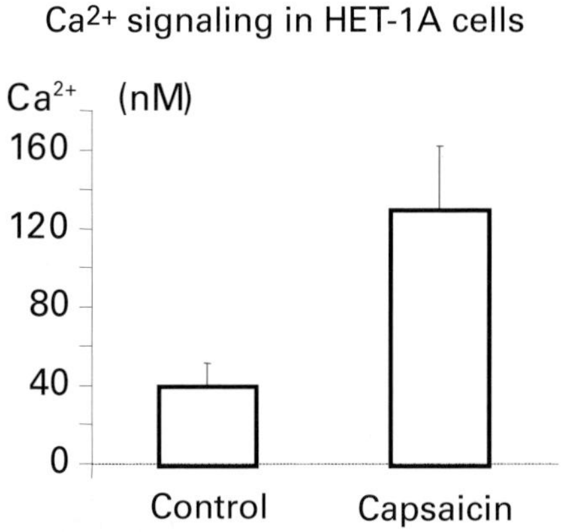

Figure 6. In fura 2-loaded HET-1A cells, capsaicin (10^{-5} M), cased a gradual increase in cytosolic Ca^{2+} levels. The values represent mean ± SEM of 10 cells after four minutes incubation.

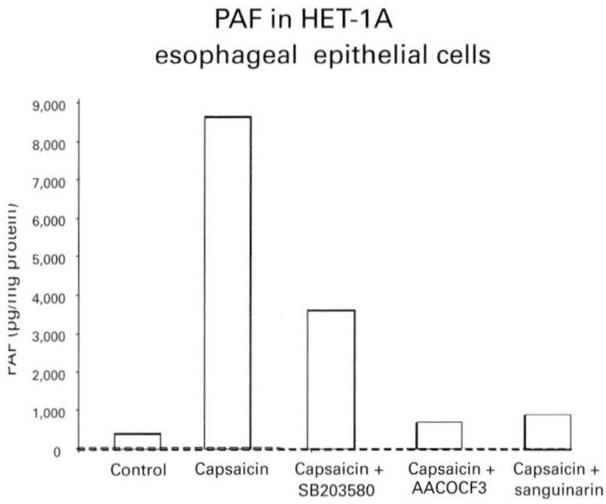

Figure 7. Production of PAF in HET-1A cells after 24 hours incubation with the TRPV1 agonist capsaicin (10^{-7} M). Capsaicin-induced PAF production was reduced by prior 30 minutes exposure to the p38 MAPK inhibitor SB203589 (10^{-5} M), and was abolished by the cPLA2 inhibitor AACOCF3 (10^{-5} M) and by the lyso-PAF acetyl-CoA transferase sanguinarin (10^{-6} M).

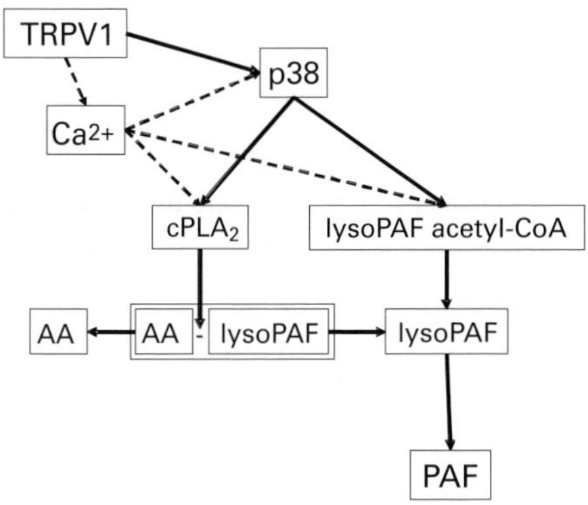

Figure 8. In this model TRPV1 receptor activates p38 MAP kinase that in turn may phosphorylate/activate cytosolic PLA_2 ($cPLA_2$), separating arachidonic acid from plasma membrane phospholipids, such as phosphatidylcholine. The remaining residue (for instance lyso-PAF) is the substrate of lyso-PAF acetyl-CoA transferase, that is also phosphorylated/activated by the p38 MAP kinase, resulting in production of PAF. The acetyltransferase catalyzing this step is regulated by phosphorylation, and by an increase in intracellular free Ca^{2+}, as occurs in HET-1A cells in response TRPV1 receptor activation by capsaicin. Thus HCl-induced activation of TRPV1 receptors and the resulting increase in cytosolic Ca^{2+}, may activate p38 MAPK, and cPLA2, resulting in activation of lysoPAF acetyl-CoA and formation of PAF.

PLA_2 ($cPLA_2$) inhibitor AACOCF3 (10^{-5} M) and by the lyso-PAF acetyl-CoA transferase sanguinarin (10^{-6} M). These data suggest a possible link between TRPV1 receptor stimulation and PAF as shown in *Figure 8*. TRPV1 receptor stimulation has been shown to stimulate p38 MAP kinase [15,16], that in turn may phosphorylate/activate $cPLA_2$,separating arachidonic acid from plasma membrane phospholipids, such as phosphatidyl-choline. The remaining residue (for instance lyso-PAF) is the substrate of lyso-PAF acetyl-CoA transferase, that is also phosphorylated/activated by the p38 MAP kinase, resulting in production of PAF. The acetyltransferase catalyzing this step is regulated by phosphorylation, and by an increase in intracellular free Ca^{2+} [17], as occurs in HET-1A cells in response TRPV1 receptor activation by capsaicin (*Figure 6*). Thus HCl-induced activation of TRPV1 receptors and the resulting increase in cytosolic Ca^{2+}, may activate p38 MAPK, and $cPLA_2$, resulting in activation of lysoPAF acetyl-CoA and formation of PAF.

We conclude that activation of TRPV1 receptors by gastroesophageal reflux and the resulting intra-esophageal low pH, causes direct non neurally mediated production of the inflammatory mediator PAF by esophageal epithelial cells.

References

1. Di Marzo V. Signalling at vanilloid TRPV1 channels. Eur Biochem 2004;271:813.
2. Di Marzo V, Blumberg PM, Szallasi A. Endovanilloid signaling in pain. Curr Opin Neurobiol 2002;12:372-9.
3. Caterina MJ, Schumacher MA, Tominaga M, Rosen TA, Levine JD, Julius D. The capsaicin receptor: a heat-activated ion channel in the pain pathway. Nature 1997;389:816-24.
4. Jordt SE, Tominaga M, Julius D. Acid potentiation of the capsaicin receptor determined by a key extracellular site. Proc Nat Acad Sci 2000;97:8134-9.
5. Matthews PJ, Aziz Q, Facer P, Davis JB, Thompson DG, Anand P. Increased capsaicin receptor TRPV1 nerve fibres in the inflamed human oesophagus. Eur J Gastroenterol Hepatol 2004;16:897-902.
6. Southall MD, Li T, Gharibova LS, Pei Y, Nicol GD, Travers JB. Activation of epidermal vanilloid receptor-1 induces release of proinflammatory mediators in human keratinocytes. J Pharmacol Exp Ther 2003;304:217-22.
7. Stander S, Moormann C, Schumacher M, et al. Expression of vanilloid receptor subtype 1 in cutaneous sensory nerve fibers, mast cells, and epithelial cells of appendage structures. Exp Dermatol 2004;13:129-39.
8. Veronesi B, Carter JD, Devlin RB, Simon SA, Oortgiesen M. Neuropeptides and capsaicin stimulate the release of inflammatory cytokines in a human bronchial epithelial cell line. Neuropeptides 1999;33:447-56.
9. Birder LA, Kanai AJ, de Groat WC, et al. Vanilloid receptor expression suggests a sensory role for urinary bladder epithelial cells. Proc Natl Acad Sci USA 2001;98:13396-401.
10. Birder LA, Nakamura Y, Kiss S, et al. Altered urinary bladder function in mice lacking the vanilloid receptor TRPV1. Nat Neurosci 2002;5:856-60.
11. Reilly CA, Taylor JL, Lanza DL, Carr BA, Crouch DJ, Yost GS. Capsaicinoids cause inflammation and epithelial cell death through activation of vanilloid receptors. Toxicol Sci 2003;73:170-81.
12. Heiner I, Eisfeld J, Halaszovich CR, et al. Expression profile of the transient receptor potential (TRP) family in neutrophil granulocytes: evidence for currents through long TRP channel 2 induced by ADP-ribose and NAD. Biochem J 2003;371:1045-53.
13. Chen CW, Lee ST, Wu WT, Fu WM, Ho FM, Lin WW. Signal transduction for inhibition of inducible nitric oxide synthase and cyclooxygenase-2 induction by capsaicin and related analogs in macrophages. Br J Pharmacol 2003;140:1077-87.
14. Cheng L, Cao W, Fiocchi C, Behar J, Biancani P, Harnett KM. In vitro model of acute esophagitis in the cat. Am J Physiol Gastrointest Liver Physiol 2005;289:G860-9.
15. Miyamoto R, Tokuda M, Sakuta T, Nagaoka S, Torii M. Expression and characterization of vanilloid receptor subtype 1 in human dental pulp cell cultures. J Endod 2005;31:652-8.
16. Mizushima T, Obata K, Yamanaka H, et al. Activation of p38 MAPK in primary afferent neurons by noxious stimulation and its involvement in the development of thermal hyperalgesia. Pain 2005;113:51-60.
17. Sakamoto H, Tosaki T, Nakagawa Y. Overexpression of phospholipid hydroperoxide glutathione peroxidase modulates acetyl-CoA, 1-O-alkyl-2-lyso-sn-glycero-3-phosphocholine acetyltransferase activity. J Biol Chem 2002;277:50431-8.

Neonatal development of protective esophageal reflexes

S.R. Jadcherla (Columbus)

Recent advances in neonatal intensive care have increased the neonatal survival. However, an increase in feeding related morbidity is also evident, the mechanisms of which remain poorly understood [1,2]. In a recent survey, it was found that 26% of the preterm infants had oromotor feeding problems [3]. In another report, 80% of the infants with neurodevelopmental concerns were challenged with aerodigestive symptoms [4]. Specifically, morbidity related to the aerodigestive tract often presents as swallowing disorders, aspiration syndromes and chronic lung disease, gastroesophageal reflux disease (GERD) and gastroduodenal dysmotility [1-4]. Therefore, the study of the developmental aspects of the esophageal function assumes importance because of the increasing prevalence of feeding disorders.

The embryological origins of the aerodigestive tract are common in that the tracheobronchial diverticulum originates from foregut sharing similar neuromotor control systems [5,6]. Primitive swallowing of amniotic fluid and esophageal peristalsis have been observed in the human fetus by 10-12 weeks gestation, although perinatal viability is attained by 22-24 weeks gestation. Post-natally, there is a reversal of functions within the lungs to sustain life. For example, ventilatory functions begin to maintain life and the circulation of amniotic fluid from the lung into the esophagus ceases. However, the esophagus continues the oropharyngeal transit functions (saliva, food, secretions from upper airway such as mucus) and also defends the airway from noxious material. The protective mechanisms by which the esophagus defends the airway are not well understood in neonates. This paper discusses the use of novel methods to evaluate basal esophageal motility and the defensive esophageal reflexes during neonatal maturation.

Basal esophageal motility during maturation

Manometry methods have been used across the age spectrum in the evaluation of gastrointestinal motility [7]. With the use of specially designed catheters and sleeve devices, others and we have performed esophageal manometry to evaluate esophageal peristalsis, upper and lower esophageal sphincter (UES and LES) functions in human neonates [7-9].

The neonatal esophagus lengthens during development in a linear fashion and the change is proportionate to the body weight and length [10]. Esophageal and LES motility characteristics in neonates have been described [7-9]. Specifically, the swallow mediated primary peristalsis improves during maturation in that the peristaltic velocity, coordination of peristaltic waveforms, and waveform characteristics change during maturation. The peristaltic velocity from proximal to distal esophagus in premature born neonates at 33 weeks corrected gestation age was noted to be 1.1 ± 0.5 cm/sec, whereas in full term gestation born neonates it was 2.4 ± 1.7 cm/sec. In contrast, in the adult, the peristaltic velocity from proximal to distal esophagus was 3.6 ± 1.1 cm/sec. It is likely that further changes occur with growth and maturation. For example, ratio of completely propagated *versus* failed propagation of peristaltic waveforms at 33 weeks corrected gestation was 72:28 (%), at full term born gestation was 77:23 (%) and in healthy adults was 99:1 (%). The UES characteristics also change with maturation in that the resting tone and relaxation characteristics are altered (*Figure 1*). Specifically, the resting UES pressure, the decrease in pressure gradient during relaxation, the duration of relaxation, duration of nadir, and the nadir pressure progressively undergo changes during maturation and are different from that of the human adult [7].

The LES resting tone generally is about 5 to 10 mmHg above the intragastric pressure and is considered adequate to maintain LES competence [11]. However, the maintenance of LES tone is rather complex and prevention of gastroesophageal reflux (GER) is also dependent on other factors such as, intragastric pressure, intraabdominal pressure, or intra-thoracic pressure. In neonates, the mechanisms for the occurrence of GER have been well described [8,9]. Similar to that in adults, transient LES relaxation (TLESR) is the most common mechanism for the occurrence of GER. However, increased intragastric pressure, hypotonic LES, and swallow induced LES relaxation also occur frequently.

In summary, the transit function of the esophagus undergoes changes during maturation with the improvement in esophageal body functions. The defensive barriers at the proximal and distal ends of the esophagus, i.e., the UES and LES also undergo modifications. It is likely that with advanced growth, further development of neuromuscular apparatus occurs and functional changes in motor function then ensue.

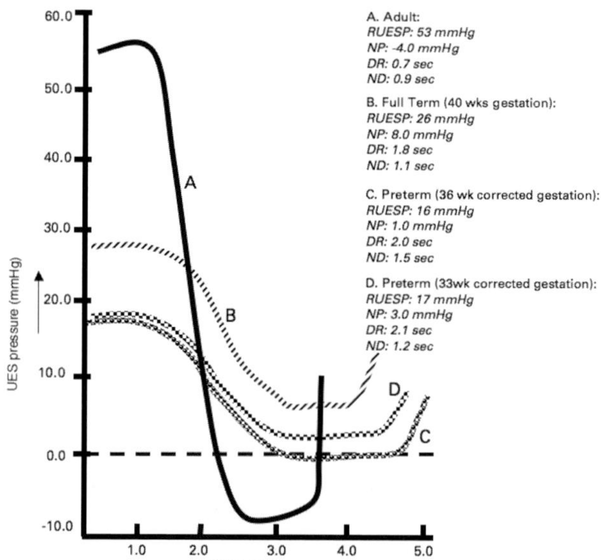

Figure 1. UES characteristics across the age spectrum.

Protective esophageal reflexes during maturation

Esophagus is the primary target during the GER events. Knowledge about the protective mechanisms by which the human neonate defends its esophagus is currently being understood. The refluxate may provoke the esophagus by virtue of its sheer volume, physical or chemical nature, osmotic properties or the extent of its retrograde transit. In any of these stimulus modes, mechanodistention of the esophagus occurs.

Recently, we have developed and validated methods to evaluate mechanostimulation induced esophageal reflexes in human neonates during maturation [12,13]. Using a specially designed esophageal manometry catheter, the effects of mid esophageal provocation and the resulting responses were evaluated. Specifically, we characterized the reflexes evoked upon infusions (*Figure 2*). Esophageal provocation resulted in local distention as evidenced by the common cavity pressure changes. Subsequently, peristaltic reflexes occurred to ensure clearance. Two types of peristaltic reflexes were noted: secondary peristalsis and esophago-deglutition reflex. The latter is similar to primary peristalsis but different in that esophageal distention resulted in a deglutition sequence. When secondary peristalsis occurred, the UES responses were: absence of contractile reflex, or presence of contractile reflex, or presence of relaxation or belch response. LES responded to esophageal distention by the presence of relaxation response. Thus in neonates, the following reflexes were recognized in response to esophageal distention:

- secondary peristalsis;
- esophago-deglutition response;
- esophago-UES-contractile reflex;

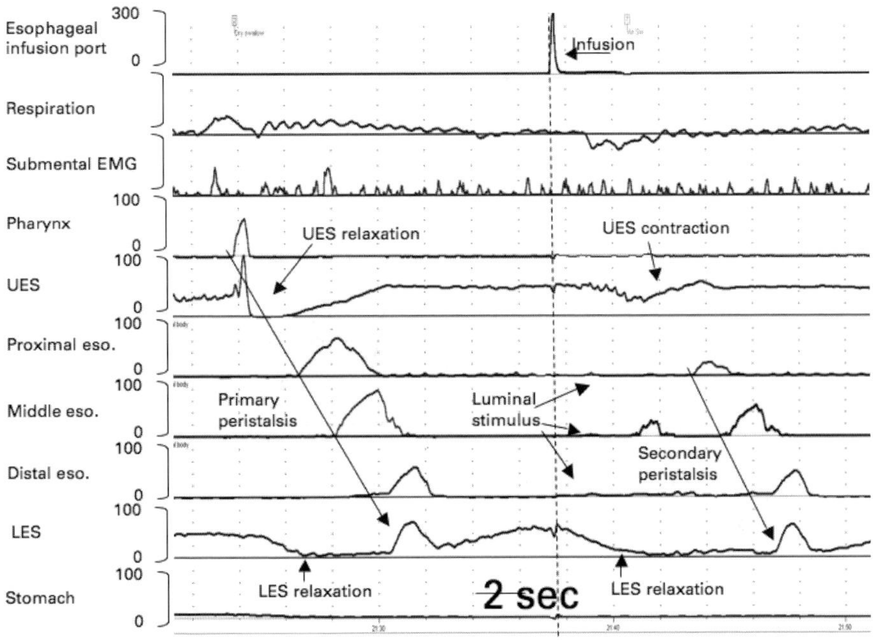

Figure 2. Effect of esophageal luminal stimulation on peristalsis, UES, and LES motility.

- esophago-UES-relaxation response;
- LES-relaxation response.

By studying the same neonates at 33 weeks and 36 weeks corrected gestational age, we observed that esophageal and UES responses were evident upon esophageal provocation at both maturational ages, and that the response characteristics improve with maturation [12].

By studying different provocative stimuli, air *versus* liquids, we found that the secondary peristalsis and the UES contractile responses were dose-volume dependent with both media. Furthermore, with liquid stimuli, completely propagated secondary peristalsis occurred with a greater peristaltic velocity compared to air stimulus [12].

By infusing graded volumes of air, sterile water (neutral medium) or apple juice (pH 3.7) at 33 weeks and 36 weeks corrected gestation ages, we tested the effects of mechanosensitive and chemosensitive media [13]. We found that the recruitment frequency and magnitude of secondary peristalsis and UES contractile reflex increased with volume increments of air and sterile water, and were similar between the media. However, with apple juice there was increased recruitment of esophago-deglutition response at 33 weeks and increased secondary peristalsis response at 36 weeks corrected gestation ages.

Clinical implications in human neonates and infants

The methods and the characteristics of the reflexes cited above may provide a reference for conditions where in foregut function may be aberrant. These methods may be of particular value in understanding the mechanism of esophageal dysfunction as in GERD, aspiration syndromes, and dysphagia in infants [14,15]. Maturation is an ongoing process, and evolving diseases may modify esophageal motor responses. Therefore, longitudinal studies may identify alteration of esophageal dysfunction resulting from modifications in disease process. The novelty of esophageal provocative manometry provides broader insight into esophageal sensory motor pathophysiology.

References

1. Kliegman RM. Neonatal technology, perinatal survival, social consequences, and the perinatal paradox. Am J Public Health 1995;85:909-13.
2. Jadcherla SR, Kliegman RM. Studies of feeding intolerance in VLBW infants: definition and significance. Pediatrics 2000;109 (3);516-7.
3. Mercado-Deane MG, Burton EM, Harlow SA, et al. Swallowing dysfunction in infants less than 1 year of age. Pediatr Radiol 2001; 31(6):423-8.
4. Field D, Garland M, Williams K. Correlates of specific childhood feeding problems. J Paediatr Child Health 2003;39(4):299-304.
5. Sadler TW. Special embryology, digestive system. In: Langman's medical embryology, Part II, 7th ed. Philadelphia: Williams and Wilkins, 1995:241-71.
6. Mansfield LE. Embryonic origins of the relation of gastroesophageal reflux disease and airway disease. Am J Med 2001;111(8A):3S-7S.
7. Jadcherla SR, Duong HQ, Hofmann C, Hoffmann RG, Shaker R. Characteristics of upper esophageal sphincter and esophageal body during maturation in healthy human neonates compared with adults. Neurogastroenterol Motil 2005;17:663-70.
8. Omari T, Snel A, Barnett C, Davidson G, Haslam R, Dent J. Measurement of upper esophageal sphincter tone and relaxation during swallowing in premature infants. Am J Physiol 1999;277:G862-6.
9. Omari TI, Barnett C, Snel A, et al. Mechanisms of gastroesophageal reflux in healthy premature infants. J Pediatr 1998;133:650-4.
10. Gupta A, Jadcherla SR. The relationship between somatic growth and in vivo esophageal segmental and sphincteric growth in human neonates. J Pediatr Gastroenterol Nut. 2006;41(1):35-41.

11. Omari, TI. Lower esophageal function in the neonate. NeoReviews 2006;7(1):e13-8.
12. Jadcherla SR, Duong HQ, Hoffmann RG, et al. Esophageal body and upper esophageal sphincter motor responses to esophageal provocation during maturation in preterm newborns. J Pediatr 2003;143:31-8.
13. Jadcherla SR, Hoffmann RG, Shaker R. Effect of maturation on the magnitude of mechanosensitive and chemosensitive reflexes in the premature human esophagus. J Pediat, 2006;141(1):77-82.
14. Jadcherla SR. Esophageal motility in the human neonate. NeoReviews 2006;7:e7-12.
15. Jadcherla SR, Rudolph CD. Gastroesophageal reflux in the preterm neonate. NeoReviews 2005;6:e87-98.

Descending control: does it influence visceral pain?

A.M. Drewes (Aalborg)

Exploring pain in the gastrointestinal tract

Diseases giving rise to visceral pain are very heterogeneous. This is partly due to the sparse and diffuse termination of visceral afferents at the central nervous system, together with the interaction between visceral pain and the somatic, autonomic and enteric nervous systems, which often blurs the clinical picture. However, descending control from higher brain centers also influence the perception of symptoms from the gut.

The sources of information for visceral pain come from the following four groups of investigations:
- animal experiments;
- experimental pain studies (volunteers and patients);
- observational studies in the clinic;
-interventional studies in the clinic.

As individual sources of information they are all limited by several biases. For example does the neurobiology of the pain system differ between the individual animal species, and this limits the interpolation of findings in animal studies to the complex clinical impression of pain in humans [1]. Experimental human pain has the advantage that the stimulus can be controlled and modulated, and the responses can be assessed quantitatively with psychophysical or neurophysiologic methods [2]. By applying the stimuli in patients, additional information about the disease mechanisms can be provided. The reaction to a single stimulus of a given modality can, however, only represent a limited fraction of the entire pain experience, and experimental pain can only to some degree mimic the clinical situation. Clinical observational studies are on the other hand limited by the heterogeneity of the clinical diseases even in patients with rather straightforward illness such as acute appendicitis. Thus, different mechanisms such as the degree of activation of the autonomous nervous system, the extent of sensitization of the peripheral nerves and the variable activation of central mechanisms differs in the individual patients. This makes it difficult to draw any firm conclusions from observational and interventional studies. However, the information obtained from these sources combined gives a rather detailed knowledge of the visceral nervous system and the interaction with other physiologic systems. Hence, knowledge about the visceral nervous system and interactions with other physiologic systems in the body can often lead the clinician to the right diagnosis. This knowledge will also give insight into pain mechanisms and lead to a better treatment approach based on logical selection of the individual therapy. This therapy should not only be targeted against the dysfunction of the organs, but also against associated symptoms relating to somatic, autonomic and other symptoms.

Methods used in human brain imaging

Brain imaging is needed to study the descending control system as this a result of brainstem activity in connection with many centers in the brain. Human studies based on positron emission tomography (PET) and magnetic resonance imaging (MRI) in healthy subjects has partly confirmed the findings regarding the pain control system in animal studies. PET can measure the cerebral blood flow after injection of a radioisotope, whereas MRI is based on the different paramagnetic properties of oxy- and deoxyhemoglobin. Subtracting maps of the relative cerebral blood volume obtained under experimental conditions and in rest will identify the brain areas active during the experiment. Painful dilatation of the esophagus was shown to be processed mainly in the anterior insular cortex and anterior cingulate gyrus in a PET study by Aziz *et al.* [3]. The anterior cingulate cortex, being a common structure of relevance in these studies, is thought to be part of the medial pain system mediating affective and emotional qualities of the pain experience [4]. Other centers such as the parietal operculum and several midbrain structures are probably also involved in the processing of visceral pain, but the specificity of these regions with respect to pain is still not settled.

PET and MRI studies have an excellent spatial resolution (2-5 mm), but a relative poor temporal resolution (minutes for PET and several seconds for MRI) as it takes some time until changes in blood flow occur and to obtain the scans [5]. Thus, these methods do not image the neuronal activity directly, but demonstrate changes in blood flow in the regions activated (or deactivated) during pain stimuli. Hence, a major problem with PET and MRI studies is the poor temporal resolution and the responses in the brain correspond to rather late events that may be non-specifically related to arousal and attention rather than pain. In contrast magnetoencephalography (MEG) and evoked cortical potentials (EPs) detect the neuronal activity in real time, with a very high temporal resolution [6-8]. When a repetitive stimulus is applied and the cortical electrical activity is averaged (time-locked to the stimulus), the stimulus evoked potentials can be extracted from the background electrical activity and is shown in shape of a waveform with different peaks. Each peak in the EP represents a synaptic event associated with the transmission of afferent information from one group of neurons to another. By recording EP or MEG from multiple sites on the scalp simultaneously, it is possible to calculate the cerebral sources generating the electromagnetic fields. However, the shortcomings are that EPs has limitations with a low spatial resolution due to distortion of the signal and overlapping of neuronal activities, and MEG suffer from lacking identification of deep and radial oriented sources [6,8,9]. Future studies such as those relying on a combination of different methods may bypass some of these problems [10].

Where MEG and EPs are recorded on the brain surface, electrical activity in assemblies of neurons in the brain (such as cellular columns) can be modeled from the surface activity. These cellular columns mimics an equivalent dipole, being a linear source (e.g., battery)

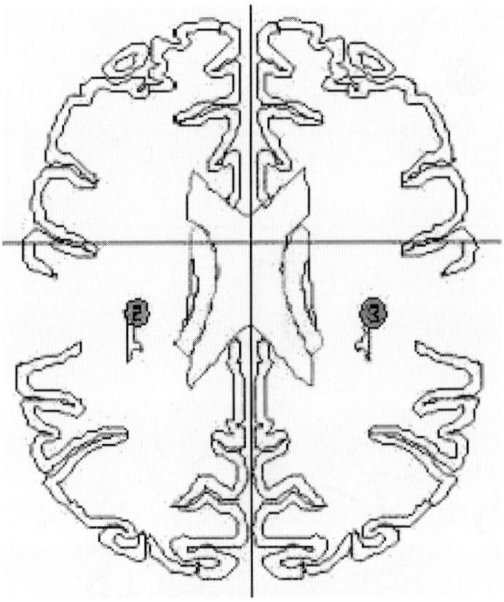

Figure 1. Locations of dipoles fitting evoked brain potentials to gut stimulation. The black dots represent the upstream brain activity in the bilateral insular region 150 ms after electrical stimulation of the rectum.

with two opposing poles [6,9]. Each dipole represents the sequential activation/ deactivation of the brain to synchronized peripheral pain stimuli. The dipoles can be projected onto the Talairach and Tournoux stereotactic brain atlas or a MRI of the subject's brain [11], and their anatomical position can be estimated (*Figure 1*) [12-15].

Pain is a complex sensation and it is difficult to separate centers dealing with pain intensity and localization from those involved in attention, emotional and motor reflexes. Most importantly many centers work in parallel during the supraspinal processing of the visceral stimuli [16]. New methods based on independent component analysis algorithms have proven capable of isolating both artifactual and neurally generated EEG sources [17]. Thus, many of the biologically plausible sources found by independent component analysis have scalp maps nearly fitting the projection of a single equivalent current dipole [18], and are therefore quite compatible with the projection to the scalp electrodes of synchronous local field activity within a connected patch of cortex. Furthermore coherence analysis makes is possible to study communication between brain centers [19]. In *Figure 2* the characteristics of such components to electrical stimulation of the distal esophagus are shown.

Brain projections of visceral pain

The major brain projections involved in visceral pain are shown in *Figure 3*. Electrophysiological and neuroanatomical studies based on animal experiments have documented the existence of afferents projecting from the viscera to the parabrachial nucleus of the pons, which relay the information to various parts of the thalamus. The afferents travel from the dorsal horn in the spinal cord *via* the spinothalamic tract to reach the thalamus and cortex. Some travel in the phylogenetically older spinoreticular tract and probably mediate arousal and autonomic responses. Other afferents ascend in the spinomesencephalic tract to reach the midbrain, are probably related to the periaquaductal gray and influencing the descending control systems as described below. Recently fibers traveling in the dorsal column have also been described. Third order neurons are thought to progress to e.g., the somatosensory cortex (sensory-discriminative component of pain), and to the limbic system (motivational-affective components of the pain) and frontal lobe (evaluative component of the pain). The insula seems play a key role in the coordination of the visceral activity [14,19] (for review, see [20] or [21]).

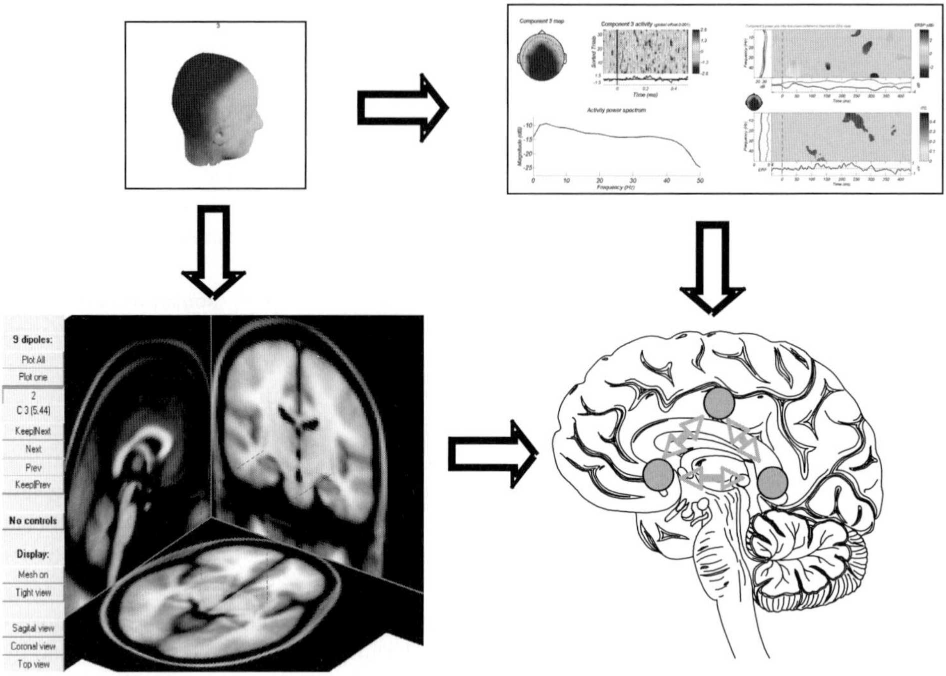

Figure 2. Independent component analysis of the surface EEG in 64 electrodes.
Top left: surface scalp map showing the interpolated projection of the component to a head model. Top right: the event related potential image consisting of 35 parallel lines representing the individual trials of the given component. The right side of this picture shows the inter-trial coherence images with the strength of phase locking of the EEG signals. This can be used in analysis of connectivity between brain centers. Bottom left: the equivalent current dipole projected into a standardized brain image. Bottom right: the connectivity analysis being an attempt to describe dynamic links between neuronal centers - "the brain web". For detailed information see [19]. (See page XIV for colour figure).

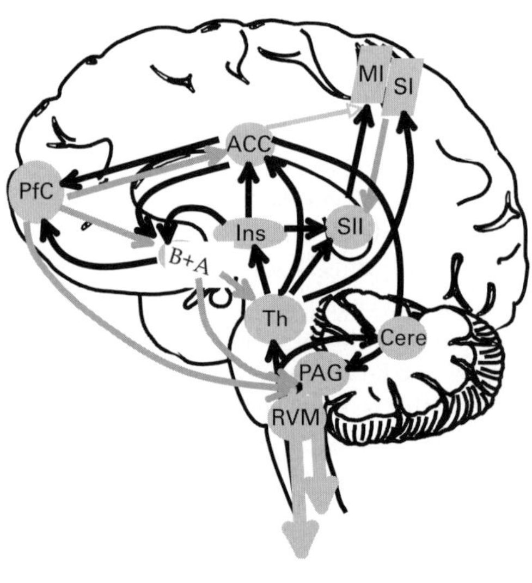

Figure 3. The supraspinal processing of visceral pain. The thalamus (Th) function as a relay centre, which convey the information to various parts of the brain. Third order neurons (black) ascend to e.g., cerebellum (Cere), the primary and secondary somatosensory cortex (SI and SII), the limbic system including anterior cingulate cortex (ACC), insula (Ins), and the prefrontal cortex (PfC). The grey lines illustrate connections to other cortical centers such as basal ganglia (B) and amygdala (A) simultaneously activated. This reflects that the neurons in the brain work "in parallel". Connections to centers such as the periaqueductal grey (PAG) and rostroventromedial medulla (RVM) are involved in descending control from the brain exerted at spinal cord neurons.

Descending control of visceral pain

The second-order neurons in the spinal cord are subject to local segmental and descending control from higher brain centers (*Figure 4*). In animal studies several groups of neurons have been identified which are controlled from such centers [22,23]. Some control systems are inhibitory, whereas others are excitatory, and the balance between the excitatory system and the inhibitory modulation could therefore determine the final interpretation of the pain.

The most important centre involved in the brain stem modulation of pain perception is the network between the periagueductal gray (PAG) and rostroventromedial medulla (RMV). Neurons in this network are able to exert bulbo-spinal inhibition at the spinal cord, a phenomenon labeled "descending noxious inhibitory control" (DNIC) (*Figure 5*). The

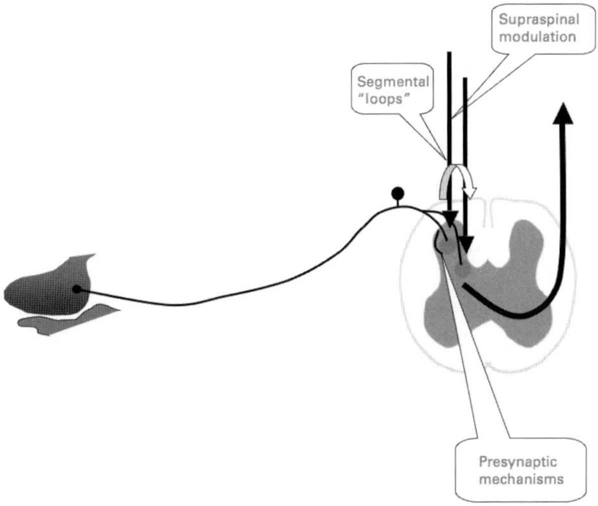

Figure 4. Local, segmental and descending control mechanisms that may modulate painful input to higher centers in the brain.

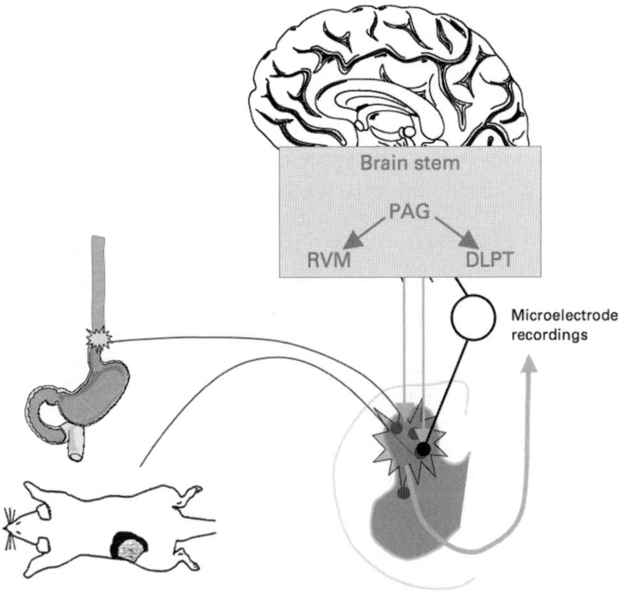

Figure 5. Schematic illustration of animal studies where direct intracellular recordings document the activity in networks between the periaqueductal grey (PAG), rostroventromedial medulla (RVM) and dorso-lateral pontomesencephalic tegmentum (DLPT) being involved in descending control of the activity in neuron at the spinal cord.

descending inhibition can be evoked by focal electrical stimulation or glutamate injections in PAG and RMV [24]. Neurons labeled as "on-cells" and "off-cells" have been identified in this network and importantly the descending control system can also be facilitatory resulting in increased pain.

Descending inhibition seems to be the major way by which the brain control pain perception. Several cortical centers are connected to the brain stem network involving PAG. Serotonergic and noradrenergic pathways project from this network to the spinal cord and form synapsis on e.g., inhibitory interneurons. The interneurons inhibit nociception by endogeneous opioids release on the projection neurons or the primary afferent in the spinal cord.

Other local mechanisms such as supraspinal modulatory effects on the cortical or thalamic level may also modulate the pain response [20,25,26]. The modulating response at the spinal neurons from higher brain centers following a visceral stimulus may result in a complex mixture of inhibition and excitation [27]. This suggests that the balance between these systems may depend on factors such as the nature, the intensity and duration of the stimulus. Recent experimental evidence supports the activation of such inhibitory systems in diseases such as chronic pancreatitis [28]. The clinical consequences of these systems may also explain the wide heterogeneity of the pain in gastrointestinal disorders.

Imaging studies support that these mechanisms are also active in humans. Dunckley *et al.* used MRI scans to study brain stem structures after painful stimulation of the rectum and lower abdominal skin [29]. Visceral as compared with somatic stimulation resulted in greater activation of nucleus cuneiformis having antinociceptive functions ~ greater descending inhibition of noxious (and subliminal) information. PAG activation correlated with anxiety ratings (which was especially increased to rectal stimulation). Wilder-Smith *et al.* [30] used a cold pressor test by immersion of the foot in ice-water for 120 seconds to activate DNIC. The cold pressor test was used during simultaneous painful dilatation of the rectum and decreased the rectal pain scores in healthy subjects but not in patients with irritable bowel syndrome (IBS). Changes in brain activation during this "counter-irritation" differed between the groups – especially in areas with strong connections to the brain stem. Hence, it was concluded that patients with IBS have abnormal endogenous pain inhibitory control (which also differed in patients with either diarrhea or constipation predominant IBS). Finally, Meyer *et al.* [31] used "connectivity analysis" in data from PET studies during painful stimulation of the rectum. They found that healthy controls and patients with ulcerative colitis activate the right lateral frontal cortex which indirectly increases DNIC. Patients with IBS on the other hand activated limbic structures that directly inhibit DNIC (*Figure 6*). Thus, there is substantial evidence that descending control systems are also

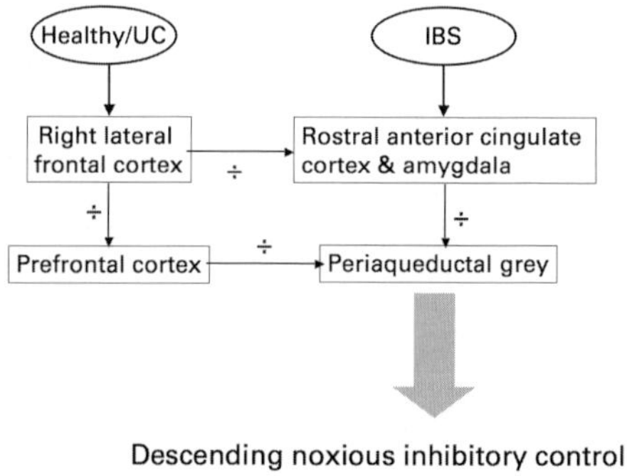

Figure 6. Connectivity analysis showing the downstream activation of different brain centers in healthy controls and patients with ulcerative colitis (UC) on the one hand, and in patients with irritable bowel syndrome (IBS) on the other. The healthy subjects and those with organic disease (UC) increase the descending inhibition at second order neurons in the spinal cord, whereas this mechanism was defect in patients with a "functional disease" (IBS). For detail see [31].

important in man. The biochemical understanding of the different mediators involved in descending control has also increased dramatically during recent years. With the development in image and signal analysis of the brain there is no doubt that new insight of descending control mechanisms will have the potential to increase our understanding and treatment of patients with visceral pain such as in esophageal diseases.

References

1. Ness TJ. Historical and clinical perspetives of visceral pain. In: Gebhart GF, ed. Visceral pain. Progress in pain research and management. Seattle: IASP Press, 1995:3-23.
2. Drewes AM, Gregersen H, Arendt-Nielsen L. Experimental pain in gastroenterology: A reappraisal of human studies. Scand J Gastroenterol 2003;38:1115-30.
3. Aziz Q, Andersson JL, Valind S, et al. Identification of human brain loci processing esophageal sensation using positron emission tomography. Gastroenterol 1997;113:50-9.
4. Mayer EA. Spinal and supraspinal modulation of visceral sensation. Gut 2000;47:iv69-iv72.
5. Hobday D,.Thompson DG. Role of functional brain imaging in gastroenterology in health and disease. Digest Liver Dis 2000;32:101-3.
6. Valeriani M, Le Pera D, Tonali P. Characterizing somatosensory evoked potential sources with dipole models: advantages and limitations. Muscle Nerve 2001;24:325-39.
7. Hollerbach S. Cerebral evoked responses to gastrointestinal stimulation in humans. Crit Rev Biomed Engin 1997;25:203-42.
8. Aziz Q,.Thompson DG. Brain-gut axis in health and disease. Gastroenterology 1998;114:559-78.
9. Bromm B, Scharein E, Vahle-Hinz C. Cortex areas involved in the processing of normal and altered pain. Prog Brain Res 2000;129:289-302.
10. Hobson AR, Furlong PL, Worthen SF, et al. Real-time imaging of human cortical activity evoked by painful esophageal stimulation. Gastroenterology 2005;128:610-9.
11. Merlet I, Garcia-Larrea L, Froment JC, Mauguiere F. Simplified projection of EEG dipole sources onto human brain anatomy. Clin Neurophysiol 1999;29:39-52.
12. Drewes AM, Rossel P, Le Pera D, Arendt-Nielsen L, Valeriani M. Dipolar source modelling of brain potentials evoked by painful electrical stimulation of the human sigmoid colon. Neurosci Lett 2004;358:45-8.
13. Drewes AM, Rossel P, Le Pera D, Arendt-Nielsen L, Valeriani M. Cortical neuroplastic changes to painful colon stimulation in patients with irritable bowel syndrome. Neurosci Lett 2005;375:157-61.
14. Drewes AM, Dimcevski G, Sami SA, et al. The "human visceral homonculus" to pain evoked in the oesophagus, stomach, duodenum and sigmoid colon. Exp Brain Res 2006;174:443-52.
15. Sami SA, Rössel P, Dimcevski G, et al. Cortical changes to experimental sensitization of the human esophagus. Neuroscience 2006;140:269-79.
16. Coghill RC. Brain mechanisms supporting the pain experience: a distributed processing system. In: Max M, ed. Pain 1999-an updated review. Seattle: IASP Press, 1999:67-76.
17. Makeig S, Westerfield M, Jung TP, et al. Functionally independent components of the late positive event-related potential during visual spatial attention. J Neurosci 1999;19:2665-80.
18. Jung TP, Makeig S, Westerfield M, Townsend J, Courchesne E, Sejnowski TJ. Analysis and visualization of single-trial event-related potentials. Hum Brain Mapp 2001;14:166-85.
19. Drewes AM, Sami SA, Dimcevski G, et al. Cerebral processing of painful oesophageal stimulation. A study based on independent component analysis of the EEG. Gut 2006;55:619-29.
20. Apkarian AV, Brüggemann J, Shi T, Airapetian LR. A thalamic model for true and referred visceral pain. In: Gebhart GF, ed. Visceral pain. Seattle: IASP Press, 1995:217-59.
21. Cechetto DF. Supraspinal mechanisms of visceral representation. In: Gebhart GF, ed. Visceral pain. Progress in pain research and management. Seattle: IASP Press, 1995:261-90.
22. Tattersall JE, Cervero F, Lumb BM. Effects of reversible spinalization on the visceral input to viscerosomatic neurons in the lower thoracic spinal cord of the cat. J Neurophysiol 1986;56:785-96.
23. Ness TJ,.Gebhart GF. Interactions between visceral and cutaneous nociception in the rat. I. Noxious cutaneous stimuli inhibit visceral nociceptive neurons and reflexes. J Neurophysiol 1991;66:20-8.
24. Ness TJ, Gebhart GF. Quantitative comparison of inhibition of visceral and cutaneous spinal nociceptive transmission from the midbrain and medulla in the rat. J Neurophysiol 1987;58:850-65.
25. Jänig W, Häbler HJ. Visceral-autonomic integration. In: Gebhart GF, ed. Visceral pain, Progress in pain research and management. Seattle: IASP Press, 1995:311-48.
26. Foreman RD. Intraspinal modulation of visceral transmission. In: Gebhart GF, ed. Visceral pain, Progress in pain research and management. Seattle: IASP Press, 1995:291-309.

27. Roza C, Laird JM, Cervero F. Spinal mechanisms underlying persistent pain and referred hyperalgesia in rats with an experimental ureteric stone. J Neurophysiol 1998;79:1603-12.
28. Dimcevski G, Schipper KP, Tage-Jensen U, et al. Hypoalgesia to experimental visceral and somatic stimulation in painful chronic pancreatitis. Eur J Gastroenterol Hepatol 2006;18:755-64.
29. Dunckley P, Wise GW, Fairhurst M, et al. A comparison of visceral and somatic pain processing in the human brainstem using functional magnetic resonance imaging. J Neurosci 2005;25:7333-41.
30. Wilder-Smith CH, Schindler D, Lovblad K, Redmond SM, Nirkko A. Brain functional magnetic resonance imaging of rectal pain and activation of endogenous inhibitory mechanisms in irritable bowel syndrome patient subgroups and healthy controls. Gut 2004;53:1595-601.
31. Mayer EA, Berman S, Suyenobu B, et al. Differences in brain responses to visceral pain between patients with irritable bowel syndrome and ulcerative colitis. Pain 2005;115:398-409.

Can esophagus sense mechanical, thermal and chemical stimuli?

H. Gregersen (Aalborg)

The ultimate goal of advanced human experimental pain research is to obtain a better understanding of the mechanisms involved in pain transduction, transmission, and perception under normal and pathophysiological conditions. Experimental approaches can be applied in the laboratory for basic studies and in the clinic to characterize patients with sensory dysfunction and/or pain in organic and functional diseases [1]. Depending on the experimental model, different central mechanisms and conditions mimicking pathological pain such as increased sensation to normal physiologic/non-painful and painful stimuli can be studied. Most previous studies have relied on relative simple mechanical or electrical stimuli. These methods are easy to apply but as discussed below they have special considerations and limitations. Therefore, new controlled and reproducible models and protocols are highly warranted.

Mechanical, thermal and chemical methods for pain stimulation of the human gastrointestinal (GI) tract are described below. Some of the existing stimulation methods seem to fulfill the above requirements but most laboratories use their own stimulation paradigms, often without the necessary standardization.

Mechanical stimulation

In the last decade, several studies have addressed the mechanical and sensory function of the esophagus by means of mechanical distension. The mechanical properties of the esophagus are important for its function and the esophagus contains mechanoreceptors at various locations in the wall, mainly in the muscle layers. Mechanical stimulation, in particular bag distension, has been widely used also to study esophageal smooth muscle tone, distensibility, secondary peristalsis, functional and organic disorders, referred pain and cerebral activation patterns and the screening of new analgesics in healthy subjects and in patients with functional esophageal disorders (see [1] for a review).

There are several ways to stimulate the esophagus mechanically. Simple and physiological methods for distension of the gut such as ingestion of well-defined meals may be useful in clinical studies. Balloon distension is, however, much more used than ingestion as mechanical stimulation method and easier to control. Newer methods based on impedance planimetry allows recording of the luminal cross-sectional area directly and estimation of the radius in the distended segment of the esophagus [2,3]. From the radius it is possible to compute the wall strain with more accuracy than from volume measurements [4]. Finally, mechanical distension combined with ultrasound methods may offer the possibility for a better anatomical characterization and computation of stress in the GI tract.

Thermal stimulation

Short lasting thermal stimuli have also been used in the human esophagus. Here they are believed to activate unmyelinated afferents in the mucosa selectively as opposed to mechanical and electrical stimuli, which activate afferents in both the superficial and deeper layers. Thermosensitive mucosal afferents in the esophagus have been demonstrated in animal studies and in the human esophagus [2,5]. Characterization of the response to stimuli in the most superficial layers of the gut may be of major importance to develop a comprehensive sensory evaluation. In recent studies the temperature of re-circulating water was continuously measured inside a balloon positioned in the esophagus [2,6]. The temperature stimuli showed a nearly linear stimulus-response relationship, demonstrating the validity of the receptor activation. *Figure 1* demonstrates the sensory response in the esophagus to thermal stimuli.

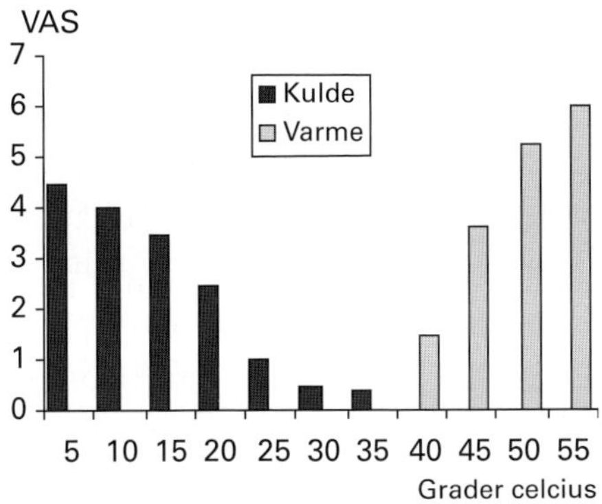

Figure 1. Sensory response to esophageal stimulation with cold and heat stimuli.

Chemical stimulation

Chemical stimulation of the GI tract more closely resembles clinical inflammation and is believed to approach the ideal experimental visceral pain stimulus. Chemical stimuli activate predominantly unmyelinated C-fibres and this may be an advantage in basic studies of differentiated nerve populations. Acid stimulation of the esophagus is the most used method to sensitize the esophagus [6-10]. The major disadvantage of chemical stimuli is that they require a relative long latency time to the onset of effects, and that they are often not reproducible when repeated. Thus, although chemical stimulation may evoke pain, the major relevance of the model is in sensitization of the visceral afferents to subsequent experimental stimulation.

Multimodal stimulation of the gastrointestinal tract

As pain is a multidimensional perception it is obvious that the reaction to a single stimulus of a given modality can represent only a limited fraction of the entire pain experience. The possibility for combining different methods for stimulation and assessment will approximate the clinical situation where many different nerves and pathways are activated. Thus, the method will give a more comprehensive and differentiated information about the nociceptive system compared to stimuli using single or a few modalities. For comprehensive experimental studies mimicking the clinical situation, a multimodal testing approach must therefore be used, where the test battery will increase the probability for activation of a range of relevant nervous mechanisms. Such sophisticated methods will be able to select the best test procedures to explore different basic aspects of pain as well as pharmacological modulations. Especially if the stimulation includes modalities known to evoke peripheral as well as central sensitization, the likelihood that a model will mimic clinical pain is high despite the non-harmful nature of the stimulation. In the GI tract difficulties with access to the organs and technical limitations of the currently available models have until now made a multimodal stimulation approach difficult. Some authors have combined mechanical and electrical stimuli [11,12] or mechanical and chemical stimuli [13,14], and in a recent study in the esophagus mechanical and electrical stimuli were combined with sensitization to acid [15]. Drewes and Gregersen recently introduced a multimodal model with combined mechanical, electrical, cold and warmth stimuli of the esophagus together with acid sensitization [2,6] (*Figure 2*). The multimodal approach gives the possibility for a differentiated stimulation of receptors in the superficial and deep layers of the esophagus. The possibility for induction of hyperalgesia with acid perfusion and evoking central phenomena such as summation, allodynia and referred pain makes the model clinically relevant with respect to increase the knowledge of peripheral and central pain mechanisms. The pain assessment should ideally also be multimodal and for example include quantitative and qualitative sensation, assessment of referred pain and neurophysiologic measurements.

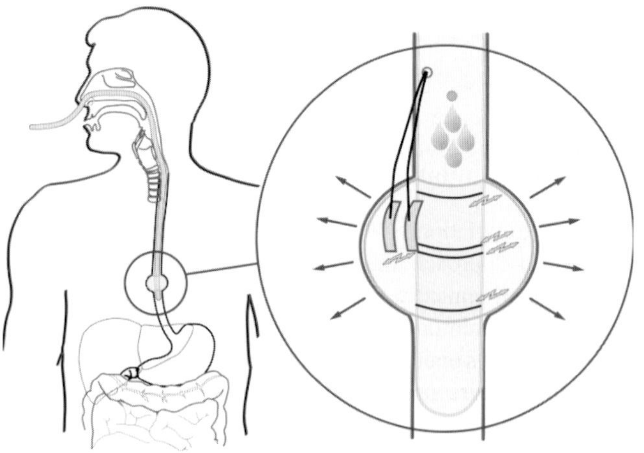

Figure 2. Probe for multimodal stimulation of the esophagus with mechanical, thermal, chemical and electrical stimulation.

Stimulation in patients with non-cardiac chest pain

Experimental pain studies in non-cardiac chest pain (NCCP) patients have the possibility to control the stimulus and assessment parameters, and thus explore the abnormal pain system in further detail. Most studies found that the sensation and pain detection thresholds to distension, electrical and acid stimuli of the esophagus were lower in NCCP patients compared with thresholds found in healthy subjects [12,15-21]. However, the reliability of the test for diagnosing NCCP has been questioned, and in some experiments only few patients had abnormal sensation [22]. There are, however, severe methodological problems relating to these studies. Early balloon distension studies were based on simple volume and pressure measurements using latex balloons. As stated in the section above "Mechanical stimulations" this caused large errors due to the deformability of latex and lack of control of the stimulation field. There are also limitations and sources of error with the systems based on volume and pressure. The use of methods based on impedance planimetry has encompassed many of these limitations. Rao *et al.* [23] used impedance planimetry and showed that patients with NCCP suffered from esophageal hyperalgesia. Furthermore the esophagus was more "irritable" than in controls, as the distensions resulted in more vigorous contractions at lower pressures. In more recent studies hyperalgesia was also found after relaxation of the smooth muscle with atropine [24], and there was evidence that the lower segments of the esophagus exhibited a higher level of sensory dysfunction compared to higher segments [25].

Central pain mechanisms

Paterson *et al.* [26] showed that repeated distensions conditioned the esophagus in NCCP resulting in higher pain scores. Probably this is a phenomenon relating to central hyperexcitability. In a recent study we used a ramp distension protocol to distend the distal esophagus in patients with NCCP before and after sensitization with acid [27]. Patients with NCCP did not seem to be more vulnerable to develop esophageal hyperalgesia to the slowly increasing mechanical distensions as compared to controls. However, there was evidence for abnormal central pain processing as there was an increased and widespread referred pain area to the mechanical stimulations and the patients were sensitive to repeated mechanical stimulation. Furthermore, after acid perfusion (believed to evoke hyperexcitability of central pathways mainly) there was a major sensitization to the distensions. Thus, it was concluded that NCCP patients showed facilitated central pain mechanisms, which may explain the character of their symptoms. This may have important implications for the diagnosis and treatment in these patients, where drugs with central effects should be used in the treatment.

Conclusions

The esophagus can sense mechanical, thermal and chemical stimuli. The responses can be measured in different ways and the stimuli can be applied independent of each other. However, a multimodal approach where stimuli are combined seems useful in studies of esophageal hypersensitivity.

References

1. Drewes AM, Gregersen H, Arendt-Nielsen L. Experimental pain in gastroenterology: a reappraisal of human studies. Scand J Gastroenterol 2003;38(11):1115-30.
2. Drewes AM, Schipper KP, Dimcevski G, et al. Multimodal assessment of pain in the esophagus: a new experimental model. Am J Physiol Gastrointest Liver Physiol 2002;283(1):G95-103.
3. Drewes AM, Pedersen J, Liu W, Arendt-Nielsen L, Gregersen H. Controlled mechanical distension of the human oesophagus: sensory and biomechanical findings. Scand J Gastroenterol 2003;38(1):27-35.
4. Gregersen H, Kassab G. Biomechanics of the gastrointestinal tract. Neurogastroenterol Motil 1996;8(4):277-97.
5. Sengupta J.N., Gebhart G.F. Gastrointestinal afferent fibers and sensation. In: Johnson L, ed. Physiology of the gastrointestinal tract, third ed. New York: Raven Press, 1994:484-519.
6. Drewes AM, Schipper KP, Dimcevski G, et al. Multi-modal induction and assessment of allodynia and hyperalgesia in the human oesophagus. Eur J Pain 2003;7(6):539-49.
7. Bernstein LM, Baker LA. A clinical test for esophagitis. Gastroenterology 1958;34:760-81.
8. Tack JF. Chest pain of oesophageal origin. In: Corazziari E, ed. Approach to the patient with chronic gastrointestinal disorders, first ed. Milano: Messaggi, 1999:153-70.
9. Drewes AM, Reddy H, Staahl C, et al. Sensory-motor responses to mechanical stimulation of the esophagus after sensitization with acid. World J Gastroenterol 2005;11:4367-74.
10. Reddy H, Arendt-Nielsen L, Staahl C, et al. Gender differences in pain and biomechanical responses after acid sensitization of the human esophagus. Dig Dis Sci 2005;50:2050-8.
11. Hollerbach S, Hudoba P, Fitzpatrick D, Hunt R, Upton AR, Tougas G. Cortical evoked responses following esophageal balloon distension and electrical stimulation in healthy volunteers. Dig Dis Sci 1998;43(11):2558-66.
12. Mehta AJ, De Caestecker JS, Camm AJ, Northfield TC. Sensitization to painful distention and abnormal sensory perception in the esophagus. Gastroenterology 1995;108(2):311-9.
13. DeVault KR. Acid infusion does not affect intraesophageal balloon distention- induced sensory and pain thresholds. Am J Gastroenterol 1997;92(6):947-9.
14. Hu WH, Martin CJ, Talley NJ. Intraesophageal acid perfusion sensitizes the esophagus to mechanical distension: a Barostat study. Am J Gastroenterol 2000;95(9):2189-94.
15. Sarkar S, Aziz Q, Woolf CJ, Hobson AR, Thompson DG. Contribution of central sensitisation to the development of non-cardiac chest pain. Lancet 2000;356:1154-9.
16. Frobert O, Arendt-Nielsen L, Bak P, Funch-Jensen P, Peder BJ. Pain perception and brain evoked potentials in patients with angina despite normal coronary angiograms 1. Heart 1996;75(5):436-41.
17. Hollerbach S, Bulat R, May A, et al. Abnormal cerebral processing of oesophageal stimuli in patients with noncardiac chest pain (NCCP). Neurogastroenterol Motil 2000;12(6):555-65.
18. Smout AJPM, Devore MS, Dalton CB, Castell DO. Cerebral potentials-evoked by esophageal distension in patients with noncardiac chest pain. Gut 1992;33(3):298-302.
19. Richter JE, Barish CF, Castell DO. Abnormal sensory perception in patients with esophageal chest pain. Gastroenterology 1986;91(4):845-52.
20. Cannon RO, III, Benjamin SB. Chest pain as a consequence of abnormal visceral nociception. Dig Dis Sci 1993;38(2):193-6.
21. Barish CF, Castell DO, Richter JE. Graded esophageal balloon distention. A new provocative test for noncardiac chest pain. Dig Dis Sci 1986;31(12):1292-8.
22. Nevens F, Janssens J, Piessens J, Ghillebert G, De Geest H, Vantrappen G. Prospective study on prevalence of esophageal chest pain in patients referred on an elective basis to a cardiac unit for suspected myocardial ischemia. Dig Dis Sci 1991;36(2):229-35.
23. Rao SS, Gregersen H, Hayek B, Summers RW, Christensen J. Unexplained chest pain: the hypersensitive, hyperreactive, and poorly compliant esophagus. Ann Intern Med 1996;124(11):950-8.
24. Rao SS, Hayek B, Summers RW. Functional chest pain of esophageal origin: hyperalgesia or motor dysfunction. Am J Gastroenterol 2001;96(9):2584-9.
25. Rao SS, Hayek B, Mudipalli R, Gregersen H. Does esophageal function vary at the striated and smooth muscle segments in functional chest pain? Am J Gastroenterol 2002;97(9):2201-7.
26. Paterson WG, Wang H, Vanner SJ. Increasing pain sensation to repeated esophageal balloon distension in patients with chest pain of undetermined etiology. Dig Dis Sci 1995;40(6):1325-31.
27. Drewes AM, Pedersen J, Reddy H, et al. Central sensitisation in patients with non-cardiac chest pain: a clinical experimental study. Scand J Gastroenterol 2006;41:640-9.

Acid sensitivity and esophageal hypersensitivity; is it peripheral or central?

A. Sharma, Q. Aziz (Salford)

Patients with functional gastrointestinal disorders (FGD) often display a heightened sensitivity to experimental gut stimulation, termed visceral hypersensitivity. For instance, Richter *et al.* demonstrated that a greater proportion of patients with non cardiac chest pain (NCCP) experienced pain to esophageal balloon distension compared to healthy controls (60% *versus* 20%) and that this occurred at smaller volumes of esophageal balloon distension [1]. This hypersensitivity seems to exist for other modes of stimuli as these patients also demonstrate hypersensitivity to chemical stimuli such as acid [2]. This heightened perception of visceral stimuli is believed to be relevant to the symptomatology of these disorders; however the factors that determine this sensitivity are incompletely understood.

In the case of functional esophageal disorders, which are often characterised by pain or heartburn, it is of prime importance to rule out acid reflux as a cause of recurrent heartburn or chest pain as symptoms may be then amenable to treatment with proton pump inhibitors (PPIs). On endoscopy however the majority of patients do not have evidence of gastroesophageal reflux disease (GERD) characterised by erosions or inflammation at the gastroesophageal junction, and so fall under the diagnostic umbrella of non-erosive reflux disease (NERD). This group can be subsequently subclassified according to the findings on pH studies into those with excessive esophageal acid exposure, those with hypersensitivity to normal levels of esophageal acid exposure ("hypersensitive esophagus"), or those with no abnormalities on pH studies ("functional heartburn" or "functional chest pain" according to symptoms). Progressing along the spectrum of these disorders, visceral hypersensitivity seems to become increasingly relevant despite the absence of abnormal mucosal features [3].

At exactly what level abnormalities exist in these patients is still under investigation, and the debate has been invigorated by evidence suggesting changes at both peripheral (tissue and primary afferent level) and central (spinal cord and above) levels. Before discussing these findings it is important to understand some basic neurophysiological concepts in nociceptive signalling, and these will be discussed.

The modulation of pain perception

Neuronal sensitisation

During tissue inflammation or injury peripheral nociceptor (pain signalling afferent) terminals become exposed to a number of immune and inflammatory mediators such as prostaglandins and cytokines which can upregulate their firing through a reduction in their transduction thresholds, a phenomenon termed "peripheral sensitisation (PS)". This modifiable synaptic activity ("synaptic plasticity") is an essential feature of the nervous system allowing it to adapt to adverse/noxious stimuli and bring about subsequent changes to facilitate avoidance of that stimulus and/or tissue healing. PS is believed to cause pain hypersensitivity at the site of injury or inflammation, resulting in a heightened awareness of painful stimuli (primary hyperalgesia), and the perception of innocuous stimuli as being painful (primary allodynia). A good example of this is when hyperalgesia and allodynia develop in sunburnt skin.

Hypersensitivity to painful and non-painful stimuli can also be demonstrated in areas surrounding the inflamed or injured tissue in somatic pain models – so called "secondary hyperalgesia" and "secondary allodynia" respectively. These phenomena are believed to result from the increase in nociceptive information arriving at the spinal cord due to PS, which subsequently increases the excitability and widens the receptive fields of dorsal horn neurones. In addition, previously silent nociceptors become recruited to further facilitate nociceptive signalling; this process is called "central sensitisation (CS)" [4]. Due to co-localisation of peripheral sensory afferent nerve terminals from the gut and skin on the same spinal dorsal horn neurones, there is heightened somatic referral of visceral sensation in the presence of CS.

Spinal and supraspinal modulation of nociceptive signalling

Even beyond the level of the spinal dorsal horn, pain signalling is subject to further modulation by spinal and supraspinal processes. Tracts that emanate from sites in the midbrain and brainstem can inhibit or excite spinal ascending nociceptive transmission by their close proximity to the central terminals of primary afferent nociceptors and dorsal horn neurons that respond to noxious stimulation, effects that are mediated *via* a number of neurotransmitters such as endogenous opioids, catecholamines and serotonin [5].

Modulation of pain sensitivity by neurohumoral factors

Mounting evidence supports the role of the autonomic nervous system (ANS) and hypothalamic-pituitary-adrenal (HPA) axis in modulating visceral sensitivity both in health and FGD. It has been demonstrated that heightened sympathetic activation in humans can increase the perception of intestinal distension [6], and both animal and human data support a vagally mediated inhibition of visceral nociceptive sensory inputs [7,8]. In irritable bowel syndrome, the administration of corticotropin releasing hormone (CRH) seems to be pro-nociceptive whereas the administration of its antagonists seems to reduce visceral perception [9].

Acid sensitivity and esophageal hypersensitivity – peripheral or central?

The role of peripheral factors

Sarkar *et al.* studied the role of acid exposure in the pathophysiology of NCCP and functional heartburn by comparing thresholds to electrically induced esophageal pain before and after 6 weeks of high-dose PPI therapy [10]. Following PPI therapy, the pain thresholds increased (34.65 ± 13.4 to 40.5 ± 12.5 mA, $p = .03$), suggesting that esophageal hypersensitivity was at least partially responsive to acid suppression. It was proposed that treatment of acid reflux removed the peripheral afferent input to the spinal cord which may in turn have reduced the degree of resultant central sensitisation. Patients with functional esophageal disorders without evidence of acid involvement have been speculated to have heightened sensation to other peripheral inputs such as bile reflux [11]. However, what determines sensitivity to esophageal chemical stimuli is far from understood, especially when one considers that even in patients with documented acid reflux on pH studies, the majority of events are not perceived [3].

In response to esophageal acid exposure, an upregulation of acid-sensitive receptors has been demonstrated which may impact on subsequent nociceptive signalling. Recently, Matthews *et al.* demonstrated that the vanilloid receptor 1 (TRPV1), a non-selective cation channel expressed by sensory nerves, was present in healthy esophageal mucosa but upregulated in patients with GERD [12]. This raises the possibility that acid-induced esophageal inflammation might, in susceptible individuals, upregulate acid-sensitive receptors such as TRPV1 and enhance visceral sensation. Whether or not these receptors play a role in the visceral hypersensitivity seen in functional esophageal disorders remains to be established.

The role of central factors

A model of human visceral pain hypersensitivity has been developed highlighting the relevance of CS in which a distal esophageal acid infusion reduces subsequent pain thresholds to electrical stimulation in the distal esophagus, the non acid exposed proximal esophagus and anterior chest wall [2]. Although the primary hyperalgesia/allodynia at the site of infusion is believed to be due to PS, the secondary hyperalgesia/allodynia in the proximal esophagus and anterior chest wall, distant to the acid infusion, is believed to be due to the sensitisation of spinal dorsal horn neurones [2].

Repeated studies with this model have demonstrated that around 20% of subjects fail to sensitise to esophageal acid infusion and there is variation in the magnitude of response (reduction in pain threshold to acid infusion) between subjects to the order of 24% [13]. Recently state anxiety has been implicated as a factor that may modulate not only baseline pain threshold reporting within the esophagus but also the degree of sensitisation to esophageal acidification within this model [14,15]. It is possible that psychological state modulates pain sensitivity and the degree of central sensitisation in response to injury by moderating descending spinal inhibitory and facilitatory influences.

The role of the ANS in modulating esophageal sensitivity has also been demonstrated. For instance, increased basal sympathetic activity and lower vagal activity, as measured by power spectral analysis of heart rate variability, are associated with increased sensitivity to esophageal acid perfusion in patients with NCCP compared with healthy matched controls [16]. In addition, the heightened sensitivity to esophageal acid infusion in GERD patients as compared to healthy controls has been shown to be associated with reduced vagal tone during the infusion [17]. These data support the concept of neurohumoral influences on the susceptibility to symptoms such as heartburn.

Psychological comorbidity such as anxiety or stress can heighten the perception of esophageal stimuli causing patients to perceive low intensity stimuli as painful [18]. Although studies have failed to demonstrate an increase in acid reflux during stressful stimuli, interventions aimed at reducing stress such as hypnosis and muscle relaxation have produced subjective improvement in reflux symptoms ratings [19].

Conclusion

The interplay between the factors that determine an individual's sensitivity to a variety of esophageal stimuli such as acid is complex, but clearly changes occur at both peripheral and central levels. The relative contribution of each of these factors in modulating sensory perception is likely to be different in the heterogeneous patient population. It seems likely that distinct phenotypes exist who manifest these abnormalities to differing degrees, such as those in whom psychological comorbidity is more prominent or those in whom chronic prior acid exposure may have resulted in upregulated TRPV1 expression and chronic central sensitisation. Further studies are required to demonstrate the interactions of peripheral and central factors in modulating pain perception and sensitivity, and this is likely to be advanced by future drug discovery such as TRPV1 antagonists.

References

1. Richter JE, Barish CF, Castell DO. Abnormal sensory perception in patients with esophageal chest pain. Gastroenterology 1986;91(4):845-52.
2. Sarkar S, Aziz Q, Woolf CJ, Hobson AR, Thompson DG. Contribution of central sensitisation to the development of non-cardiac chest pain. Lancet 2000;356(9236):1154-9.
3. Fass R, Tougas G. Functional heartburn: the stimulus, the pain, and the brain. Gut 2002;51(6):885-92.
4. Mayer EA, Gebhart GF. Basic and clinical aspects of visceral hyperalgesia. Gastroenterology 1994;107(1):271-93.
5. Millan MJ. Descending control of pain. Prog Neurobiol 2002;66(6):355-474.
6. Iovino P, Azpiroz F, Domingo E, Malagelada JR. The sympathetic nervous system modulates perception and reflex responses to gut distention in humans. Gastroenterology 1995;108(3):680-6.
7. Randich A, Gebhart GF. Vagal afferent modulation of nociception. Brain Res Brain Res Rev 1992;17(2):77-99.
8. Diop L, Riviere PJ, Pascaud X, Dassaud M, Junien JL. Role of vagal afferents in the antinociception produced by morphine and U-50,488H in the colonic pain reflex in rats. Eur J Pharmacol 1994;257(1-2):181-7.
9. Fukudo S, Nomura T, Hongo M. Impact of corticotropin-releasing hormone on gastrointestinal motility and adrenocorticotropic hormone in normal controls and patients with irritable bowel syndrome. Gut 1998;42(6):845-9.
10. Sarkar S, Thompson DG, Woolf CJ, Hobson AR, Millane T, Aziz Q. Patients with chest pain and occult gastroesophageal reflux demonstrate visceral pain hypersensitivity which may be partially responsive to acid suppression. Am J Gastroenterol 2004;99(10):1998-2006.
11. Siddiqui A, Rodriguez-Stanley S, Zubaidi S, Miner PB Jr. Esophageal visceral sensitivity to bile salts in patients with functional heartburn and in healthy control subjects. Dig Dis Sci 2005;50(1):81-5.
12. Matthews PJ, Aziz Q, Facer P, Davis JB, Thompson DG, Anand P. Increased capsaicin receptor TRPV1 nerve fibres in the inflamed human oesophagus. Eur J Gastroenterol Hepatol 2004;16(9):897-902.
13. Willert R. Receptor mechanisms mediating human oesophageal hypersensitivity [PhD Report]. Manchester: University of Manchester; 2005.
14. Worthen SF HJ, Aziz Q, Hobson AR. Effect of anxiety on the sensory and perceptual characteristics of visceral and somatic sensation. Gut 2005;54(suppl 2):A19.
15. Sharma A AQ, Delaney C, Hobson AR. The magnitude of visceral pain hypersensitivity after distal oesophageal acidification correlates with pre-study anxiety state scores. Gastroenterology 2006;130 (suppl 2):880.
16. Tougas G, Spaziani R, Hollerbach S, Djuric V, Pang C, Upton AR, et al. Cardiac autonomic function and oesophageal acid sensitivity in patients with non-cardiac chest pain. Gut 2001;49(5):706-12.
17. Chen CL, Orr WC. Autonomic responses to heartburn induced by esophageal acid infusion. J Gastroenterol Hepatol 2004;19(8):922-6.
18. Bradley LA, Richter JE, Pulliam TJ, Haile JM, Scarinci IC, Schan CA, et al. The relationship between stress and symptoms of gastroesophageal reflux: the influence of psychological factors. Am J Gastroenterol 1993;88(1):11-9.
19. McDonald-Haile J, Bradley LA, Bailey MA, Schan CA, Richter JE. Relaxation training reduces symptom reports and acid exposure in patients with gastroesophageal reflux disease. Gastroenterology 1994;107(1):61-9.

What is the role of mucosal barrier in acid-induced pain?

R.C. Orlando (Chapel Hill)

The esophageal mucosal barrier (EMB) is a defensive process by which the esophagus protects itself and the organism from injury by noxious luminal substances. Further and more specifically the EMB is created around and for the protection of the esophageal epithelium which comes into daily contact with a variety of noxious products that arrive by ingestion, regurgitation or reflux. The phenomenon of gastroesophageal reflux appears, by far, to pose the greatest risk of injury since it brings the epithelium into repeated contact with high concentrations of gastric acid. As defense against acid injury, the EMB is depicted as having both structural and functional components [1]. Among the most important structural components are the apical and basolateral membranes of the cell and the apical junctional complex consisting of both tight junctions and zonula adherens that regulate the permeability of ions and molecules passing between cells. Among the most important functional components are intracellular and intercellular buffers for acid, integral membrane proteins for control of intracellular pH, and the blood supply for delivery of oxygen and nutrients and removal of metabolic byproducts and waste [2] (*Figure 1*).

Together the interplay between the structural and functional elements of esophageal epithelium create an electrically tight, stratified squamous epithelium that remains healthy

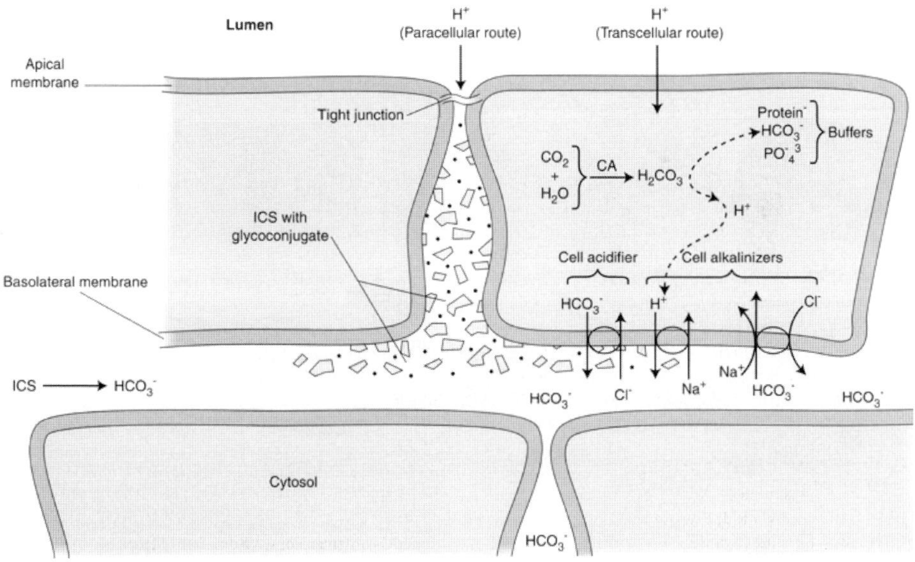

Figure 1. The esophageal mucosal barrier, also referred to as tissue resistance, comprises structural and functional elements. Structures including the cell membrane and apical intercellular junctional complex limit the rate of diffusion of luminal acid (H^+) into and between the epithelial cells, respectively. Functional defenses include intracellular and extracellular buffers and processes that extrude H^+ from the cytosol (e.g. basolateral membrane Na^+/H^+ exchanger and Na^+-dependent Cl^-/HCO_3^- exchanger). CA = carbonic anhydrase; ICS = intercellular space. (Modified from [2]).

despite the repeated daily contact with refluxed gastric acid and components of meals, particularly alcohol, heat and hypertonicity. And, further, the capacity of the EMB to resist injury by contact with luminal acid is considerable, as evidenced by the ability to prevent the occurrence of heartburn during physiologic acid reflux observed on 24-hour esophageal pH monitoring and during the Bernstein (esophageal acid perfusion) test. Esophageal pH monitoring demonstrates that the healthy esophagus tolerates intermittent acidification to levels below pH 4.0 for ~ 5% of the time or 1.2 hours per day while during the Bernstein test, continuous perfusion of the healthy esophagus with 0.1N HCl for up to 30 minutes produces no symptoms [3,4]. The reason for this is that the intact (undamaged) esophageal epithelium provides an effective barrier that limits acid's access to the senory nerves within the esophageal wall.

Support for the concept that the EMB represents one of the final arbiters of symptoms in those with gastroesophageal reflux disease (GERD) is shown by the elicitation of heartburn in GERD subjects undergoing the Bernstein test [4-6]. The reason for this is because heartburn requires luminal acid to contact a "damaged" esophageal epithelium – eliciting symptoms when acid diffuses across the epithelium in sufficient quantities to activate chemosensitive nociceptors within the organ. Lowering pH in the vicinity of the nociceptor in turn sends the signal to the central nervous system (CNS) for the conscious perception of heartburn [7] (*Figure 2*). In healthy subjects no symptoms are elicicted during the Bernstein test because acid backdiffusion across the intact EMB is limited and

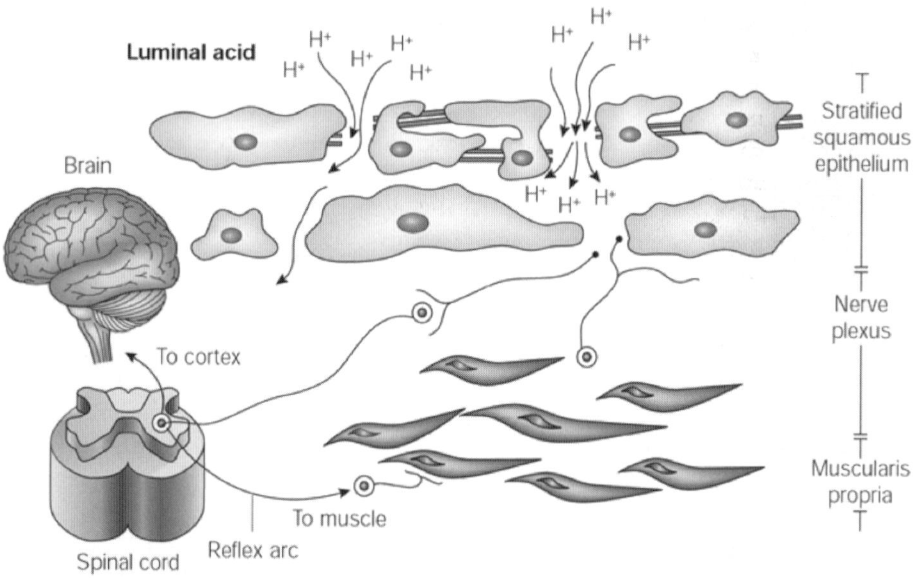

Figure 2. The presence of abnormal tissue resistance – demonstrated by defects within the intercellular junctional complex between cells of the surface layers of esophageal (stratified squamous) epithelium – is shown to enable the ready diffusion of refluxed gastric acid (H^+) into the intercellular space. Within this space, it encounters and activates chemosensitive nociceptors whose signals are transmitted *via* the spinal cord to the brain for symptom (heartburn) perception. Activation of the same nociceptors are also capable of initiating a short reflex arc to esophageal (longitudinal) smooth muscle as means of precipitating a sustained esophageal contraction. (Modified and reprinted with permission from [7]).

insufficient for nociceptor activation. Consistent with this concept are findings on functional magnetic resonance imaging of CNS activity during esophageal acid perfusion in healthy and GERD subjects [8]. The findings revealed that acid perfusion triggers a signal to the same areas of CNS, but the signals in GERD were more rapid in onset and greater in magnitude than in healthy subjects – differences which likely account for heartburn in GERD subjects and absence of heartburn in healthy subjects during esophageal acid perfusion.

The nature of the break in the EMB responsible for heartburn appears clearer now that a lesion known as "dilated intercellular spaces" has been demonstrated in patients with both erosive and non-erosive reflux disease (NERD) [9-11] (*Figure 3*). This lesion correlates with the symptom of heartburn in GERD and with its resolution upon treatment with proton pump inhibitors [12]. Moreover, the lesion correlates with heartburn irrespective of whether the acid contact time on 24-hour pH monitoring is found to be normal or abnormal [13]. The reason for this correlation is because "dilated intercellular spaces" occurs when there is damage to the apical junctional complex between squamous cells which allows the shunt (paracellular) pathway within the tissue to be highly permeable to luminal contents. Diffusion of luminal contents across the damaged apical junctional complex accounts for dilated spaces by creation of osmotic gradients for water movement through the epithelium's paracellular pathway [14].

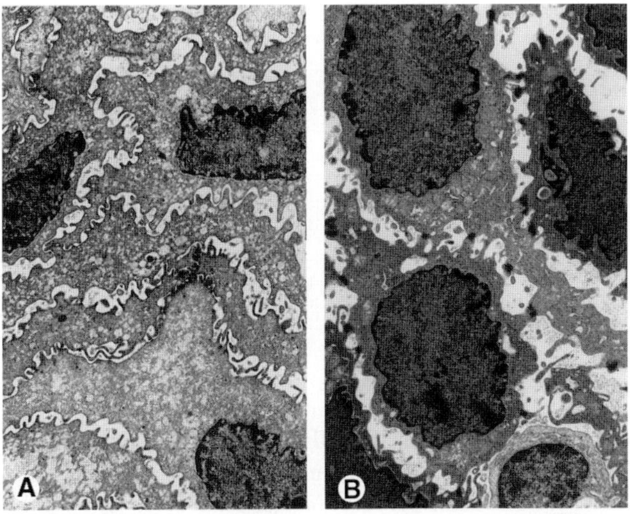

Figure 3. Transmission electron micrographs showing the differences in size of the intercellular spaces for normal (**A**) and non-erosive acid-damaged (**B**) esophageal epithelia. X 9000 (Reprinted with permission from [7]).

In summary, the EMB plays an essential role in acid-induced esophageal pain by virtue of its ability to restrain refluxed (luminal) acid from accessing the sensory nerves within the esophageal wall. An intact EMB explains the lack of symptoms in healthy subjects during physiologic reflux and during the Bernstein test while a damaged EMB — characterized by dilated intercellular spaces and "leaky" shunt pathway in esophageal epithelium – explains the occurrence of heartburn in GERD subjects spontaneously and during the Bernstein test.

References

1. Orlando RC. Pathophysiology of gastroesophageal reflux disease: esophageal epithelial resistance. In: Castell DO, Richter JE,eds. The esophagus. Philadelphia: Lippincott Williams & Wilkins, 2004:421-33.
2. Orlando RC. Reflux esophagitis. In: Yamada T, Alpers D, Owyang C, et al., eds. Textbook of gastroenterology. Philadelphia: JB Lippincott Williams & Wilkins, 1999:1235-63.
3. Galmiche JP, Scarpignato C. Esophageal pH monitoring. In: Scarpignato C, Galmiche JP, eds. Functional investigation in esophageal disease. Frontiers of gastrointerstinal research. Basel: Karger, 1994;22:71-108.
4. Bernstein LM, Baker LA. A clinical test for esophagitis. Gastroenterology 1958;34:760-81.
5. Bernstein LM, Fruin RD, Pacini R. Differentiation of esophageal pain from angina pectoris: role of the esophageal acid perfusion test. Medicine (Baltimore) 1962;41:143-62.
6. Richter JE. Provocative tests in esophageal diseases. In: Scarpignato C, Galmiche JP, eds. Functional investigation in esophageal disease. Frontiers of gastrointerstinal research. Basel: Karger, 1994;22:188-208.
7. Barlow WJ, Orlando RC. The pathogenesis of heartburn in nonerosive reflux disease: a unifying hypothesis. Gastroenterology 2005;128:771-8.
8. Kern M, Hofmann C, Hyde J, Shaker R. Characterization of the cerebral cortical representation of heartburn in GERD patients. Am J Physiol Gastrointest Liver Physiol 2004;286:G174-81.
9. Tobey NA, Carson JL, Alkiek RA, Orlando RC. Dilated intercellular spaces: a morphological feature of acid reflux—damaged human esophageal epithelium. Gastroenterology 1996;111:1200-5.
10. Solcia E, Villani L, Luinetti O, et al. Altered intercellular glycoconjugates and dilated intercellular spaces of esophageal epithelium in reflux disease. Virchows Arch 2000;436:207-16.
11. Villanacci V, Grigolato PG, Cestari R, et al. Dilated intercellular spaces as markers of reflux disease: histology, semiquantitative score and morphometry upon light microscopy. Digestion 2001;64:1-8.
12. Calabrese C, Bortolotti M, Fabbri A, et al. Reversibility of GERD ultrastructural alterations and relief of symptoms after omeprazole treatment. Am J Gastroenterol 2005;100:537-42.
13. Caviglia R, Ribolsi M, Maggiano N, et al. Dilated intercellular spaces of esophageal epithelium in nonerosive reflux disease patients with physiological esophageal acid exposure. Am J Gastroenterol 2005;100:543-8.
14. Tobey NA, Hosseini SS, Argote CM, Dobrucali AM, Awayda MS, Orlando RC. Dilated intercellular spaces and shunt permeability in nonerosive acid-damaged esophageal epithelium. Am J Gastroenterol 2004;99:13-22.

Can non-acid reflux cause esophageal symptoms?

F. Fornari, D. Sifrim (Leuven)

Non-acid reflux has been defined as reflux episodes with a nadir pH > 4. A more precise classification categorizes these episodes as weakly acidic reflux (nadir pH 4-7) and weakly alkaline reflux (nadir pH > 7) [1], with the former representing most events of non-acid reflux. Whilst the well known acid reflux (nadir pH < 4) has an established role on the generation of esophageal symptoms [2-4], non-acid reflux has recently gained attention with the employment of combined impedance and pH monitoring, and its involvement with esophageal symptoms is under investigation.

The studies focused on non-acid reflux have been performed in patients with symptoms of gastroesophageal reflux disease (GERD) evaluated "off" and "on" proton pump inhibitors (PPIs). For this purpose, patients have been studied with combined impedance-pH monitoring, able to detect acid and non-acid reflux. The occurrence of GERD symptoms during impedance-pH monitoring provides the opportunity to identify episodes of non-acid reflux possible associated with symptoms. Thus, a reflux-symptom association (R^+S^+) has been established when GERD symptom started in the 2-min period following an episode of reflux [5]. Different statistical models have been employed to express the magnitude of reflux-symptom association, including symptom association probability (SAP) and symptom index (SI).

Initial impedance-pH studies showed that in patients with typical GERD symptoms (heartburn and acid regurgitation) studied off PPIs, non-acid reflux accounted for a minority of heartburn preceded by reflux, suggesting that heartburn is mainly associated with traditional acid reflux [6]. Additionally, in non-erosive reflux disease (NERD) patients evaluated off PPIs, non-acid reflux was more often associated with regurgitation than with heartburn, however accounting for a minority of these symptomatic episodes [7]. In a recent study, non-acid reflux was implicated on the generation of 44% of GERD symptoms of patients with SAP+ evaluated off PPIs, being belch and cough the most prevalent symptoms [8]. In patients on PPIs, the impact of non-acid reflux on symptom generation was higher than acid reflux, accounting for 86% of symptoms in patients with SAP+, particularly associated with regurgitation and cough.

A study in patients with persistent GERD symptoms despite the use of PPIs showed that non-acid reflux preceded the majority (77%) of R^+S^+ events analyzed by means of SI [9]. When discriminated by typical and atypical GERD symptoms, non-acid reflux preceded 73% and 86% of these symptomatic events, respectively.

The relationship between non-acid reflux and unexplained chronic cough has been investigated in our laboratory [10]. Using an objective method to detect cough and reflux (manometry combined with impedance-pH), non-acid reflux was implicated as a potential cause of cough in 24% of patients whereas acid reflux was found implicated in 45% of patients.

Based on these evidences, non-acid reflux seems to have a clear impact on the generation of either typical or atypical GERD symptoms, particularly in patients poorly responsive to acid-suppressive therapy. The ability of non-acid reflux to cause symptoms may be explained by hypersensitivity to reflux-associated esophageal distension or the action of components other than acid, including pepsin and bile acids. In favour of the latter hypothesis, experimental studies performed in our laboratory showed that esophageal mucosal perfusion with non-acid solutions containing small amounts of bile acids is able to provoke increased mucosa permeability, a phenomenon likely related with symptom genesis [11].

From the clinical point of view, the judicious use of impedance-pH monitoring and reflux-symptom association in the identification of patients with non-acid reflux as a possible cause of esophageal symptoms might improve therapeutic outcomes. In addition, objective methods for detection of symptoms during impedance-pH studies have been developed and considered fundamental for properly selection of patients. Nevertheless, outcome studies are still needed to prove the real impact of non-acid reflux on the generation of esophageal symptoms.

References

1. Sifrim D, Castell D, Dent J, Kahrilas PJ. Gastro-oesophageal reflux monitoring: review and consensus report on detection and definitions of acid, non-acid, and gas reflux. Gut 2004;53:1024-31.
2. Baldi F, Ferrarini F, Longanesi A, Ragazzini M, Barbara L. Acid gastroesophageal reflux and symptom occurrence. Analysis of some factors influencing their association. Dig Dis Sci 1989;34:1890-3.
3. Cicala M, Emerenziani S, Caviglia R, et al. Intra-oesophageal distribution and perception of acid reflux in patients with non-erosive gastro-oesophageal reflux disease. Aliment Pharmacol Ther 2003;18:605-13.

4. Fass R, Tougas G. Functional heartburn: the stimulus, the pain, and the brain. Gut 2002;51:885-92.
5. Lam HG, Breumelhof R, Roelofs JM, van Berge Henegouwen GP, Smout AJ. What is the optimal time window in symptom analysis of 24-hour esophageal pressure and pH data? Dig Dis Sci 1994;39:402-9.
6. Sifrim D, Tack J, Holloway R, Silny J, Janssens J. Heartburn during ambulatory 24-hs pH-impedance recordings in patients with reflux disease "off" medication. Gastroenterology 2002;122:432.
7. Emerenziani S, Cicala M, Zhang X, et al. Weakly acidic reflux in endoscopy negative reflux disease. Gastroenterology 2005;128:A519.
8. Zerbib F, Duriez A, Roman S, Capdepont M, Mion F. Determinants of gastro-oesophageal reflux perception in patients with persistent symptoms despite proton pump inhibitors. Gut 2008;57:156-60.
9. Mainie I, Tutuian R, Shay S, et al. Acid and non-acid reflux in patients with persistent symptoms despite acid suppressive therapy: a multicentre study using combined ambulatory impedance-pH monitoring. Gut 2006;55:1398-402.
10. Blondeau K, Dupont LJ, Mertens V, Tack J, Sifrim D. Improved diagnosis of gastro-oesophageal reflux in patients with unexplained chronic cough. Aliment Pharmacol Ther 2007;25:723-32.
11. Farre R, van Malenstein H, de Vos R, et al. Weakly acidic solutions containing pepsin and bile acids can increase significantly esophageal mucosa permeability. Gastroenterology 2007;132:A274-5.

Targeting $GABA_B$ and glutamate receptors: is it the way to go for treating esophageal symptoms?

A. Lehmann (Mölndal)

γ-aminobutyric acid (GABA) and glutamate are the major inhibitory and excitatory, respectively, transmitters in the central nervous system (CNS). Their role in neurotransmission is, however, not confined to the CNS. In the periphery, glutamate is abundantly present while the localization of GABA is more restricted. In the foregut, GABA is found in gastric D-cells [1] and in subpopulations of gastric myenteric neurons [2]. There are no reports on the presence of GABA or its synthesizing and degrading enzymes in the esophagus and there are no functional $GABA_B$ receptors in the lower esophageal sphincter (LES) [3]. Likewise, very little is known about markers for glutamatergic transmission in this region. However, isolated reports indicate that one subtype of glutamate receptors (the N-methyl-D-aspartate [NMDA] receptor) may be expressed in rat esophageal intrinsic neurons [4] and in the rabbit LES [5].

Before addressing the question whether there may be a role for $GABA_B$ and glutamate receptors in the treatment of esophageal symptoms, it is appropriate to review the complexity of the receptors. GABA receptors are subdivided into $GABA_A$ and $GABA_B$ subtypes [6]. Whilst the former is an ionotropic receptor (ligand-gated ion channel responsible for fast synaptic transmission), the latter belongs to the G-protein coupled receptor superfamily. In contrast to the $GABA_A$ receptor which is assembled from a number of subunits, the $GABA_B$ receptor only contains two subunits, $GABA_{B(1)}$ and $GABA_{B(2)}$. Both subunits must be present for the receptor to be functional, and there are splice variants of both $GABA_{B(1)}$ and $GABA_{B(2)}$. Despite several observations indicative of pharmacological subtype receptor selectivity, studies on recombinant $GABA_B$ receptors have failed to find compounds selective for different splice variants [7].

An even greater diversity is found in the glutamate receptor family which also can be divided into ionotropic and metabotropic receptors [8]. The ionotropic receptors are comprised by the NMDA, kainate and AMPA subfamilies, each consisting of various subunits [8]. Metabotropic glutamate receptors are substantially more complex than the $GABA_B$ receptors in that they form three subdivisions (mGluR groups I-III) encoded by eight different genes (mGluR1-8) [9].

Pharmacology of $GABA_B$ and glutamate receptors

As mentioned above, the options to modulate the $GABA_B$ receptor are limited. The only clinically used compound acting on this receptor is the agonist baclofen (Lioresal®), a myorelaxant used to treat spasticty. A number of antagonists are available but despite considerable efforts of pharmaceutical companies, no $GABA_B$ antagonist has been launched in the marketplace. An exciting development in $GABA_B$ pharmacology is currently taking place. Some years ago, Novartis reported that one compound, CGP7930, acts as a positive allosteric modulator [10]. Such drugs do not have any intrinsic activity at the receptor but enhance the effect of an agonist. They have the distinct advantage over agonists that they only strengthen signaling where the receptor is tonically active. Therefore, side-effects associated with general stimulation of receptors can be expected to be reduced.

Several tools exist to alter glutamatergic transmission but very few compounds are used clinically, and none of those are selective for glutamatergic transmission. The dissociative anesthetic ketamine is an NMDA antagonist but it also interacts with several other transmitter receptors and ion channels [11]. Dextromethorphan, an antitussive, can also antagonize NMDA receptors but is not selective for this receptor [12]. Riluzole, used to ameliorate symptoms in amyotrophic lateral sclerosis, inhibits release of glutamate but may have effects on other transmitter systems as well [13]. No drugs acting on mGluRs have been approved for human use.

From a drug development perspective, mGluRs are more attractive than iGluRs. Ionotropic glutamate (and GABA) receptors are responsible for fast neurotransmission and disruption of these systems is often associated with marked side-effects. In contrast, mGluRs serve a modulating function and changes in their activity is less likely to produce side-effects.

Reduction of esophageal symptoms by $GABA_B$ and glutamate receptor ligands

Stimulation of esophageal afferents is the first link in a chain of events leading to perception of symptoms. In principle, any effect of drugs attributable to inhibition of esophageal afferents may be primary, i.e. a direct inhibition, or secondary, i.e. blockade of events that trigger afferent activation.

There is ample evidence that targeting of $GABA_B$ and glutamate receptors may ameliorate esophageal symptoms through indirect mechanisms. More specifically, modulation of these receptors has been shown to inhibit transient LES relaxations (TLESRs) [14], the major cause of gastroesophageal reflux. TLESRs are known to be triggered by excitation of gastric vagal mechanoreceptors [15], and drugs suppressing TLESRs frequently block this event, but it cannot be excluded that direct effects on nociceptive esophageal afferents also may afford therapeutic effects.

Table I. Effects of glutamate and $GABA_B$ receptor ligands on TLESRs.

Receptor	Species	Compounds	Effect	Ref.
NMDA	Dog, human	CGS 19755 Dextromethorphan	Variable Weak inhibition	[20] [19]
Glutamate receptors	Human	Riluzole (glutamate release inhibitor)	Weak inhibition	[19]
mGluR5	Dog, ferret	MPEP, MTEP (antagonists)	Inhibition	[21,22]
mGluR group I	Ferret	DHPG (non-selective agonist)	Weak stimulation	[22]
mGluR group II	Ferret	2R,4R-APDC (non-selective agonist)	No effect	[22]
mGluR group III	Ferret	L-AP4 (non-selective agonist), S-3,4-DCPG (mGluR8-selective agonist)	Inhibition	[22]
$GABA_A$	Dog, ferret	Muscimol, THIP, isoguvacine (agonists), diazepam (allosteric enhancer)	Variable inhibition	[28,29]
$GABA_B$	Dog, ferret, cat, human	Baclofen, CGP44532, SK&F97541	Inhibition	[23,28, 30-33]

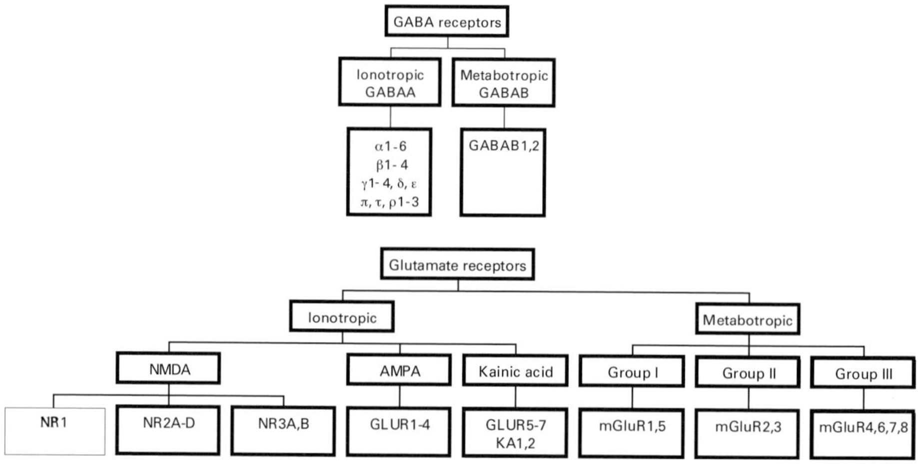

Figure 1. Overview of GABA and glutamate receptors.

Reduction of esophageal symptoms through inhibition of transient lower esophageal sphincter relaxations

First, it must be mentioned that there are very few reports on symptomatic improvement of esophageal symptoms during treatment affecting $GABA_B$ receptors, and none relating to glutamatergic drugs. Any discussion on therapeutic effects of glutamate receptor ligands at this stage therefore has to be speculative and based on extrapolation of data from preclinical studies. However, the strong association between TLESRs and reflux [15], and between

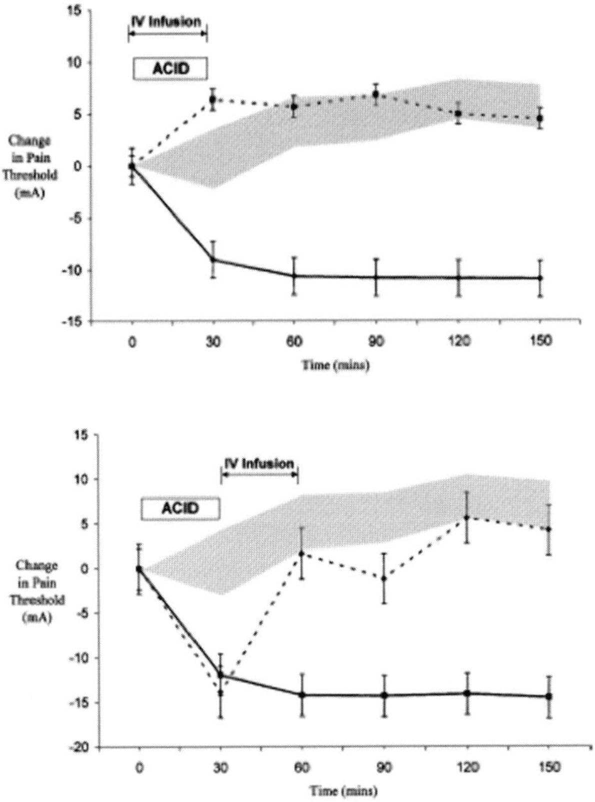

Figure 2. Effects of ketamine on hypersensitivity of the upper esophagus to electrical stimulation induced by perfusion of the lower esophagus with acid. Upper panel: ketamine (interrupted line) given during acid infusion prevents development of hypersensitivity (solid line; placebo). Lower panel: ketamine administered after acid perfusion reverses hypersensitivity. (Reprinted from [27], with permission from the American Gastroenterological Association).

reflux and esophageal symptomatology, suggests that there is a good chance that preclinical and phase I results will translate into clinical benefit.

Baclofen has repeatedly been demonstrated to inhibit TLESRs in experimental animals and in both healthy subjects and gastroesophageal reflux disease (GERD) patients [14]. Of the 5 studies published on the effects of baclofen on esophageal symptoms, 4 have been positive [14]. The interpretation of the negative study is hampered by a low level of symptoms in the placebo arm. A therapeutic effect of baclofen has been observed both in general GERD populations [16] and in selected patients such as proton pump inhibitor (PPI)-resistant patients in which bile reflux may be responsible for symptoms [17] as well as in neurologically impaired children whose main quantifiable symptom is emesis [18]. All of these studies are limited by small sample sizes.

While the role of glutamate receptors in esophageal symptom production through reduction in TLESR incidence has not been reported to date, there are several indications that activation or inhibition of these receptors may have a role to play. Clinical studies have shown that both riluzole and dextromethorphan have a weak inhibitory effect on TLESRs in healthy individuals [19]. Given the lack of selectivity of these drugs, it can only be speculated that the effects occur through glutamate release inhibition and NMDA antagonism, respectively. The effects of CGS19755 (a competitive NMDA blocker) on TLESRs in dogs were variable [20]. Recently, group I and III of the mGluRs have been implicated in TLESR inhibition in laboratory animals. The selective mGluR5 antagonist

MPEP affords potent inhibition of TLESRs in dogs [21] and ferrets [22], and a non-selective group III agonist as well as a selective mGluR8 agonist attenuate TLESRs incidence in ferrets [22].

Reduction of symptoms through direct inhibition of sensory pathways

Whereas the assumption that GERD symptoms can be treated with $GABA_B$ and glutamate ligands by virtue of their inhibition of TLESRs is reasonably well founded, very few studies have addressed the question if such compounds can have a direct effect on symptoms. As far as $GABA_B$ is concerned, a lateral finding in one study suggests that nausea and heartburn produced by gastric distension are mitigated by baclofen [23]. Whether this effect relates to actions on gastric afferents is unknown, but stimulation of the receptor is known to inhibit mechanosensitive gastroesophageal afferents [24], so a direct effect is possible. All three groups of mGluRs have been found to be involved in gastroesophageal afferent signaling in mice and ferrets. Agonists of group II and III, and an antagonist of group I, produce inhibition of firing during mechanical stimulation [25]. Similarly, iGluR ligands consistently affect gastroesophageal afferents, and here, agonists of the different subtypes of receptors are excitatory while antagonists are inhibitory [26]. Taken together, it is conceivable that mGluR agonists/antagonists, and iGluR antagonists, may reduce esophageal symptoms through their actions on primary afferents, but this proposal remains conjectural at present.

The most convincing evidence for a role for glutamate receptors in esophageal symptoms comes from a study of Willert *et al.* [27]. They studied healthy volunteers in which hypersensitivity to electrical stimulation of the upper esophagus was induced by distal esophageal acid perfusion. When ketamine, the nonselective NMDA antagonist, was administered before acid perfusion, sensitization was prevented. In addition, ketamine could reverse established hypersensitivity. The authors suggested that the effect was central since a peripheral effect would probably not overcome direct electrical stimulation of afferents.

In conclusion, there are several preclinical and some clinical findings that hold promise for successful targeting of $GABA_B$ and glutamate receptors to reduce esophageal symptoms, at least those associated with GERD. With regard to glutamate receptors, the metabotropic subtypes are more appealing from a drug discovery perspective than the ionotropic ones simply because they are less likely to produce adverse events. However, the tolerance for side-effects in a benign albeit troublesome disease such as GERD is low. As new compounds emerge which can fine-tune the receptors more precisely, we will learn if they can achieve an acceptable therapeutic index.

References

1. Davanger S, Hjelle OP, Babaie E, et al. Colocalization of gamma-aminobutyrate and gastrin in the rat antrum: an immunocytochemical and in situ hybridization study. Gastroenterology 1994;107:137-48.
2. Tsai LH, Tsai W, Wu JY. Action of myenteric GABAergic neurons in the guinea pig stomach. Neurochem Int 1993;23:187-93.
3. Blackshaw LA, Smid SD, O'Donnell TA, Dent J. GABA(B) receptor-mediated effects on vagal pathways to the lower oesophageal sphincter and heart. Br J Pharmacol 2000;130:279-88.
4. Robertson BS, Satterfield BE, Said SI, Dey RD. N-methyl-D-aspartate receptors are expressed by intrinsic neurons of rat larynx and esophagus. Neurosci Lett 1998;244:77-80.

5. Kohjitani A, Funahashi M, Miyawaki T, Hanazaki M, Matsuo R, Shimada M. Peripheral N-methyl-D-aspartate receptors modulate nonadrenergic noncholinergic lower esophageal sphincter relaxation in rabbits. Anesth Analg 2005;101:1681-8.
6. Chebib M, Johnston GA. The 'ABC' of GABA receptors: a brief review. Clin Exp Pharmacol Physiol 1999;26:937-40.
7. Bettler B, Kaupmann K, Mosbacher J, Gassmann M. Molecular structure and physiological functions of GABA(B) receptors. Physiol Rev 2004;84:835-67.
8. Simeone TA, Sanchez RM, Rho JM. Molecular biology and ontogeny of glutamate receptors in the mammalian central nervous system. J Child Neurol 2004;19:343-60.
9. Schoepp DD, Jane DE, Monn JA. Pharmacological agents acting at subtypes of metabotropic glutamate receptors. Neuropharmacology 1999;38:1431-76.
10. Urwyler S, Mosbacher J, Lingenhoehl K, et al. Positive allosteric modulation of native and recombinant gamma-aminobutyric acid(B) receptors by 2,6-Di-tert-butyl-4-(3-hydroxy-2,2-dimethyl-propyl)-phenol (CGP7930) and its aldehyde analog CGP13501. Mol Pharmacol 2001;60:963-71.
11. Kohrs R, Durieux ME. Ketamine: teaching an old drug new tricks. Anesth Analg 1998;87:1186-93.
12. Tortella FC, Pellicano M, Bowery NG. Dextromethorphan and neuromodulation: old drug coughs up new activities. Trends Pharmacol Sci 1989;10:501-7.
13. Westphalen RI, Hemmings HC Jr. Selective depression by general anesthetics of glutamate versus GABA release from isolated cortical nerve terminals. J Pharmacol Exp Ther 2003;304:1188-96.
14. Lehmann A. Inhibitors of transient lower esophageal sphincter relaxations ("reflux inhibitors") in the future treatment of GERD. Gastroenterol Hepatol Ann Rev 2006;1:109-17.
15. Mittal RK, Holloway RH, Penagini R, Blackshaw LA, Dent J. Transient lower esophageal sphincter relaxation. Gastroenterology 1995;109:601-10.
16. Ciccaglione AF, Marzio L. Effect of acute and chronic administration of the GABA B agonist baclofen on 24 hour pH metry and symptoms in control subjects and in patients with gastro-oesophageal reflux disease. Gut 2003;52:464-70.
17. Koek GH, Sifrim D, Lerut T, Janssens J, Tack J. Effect of the GABAB agonist baclofen in patients with symptoms and duodeno-gastro-oesophageal reflux refractory to proton pump inhibitors. Gut 2003;52:1397-402.
18. Kawai M, Kawahara H, Hirayama S, Yoshimura N, Ida S. Effect of baclofen on emesis and 24-hour esophageal pH in neurologically impaired children with gastroesophageal reflux disease. J Pediatr Gastroenterol Nutr 2004;38:317-23.
19. Hirsch DP, Tytgat GN, Boeckxstaens GE. Is glutamate involved in transient lower esophageal sphincter relaxations? Dig Dis Sci 2002;47:661-6.
20. Lehmann A, Brändén L. Effects of antagonism of NMDA receptors on transient lower esophageal sphincter relaxations in the dog. Eur J Pharmacol 2001;431:253-8.
21. Jensen J, Lehmann A, Uvebrant A, et al. Transient lower esophageal sphincter relaxations in dogs are inhibited by a metabotropic glutamate receptor 5 antagonist. Eur J Pharmacol 2005;519:154-7.
22. Frisby CL, Mattsson JP, Jensen JM, Lehmann A, Dent J, Blackshaw LA. Inhibition of transient lower esophageal sphincter relaxation and gastroesophageal reflux by metabotropic glutamate receptor ligands. Gastroenterology 2005;129:995-1004.
23. Lee KJ, Vos R, Janssens J, Tack J. Differential effects of baclofen on lower oesophageal sphincter pressure and proximal gastric motility in humans. Aliment Pharmacol Ther 2003;18:199-207.
24. Smid SD, Young RL, Cooper NJ, Blackshaw LA. GABA(B)R expressed on vagal afferent neurones inhibit gastric mechanosensitivity in ferret proximal stomach. Am J Physiol 2001;281:G1494-501.
25. Page AJ, Young RL, Martin CM, et al. Metabotropic glutamate receptors inhibit mechanosensitivity in vagal sensory neurons. Gastroenterology 2005;128:402-10.
26. Slattery JA, Page AJ, Blackshaw LA. Ionotropic glutamate receptor modulation of vagal afferent mechanosensitivity in mouse. Gastroenterology 2005;128:A495.
27. Willert RP, Woolf CJ, Hobson AR, Delaney C, Thompson DG, Aziz Q. The development and maintenance of human visceral pain hypersensitivity is dependent on the N-methyl-D-aspartate receptor. Gastroenterology 2004;126:683-92.
28. Blackshaw LA, Staunton E, Lehmann A, Dent J. Inhibition of transient LES relaxations and reflux in ferrets by GABA receptor agonists. Am J Physiol 1999;277:G867-74.
29. Beaumont H, Pierrou S, Jönsson-Rylander AC, et al. The role of GABAA receptors in the control of transient lower esophageal sphincter relaxations (TLESRs) in the dog. Neurogastroenterol Mot 2006;in press.
30. Lehmann A, Antonsson M, Bremner-Danielsen M, Flärdh M, Hansson-Brändén L, Kärrberg L. Activation of the GABAB receptor inhibits transient lower esophageal sphincter relaxations in dogs. Gastroenterology 1999;117:1147-54.
31. Liu J, Pehlivanov N, Mittal RK. Baclofen blocks LES relaxation and crural diaphragm inhibition by esophageal and gastric distension in cats. Am J Physiol 2002;283:G1276-81.
32. Lidums I, Lehmann A, Checklin H, Dent J, Holloway RH. Control of transient lower esophageal sphincter relaxations and reflux by the GABAB agonist baclofen in normal subjects.. Gastroenterology 2000;118:7-13.
33. van Herwaarden MA, Samsom M, Rydholm H, Smout AJ. The effect of baclofen on gastro-oesophageal reflux, lower oesophageal sphincter function and reflux symptoms in patients with reflux disease. Aliment Pharmacol Ther 2002;16:1655-62.

Achalasia and esophageal pain: what is the prevalence and possible mechanism?

A.M. Drewes (Aalborg)

The burden of pain in achalasia

Visceral pain is very frequent both in the normal population and in the clinic [1]. Pain is also a major symptom in achalasia and is present in approximately 70% of the patients (*Figure 1*) [2,3]. The reason for the pain is most likely related to acid reflux, dilatation of the esophagus and fermentation of food in the organ [4]. More importantly the pain is often atypical and may overshadow more traditional symptoms such as dysphagia and regurgitation leading to a delay in diagnosis. Diseases giving rise to visceral pain are often difficult to diagnose. This is partly due to the sparse and diffuse termination of visceral afferents at the central nervous system (CNS), together with the interaction between visceral pain and the somatic, autonomic and enteric nervous systems, which often blurs the clinical picture. Hence, complaints related to the autonomic nervous system and symptoms related to referred pain to somatic structures can easily change the clinical impression of the patient. For example are the symptoms due to gastrointestinal diseases initially often vague and concomitant complaints related to e.g., enteric dysfunction (nausea, constipation, etc.) are frequently the major complains. Referred pain to e.g., the abdomen and back can be dominating symptoms in patients with diseases of the esophagus, and hence may the diseased organs be overlooked at the first visit, especially if the symptoms are intermittently present. Thus, to understand the symptoms in achalasia knowledge about the visceral pain system is important.

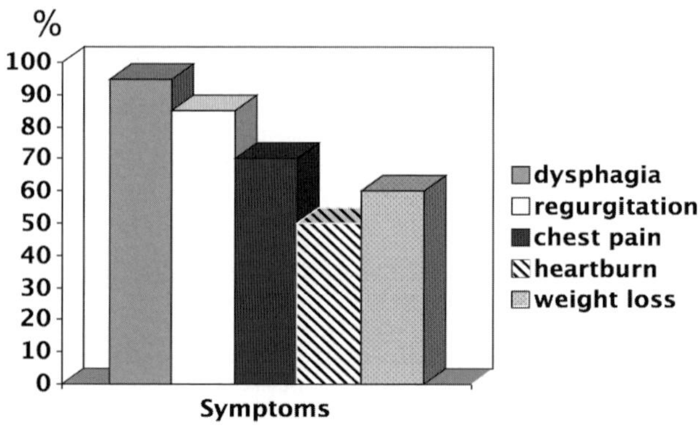

Figure 1. The prevalence of different symptoms in achalasia. Approximately 70% suffers from pain.

Pain physiology

The activity in the visceral organs does normally not reach the higher brain centers, except from information due to filling of the esophagus, stomach, rectum and bladder. However, when the organs are potentially in danger – such as due to diseases – symptoms such as discomfort and pain are reported. The feeling is typically vague and difficult to characterize, and is often quite distinct from what is felt during noxious diseases of the somatic system. That visceral pain is different from the somatic counterpart is mainly explained by the different anatomical structures of the two systems (*Figure 2*). All histological specified layers of the organs seem to be innervated by sensory afferents, although the density and specificity seems to differ in the individual layers and organs. The reproductive organs, the esophagus and rectum also have a somatic innervation. The importance of this innervation is not known, although the rectum has more complex functions than most other viscera and may need a more differentiated innervation. The peritoneum and parietal serous membranes of the lungs and heart have their own parietal nerve supply, which is organized like the skin [5]. Hence, pain from these structures gives a distinct, intense and localized pain, which is comparable to the pain evoked by skin lesions.

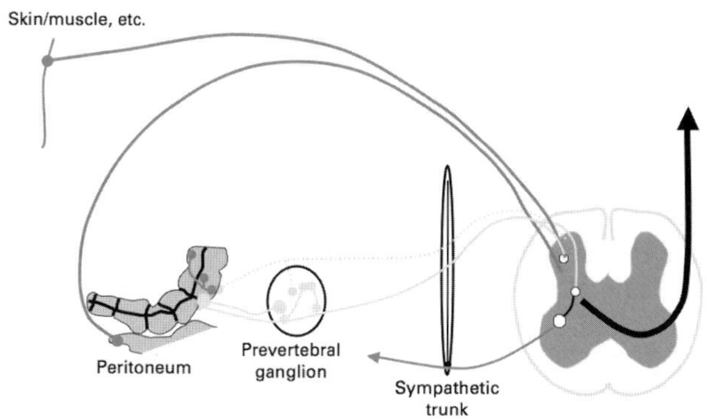

Figure 2. The afferent nerve supply of the gut. "True" visceral afferents (grey) innervate the gut and most run temporarily together with either the sympathetic (most pain mediating fibers) or parasympathetic nerves to enter the spinal cord. During inflammation "silent afferents" (dashed line) may become activated and contribute to the sensory response. The peritoneum and parietal serous membranes of the lungs and heart has their own parietal nerve supply, which is organized like the somatic structures (black afferents).

The afferent nerves from the esophagus do primarily project to the spinal cord or brain stem, but can also send information to the viscera by extra-central reflexes with the autonomic/enteric nerves. The visceral afferents are integrated into the autonomic nervous system. Hence, the spinal visceral innervation where the afferents travel together with the sympathetic nerves is to some degree segmental organized, whereas fibers traveling together with the parasympathetic system ascend *via* the vagal nerves to the nodose ganglia and terminate in the brainstem. The autonomic nerves exert mainly secretory and trophic integrity together with control of motility (for further information see [6]). In the major parts of the gut these integrative systems are under normal circumstances automatic and are not influenced by the CNS. In the esophagus, however, initiation of swallowing can be under voluntary control, as the upper part of the organ has a somatic innervation. Most afferents mediating conscious sensory information travel together with the sympathetic nerves, whereas those traveling together with the parasympathetic nerves mainly are involved in secretion, motor and regulatory reflexes that does not reach consciousness. In the esophagus, however, nerves traveling together with the vagal nerves may also signal pain, and there is increasing evidence for pain transmission *via* vagal afferents from other segments of the gut [7]. The complex anatomy gives possibility for cross-talk with the autonomic nervous system at several peripheral and central levels. Thus, excitation of visceral afferent neurons may not only elicit pain and discomfort, but also induce protective spinal and extra-spinal reflexes as well as peripheral changes of target organ responses. This can explain the changes in blood pressure, heart rate, sweating, nausea, vomiting and piloerection typically evoked by visceral pain.

The enteric nervous system is closely related to the CNS and the autonomic nervous system [8]. It has a neural network within the myenteric and submucous plexus, and is a local minibrain with reflexes and a library of information for different patterns of gut behaviour. Motility changes are frequently seen during anxiety and stress, and interactions between the emotional state and the enteric nervous system can be seen as changes in abdominal pain, nausea and altered secretion/absorption.

In the spinal cord the nociceptive afferents terminate mostly in laminae I and V [9]. The visceral afferents converge on a large scale with neurones in lamina I and V that receive input from superficial and deep somatic tissue as well as other viscera (*Figure 3*). Accordingly, in the thoracic spinal cord more that 75% of all neurons receive both somatic and visceral information, being contrasted by the actual number of visceral afferents (5-15% of the inflow) entering the dorsal roots [10]. The low density of sensory innervation may therefore explain why large areas of the gut appear to be relatively insensitive to pain stimuli. The visceral afferent terminals are widely distributed at the spinal level and some organs have a spinal representation spreading to multiple segmental levels [7]. For example the esophagus is innervated craniocaudally from the first cervical to the second lumbar segments [10]. Therefore a few visceral afferent fibers can activate many neurons through the extensive functional convergence [11], and this wide activation of the CNS may explain the diffuse and unpleasant nature of visceral pain. The poor localization of symptoms from the esophagus was demonstrated in a clinical study by [12]. The subjective localization of dysphagia in 101 patients was reviewed after they have been investigated with endoscopy and manometry. Patient localization to the proximal esophagus was accurate in only 1.8% of cases! Mid-esophageal localization was never related to mid-esophageal anatomic pathology, whereas distal localization was correct in 80%.

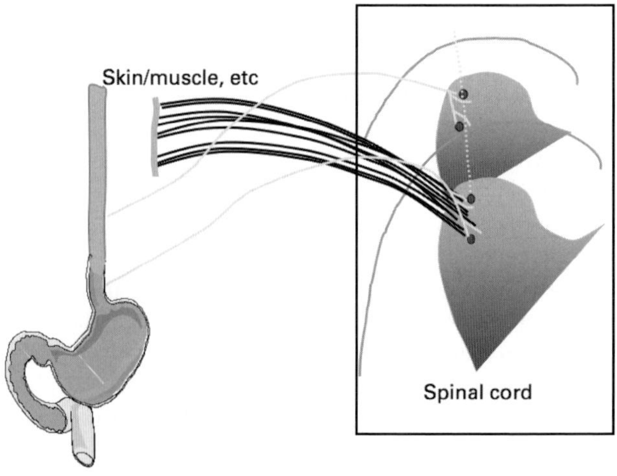

Figure 3. The innervation of the viscera is very sparse compared to the somatic system. On the other hand most visceral afferents converge with neurons that receive input from superficial and deep somatic tissue as well as other viscera. The diffuse and widespread innervation of the spinal cord may to some degree explain the unpleasant nature of visceral pain.

Pain originating in the gut is typically felt in areas remote from the organ as referred pain. This clinical experience is supported in experimental studies where localized stimuli of the esophagus, stomach small and large intestine may be projected somatic areas far from the gut focus [13,14]. The referred pain area is a proxy of central hyperexcitability. This area is often enlarged in patients with organic diseases of the esophagus (*Figure 4*). Primary allodynia/hyperalgesia together with central hyperexcitability can by itself adequately explain the pain associated with inflammatory conditions as well as that in functional disorders [15,16]. Thus, after the peripheral stimulation (such as inflammation due to reflux) subsides, sensitized second order neurons continue to fire, and for example subthreshold regulatory stimuli are still perceived as painful.

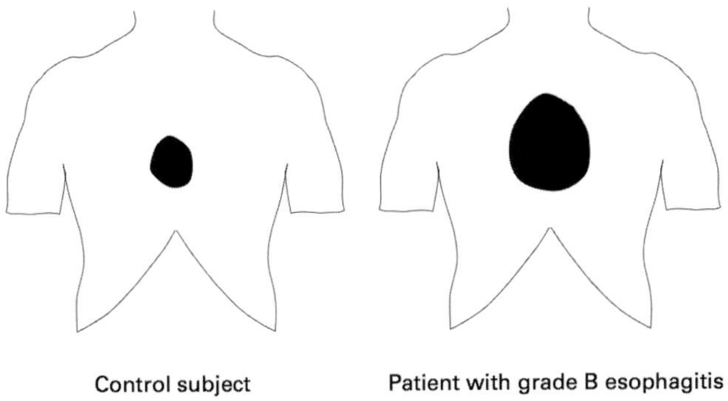

Figure 4. Referred pathways may be activated by impulses converging from visceral pathways to central neurons also receiving somatic input. The activity in these central neurons may be interpreted by the patient as somatic pain. As illustrated the referred pain to electrical stimulation of the esophagus in patients with esophagitis is typically much larger than in healthy controls.

In the context of algogenic processes from internal organs, an important role is also to be attributed to the so-called phenomena of viscero-visceral hyperalgesia. Viscero-visceral hyperalgesia is a complex form of hypersensitivity which is likely to be explained by more than one mechanism. Since this phenomenon takes place preferentially between visceral organs which share, at least in part, their central projection, it is plausible that phenomena of central sensitization play an important role.

During diseases such as achalasia sensitization of the peripheral and mainly central neuronal pathways probably take place. Peripheral nociceptor sensitization underlies the hyperalgesia that develop immediate around an injury site. Central rather that peripheral sensitization is thought to be accountable for many of the symptoms seen in diseases of the gut. Neurophysiologically, central sensitization is characterized by increased spontaneous activity, decreased firing threshold and expansion of the receptive fields of dorsal horn neurons [17]. In diseases of the chest organs such central hyperexcitability, as well as alterations in supraspinal descending modulation, may explain the increase the sensation to painful stimuli (hyperalgesia) and to stimuli that are normally not perceived as pain (allodynia) [17]. Under some circumstances the central hyperexcitability seems to outlive the presence of the primary focus [18]. Experimentally studies using electrical and mechanical stimuli have indicated that acid perfusion of the esophagus results in peripheral as well as central sensitization of the nervous system [19-21]. This probably reflects central neuroplastic changes evoked by the peripheral sensitization as have also been shown in somatic studies. Thus, it is likely that in patients with latent reflux this sensitization and visceral hyperalgesia may persist after the local injury has healed, leading to e.g., functional or "non-cardiac chest pain".

The course of chest pain in achalasia

Eckard *et al.* [2] followed 101 patients with achalasia for 18 years, where 63% initially had chest pain. Over the years improvement in chest pain frequency occurred, but a significant proportion still had unimproved chest pain. However, it is unpredictable which patients improve, and most importantly no relationship exists between manometric/radiologic findings and the symptoms in achalasia [22]. Eckard *et al.* also investigated the probability of chest pain after effective therapy relieving dysphagia and regurgitation. Episodic chest pain persisted in 40% despite disappearance of the other symptoms, pointing towards more complex pathophysiology behind the pain in achalasia patients [2]. The same authors found that there was a delay of ~ 5 years before the right diagnosis was found, predominantly due to misinterpretation of the typical findings by the physician. Among 87 patients, 15% consulted five or more physicians before the presence of an esophageal motility disorder was suspected [23]. This also reflects the importance of abnormal representations of visceral pain in the clinic.

Explanations for the pain in achalasia

The reason for the pain in achalasia is believed to be regurgitation of acid, dilatation and fermentation of food. However, Echardt *et al.* found no relation between the severity of chest pain on the one hand and dysphagia, esophageal morphology and function on the other. Thus, they concluded that mechanical factors are unlikely causes of chest pain [2]. Achalasia is a neurogenic disorder with loss of inhibitory nitrinergic neurons in the myenteric plexus of the esophagus [24]. In other diseases with destruction of the nerves such as after spinal cord injury, post-herpetic and diabetic neuropathy, pain is a frequent complication with stimulus-independent and stimulus-evoked pain features [25]. It is therefore plausible that neuropathic pain may contribute to the pain in achalasia. In other diseases of the gut such as chronic pancreatitis there is evidence for features of neuropathic pain. Histological findings in the pancreas in these patients have revealed an increase in the number and diameter of pancreatic nerve fibers and in the amount of neurotransmitters. These findings are also seen after neuronal lesions in other tissues and have supported that neurogenic inflammation plays a key role in the pain pathogenesis [26]. Some of the mechanisms in neuropathic pain are outlined in *Figure 5*. Typically the cause of pain is a mixture of sensitization of nociceptors terminals, loss of cells and axons, spontaneous firing of damaged afferents and loss of central inhibition amongst other mechanisms [25].

In pancreatitis hypoalgesia to stimulation of the upper gut is a cardinal feature in experimental studies [27]. Hypoalgesia was also seen in the only experimental study of achalasia [28]. Therefore the pain in pancreatitis and achalasia may share at least some mechanisms. The reason for the hypoalgesia to experimental stimulation may be increased inhibition from midbrain structures counteracting the increased afferent barrage from peripheral afferents with spontaneous firing such as in neuropathic pain. In the clinic neuropathic pain is typically characterized by stimulus-independent pain which is typically shooting, lancinating or burning, and stimulus-evoked pain that has features of allodynia

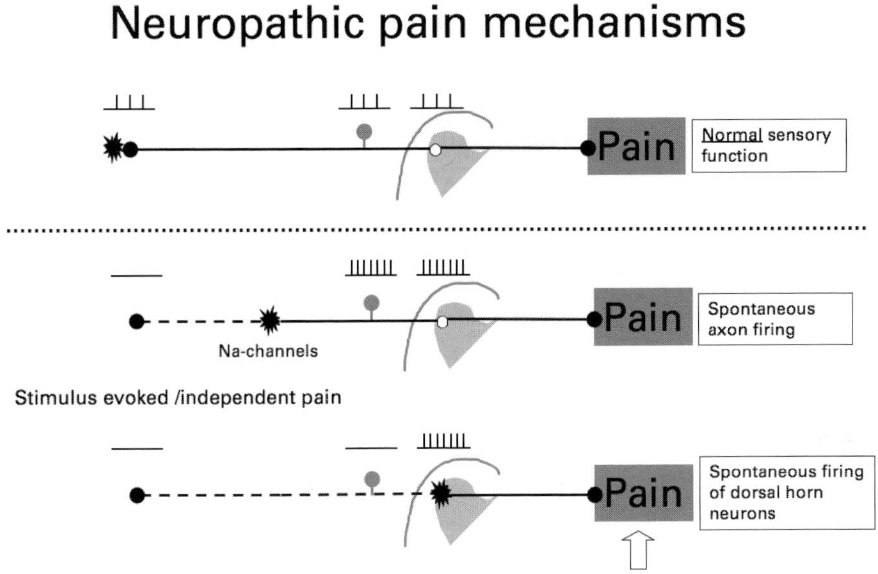

Figure 5. The normal sensory function mediating pain to the central nervous system is illustrated in the top figure. Below the stippled line some mechanisms for neuropathic pain are outlined. After nerve injury sodium channels may accumulate at the neuroma site and ectopic action potentials are interpreted as pain. The secondary neurons in the central nervous system can also fire spontaneously due to reduced activity of the normal inhibitory mechanisms. Furthermore GABA and opioids receptors are typically downregulated. These mechanisms may work at a segmental level in the spinal cord or can involve descending pathways from the brain stem.

and hyperalgesia. Such features are also seen in pain arising from the esophagus, and hence increased sensitivity to e.g., food and acid in the esophagus may be a clinical finding. However, no studies have systematically investigated the sensory profile in achalasia with more advanced methods [29] and more clinical, epidemiological and experimental studies are highly warranted to understand the symptoms and improve treatment of these difficult patients.

References

1. Sandler RS, Stewart WF, Liberman JN, Ricci JA, Zorich NL. Abdominal pain, bloating, and diarrhea in the United States: prevalence and impact. Dig Dis Sci 2000;45:1166-71.
2. Eckardt VF, Stauf B, Bernhard G. Chest pain in achalasia: patient characteristics and clinical course. Gastroenterology 1999;116:1300-4.
3. Eckardt VF, Kohne U, Junginger T, Westermeier T. Risk factors for diagnostic delay in achalasia. Dig Dis Sci 1997;42:580-5.
4. Patti MG, Arcerito M, Tong J, et al. Importance of preoperative and postoperative pH monitoring in patients with esophageal achalasia. J Gastrointest Surg 1997;1:505-10.
5. Bonica JJ. Anatomic and physiologic basis of nociception and pain. In: Bonica JJ, ed. The management of pain. Philidelphia: Lea and Febiger, 1990:1186-213.
6. Jänig W, Häbler HJ. Visceral-autonomic integration. In: Gebhart GF, ed. Visceral pain, progress in pain research and management. Seattle: IASP Press, 1995:311-48.
7. Bielefeldt K, Christianson JA, Davis BM. Basic and clinical aspects of visceral sensation: transmission in the CNS. Neurogastroenterol Motil 2005;17:488-99.

8. Wood JD, Alpers DH, Andrews PL. Fundamentals of neurogastroenterology. Gut 1999;45:II6-II16.
9. Cervero F,.Laird JM. Visceral pain. Lancet 1999;353:2145-8.
10. Sengupta JN, Gebhart GF. Gastrointestinal afferent fibers and sensation. In: Johnson L, ed. Physiology of the gastrointestinal tract. New York: Raven Press, 1994:484-519.
11. Giamberardino MA,Vecchiet L. Pathophysiology of visceral pain. Curr Rev Pain 1996;1:23-33.
12. Roeder BE, Murray JA, Dierkhising RA. Patient localization of esophageal dysphagia. Dig Dis Sci 2004;49:697-701.
13. Drewes AM, Schipper KP, Dimcevski G, et al. Multimodal assessment of pain in the esophagus: a new experimental model. Am J Physiol Gastrointest Liver Physiol 2002;283:G95-103.
14. Drewes AM, Rossel P, Le Pera D, Arendt-Nielsen L, Valeriani M. Cortical neuroplastic changes to painful colon stimulation in patients with irritable bowel syndrome. Neurosci Lett 2005;375:157-61.
15. Drewes AM, Pedersen J, Reddy H, et al. Central sensitisation in patients with non-cardiac chest pain: a clinical experimental study. Scand J Gastroenterol 2006;41:1-10.
16. Drewes AM, Reddy H, Pedersen J, Funch-Jensen P, Gregersen G, Arendt-Nielsen L. Multimodal pain stimulations in patients with grade B oesophagitis. Gut 2006;55:926-32.
17. Coderre TJ, Katz J, Vaccarino AL, Melzack R. Contribution of central neuroplasticity to pathological pain: review of clinical and experimental evidence. Pain 1993;52:259-85.
18. Gebhart GF. Visceral pain-peripheral sensitisation. Gut 2000;47:iv54-5.
19. Sarkar S, Aziz Q, Woolf CJ, Hobson AR, Thompson DG. Contribution of central sensitisation to the development of non-cardiac chest pain. Lancet 2000;356:1154-9.
20. Drewes AM, Schipper K-P, Dimcevski G, et al. Multi-modal induction and assessment of allodynia and hyperalgesia in the human oesophagus. Eur J Pain 2003;7:539-49.
21. Sami SA, Rössel P, Dimcevski G, et al. Cortical changes to experimental sensitization of the human esophagus. Neuroscience 2006;140:269-79.
22. Blam ME, Delfyett W, Levine MS, Metz DC, Katzka DA. Achalasia: a disease of varied and subtle symptoms that do not correlate with radiographic findings. Am J Gastroenterol 2002;97:1916-23.
23. Eckardt VF, Kohne U, Junginger T, Westermeier T. Risk factors for diagnostic delay in achalasia. Dig Dis Sci 1997;42:580-5.
24. Park W,Vaezi MF. Etiology and pathogenesis of achalasia: the current understanding. Am J Gastroenterol 2005;100:1404-14.
25. Woolf CJ, Mannion RJ. Neuropathic pain: aetiology, symptoms, mechanisms, and management. Lancet 1999;353:1959-64.
26. Di SP, di Mola FF, Di FC, et al. Expression of interleukin 8 (IL-8) and substance P in human chronic pancreatitis. Gut 2000;47:423-8.
27. Dimcevski G, Schipper KP, Tage-Jensen U, et al. Hypoalgesia to experimental visceral and somatic stimulation in painful chronic pancreatitis. Eur J Gastroenterol Hepatol 2006;18:755-64.
28. Brackbill S, Shi G, Hirano I. Diminished mechanosensitivity and chemosensitivity in patients with achalasia. Am J Physiol Gastrointest Liver Physiol 2003;285:G1198-203.
29. Drewes AM, Gregersen H, Arendt-Nielsen L. Experimental pain in gastroenterology: a reappraisal of human studies. Scand J Gastroenterol 2003;38:1115-30.

Mechanisms of reflux-induced signs and symptoms in non-acid reflux

F. Pace, S. Pallotta, P. Molteni (Milan)

Although acid reflux is considered the most relevant pathogenetic factor in gastroesophageal reflux disease (GERD), the nonacid component of the refluxate may play a role in inducing reflux symptoms and esophageal damage. As an example, it is well known that pepsin, even in small amounts, may greatly increase both the microscopic and macroscopic esophageal mucosal damage due to acid [1-3]. Most studies on nonacid reflux have focused on the importance of duodenogastroesophageal reflux (DGER) in the generation of esophageal damage, complications of GERD, and recently also persisting symptoms despite apppropriate antisecretory treatment [4]. Thus, biliary reflux has been shown to have a synergistic role with acid in some patients with Barrett's esophagus [5,6], in complicated esophagitis [7], and in GERD patients refractory to proton pump inhibitors (PPIs) [8]. Beside these observations, esophageal exposure to isolated bile reflux has been shown to be responsible for reflux esophagitis or Barrett's development in patients without gastric acid secretion, i.e. after total gastrectomy [9,10].

However, as recognized by others [4], substantiation of the role of DGER has been hampered by the lack of a "true" gold standard by which it can be measured; in fact, many methods have been proposed in the recent past, each one with its one advantages and disadvantages.

Historically, DGER has been thought to be measurable by scintigraphy, endoscopy, gastric aspiration techniques, ambulatory gastric pH monitoring and more recently by endoluminal spectrophotometric techniques (Bilitec™) and impedance monitoring [4]; notably, only the last three methods will allow continuous and physiological measurements to be performed. However, the pH-metric identification of esophageal pH > 7 as a marker of DGER, as proposed by Pellegrini and DeMeester [11], is confounded by several problems, and may be in fact considered a misnomer [12]; as an example, no correlation can be found between precentage of total time with pH > 7 and bile reflux, as measured by a combined ambulatory pH and bilirubin device (Bilitec™) [6].

The latter, i.e., a device which allows combined bilirubin monitoring (Bilitec") with pH monitoring, originally proposed by Bechi *et al.* [13], provides the most accurate information available with regard to DGER in humans [4].

Recently, a new technique has been introduced to study bolus movements in hollow organs like the esophagus, i.e. the intraluminal impedance monitoring (IIM), which allows detection of gastroesophagal reflux based on changes in resistance to electrical current flow between two or more electrodes, when a liquid and/or gas bolus moves between them [14]. The present literature contains different definitions of "non-acid" reflux, which has been used either to indicate DGER events detected at Bilitec™ monitoring [4] or reflux events diagnosed by IIM when no change in pH occurs, or a pH fall of less than 1 pH unit [15].

To our knowledge, no study using the two techniques simultaneously has been conducted so far. We therefore planned a study to verify the hypothesis that no correlation could exist between non-acid reflux episodes, as detected by IIM and biliary reflux episodes, as detected by Bilitec™.

We choose to simultaneously perform the two tests in a heterogeneous group of GERD patients, namely 20 patients refractory to PPI therapy or with atypical symptoms. Furthermore, some of them were on and some other were off PPI therapy during the tests. Details of the study can be found elsewhere [16].

Under these conditions, it turned out that no correlation at all can be found between the two methods as far as detection and identification of non-acid *versus* biliary reflux episodes is concerned. Intuitively, the main explanation for this observation is the fact, that at least in the intact human stomach, biliary reflux may occur at different pH values, including acid ones [4], and therefore the pH change during reflux cannot allow the presence of bile acids in the refluxate to be suspected. Thus, similarly to what has already been established with pH-metry, when it was proposed and then refused to use pH > 7 as marker of DGER, the only possibility to confidently identify a biliary content in the refluxate is a direct method to be used, such as esophageal aspiration with subsequent chemical analysis [17] or "*in situ*" spectrophotometric determination of bilirubin content [13], but cannot be deduced by indirect methods, such as IIM.

The practical consequence of our study is that, despite the fact that IIM offers the "opportunity to conceive gastroesophageal reflux more broadly, both in terms of frequency and characteristics of the refluxate" [18], it cannot describe its composition, in particular in terms of biliary content, which can only be afforded by esophageal bilirubin concentration monitoring. Both techniques will be ultimately required in order to characterize a non-acid reflux episod in its physico-chemical essence.

In conclusion, our study has confirmed that biliary reflux and non-acid reflux as detected respectively by Bilitec™ and by IIM are two distinct phenomena, which need different techniques to be assessed in humans.

References

1. Goldberg HI, Dodds WJ, Gee S, Montgomery C, Zborlaske FF. Role of acid and pepsin in acute experimental esophagitis. Gastroenterology 1969;56:223-30.
2. Johnson LF, Harmon JW. Experimental esophagitis in a rabbit model. J Clin Gastroenterol 1986;8:26-44.
3. Zaninotto G, Di Mario F, Costantini M, et al. Oesophagitis and pH of refluxate: an experiemental and clinical study. Br J Surg 1992;79:161-4.
4. Katz PO. Review article: the role of non-acid reflux in gastro-oesopahgeal reflux disease. Aliment Pharmacol Ther 2000;14:1539-51.
5. Attwood SEA, DeMeester TR, Bremner CG, Barlow AP, Hinder RA. Alkaline gastro-esophageal reflux: implications in development of complications in Barrett's columnar lined lower esophagus. Surgery 1989;106:764-70.
6. Champion G, Richter JE, Vaezi MF, Singh S, Alexander R. Duodenogastroesophageal reflux: relationship to pH and importance in barrett's esophagus. Gastroenterology 1994;107:747-54.
7. Robertson D, Aldersley M, Shepherd H, et al. Patterns of acid reflux in complicated oesophagitis. Gut 1987;28:1484-8.
8. Tack J, Koek G, Demedts I, Sifrim D, Janssens J. Gastroesophageal reflux disease poorly responsive to single-dose proton pump inhibitors in patients without Barrett's esophagus: acid reflux, bile reflux or both? Am J Gastroenterol 2004;99:981-8.
9. Yumiba T, Kawahara H, Nishikawa K, Inoue Y, Ito T, Matsuda H. Impact of esophageal bile exposure on the genesis of reflux esophagitis in the absence of gastrica acid after total gastrectomy. Am J Gastroenterol 2002;97:1647-52.
10. Taha AS, Angerson WJ, Morran CG. Reflux and Barrett's oesophagitis after gastric surgery- long-term follow-up and implications for the roles of gastric acid and bile in oesophagitis. Aliment Pharmacol Ther 2003;17:547-52.
11. Pellegrini CA, DeMeester TR, Wernly JA, Johnson LF, Skinner DB. Alkaline gastroesophageal reflux. Am J Surg 1978;75:177-84.
12. Vaezi MF, Richter JE. Importance of duodeno-gastro-esophageal reflux in the medical outpatient practice. Hepato-gastroenterol 1999;46:40-7.
13. Bechi P, Paucciani F, Baldini F, et al. Long-term ambulatori enterogastric reflux monitoring system. Validation of a new fiberoptic technique. Dig Dis Sci 1993;38:1297-306.
14. Silny J. Intraluminal multiple electrical impedance procedure for measurement of gastro-intestinal motility. J Gastrointest Motil 1991;3:151-62.
15. Vela M, Camacho-Lobato L, Srinivasan R Tutuian R, Katz PO, Castell DO. Simultaneous intraesophageal impedance and pH measurement of acid and non-acid gasrtoesophageal reflux: effect of omeprazole. Gastroenterology 2001;120:1599-606.
16. Pace F, Sangaletti O, Pallotta S, Molteni P, Porro GB. Biliary and non-acid reflux are two distinct phenomena: a comparison between 24-h multichannel intraesophageal impedance and bilirubin monitoring, Scand J Gastroenterol 2007;42:1031-9.
17. Stein HJ, Kauer WHK, Feussner H, et al. Bile acids as components of the duodenogastric refluxate: detection, relationship to bilirubin, mechanism of injury and clinical relevance. Hepatogastroenterol 1999;46:66-73.
18. Sifrim D, Castell D, Dent J, Kahrilas PJ. Gastro-oesophageal reflux monitoring: review and consensus report on detection and definitions of acid, non-acid and gas reflux. Gut 2004;53:1024-31.

Globus – what causes that sensation?

I.J. Cook (Sydney)

Definition and epidemiology

Globus is extremely common being reported in 7-46% of the general population [1-4]. The symptom in healthy individuals who are not seeking health care for it shares an equal prevalence between males and females [2,5] but there is a higher prevalence of females among those seeking health care for globus [6]. Typically the symptom is described as a sense of a lump or retained food bolus or tightness in the throat. A range of other foreign body-like descriptors are volunteered by patients including a sense of retained particulate matter, mucus accumulation or a restrictive or choking sensation. There are additional qualifiers on which there seems to be broad agreement. The symptom is non-painful, frequently improve with eating, and is frequently episodic [2,6-8]. Conversely, there are a number of features which most would agree incompatible with the diagnosis such as constant or intermittent pain or weight loss [2,9]; dysphagia or odynophagia [7,10]. The most recent consensus-derived definition of globus forms part of the Rome III criteria for functional disorders (*Table I*) [11].

Table I. Rome III definition of globus.

1. Persistent or intermittent, non-painful, sensation of a lump or foreign body in the throat or neck
AND
2. Occurrence of the sensation between meals
AND
3. Absence of dysphagia or odynophagia
AND
4. Absence of evidence that gastroesophageal acid reflux is the cause of the symptoms
AND
5. Absence of histopathology-based esophageal motility disorders (e.g. achalasia, diffuse esophageal spasm)

Aetiology

A number of conditions have been reported to be associated with globus including hiatal hernia, cervical osteophytes, cricopharyngeal bar, cervical web, peptic ulcer and gallstones. However, the prevalence of such findings varies dramatically among such studies [9,12,13]. A well designed prospective analysis of 77 consecutive cases found normal radiographic examinations in 53% and hiatus hernias in only 13% [14]. Hiatal hernia is unlikely to have aetiological significance as the reported prevalence of hiatus hernia in uncontrolled studies of globus patients (30-50%) [9-13] is comparable to that estimated in the general population [15,16]. The cricopharyngeal bar, found in up to 17% of individuals undergoing contrast radiography [17,18], is no more prevalent in globus [9]. In summary, there is no good evidence to attribute globus to any local anatomical abnormality.

A range of plausible mechanisms have been proposed to explain globus including gastroesophageal reflux (GER), esophageal dysmotility, cricopharyngeal spasm, reflexive hypercontraction of the cricopharyngeus in response to oesophageal stimuli (eg acid or distension), deglutitive pharyngeal motor dysfunction, and reflexive cough or habitual throat clearing in response to esophageal acidification.

Cricopharyngeal hypertonicity was initially suspected when an early study, using a posteriorly oriented perfused catheter and pull-through technique, found higher resting upper esophageal sphincter (UES) pressures when compared with controls [19]. However, UES pressure is labile and both responsive to emotional stress and to local physical stimulation. Hence this finding may better reflect an abnormal response to the mechanical stimulation induced by the pull-through itself [20]. Accordingly, subsequent studies, either using stationary sleeve sensors [5,21] or non-perfused manometric catheters and a station pull-through technique to measure UES tone [5,22], found no difference in resting UES pressure in globus compared with controls. The notion that UES hyper-reactivity might be implicated in globus was formally evaluated in response to stimuli known to augment sphincter tone. Although the symptom of globus is anecdotally precipitated by deep emotion, and although the UES normally contracts in response to emotional stress, such stress-induced augmentation in UES tone in these patients is normal [21]. Additionally, UES pressure augmentation in response to esophageal balloon distension was comparable to that of controls [23].

Based on videoradiographic and most manometric assessments, the pharyngeal swallow mechanism is normal in globus [12,24]. This is not surprising as these patients do not have dysphagia and symptoms generally improve during eating.

Another hypothesis that has been explored is that esophageal motor or sensory dysfunction accounts globus. A tertiary referral centre which carefully examined physiological and psychometric variables in globus patients reported approximately 25% of those presenting with globus to have manometrically proven achalasia [24,25]. However, 21 of 24 of such patients had one or more of the typical symptoms of achalasia when questioned after the diagnosis was made. Furthermore, this is not a consistent finding among other studies. Other motor disorders, including diffuse esophageal spasm and non-specific motor disorders have been reported in a proportion of patients [26-28] although the prevalence among such studies varies widely [5] (*Table II*). One controlled study found no difference in the prevalence of these motility abnormalities (25%) between patients and controls [28]. On the basis of current evidence, it is possible that esophageal dysmotility

Table II. Studies examining esophageal motor function in patients with globus. Only one study examined controls (with non-ulcer dyspepsia).

Author	Study design	n	Achalasia	DES	NSEMD	Aperistalsis
Wilson 1987	Uncontrolled	47	0%	2%	0%	0%
Linsell 1987	Uncontrolled	18	0%	11%	11%	0%
Moser 1991	Uncontrolled	30	23%	3%	23%	0%
Farkkila 1994	Uncontrolled	21	0%	0%	29%	0%
Leelamanit 1997	Uncontrolled	111	0%	0%	20%	20%
Hill 1997	Controlled	26	0%	4%	15%	4%

might have globus as one of its manifestations, but there is certainly no esophageal motor pattern which characterises globus and the majority of globus sufferers do not have significant esophageal dysmotility.

A popular, but unsubstantiated hypothesis, is that GER accounts for globus. Unfortunately, the evidence for a causative link between GER disease (GERD) and globus is sparse. However, there is a little epidemiological evidence supporting a potential causative link. A population survey in Olmstead county found a prevalence for heartburn or regurgitation of 42% and for globus of 7%. More relevant, the odds ratio of someone with reflux symptoms experiencing globus was 1.9 (95% CI, 1.0-3.6) times that of someone without reflux symptoms [3].

Pooling data from studies utilising ambulatory 24-hour pH monitoring, increased esophageal acid exposure is present in around one third of patients with globus [12,27-33]. The two key issues, however, are whether GERD is over-represented in globus compared with appropriate controls and whether esophageal acidification causes the symptom. There are only two adequately controlled studies that addressed these issues and they report conflicting results [12,28]. Wilson *et al.* found that 24-hour esophageal acid profile did not differ between those with globus and appropriate controls nor was there any temporal relationship identified between globus sensation and actual reflux events [12]. Hill *et al.*, in a Chinese population, found an abnormal pH profile in a significantly higher proportion (31%) of globus patients compared with 5% of controls [28].

Establishing a dose-response relationship between acid reflux and globus is not practical. The best method, albeit indirect, to determined such a relationship is to examine the responsiveness of the symptom to potent acid suppression. Timon *et al.* found that neither the presence of heartburn, independent evidence of reflux nor medical antireflux therapy had any significant impact on the likelihood of symptom resolution [34]. Unfortunately there is only one randomised controlled trial of antisecretory therapy (cimetidine) for globus [35] which concluded no benefit. The remaining efficacy data, including three trials examining response to proton pump inhibitors (PPIs), is uncontrolled (*Table III*). Response rates vary among studies from 25%-38% with overall response being comparable to expected placebo response or natural symptom resolution rate over time. A randomised controlled trial of high dose PPI is required, but the there is no currently available high level evidence supporting acid suppressive therapy in globus. These data do not support the hypothesis that globus is reflux-related.

Table III. Summary of clinical trials of acid suppressive therapy the in treatment of globus.

Author	Study design	n	Drug	Response
Kibblewhite 1990	Controlled (non rand.)	20	Cimetidine *versus* placebo	30% *versus* 25% (NS)
Timon 1991	Uncontrolled	73	Cimetidine or antacids	25%
Curran 1995	Uncontrolled	21	Cimetidine	30%
Hill 1997	Uncontrolled	26	Omeprazole 20 mg	20%
Chevalier 2003	Uncontrolled	13	Omeprazole 40 mg	38%
Tokashidi 2002	Uncontrolled	25	Lansoprazole 30 mg	33%

Could globus represent a form of visceral hypersensitivity? Again the data is limited, but consistent with this notion. A study examining the sensory responses to esophageal distension found that balloon distension of the mid esophagus reproduced globus sensation in 80% of patients and did so at significantly lower balloon volumes that were required to produce discomfort in controls [23]. Hence, perception of esophageal distension appears to be heightened in this population.

Is globus a psychological disorder? A number of studies have demonstrated higher levels of anxiety and depression, greater introversion and neuroticism in those seeking medical attention for globus when compared with healthy controls [21,36-39]. However, psychoneurosis been not been causally linked to the symptom and may simply reflect health care seeking behaviour or self-referral bias as less than 10% of sufferers seek medical advice for it. For example, using the DSM III-R criteria a psychiatric diagnosis can be attached to 25%-60% of these patients [24,27], but these studies revealed no more anxiety and depression than was found in patients in a general medical outpatient clinic [24,34]. Therefore, there is no psychometric or personality profile that is specific for globus, nor is it necessary for such abnormalities to be present in all sufferers.

Summary

There is no good evidence to implicate pharyngeal or cricopharyngeal dysfunction in globus. Visceral hypersensitivity (probably esophageal) is currently the most plausible cause of globus. Sensitivity to esophageal acidification probably accounts for the minority of cases. Esophageal afferent responses to other stimuli such as non-acid refluxate, distension or contraction deserve further systematic evaluation.

References

1. Drossman DA, Li Z, Andruzzi E, et al. US householders survey of functional gastrointestinal disorders: prevalence, sociodemography and health impact. Dig Dis Sci 1993;38:1569-80.
2. Thompson W, Heaton K. Heartburn and globus on apparently healthy people. CMA J 1982;126:46-8.
3. Locke GR, Talley NJ, Fett SL, Zinsmeister AR, Melton LJ. Prevalence and clinical spectrum of gastroesophageal reflux: a population-based study in Olmsted County, Minnesota. Gastroenterology 1997;112:1448-56.
4. Ruth M, Mansson I, Sandberg N. The prevalence of symptoms suggestive of esophageal disorders. Scand J Gastroenterol 1991;26:73-81.
5. Wilson J, Pryde A, Piris J, et al. Pharyngoesophageal dysmotility in globus sensation. Arch Otolaryngol Head Neck Surg 1989;115:1086-90.
6. Batch AJG. Globus pharyngeus (part I). J Laryngol Otol 1988;102:152-8.
7. Deary IJ, Wilson JA, Harris MB, MacDougall G. Globus pharyngis: development of a symptom assessment scale. J Psychosom Res 1995;39:203-13.
8. Rowley H, O'Dwyer TP, Jones AS, Timon CI. The natural history of globus pharyngeus. Laryngoscope 1995;105:1118-21.
9. Malcomson K. Radiological findings in globus hystericus. Br J Radiol 1966;39:583-6.
10. Ravich WJ, Wilson RS, Jones B, Donner MW. Psychogenic dysphagia and globus: reevaluation of 23 patients. Dysphagia 1989;4:35-8.
11. Galmiche JP, Clouse RE, Balint A, et al. Functional esophageal disorders. Gastroenterology 2006;130:1459-65.
12. Wilson J, Heading R, Maran A, Pryde A, Piris J, Allan P. Globus sensation is not due to gastro-oesophageal reflux. Clin Otolaryngol 1987;12:271-5.
13. Delahunty J, Ardran G. Globus hystericus - a manifestation of reflux oesophagitis? J Larngol Otol 1970;84:1049-55.
14. Mair IW, Schroder KE, Modalsli B, Maurer HJ. Aetiological aspects of the globus symptom. J Laryngol Otol 1974;88:1033-40.
15. Dyer WH, Pridie RB. Incidence of hiatus hernia in asymptomatic subjects. Gut 1968;9:696-9.
16. Wienbeck M, Barnert J. Epidemiology of reflux disease and reflux esophagitis. Scand J Gastroenterol 1989;156:7-13.

17. Clements JL, Cox GW, Torres WE, Weens HS. Cervical esophageal webs: a roentgen anatomic correlation. AJR 1974;121:221-31.
18. Curtis DJ, Cruess DF, Berg T. The cricopharyngeal muscle: a videorecording review. AJR 1984;142:497-500.
19. Watson W, Sullivan S. Hypertonicity of the cricopharyngeal sphincter: a cause of globus sensation. Lancet 1974;2:1417-9.
20. Cook IJ, Dent J, Shannon S, Collins SM. Measurement of upper esophageal sphincter pressure: effect of acute emotional stress. Gastroenterology 1987;93:526-32.
21. Cook IJ, Dent J, Collins SM. Upper esophageal sphincter tone and reactivity to stress in patients with a history of globus sensation. Dig Dis Sci 1989;34:672-6.
22. Linsell J, Anggiansah A, Owen W. Manometric findings in patients with the globus sensation. Gut 1987;28:A1378.
23. Cook I, Shaker R, Dodds W, Hogan W, Arndorfer R. Role of mechanical and chemical stimulation of the esophagus in globus sensation. Gastroenterology 1989;96:A99.
24. Moser G, Wenzel-Abatzi TA, Stelzeneder M, et al. Globus sensation: pharyngoesophageal function, psychometric and psychiatric findings, and follow-up in 88 patients. Arch Intern Med 1998;158:1365-73.
25. Moser G, Vacariu-Granser G, Schneider C, et al. High incidence of esophageal motor disorder in consecutive patients with globus sensation. Gastroenterology 1991;101:1512-21.
26. Leelamanit V, Geater A, Sinkitjaroenchai W. A study of 111 cases of globus hystericus. J Med Assoc Thailand 1996;79:460-7.
27. Farkkila MA, Ertama L, Katila H, Kuusi K, Paavolainen M, Varis K. Globus pharyngis, commonly associated with esophageal motility disorders. Am J Gastroenterol 1994;89:503-8.
28. Hill J, Stuart RC, Fung HK, et al. Gastroesophageal reflux, motility disorders, and psychological profiles in the etiology of globus pharyngis. Laryngoscope 1997;107:1373-7.
29. Ott DJ, Ledbetter MS, Koufman JA, Chen MY. Globus pharyngeus: radiographic evaluation and 24-hour pH monitoring of the pharynx and esophagus in 22 patients. Radiology 1994;191:95-7.
30. Corso MJ, Pursnani KG, Mohiuddin MA, et al. Globus sensation is associated with hypertensive upper esophageal sphincter but not with gastroesophageal reflux. Dig Dis Sci 1998;43:1513-7.
31. Curran AJ, Barry MK, Callanan V, Gormley PK. A prospective study of acid reflux and globus pharyngeus using a modified symptom index. Clin Otolaryngol Allied Sci 1995;20:552-4.
32. Woo P, Noordzij P, Ross JA. Association of esophageal reflux and globus symptom: comparison of laryngoscopy and 24-hour pH manometry. Otolaryngol Head Neck Surg 1996;115:502-7.
33. Chevalier JM, Brossard E, Monnier P. Globus sensation and gastroesophageal reflux. Eur Arch Oto-Rhino-Laryngol 2003;260:273-6.
34. Timon C, O'Dwyer T, Cagney D, Walsh M. Globus pharyngeus: long-term follow-up and prognostic factors. Ann Otol Rhinol Laryngol 1991;100:351-4.
35. Kibblewhite DJ, Morrison MD. A double-blind controlled study of the efficacy of cimetidine in the treatment of the cervical symptoms of gastroesophageal reflux. J Otolaryngol 1990;19:103-9.
36. Puhakka H, Lehtinen V, Aalto T. Globus hystericus - a psychosomatic disease? J Laryngol Otol 1976;90:1021-6.
37. Pratt LW, Tobin WH, Gallagher RA. Globus hystericus - office evaluation by psychological testing with the MMPI. Laryngoscope 1976;86:1540-51.
38. Deary IJ, Smart A, Wilson JA. Depression and "hassles" in globus pharyngis. Br J Psychiatry 1992;161:115-7.
39. Deary IJ, Wilson JA, Kelly SW. Globus pharyngis, personality, and psychological distress in the general population. Psychosomatics 1995;36:570-7.

Reflux induced esophageal distension: does it cause heartburn/pain?

N.A. Tipnis (Milwaukee)

Acid reflux is an important cause of heartburn symptoms. However, there is poor correlation of heartburn symptoms with acid reflux and only 5-10% of acid reflux events result in heartburn symptoms on ambulatory pH monitoring [1-3]. Furthermore, some individuals continue to feel heartburn symptoms inspite of adequate acid suppression [4]. The reason for these observations is unclear.

Investigators have observed that balloon distension of the esophagus reproduces heartburn and chest pain symptoms in healthy individuals, gastroesophageal reflux disease (GERD) and non-cardiac chest pain patients [5,6]. Correlating these observations with gastroesophageal reflux (GER) events, it may be that the majority of GER events may be small while those that produce symptoms may be large. Using high-frequency intraluminal ultrasonography (HFIUS), esophageal distension can be measured by determining the cross-sectional area (CSA) of the esophagus during spontaneous GER events [7].

In a study of 10 healthy individuals and 10 heterogeneous GERD subjects, esophageal distension during spontaneous GER was determined using a combined HFIUS/multiple intraluminal impedance (MII)/pHmetry/esophageal manometry technique [8]. This combined technique allowed correlation of esophageal CSA with reflux acidity and symptoms. The effect of acid suppression therapy with esomeprazole was also evaluated.

A total of 109 reflux episodes in healthy individuals and 120 reflux episodes in GERD subjects were identified using the combined technique during a 2 hour post-prandial recording period. Most GER events were acidic (76% in healthy individuals and 88% in GERD subjects), liquid in composition (98% in healthy individuals and 82% in GERD subjects) and reached the proximal esophagus (92% in healthy individuals and 94% in GERD subjects). The range of esophageal CSA during reflux events was broad and ranged from 132 to 356 mm^2 in healthy individuals and from 68 to 521 mm^2 in GERD subjects.

Because of variability in the number of GER observation recorded for each individual, the mean esophageal CSA for each individual was determined. The mean esophageal CSA for each evaluated condition was then determined from the individual means. GERD subjects had a greater mean esophageal CSA compared during spontaneous reflux events compared to healthy individuals (271 ± 71 mm^2 *versus* 163 ± 56 mm^2, $p = 0.001$). In healthy individuals with both acid and non-acid reflux episodes, non-acid reflux events resulted in a larger mean esophageal CSA compared to acid reflux events. There was no difference between acid and non-acid reflux events in GERD subjects.

In GERD subjects, 15 GER episodes were associated with regurgitation, 28 with heartburn, 8 with chest pain and the remainder asymptomatic. Healthy controls experienced no symptoms. GER induced esophageal distension was greater for events associated with chest pain compared to asymptomatic events, but did not reach significance (459 ± 40 mm^2 *versus* 268 ± 70 mm^2, $p = 0.058$). There was no difference between events that were asymptomatic compared to those associated with regurgitation (290 ± 110 mm^2) or heartburn (271 ± 67 mm^2). Acid suppression therapy did not alter GER induced esophageal distension, but converted observed GER to predominantly non-acid events, decreased reflux frequency and decreased associated symptoms.

Two subjects were observed to have a cycling pattern of GER (*Figure 1*). These two subjects had larger GER induced esophageal distensions compared to typical GERD and healthy individuals (*Figure 2*). The cycling GER subjects accounted for approximately 50% of GER related symptoms compared to typical GER subjects prior to acid suppression therapy and all symptoms while on acid suppression therapy.

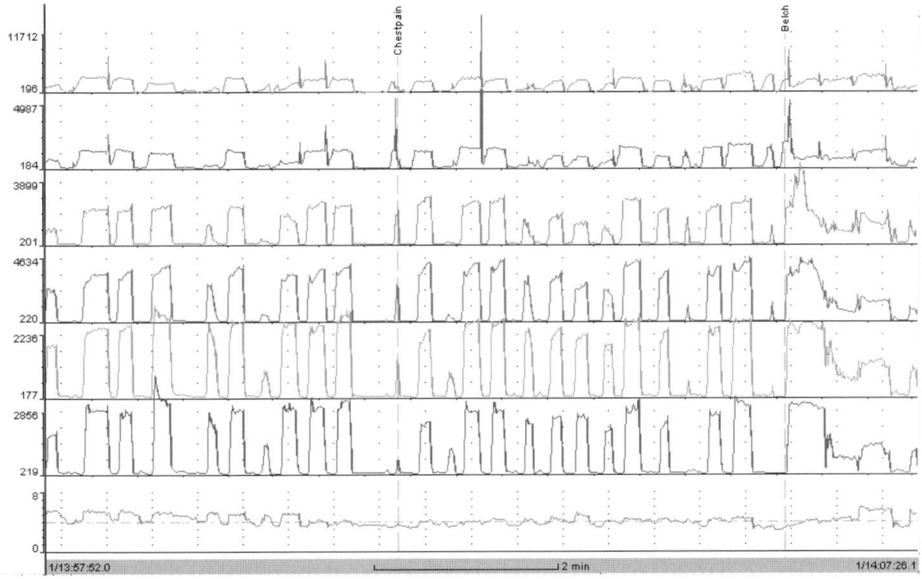

Figure 1. Example of MII/pH tracing from a subject with cycling GER. Note the repetitive, closely spaced GER episodes over a 10 minute tracing period.

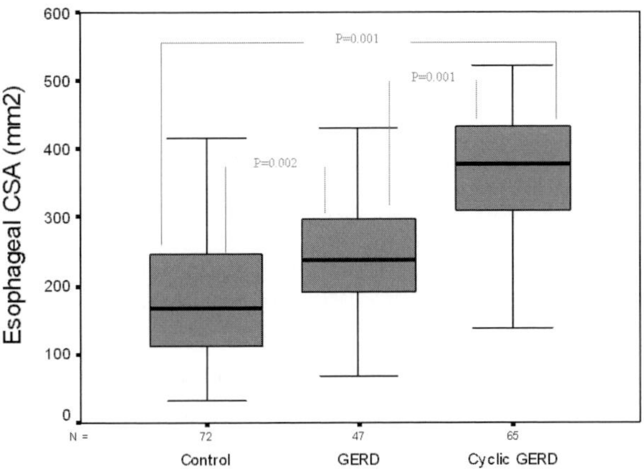

Figure 2. Comparison of peak esophageal CSA during spontaneous GER. Esophageal CSA was greater in cycling GER subjects compared to GER and healthy individuals. Esophageal CSA was also greater for GER subjects compared to healthy individuals.

Discussion

Using HFIUS to evaluate the effects of spontaneous GER on esophageal CSA, Tipnis *et al.* [8] found that there is a greater degree of esophageal distension in GER subjects compared to controls. This finding is consistent with other studies using fluoroscopy or balloon distension that demonstrated that the esophagus is more compliant in GERD subjects [9-11]. However, the Tipnis *et al.* study also found that there is no difference in esophageal distension between asymptomatic GER events compared to ones associated with regurgitation or heartburn. The amount of esophageal distension observed during spontaneous GER events was smaller than those used in balloon distension studies; therefore, distension during spontaneous GER may not have been sufficient to result in symptoms.

Other stimuli such as sustained esophageal contraction [12] or esophageal hypersensitivity may be important to the genesis of GER associated symptoms. Repetitive infusions of acid into the esophagus results in increased sensitivity to electrical and mechanical stimulation of the esophagus and reporting of stronger heartburn symptoms compared to isolated infusions [13-15]. Also, repeated esophageal distensions reduced the threshold for esophageal symptoms [16]. Therefore, a summation of multiple stimuli may be important to the production of GER related symptoms rather than a single noxious event.

References

1. Steinbach J, Fass R, Mittal RK. Assessment of relationship between acid reflux and heartburn using receiver operating characteristic curves. Gastroenterol.Clin North Am 2002;31:S45-58.
2. Taghavi SA, Ghasedi M, Saberi-Firoozi M, et al. Symptom association probability and symptom sensitivity index: preferable but still suboptimal predictors of response to high dose omeprazole. Gut 2005;54:1067-71.
3. Breumelhof R, Smout AJ. The symptom sensitivity index: a valuable additional parameter in 24-hour esophageal pH recording. Am.J.Gastroenterol 1991;86:160-4.
4. Vela MF, Camacho-Lobato L, Srinivasan R, Tutuian R, Katz PO, Castell DO. Simultaneous intraesophageal impedance and pH measurement of acid and nonacid gastroesophageal reflux: effect of omeprazole. Gastroenterology 2001;120:1599-606.
5. Takeda T, Nabae T, Kassab G, Liu J, Mittal RK. Oesophageal wall stretch: the stimulus for distension induced oesophageal sensation. Neurogastroenterol Motil 2004;16:721-8.
6. Fass R, Naliboff B, Higa L, et al. Differential effect of long-term esophageal acid exposure on mechanosensitivity and chemosensitivity in humans. Gastroenterology 1998;115:1363-73.
7. Rhee PL, Liu J, Puckett JL, Mittal RK. Measuring esophageal distension by high-frequency intraluminal ultrasound probe. Am J Physiol Gastrointest Liv Physiol 2002;283:G886-92.
8. Tipnis NA, Rhee TL, Mittal RK. Distension during gastro-esophageal reflux: effects of acid inhibition and correlation with symptom. Am J Physiol Gastrointest Liver Physiol 2007;293:G469-74.
9. Pandolfino JE, Shi G, Trueworthy B, Kahrilas PJ. Esophagogastric junction opening during relaxation distinguishes nonhernia reflux patients, hernia patients, and normal subjects. Gastroenterology 2003;125:1018-24.
10. Jenkinson AD, Scott SM, Yazaki E, et al. Compliance measurement of lower esophageal sphincter and esophageal body in achalasia and gastroesophageal reflux disease. Dig Dis Sci 2001;46:1937-42.
11. Mearin F, Vasconez C, Zarate N, Malagelada JR. Esophageal tone in patients with total aperistalsis: gastroesophageal reflux disease versus achalasia. Am J Physiol Gastrointest Liver Physiol 2000;279:G374-9.
12. Pehlivanov N, Liu J, Mittal RK. Sustained esophageal contraction: a motor correlate of heartburn symptom. Am J Physiol Gastrointest Liver Physiol 2001;281:G743-51.
13. Bhalla V, Liu J, Puckett JL, Mittal RK. Symptom hypersensitivity to acid infusion is associated with hypersensitivity of esophageal contractility. Am J Physiol Gastrointest Liver Physiol 2004;287: G65-71.
14. Sarkar S, Aziz Q, Woolf CJ, Hobson AR, Thompson DG. Contribution of central sensitisation to the development of non-cardiac chest pain. Lancet 2000;356:1154-9.
15. Sarkar S, Hobson AR, Furlong PL, Woolf CJ, Thompson DG, Aziz Q. Central neural mechanisms mediating human visceral hypersensitivity. Am J Physiol Gastrointest Liver Physiol 2001;281:G1196-202.
16. Nguyen P, Castell DO. Stimulation of esophageal mechanoreceptors is dependent on rate and duration of distension. Am J Physiol 1994;267:G115-8.

Translating esophageal mechanics and sensation into clinical applications

H. Gregersen (Aalborg)

The main function of the esophagus is mechanical, transporting fluid and food from the pharyngeal cavity to the stomach. Dysfunction of the esophagus due to known or unknown causes may result in symptoms like heartburn and pain. To understand the pathogenesis of the symptoms, it is important to be able to measure the symptoms in a reliable way and to develop clinical applicable test methods where the stimulus can be controlled. Development of new reliable and accurate methods may help to subgroup patients with apparent "heterogeneous" functional disease such as un-explained chest pain or non-erosive reflux disease. Subgrouping based on stimulus-specific symptoms will aid treatment of individual patients and aid development of new targeted drugs. However, the path from idea to regulatory approval and clinical acceptance of new technologies is long, cumbersome and expensive. Therefore, many techniques continue to be research tools that never reach the gastrointestinal (GI) diagnostics laboratories.

Methods such as manometry, radiography, and to some extent balloon distension have been used for a number of years to study esophageal function. In recent years manometry has been further developed into high-resolution manometry and other techniques as intraluminal impedance and endoscopic ultrasonography are now also used in esophageal function laboratories. However, for clinical applications and for mimicking symptoms, there is a rationale for development of techniques that challenges the esophagus, e.g. mechanical stimulation by distending a bag where the size of the bag and the sensory response can be measured.

In this context focus will be on two technologies based on bag distension and cross-sectional area of the distending bag measured using impedance planimetry. In recent years impedance planimetry has been further developed into the functional luminal imaging probe (FLIP) and the multimodal stimulation probe. It can be expected that these techniques will be further modified and made commercial within a short time frame.

Functional lumen imaging probe

Impedance planimetry has recently been further developed into multi-electrode systems for the purpose of measuring up to eight cross-sections inside a saline filled bag in the esophagogastric junction (EGJ) [1,2] (*Figure 1*). Until now, FLIP is the first technique to give a clear semi-3D outline of the geometric profile of the sphincter at various levels of distension (*Figure 2*). The closely spaced CSA measurement allow the reconstruction of the geometry and this in turn allows the generation of images which represent the sphincter lumen when the sphincter is physiologically active. This provides valuable data on the competence of the sphincter. The EGJ is the barrier mechanism that prevents the refluxing of stomach contents into the esophagus. The closing off must be related to a narrowing of the lumen which can be represented by CSAs measured in this region. Hence, FLIP could represent a major step forward in the diagnosis, monitoring and evaluation of diseases such

Figure 1. The functional luminal imaging probe with electrodes for eight cross-sectional area measurements in the esophagogastric junction. P1 and P2 illustrate the side holes for pressure measurements, EE are the two excitation electrodes and SE are the sensing electrodes. The system is currently being extended to 16-channels. (Courtesy of Dr. McMahon).

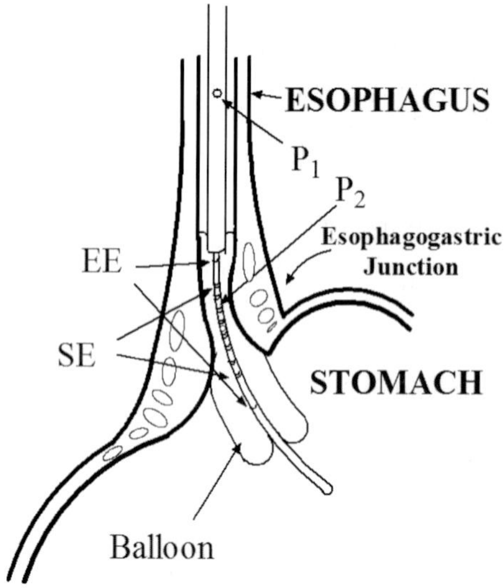

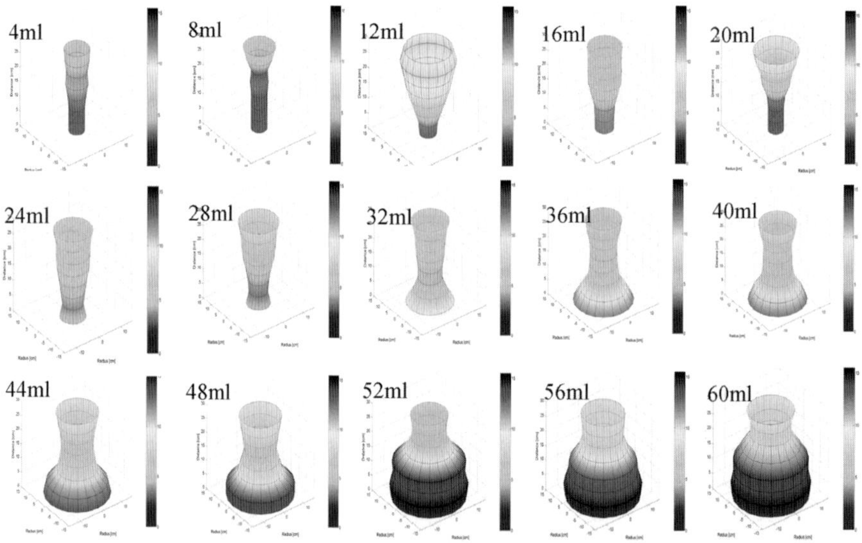

Figure 2. Reconstruction of the geometry of the esophago-gastric junction from a healthy subject shown at various bag fill volumes. The color represents radii (mm). Modified from a previous publication. (Courtesy of Dr. McMahon). (See page XIV for colour figure).

as gastroesophageal reflux disease where an ineffective junction allows acid from the stomach to travel back up into the esophagus..

Recent preliminary studies suggest that the technique has a role in assisting with drug therapy and surgical therapies for reflux.

Multimodal probe

The reaction to a single stimulus of a given modality only represents a limited fraction of the entire pain experience because pain is a multidimensional perception. Combining different methods for stimulation and assessment will approximate the clinical situation where different nerves and pathways are activated. Thus, multimodal stimulation will provide more comprehensive and differentiated information about the nociceptive system compared to stimuli using single or a few modalities [3]. A multimodal testing approach must therefore be used where the test battery will increase the probability for activation of a range of relevant nervous mechanisms. Such sophisticated methods will be able to select the best test procedures to explore different basic aspects of pain as well as pharmacological modulations.

Within the last decade Drewes and Gregersen introduced several multimodal models combining chemical, mechanical, electrical, cold and warmth stimuli to assess the sensation of the esophagus together with acid sensitization [4]. The model has been used in to unravel the pain mechanisms in different patients and in drug research. Mechanical stimulation is achieved with impedance planimetric bag distension. Thermal stimulation is achieved by recirculating fluid inside the bag with concomitant measurement of temperature. Chemical and electrical stimulation is achieved be means of side holes placed proximal to the bag and by electrodes on the outside of the bag. Sensitization with acid was added to the protocol to evoke hyperalgesia [4-7] (*Figure 3*).

The multimodal approach gives the possibility for a differentiated stimulation of receptors in the superficial and deep layers of the esophagus. The possibility for induction of hyperalgesia with acid perfusion and evoking central phenomena such as allodynia and

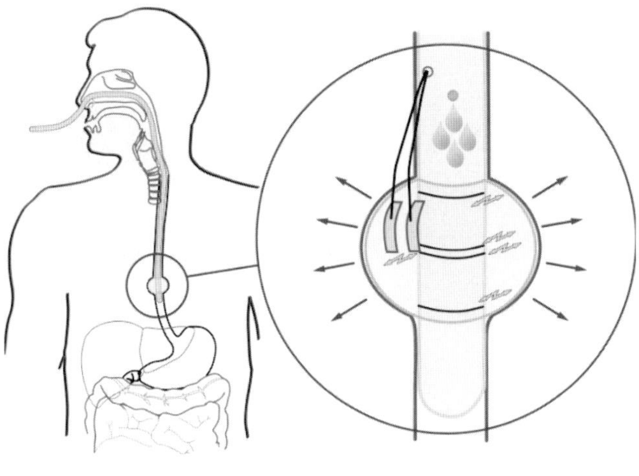

Figure 3. The multimodal probe assembly for mechanical, thermal, chemical and electrical stimulation of the esophagus.

referred pain makes the model clinically relevant with information on peripheral and central symptom mechanisms. Ideally the symptom assessment should also be multimodal including quantitative and qualitative sensation, assessment of referred pain and neurophysiologic measurements [6].

References

1. McMahon BP, Frokaer JB, Drewes AM, Gregersen H. A new measurement of oesophago-gastric junction competence. Neurogastroenterol Motil 2004;16:543-6.
2. McMahon B, Frokjaer J, Liao D, Kunwald P, Drewes A, Gregersen H. A new technique for evaluating sphincter function in visceral organs: application of the functional lumen imaging probe (FLIP) for the evaluation of the oesophago-gastric junction. Physiol Meas 2005;26:823-36.
3. Staahl C, Drewes AM. Experimental human pain models: a review of standardised methods for preclinical testing of analgesics. Basic Clin Pharmacol Toxicol 2004;95:97-111.
4. Drewes AM, Gregersen H, Arendt-Nielsen L. Experimental pain in gastroenterology: a reappraisal of human studies. Scand J Gastroenterol 2003;38:1115-30.
5. Drewes AM, Schipper KP, Dimcevski G, et al. Multimodal induction and assessment of allodynia and hyperalgesia in the human oesophagus. Eur J Pain 2003;7:539-49.
6. Drewes AM, Gregersen H. Multimodal pain stimulation of the gastrointestinal tract. World J Gastroenterol 2006;12:2477-86.
7. Drewes AM, Reddy H, Staahl C, Pedersen J, Funch-Jensen P, Arendt-Nielsen L, Gregersen, H. Sensory-motor responses to mechanical stimulation of the esophagus after sensitization with acid. World J Gastroenterol 2005;11:4367-74.

Brain - Foregut connections

What are the effects and implications of electrical stimulation of the esophagus on cerebral evoked potentials?

A.R. Hobson (Harlow)

Sensory signals from gastrointestinal (GI) afferents encode a wide range of peripheral activity. These signals predominantly help regulate our homeostatic balance and influence motility, secretion and appetite [1]. Most of these signals are subliminal, rarely reaching our consciousness, liminal sensations however such as satiety and fullness, along with supraliminal sensations such as pain complete this sensory spectrum. All of these sensations invoke activity in a complex array of cortical and subcortical structures *via* projections from both vagal and spinal visceral afferents.

Assessment of brain-gut signaling often requires delivery of an exogenous stimulus followed by observation of changes in neural and behavioral measures. The modality and characteristics of this exogenous stimulus is dependent on the mechanism or physiological process under observation and the most important factor when designing an experimental protocol to assess GI sensation is to have a clear hypothesis regarding the biological question that to be addressed [2].

The GI tract contains afferents that encode a wide range of intensities and modalities of stimulation including electrical, mechanical, thermal and chemical (including nutrient) stimuli [3]. Choosing the correct stimulation method or interpreting differential responses to multiply stimuli may be extremely important in delineating pathological mechanisms.

For instance, electrical stimulation is often thought of as non-physiological and therefore of limited use in assessing GI sensation. However, it is exactly because electrical stimulation bypasses the peripheral receptor that it is so useful, as it acts on the primary afferent directly allowing exploration of predominantly central afferent excitability. In contrast, it is known that "silent" nociceptors become active in inflammatory conditions and the fact that electrical stimulation would activate these regardless of the presence or absence of a peripheral insult renders this modality inadequate. If one wished to determine the presence of peripheral sensitization at the sensory receptor level in inflammatory conditions, then stimuli such as thermal, chemical and mechanical are the modalities of choice as has demonstrated in previous studies [4].

One of the major advantages in using electrical stimulation is the the asessment of central afferent pathway sensitivty using cerebral (cortical) evoked potentials (CEP). Neurophysiologists have used evoked potentials to study somatosensory, visual, auditory and pain pathways for half a century [5]. This technique involves the brief presentation of a sensory stimulus which is time and phase locked to the recording of the electroencephalogram (EEG) *via* surface electrodes placed on the scalp. The event-related signal is small in amplitude but occurs at the same moment in time following each stimulus, whilst the large amplitude background EEG is occurs randomly. In order to extract the desired signal, repeated stimuli are given and the subsequent brain activity averaged. This reduces the unwanted EEG whilst enhancing the event-related evoked potentials (EP) [6].

Frieling *et al.* were the first to record EP responses to esophageal stimulation and they, along with other investigators suggested that the esophageal evoked response (EEP) was predominantly mediated *via* vagal afferent pathways [7]. However, further studies have shown that the stimulus response characteristic of the visceral EP points to mediation *via* by both spinal and vagal afferents. Frieling also recorded these responses from the recto-sigmoid [8], and subsequently it has been demonstrated that EP's can be recorded in response to stimulation throughout the GI tract [9].

A comparison of EEP elicited by electrical and mechanical stimulation showed that both responses were mediated by thinly myelinated Aδ-fibers, both produced responses of identical morphology (*Figure 1*) and that the latency difference between the first mechanical and electrical EEP component of ~ 50 ms was due to the physical delay encountered during balloon inflation not activation of different fiber types [10]. This is not to say that unmyelinated C-fibers are not activated by esophageal stimulation, just that they do not contribute to the early response complex recorded with EEP [10].

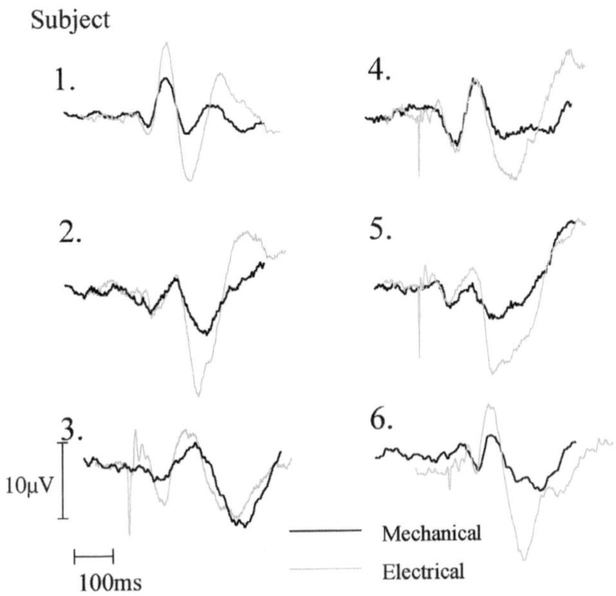

Figure 1. This figure shows the raw data for mechanical and electrical stimulation in six subjects. Each trace represents the average of 200 esophageal stimuli acquired at a stimulation intensity that was 75% of the subjects pain threshold. In order to demonstrate the similarities of morphology and inter-peak latencies, the authors have superimposed the traces and the P1 peaks have been aligned to compensate for the differences in peak latency. This also demonstrates the smaller amplitude CEP components acquired with mechanical stimulation. (Reproduced from [10] with permission.)

Importantly, the amplitude of mechanically evoked EEP was smaller than that seen to electrical stimulation. It is known that the amplitude of the EEP increases with increased afferent recruitment. These amplitude differences could therefore be explained by the fact that mechanical stimulation is specific to mechanosensitive afferent receptors whilst electrical stimulation activated all afferents regardless of modality, hence leading to greater afferent recruitment [10].

A major advantge of using electrical stimultaion comes from the fact that the instanataneous onset of the stimulus coupled with ease of control and reliability of the stimulus response characteristics reduces the intra and inter individual differences of the CEP response. This is critically important especially when studying clinical populations, for instance, where group heterogeniety may already introduce considerable variability into the data set. On a more practical level, mechanical stimuluation requires the design and construction of a purpose built inflation device [11], as none are available at present, and intraluminal balloons often fail mid-study under the pressure of long trains of distension. However, an important caveat to consider when using electrical stimulation, particularly in the esophagus, is the effects on cardiac pacing and the safety of the intervention should be of paramount concern.

Cardiologists have used trans-esophageal electrical stimulation to pace the heart for many years. Much of the work has concentrated on the effects of electrode configuration, position and stimulus characteristics on ventricular and/or atrial capture. In short, bipolar ring electrodes with minimal inter-electrode distance (< 2 cm) ensure that the given current stays relatively localised to esophageal tissue. However, if the duration of the stimulus is sufficiently long, then more energy is dispersed into the tissue and this can spread to adjacent structures including cardiac muscle (which is often less than 1 cm away from the distal esophageal region being stimulated) causing atrial capture. In Cochrane *et al.* study, a 9 ms duration stimulus achieved atrial capture in over 80% of stimulated patients [12]. It was also reported in Frobert's early EEP work that at stimulation intensities of up to 70 mA (duration 1 ms in this case) transient atrial capture was observed in 2 subjects [13]. However, in most studies, the stimulus duration used to elicit EEP has been around 200 μsec and no adverse cardiac events have been recorded [14]. Nonetheless, it is very important that ECG is carefully monitored as routine, when applying electrical stimulation in the esophagus.

In conclusion, electrical stimulation provides a robust activation of GI afferents and is ideal for studying central afferent pathway sensitivity especially when using sensitive and objective neurophysiological techniques such as CEPs. This technique provides complementary information to that gained from other stimulation modalities and used together one can begin to build a detailed profile of visceral sensory responsiveness in health and in a broad rage of patients with GI disease. This will lead to a better understanding of the underlying mechanism of GI sensory dysfunction and to a mechanistic approach to drug therapies in this difficult area.

References

1. Roman C, Gonella J. Extrinsic control of digestive tract motility. In: Johnson L, ed. Physiology of the GI tract. New York: Raven, 1987:503-53.
2. Hobson AR, Aziz Q, Furlong PL, Barlow JD, Bancewicz J, Thompson DG. Comparison of cortical potentials evoked by mechanical and electrical stimulation of the human oesopahgus. Gastroenterology 1998;A-1130.

3. Sengupta JN, Gebhart GF. Gastrointestinal afferent fibres and sensation. In: Holle GE, ed. Physiology of the gastrointestinal tract. New York: Raven Press, 1992:483-519.
4. de Caesteker JS, Pryde AHRC. Comparison of intravenous edrophonium and oesophageal acid perfusion during oesopahgeal manometry in patients with non-cardiac chest pain. Gut 1989;29:1029-34.
5. Desmedt JE. Somatosensory CEP in man. In: Cobb WA, ed. Handbook of electroencephalography and neurophysiology. Amsterdam: Elsevier, 1971:55-82.
6. Jones S. Somatosensory evoked potentials : the normal waveform. In: AM H, ed. Evoked potentials in clinical testing. Churchill Livingston, 1982:393-429.
7. Frieling T, Enck P, Wienbeck M. Cerebral responses evoked by electrical stimulation of the esophagus in normal subjects. Gastroenterology 1989;97:475-8.
8. Frieling T, Enck P, Wienbeck M. Cerebral responses evoked by electrical stimulation of rectosigmoid in normal subjects. Dig Dis Sci 1989;34:202-5.
9. Hobday DI, Hobson AR, Sarkar S, Furlong PL, Thompson DG, Aziz Q. Cortical processing of human gut sensation: an evoked potential study. Am J Physiol Gastrointest Liver Physiol 2002;283:335-9.
10. Hobson AR, Sarkar S, Furlong PL, Thompson DG, Aziz Q. A cortical evoked potential study of afferents mediating human esophageal sensation. Am J Physiol Gastrointest Liver Physiol 2000;279:139-47.
11. Hobson AR, Sarkar S, Furlong PL, Thompson DG, Aziz Q. Identification of the optimal parameters for recording cortical potentials evoked by mechanical stimulation of the human oesophagus. Neurogastroenterol Motil 2000;12:163-71.
12. Cochrane DJ, McEneaney DJ, Dempsey GJ, Anderson JM, Adgey AA. An esophageal and gastric approach to ventricular pacing. Pacing Clin Electrophysiol 1995;18:28-33.
13. Frobert O, Arendt-Neilsen L, Bak P, Funch-Jensen P, Bagger J. Electrical stimulation of the oesophageal mucosa, perception and brain potentials. Scan j gastro 1994;29:776-81.
14. Hobson AR, Aziz Q, Furlong PL, Barlow JD, Bancewicz J, Thompson DG. Identification of the optimal parameters for recording cortical evoked potentials to human oesophageal electrical stimulation. Neurogastroenterol Mot 1998;10:421-30.

How can stresses and strains at the receptor sites be measured?

H. Gregersen (Aalborg)

The biomechanics of the esophagus is not well understood despite the fact that the esophagus has a mechanical function [1,2]. Consequently, the stimuli for the mechanosensitive receptors are not understood as well. Stresses and strains, i.e. force-deformation relations are important concepts in biomechanics. The stress-strain relation determines the tissue stiffness, breaking strength, etc. Many artificial (engineered) materials express simple stress-strain relations because the material is homogeneous, behaves in an isotropic manner and show infinitesimal deformation even at large stresses. However, biological tissues such as the wall of the esophagus differ in several ways from the usual engineering materials that exhibit such behavior. Specifically, the gastrointestinal (GI) wall possesses or exhibits:

- complex geometry;
- a layered structure;
- heterogeneous materials;
- viscoelastic behavior, in that the tissue has the mechanical properties of both solids and fluids;
- anisotropic mechanical behavior (behavior that differs in one direction or dimension from another);

- behaviors in which large deformations produce non-linear stress-strain curves;
- the intrinsic active properties of muscle cells and their associated nerves.

Hence, stresses and strains are not easy to access.

The esophageal wall contains mechanosensitive receptors at various locations inside the wall. These receptors are important for the motor and sensory functions of the esophagus. It has been a common mistake in GI distension studies to consider the mechanoreceptors to be pressure receptors, volume receptors or tension receptors. Strain or stress are more likely candidates as the direct receptor stimulus since the receptors will experience the deformation and force in their vicinity rather the pressure and volume in the lumen [2,3].

Definition of mechanical stress and strain

In order to understand mechanoreceptor responses and mechanical stresses and strains, we need to define these terms. Stress is force per unit cross-sectional area ($\sigma = \frac{F}{A}$) with units of Pa or N m^{-2}. The force may be applied perpendicular to the surface, representing the bolus pressure (normal stress) exerted on the wall, or parallel to the surface, representing the force exerted by the fluid flow (shear stress) on the wall. Normal stresses may be either compressive or tensile. A force may be applied in any direction and can induce stresses and strains in various directions. At any given point in the body, the state of stress is described by a stress tensor that consists of three normal stresses and six shear stresses, three of which are independent. In a cylindrical tube, we deal with radial, circumferential and longitudinal components of stress in the respective directions. These are the normal components of stress in the wall of the cylinder (*Figure 1*). The stress components are obviously difficult to determine in biological studies. This article will not deal with these complex issues (the reader is referred to [2-4] for further reading on stresses) but will rather give examples of simple La Place stresses that have been used in studying the esophagus. La Place's law is an example of one of the simplest equations to be used for stress calculations.

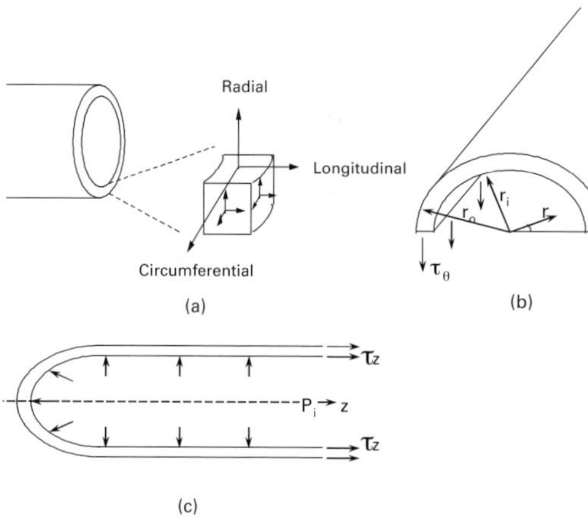

Figure 1. A pressurized cylindrical tube and sphere. **(a)** An infinitesimal element of the cylindrical tube showing the radial, longitudinal and circumferential directions. **(b)** A free-body diagram of half the tube cut parallel to the central axis. **(c)** A free-body diagram of the tube cut perpendicular to the central axis. The longitudinal, radial and circumferential directions are symbolized by z, r and θ. The pressure P from a bolus or a distending balloon induces a normal stress that will stretch the tube in the circumferential direction and cause radial compression (a thinner wall). Longitudinal extension may also occur. A moving bolus will also cause shear stresses in the mucosa.

Using La Place's law we will assume that the GI tract is a thin-walled cylindrical pressure vessel. In the following, we shall consider the circumferential stress, also called the hoop stress. In tubular organs, the major tensile stress induced by distension is in the circumferential direction. During luminal pressure loading, the equilibrium condition requires that the force in the intestinal wall in the circumferential direction to be balanced by the force in the intestinal lumen contributed by the inflation pressure. When the geometry is cylindrical, it can be shown that the average circumferential wall stress is $\tau_\theta = \frac{pr_i}{h}$ (1) where p, r_i, and h are the transmural pressure, internal radius, and wall thickness, respectively. This formula is commonly known as Laplace's law which is base don several assumptions. If the deformation is expressed in terms of Green strain (large deformation theory with reference to the initial state), the stress must be expressed as a commensurate measure and should, in that case, be expressed as Kirchhoff stress $S_\theta = \frac{\mathrm{Pr}_i}{h\,\lambda_\theta^2}$ (2) where λ is the circumferential stretch ratio (circumferential length when the segment is pressurized divided by the circumferential length when unloaded).

The term "deformation" refers to a change in the shape of a continuum (a continuous distribution of matter in space) between some initial (undeformed) configuration and a subsequent (deformed) configuration. Deformation can take many forms; for example, when we pull on a strip of tissue, it stretches, and if we inflate a tubular organ, it distends. To be able to describe such deformations quantitatively, the strain measures must be introduced. A force may be applied in any direction and can induce strains in any direction. On any surface, the strain may be perpendicular to the surface (normal strain), or parallel to the surface, such as the strain exerted on the wall of a viscus by the flow of fluid (shear strain). At any given point in the body, the state of strain is described by a strain tensor that consists of three normal strains and six shear strains, three of which are independent (as shown in *Figure 1* for stress).

Strains can be defined in several different ways. For simplicity, consider a tissue strip of tissue of initial length L_0 (*Figure 2*). If we stretch it to length L, the change in length can be described by several dimensionless ratios such as:

Stretch ratio $\lambda = \frac{L}{L_0}$, Cauchy strain $\in = \frac{L - L_0}{L_0}$, Green's strain $\mathrm{E} = \frac{L^2 - L_0^2}{2L_0^2}$ (3).

Thus, for a continuum subjected to finite deformation, strains can be defined in several different ways in relation to the deformation gradient. The selection of the proper strain measures is dictated primarily by the stress-strain relationship. The strains can be computed for all surfaces or interfaces between layers where the geometric data can be obtained. The measures are dimensionless. This is advantageous since it eliminates the absolute length

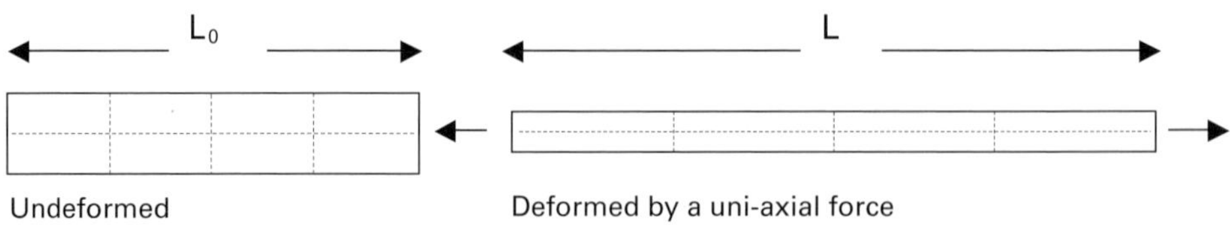

Figure 2. Simple extension of a bar with undeformed length (L_0) at resting state and length L at deformed state caused by a uni-axial force. The force induced a positive (tensile) strain. A force in the opposite direction will induce a negative (compressive) strain.

and any system of units from consideration. In Eqs. 3, the strain measures are expressed as a fraction of the initial length (Lagrangian strains). Either one of these strain measures is useful. In infinitesimal elongations, the strain measures are equal. However, in finite elongations, they are different which easily can be shown by examples. The Cauchy strain is especially useful in the linearized theory of elasticity, which is valid when $\in$ is infinitesimal. For finite deformations, strain defined by Green is more conveniently related to stress. One strain measure can readily be transformed into another.

The strain measures can be used readily for the study of organs of complex configuration, so long as the geometric data can be obtained. In the case of the GI tract, let us, for simplicity, consider a straight circular cylindrical tube of homogenous material. We may refer to radial, circumferential and longitudinal components of strain in the respective directions, as defined before. These are the normal components of strain in the wall of the cylinder. During luminal pressure loading (distension) the circumferential length increases (tensile circumferential strain), the wall thickness decreases (compressive radial strain) and compression or elongation may occur in the longitudinal direction (dependent on the material properties). During contraction of the circumferential muscle layer, the circumferential strain will be compressive (negative) and the wall will become thicker.

How to obtain strain and stress data

As emphasized above, the stress and strain can not be measured, rather they must be computed, and the direction and location need to be taken into account. Furthermore, since the wall in geometrically complex, layered and heterogeneous, we need numerical analysis for computation of stresses and strains in the vicinity of the receptors.

Nevertheless we are often left with less advanced methods and we have to rely on the measurements that can be obtained. Stresses averaged across the wall can be determined if the transmural pressure, the luminal radius and the wall thickness is known. These can be determined using distension with concurrent manometry and imaging such as ultrasonography and magnetic resonance imaging (MRI). Especially endoluminal ultrasonography is of interest because it can display the luminal geometry and the wall layers. Also new techniques such as strain rate imaging may have a future potential for characterizing receptor stimuli.

Thoughts on the receptor stimulus

If the simple and inappropriate views of the receptors being pressure and volume receptors are not considered, then we are left with stresses and strains as the direct stimuli. Many authors seem to confuse stress and tension and a school has existed for many years that considered tension to be important. However, tension cannot be the direct stimulus because tension does not take the wall thickness and the location of the receptors in the wall into account. Considering mechanical and receptor kinematic properties, strain is a more relevant parameter than stress. In fact it seems much more likely that is receptor is designed to sense deformation rather than a complex parameter as the stress. In fact some receptors have been described as stretch sensitive ion channels, i.e. the opening of the channel will depend on the degree of deformation. Recent studies in humans have provided evidence that circumferential strain is an important determinant of mechanoreceptor mediated responses [5-8].

References

1. Brasseur JG. Mechanical studies of the esophageal function. Dysphagia 1993;8:384-6.
2. Gregersen H. Biomechanics of the gastrointestinal tract. Springer Verlag 2002.
3. Gregersen H, Kassab GS. Biomechanics of the gastrointestinal tract. Neurogastroenterol Motil 1996;8:277-97.
4. Fung YC. Biomechanics. Mechanical properties of living tissues, 2nd ed. New York: Springer-Verlag, 1993.
5. Gao C, Arendt-Nielsen L, Liu W, Petersen P, Drewes AM, Gregersen G. Sensory and biomechanical responses to ramp-controlled distension of the human duodenum. Am J Physiol 2003;284:G461-71.
6. Barlow JD, Gregersen H, Thompson DG. Identification of biomechanical factors associated with the perception of distension in the human esophagus. Am J Physiol 2002;282:G683-9.
7. Drewes AM, Pedersen J, Liu W, Arendt-Nielsen L, Gregersen H. Controlled mechanical distension of the human oesophagus: sensory and biomechanical findings. Scand J Gastroenterol 2003;38(1):27-35.
8. Petersen P, Gao C, Arendt-Nielsen L, Gregersen H, Drewes AM. Pain intensity and biomechanical responses during ramp-controlled distension of the human rectum. Dig Dis Sci 2003;48:1310-6.

What is the relationship between cerebral neuronal activation and responses and mechanical behaviour of the pharynx and esophagus?

A. Schindler (Milan)

There is both clinical and scientific evidence that cerebral neuronal activation influences the mechanical behaviour of the pharynx and of the esophagus. However, the exact relationship between cerebral neuronal activation and the foregut responses is still a matter of debate. Different approaches have shown that a large number of areas within the central nervous system (CNS) take part in the swallowing mechanism; each of them may influence the mechanical behaviour of both the pharynx and the esophagus.

Two regions of the CNS appeared to have a role in the control of swallowing: the brain stem and the supramedullary areas [11,29]. The brain stem is responsible for the reflex part of the swallowing mechanism: both the sensory and motor nuclei of the cranial nerves involved in swallowing as well as the interneurons connecting them lie in this part of the CNS; moreover the sequential and rhythmic patterns of swallowing are generated by a group of neurons of the medulla oblongata, called central pattern generator (CPG). The brain stem sequential activity may be triggered or modulated by the supramedullary regions including the supplementary motor area, the pre- and post-central gyri, the insula, the anterior cingulated gyrus, the basal ganglia and the cerebellum (*Figure 1*).

A large number of oral and pharyngeal reflexes are controlled by the neuronal connections of the brain stem and play a vital role in the complex behaviour of swallowing (*Table I*); these reflexes modify motoneurons' activity, that receive synaptic input from higher centers, and function as supporting networks of neurons assisting in the control of complex motor responses, such as speech, intra-oral transport of food, chewing and swallowing [38].

From a theoretical point of view, cerebral neuronal activation may have two consequences: modify pharyngeal and esophageal muscle tone, increasing or decreasing it,

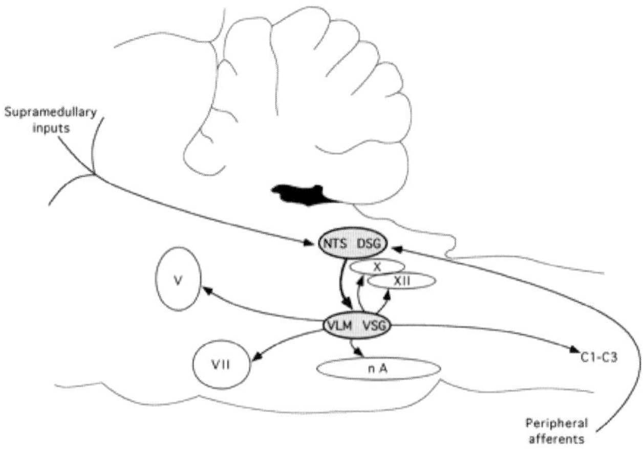

Figure 1. Diagram of the brain stem mechanism involved in swallowing; supramedullary inputs may influence the activity of the central pattern generator (CPG). The CPG includes two main groups of neurons located within the medulla oblongata: a dorsal swallowing group (DSG), located within the nucleus tractus solitarii (NTS) and a ventral swallowing group (VLM) adjacent to the nucleus ambigus (nA). The CPG activate the motor nuclei involved in the swallowing reflex.

and induce or inhibit complex behaviour, such as swallowing. Different models can be used to analyse the relationship between cerebral activation and pharyngeal and esophageal responses: swallowing modifications in patients with CNS diseases, neuronal stimulation/inhibition in animal models, neuroimgaging and electrophysiological studies in human subjects, swallowing modifications in developing or aging subjects.

Pharyngeal and esophageal behaviour modifications in patients with cerebral diseases

It is well known that a large number of CNS diseases can disrupt the swallowing mechanism; knowing the areas within the CNS disrupted by each disease and their characteristic of dysphagia, it is possible to infer the role of these area in the swallowing mechanism.

The modifications induced by cortical neuron death on swallowing has been studied in patients following stroke [17,19,22]. It appeared that the swallowing musculature is somatotopically represented on the motor and pre-motor cortex of both hemispheres, but displays asymmetry, independent of handness [17]. Besides, the dysphagia was associated with a smaller electromyographic pharyngeal response after supratreshold transcranialmagneto-electric stimulation (TMS) of the affected hemisphere [19] and the recovery of swallowing depended on compensatory reorganization of the undamaged hemisphere [22].

Electrophysiological studies of patients with amyotrophic lateral sclerosis (ALS) showed that the triggering of the swallowing reflex for the voluntarily initiated swallow is abolished and the cricopharyngeal spincter muscle becomes hyper-reflexic and hypertonic [9]. Both of these finding have been interpreted as the degeneration of the excitatory and inhibitory corticobulbar pyramidal fibres. Similar findings have been reported in patients with suprabulbar palsy with lacunar infarct [8], while data from normal subjects support these findings [10].

Dysphagia in Parkinson's disease represent a pathological model of the basal ganglia involvement in the swallowing mechanism. In an electrophysiological study, Parkinson's

Table I. Oral and pharyngeal reflexes: sensory input, motor output and effect of each reflex are shown.

Type of reflex	Sensory input	Motor ouput	Effect
Tongue-tongue reflex	Touching tongue	Hypoglossal motoneurons	Tongue tipe orients toward stimulus
Lip-lip reflex	Tap upper lip	Facial motoneurons	Lip muscles contract
Oral-lip reflex	Intra-oral pressures	Facial motoneurons	Excite lip muscles
Tongue-facial reflex	Hypoglossal nerve	Facial motoneurons	Excite facial muscles
Lingual-hypoglossal reflex	Lingual nerve or mechanical stimulation of tongue	Hypoglossal motoneurons	Excite or inhibit different tongue muscles
Masseter-hypoglossal reflex	Masseteric nerve	Hypoglossal motoneurons	Inhibit tongue muscles and excite tongue-protruding muscles
Inferior alveolar-hypoglossal reflex	Inferior alveolar nerve	Hypoglossal motoneurons	Inhibit both tongue-protruding and retrusive muscles
Glossopharyngeal-hypoglossal reflex	Glossopharyngeal nerve	Hypoglossal motoneurons	Excite protrusive muscle/some intrinsic muscles and inhibit retrusive muscles
Jaw-hypoglossal reflex	Rotating jaw open	Hypoglossal motoneurons	Opening jaw increases tongue-protruding
Temporalis-hypoglossal reflex	Temporalis muscle	Hypoglossal motoneurons	Streching temporalis increases styloglossus activity
Taste-hypoglossal reflex	Glucose to tongue	Hypoglossal motoneurons	Lateral tongue movement to side o stimulus
Oral/jaw-closing muscles reflex	Oral region	Trigeminal motoneurons	Primarily inhibiting jaw-closing muscles
Jaw-opening reflex	Oral region	Trigeminal motoneurons	Jaw lowers
Periodontal-masseteric reflex	Periodontal region	Trigeminal motoneurons	Jaw lowers
Lateral mandibular reflex	Rapid pressure on incisor	Trigeminal motoneurons	Jaw moves to contralateral side
Gag reflex	Oropharyngeal region	Nucleus ambiguus, trigeminal and hypoglossal motoneurons	Expulsion movements
Apneic reflex	Lingual nerve, water on laryngeal surface of epiglottis	Phrenic and nucles ambiguous motoneurons	Cessation of breathing
Aspiration reflex	Trigeminal nerve branches, glossopharyngeal branches	Phrenic motoneurons	Brief inspiratory burst
Respiration reflexes	Pharyngeal region	Intercostal motoneurons, autonomic ganglionic neurons	Forced expiration, bronchi secretions and constriction
Cardiovascular reflexes	Pharyngeal region	Autonomic ganglionic neurons	Bradycardia

disease patients showed a prolongation of the pharyngeal reflex time, due to slowness of the sequential muscle movements, while the cricopharyngeal muscle appeared electrophysiologically normal [10].

Dystonias are generally considered movement disorders due to basal ganglia involment; it has been recently reported that patients with craniocervical dystonia show prolongation of laryngeal relocation times, delay of the triggering time to swallowing reflex and, at least in some patients, hyperreflexive cricopharyngeal muscle.

Cerebral neuronal stimulation in animal models

The study of swallowing cerebral control in animal models has a more than 30 years history and allowed the definition of different circuits within the brainstem and the supramedullary regions involved in deglutition [5,29].

The sheep has been used to study the CPG and its regulation by cortical centres [2,6,32]. It appeared that stimulation of the chewing area, within the fronto-orbital cortex, inhibit the CPG and suppress the muscular activity of the pharynx and of the esophagus [2,32]. Moreover, muscarinic receptors appear to control the primary peristalsis of the esophagus, but not the oropharyngeal component [6].

The role of different molecules in brain stem swallowing regulation has been investigated also in the rat [12,31,41,42]. It has been shown that monoamines (serotonin, noradrenaline) inhibit the swallowing reflex [31]; besides noadrenergic neurons of the nucleus of the solitary tract inhibit the dorsal motor nucleus [41,42]. More recently it was demonstrated that leptin, a hormone regulating feeding behaviour and energy balance, inhibits swallowing [12].

The role of different brain areas on swallowing has been studied in the cat [23,33,48]. The basal forebrain, together with amigdalar and hypothalamic components, appeared to facilitate the swallowing reflex [48]. More recently it has been proved that light TMS of the cortex evoked short latency electromyographic responses of pharyngeal and esophageal muscles, while higher intensity stimulation induced swallowing activity, suggesting an oligosynaptic projection from cortex to swallowing muscles with the need for greater cortical motorneuron activation to induce swallowing [23]. In the cat it has also been analyzed the role of different nucleus tractus solitarius subnuclei in the pharyngeal and esophageal phase of swallowing [33].

The monkey (*Macaca fascicularis)* is a well studied model to analyze the relationship between cortical stimulation and both mastication and swallowing [25,27,34,35,40,49,50]. It has been demonstrated that the tongue primary motor cortex plays a role in both swallowing and other trained motor behaviour [34]; besides, the regions that trigger swallowing have been found: the face motor cortex, the primary somatosensory cortex, the cortical masticatory area (CMA) and the white matter underlying the CMA and frontal operculum [35]. In most of the areas, the electrophysiological stimulation induced not only swallowing, but also other oro-facial responses. Cortical inactivation through cold block showed that while blocking the CMA markedly affected the ability to carry out swallowing [40], inactivation of the somatosensory cortex as well as of the primary motor cortex, preserve swallowing [49,50]. In summary while different cortical region can induce swallowing if stimulated electrophisiologically, only the CMA seem to play a vital role in deglutition.

Neuroimaging and electrophysiological studies in human subjects

Positron emission tomography (PET), functional magnetic resonance imaging (fMRI), TMS, magnetoencefalography (MEG), have been used in the last ten years to study the cerebral neuronal activation in awake normal human subjects; a lot of information concerning the role of cortical and subcortical areas in voluntary and automathic swallowing are now available.

Different neuroimaging studies showed that in the adult normal human subjects different cortical and subcortical areas come in to play: bilateral caudolateral sensorimotor cortex (Broadman's area – BA – 3,4 and 6), anterior insula (BA 16), orbitofrontal cortex (BA 11), mesial premotor cortex (BA 6 and 24), amygdala (BA 34), anterior cingulated gyrus, putamen, globus pallidus, substantia nigra and cerebellum [20,21,45,51]. Further investigation through fMRI allowed to understand that, even if most of the swallow-related cortical acitivty maps are not specific to swallowing [30], a difference between automatic and volitional swallowing in cerebral activation is present [36,46]; in particular the anterior cingulated cortex, together with the pre- and post-central giri are involved in voluntary swallowing. Applying statistical analysis to different brain regions activation seen through fMRI, five functional modules have been suggested:

- sensorimotor areas and cingulated cortex, establishing a sensorimotor output for which other areas converge;
- inferior frontal gyrus, corpus callosum, basal ganglia and thalamus, involved in movement planning and implementation to other voluntary motor behaviours;
- premotor cortex and posterior parietal cortex, serving to integrate sensory information about the bolus with the internal representation of swallowing movements;
- cerebellum, whose role is to facilitate modulation of the internal representation for swallowing and coordination among the multiple effectors and effectors states during swallowing;
- insula, recruited for synchronizing the kinematics of the movements [39].

The role of different cortical areas in the swallowing mechanism has been studied through electrophysiological approaches. The cerebral activation in volitional swallowing has been assessed through movement-related cortical potentials [26,43]; it appeared that activation of the supplementary motor cortex precedes the onset of volitional swallowing. TMS stimulation studies demonstrated that trigeminal and vagus stimulation as well as swallowing facilitate corticalbulbar pathways [10,13,18].

More recently the temporospatial sequence of cerebral loci activation was studied through MEG [1,7,14,16,47]. It was demonstrated that the supplementary motor area and the anterior cingulated gyrus are activated before swallowing [1,47]; while the insula and the frontal operculum activate only during the preparation and the execution of volitional swallowing, sensorymotor cortex are involved in both reflexive and voluntary swallowing execution [7]. Finally, it has been shown that pharyngeal stimulation activates caudolateral sensory and motor cortical areas, which prime superior sensorimotor cortex, thus facilitating cortico-bulbar projections [14,16].

Swallowing behaviour in developing and aging human subjects

The study of swallowing behaviour in developing and aging human subjects is in its infancy [24,37]; nonetheless, insightful information can be drawn following this approach, since in both the child and the old the connections between supramedullary and brainstem regions strongly differs from that present in adulthood.

The cerebral and brainstem pathways involved in oral-motor function and swallowing undergo developmental maturation. By 40 week's gestation, myelination of the reticular formation around the nucleus ambiguous and the nucleus tractus solitarius commences and continues through early infancy; it is interesting that these myelination patterns occur at a time in which more voluntary aspects of feeding and swallowing appear. The process of increasing suprabulbar control of oral feeding is illustrated by the recognized diminution of infant oral reflexes during the first year of life and by increased sucking and swallowing rates and larger volumes per suck with increasing age [3]. Besides, it is well known that the infant animal is unable to discharge its motor fibers to the muscles active in pharyngeal swallowing with a high short frequency, but elicits a slow, prolonged discharge [44]. We might therefore speculate that suprabulbar stimulation, acquired during the first year of life development, play an active role in triggering the swallowing reflex, while inhibiting other oral and pharyngeal reflexes, thus allowing the deglutition of several boli in less time. The preliminary neuroimaging study of swallowing in children [24] does not show evidence in favour or against this speculation, but opens the door to further understanding of the cerebral activation during swallowing in the developmental age.

Different lines of research suggest the possibility that the neural processing of motor performances is altered as a function of normal aging [4]; yet, age-related changes in swallowing physiology have been reported, including delayed pharyngeal triggering and upper esophageal sphincter opening [15]. Even if different factors are involved in the swallowing aging, including decreased muscle strength and sensory receptors activity, a possible role of the different cerebral neuronal activation, recently reported [37], exist.

Conclusion

In conclusion clinical and scientific data demonstrated that the cerebral activation in swallowing is extremely complex. The reflexes within the brainstem provide the underlying framework of neural control upon which more complex motor responses can build and recruit in a functional framework; cortical activation facilitate or inhibit brainstem reflexes, and favour pharyngeal and esophageal contraction, but a complex network of different cortical and subcortical regions is necessary to coordinate movement planning and implementation to other voluntary motor behaviours, integrate sensory information about the bolus with the internal representation of swallowing movements and facilitate modulation of the internal representation for swallowing and coordination among the multiple effectors and effectors states during swallowing.

References

1. Abe S, Wantanabe Y, Shintani M, et al. Magnetoencefalographic study of the starting point of voluntary swallowing. Cranio 2003;21:46-9.
2. Amri M, Lamkadem M, Car A. Effects of lingual and chewing cortex stimulation upon activity of the swallowing neurons located in the region of the hypoglossal motor nucleus. Brain Res 1991;548:149-55.
3. Arvedson JC, Brodsky L. Anatomy, embryology, physiology and normal development. In: Pediatric swallowing and feeding: assessment and management, 2nd ed. Albany: Singular Thompson Learning, 2002:13-79.
4. Calautti C, Serrati C, Baron JC. Effects of age on brain activation during auditory-cued thumb-to-index opposition: a positron emission tomography study. Stroke 2001;32:139-46.
5. Car A. La commande corticale de la déglutition. I: sa vie d'expression. J Physiol 1973;66:531-55.
6. Car A, Roman C, Zoungrana OR. Effects of atropine on the central mechanism of deglutition in anesthetized sheep. Exp Brain Res2002;142:496-503.
7. Dziewas R, Soros P, Ishii R, et al. Neuroimage 2003;20:135-44.
8. Erketin C, Aydogdu I, Tarlaci S, Turman AB, Kiylioglu N. Mechanism of dysphagia in suprabulbar palsy with lacunar infarct. Stroke 2000;31:1370-6.
9. Erketin C, Aydogdu I, Yuceyar N, Kiylioglu N, Tarlaci S, Uludag B. Pathophysiological mechanism of oropharyngeal dysphagia in ALS. Brain 2000;123:125-40.
10. Ertekin C, Turman B, Tarlaci S, et al. Cricopharyngeal pphincter muscle responses to transcranial magnetic stimulation in normal subjects and in patients with dysphagia. Clin Neurophysiol 2001;112:86-94.
11. Ertekin C, Aydogdu I. Neurophysiology of swallowing. Clin Neurophysiol 2003;114:2226-44.
12. Felix B, Jean A, Roman C. Leptin inhibits swallowing in rats. Am J Physiol Reg Integr Comp Physiol 2006;291:657-63.
13. Fraser C, Rothwell J, Power M, Hobson A, Thompson D, Hamdy S. Differntial changes in human pharyngoesophageal motor excitability induced by swallowing, pharyngeal stimulation, and anesthesia. Am J Physiol Gastrointest Liver Physiol 2003;285:G137-44.
14. Furlong PL, Hobson AR, Aziz Q, et al. Dissociating the spatio-temporal characteristics of cortical neuronal activity associated with human volitional swallowing in the healthy adult brain. Neuroimage 2004;22:1447-55.
15. Gleeson DCL. Oropharyngeal swallowing and aging: a review. J Comm Disord 1999;32:373-396.
16. Gow D, Hobson AR, Furlong P, Hamdy S. Characterising the central mechanism of sensory modulation in human swallowing motor cortex. Clin Neurophysiol 2004;115:2382-90.
17. Hamdy S, Aziz Q, Rothwell JC, et al. The cortical topography of human swallowing musculature in health and disease. Nat Med 1996;2:1217-24.
18. Hamdy S, Aziz Q, Rothwell JC, Hobson A, Barlow J, Thompson DG. Cranial nerve modulation of human swallowing motor pathways. Am J Physiol 1997;272:G802-8.
19. Hamdy S, Aziz Q, Rothwell JC, et al. Explaining oropharyngeal dysphagia after unilateral hemispheric stroke. Lancet 1997;350:686-92.
20. Hamdy S, Rothwell JC, Brooks DJ, Bailey D, Aziz Q, Thompson DG. Identification of the cerebral loci processing human swallowing with H2O PET activation. J Neurophysiol 1999;81:1917-26.
21. Hamdy S, Mikulis DJ, Crawley A, et al. Cortical activation during human volitional swallowing: an event-related fMRI study. Am J Physiol 1999;277:G219-25.
22. Hamdy S, Rothwell JC, Aziz Q, Thompson DG. Organization and reorganization of human swallowing motor cortex: implications for recovery after stroke. Clin Sci 2000;98:151-7.
23. Hamdy S, Xue S, Valdez D, Diamant NE. Induction of cortical swallowing activity by transcranial magnetic stimulation in the anaesthetized cat. Neurogastroenterol Mot 2001;13:65-72.
24. Hartnick C, Rudolph C, Willging JP, Holland SK. Functional magnetic resonance imaging of the paediatric swallow: imaging the cortex and brainstem. Laryngoscope 2001;111:1183-91.
25. Huang CS, Hiraba H, Murray GM, Sessle BJ. Topographical distribution and functional properties of cortically induced rhythmical jaw movements in the monkey (Macaca fascicularis). J Neurophysiol 1989;61:635-50.
26. Huckabee ML, Deecke L, Cannito MP, Gould HJ, Mayr W. Cortical control mechanisms in volitional swallowing: the Bereitschaftpotential. Brain Topog 2003;16:3-17.
27. Huang CS, Hiraba H, Sessle BJ. Input-output relationship of the primary face motor cortex in the monkey (Macaca fascicularis). J Neurophysiol 1989;61:350-62.
28. Huang CS, Sirisko MA, Hiraba H, Murray GM, Sessle BJ. Organization of the primate face motor cortex as revealed by intracortical microstimulation and electrophysiological identification of afferent inputs and corticobulbar projections. J Neurophysiol 1988;796-818.
29. Jean A. Brain stem control of swallowing: neuronal network and cellular mechanism. Physiol Rev 2001;81:929-69.
30. Kern M, Birn R, Jaradeh S, et al. Swallow-related cerebral cortical activity maps are not specific to deglutition. Am J Physiol Gastrointest Liver Physiol 2001;280:G531-8.
31. Kessler JP, Jean A. Inhibitory influence of monoamines and brainstem monoaminergic regions on the medullary swallowing reflex. Neurosci Lett 1986;65:41-6.

32. Lamkadem M, Zoungrana OR, Amri M, Car A, Roman C. Stimulation of the chewing area of the cerebral cortex induces inhibitory effects upon swallowing in sheep. Brain Res 1999;832:97-111.
33. Lang IM, Dean C, Medda BK, Aslam M, Shaker R. Differential activation of medullary vagal nuclei during different phases of swallowing in the cat. Brain Res 2004;1014:145-63.
34. Martin RE, Murray GM, Kemppainen P, Masuda Y, Sessle BJ. Functional properties of neurons in the primate tongue primary motor cortex during swallowing. J Neurophysiol 1997;1516-30.
35. Martin RE, Kemppainen P, Masuda Y, Yao D, Murray G, Sessle BJ. Features of cortically ecoked swallowing in the awake primate (Macaca fascicularis). J Neurophysiol 1999;82:1529-41.
36. Martin RE, Goodyear BG, Gati JS, Menon RS. Cerebral cortical representation of automatic and volitional swallowing in humans. J Neurophysiol 2001;85:938-50.
37. Martin R, Barr A, MacIntosh B, et al. Cerebral cortical processing of swallowing in older adults. Exp Brain Res 2007;176:12-22.
38. Miller AJ. Oral and pharyngeal reflexes in the mammalian nervous system: their diverse range in complexity and their pivotal role of the tongue. Crit Rev Oral Biol Med 2002;13:409-25.
39. Mosier K, Bereznaya I. Parallel cortical networks for volitional control of swallowing in humans. Exp Brain Res 2001;140:280-9.
40. Narita N, Yamamura K, Yao D, Martin RE, Sessle BJ. Effects of functional disruption of lateral pericentral cerebral cortex on primate swallowing. Brain Res 1999;824:140-5.
41. Rogers RC, Hermann GE, Travagli RA. Brainstem pathways responsible for oesophageal control of gastric motility and tone in the rat. J Physiol 1999;514:369-83.
42. Rogers RC, Travagli RA, Hermann GE. Noradrenergic neurons in the rat solitari nucleus partecipate in the esophageal-gastric relaxation reflex. Am j PHysiol Regul Integr Com Physiol 2003;285:R479-89.
43. Satow T, Ikeda A, Yamamoto J, et al. Role of primary sensorimotor cortex and supplementary motor area in volitional swallowing: a movement-related cortical potential study. Am J Physiol Gastrointest Liver Physiol 2004;287;G459-70.
44. Sumi T. Coordination of neuronal organization of respiratory and deglutition: its change with post-natal maturation. In: Bosma JF, Showacre J, eds. Development of upper respiratory anatomy and function. Bethesda: National Institute of Health, 1975:145-59.
45. Suzuki M, Asada Y, Ito J, Hayashi K, Inoue H, Kitano H. Activation of cerebellum and basal ganglia on volitional swallowing detected by functional magnetic resonance imaging. Dysphagia 2003;18:71-7.
46. Toogood JA, Barr AM, Stevens TK, Gati JS, Menon RS, Martin RE. Discrete functional contributions of cerebral cortical foci in voluntary swallowing: a functional resonance imaging (fMRI) "go-no-go" study. Exp Brain Res 2005;161:81-90.
47. Watanabe Y, Shinichi A, Ishikawa T, Yamada Y, Yamane G. Cortical regulation during the early stage of initiation of voluntary swallowing in humans. Dysphagia 2004;19:100-8.
48. Weerasuriya A, Bieger D, Hockman CH. Basal forebrain facilitation of reflex swallowing in the eat. Brain Res 1979;174:119-33.
49. Yamamura K, Narita N, Yao D, Martin RE, Masuda Y, Sessle BJ. Effects of refversible bilateral inactivation of face primary motor cortex on mastication and swallowing. Brain Res 2002;944:40-55.
50. Yao D, Yamamura K, Narita N, Murray GM, Sessle BJ. Effects of reversible cold block of face primary somatosensory cortex neuronal activity. Somatosens Motor Res 2002;19:261-71.
51. Zald DH, PArdo JV. The functional neuroanatomy of voluntary swallowing. Ann Neurol 1999;46:281-6.

How does the larynx protect itself from acid regurgitation?

E. Brossard (Lausanne)

The three main functions of the larynx are: protection of airways, breathing and phonation. The protective function is entirely reflexive and involuntary, whereas both breathing and phonation are initiated voluntarily but regulated involuntarily. Because of the low position of the larynx in the human neck, there is an increased risk of pulmonary contamination by swallowed bolus as well as by regurgitated material.

Closure of vocal cords provides most of the lower airway protection. The epiglottis directs swallowed food laterally into the hypopharynx and the elevation of the larynx through contraction of pharyngeal muscles during deglutition enhances the protection against aspiration.

The laryngeal mucosa is not adapted to acid exposure. Differents mechanisms protect the larynx against acid reflux. Shaker has extensively studied the physiological barriers (upper and lower esophageal sphincters – UES and LES) and response mechanisms (different reflexes) which prevent the gastric content to reach the larynx [1].

Both LES and UES are the main sphincters that protect the larynx against gastroesophageal reflux (GER). These protective mechanisms are maintained without the need of stimulation. The UES resting pressure is variable and decreases during sleep and with age, and may, in some circumstances, be overcome by acid reflux [2].

A second group of protective mechanisms are those who become active in case of stimulation of different origins. These mechanisms include bolus clearance phenomenon (secondary peristalsis) and vasovagal reflexes. Among the multiple reflexes that protect the larynx from acid reflux, esophagoglottal reflex and esophago-UES contractile reflex are the two most important.

The **esophagoglottal reflex** is triggered by stretch receptors located along the esophagus. This reflex is enhanced more frequently, in the proximal esophagus, due to the distribution of vagal afferents fibers and the concomitant innervation by the recurrent laryngeal nerve [3]. A study on feline model showed that this reflex is significantly altered by acute experimental esophagitis [4].

The **esophago-UES contractile reflex**, normally triggered by a segmental distension of the esophagus, could also play a role in response to esophageal acidification. Some studies report an increase pressure in the UES after esophageal acid reflux events [5].

Koufman has reported that acid alone is relatively armless to laryngeal mucosa under physiological condition. In high concentration and in the presence of pepsin, the incidence of mucosal lesions is increased [6]. In a recent study, he investigated the presence of pepsin in laryngeal biopsies from patients with laryngopharyngeal reflux (LPR) and the expression of E-Cadherin and carbonic anhydrase [7].

E-Cadherin is a cell adhesion protein of the intercellular junctional complex. This protein plays an important role in mucosal integrity and barrier function. Pepsin is thought to digest the intercellular structures and destruct the mucosal barrier. In the Koufman study, intracellular pepsin was found in LPR patients, not in controls. E- Cadherin expression was reduced in LPR patients. It is not clear if the changes in E-Cadherin were secondary to acidified pepsin or to inflammatory process.

Carbonic anhydrase isoenzyme III (CA III) is an enzyme which regulates the pH and the fluid balance. CA III is responsible for the endogenous bicarbonate secretion by the esophagus mucosa.

In the Koufman study, CA III is increased in inflamed esophageal epithelia but not in laryngeal mucosa in response to LPR. The CA III expression is reduced in vocal cords and ventricle of the larynx, meaning a reduced ability to provide a bicarbonate barrier against reflux. In the posterior commissure of the larynx, the CA III expression is maintained. This could explain a certain degree of resistance of this part of the larynx to acid reflux.

Conclusions

In addition to the different mechanisms which prevent the entry of gastric content into the larynx, laryngeal epithelial cell defenses seem to play a role in the ability of the larynx to defend itself from acid reflux. Eventhough these mechanisms have been very well documented on healthy patients, there is a need for further investigations on patients with proven LPR.

New investigation tools like Impedance-pH metry will probably help us to better understand the role of all kind of refluxate in the pathogenesis of GER and its effect on laryngeal damages [8].

References

1. Shaker R. Airway protective mechanisms: current concepts. Dysphagia 1995;10:216-27.
2. Ulualp SO, Toohill RJ. Laryngopharyngeal reflux: state of the art diagnosis and treatment. Otolaryngol Clin North Am 2000;33-4:785-801.
3. Shaker R, Dodds WJ, Ren J, Hogan WJ, Arndorfer RC. Esophagoglottal closure reflex: a mechanism of airway protection. Gastroenterology 1992;102:857-61.
4. Ren J, Shaker R, Medda B, Bonnevier J, Kern M, Dunn B. Effect of acute esophagitis on the esophagoglottal reflex in a feline model. Gastroenterology 1995;108(4):A 677.
5. Kahrilas PJ, Dodds WJ, Dent J, Haeberle B, Hogan WJ, Arndorfer RC. Effect of sleep, spontaneous gastroesophageal reflux and meal on upper esophageal sphincter pressure in normal humans volunteers. Gastroenterology 1987;92:466-71.
6. Koufman JA. The otolaryngologic manifestation of gastroesophageal reflux disease. Laryngoscope 1991;101:1-78.
7. Gill AG, Johnston N, Buda A, et al. Laryngeal epithelial defenses against laryngopharyngeal reflux: investigations of E-cadherin, carbonic anhydrase isoenzyme III and pepsin. Ann Otol Rhinol Laryngol 200 ;114(12):913-21.
8. Sifrim D. Acid, weakly acidic and non-acid gastro-oesophageal reflux :differences, prevalences and clinical relevance. Eur J Gastroenterol Hepatol 2004;16:823-30.

Do we know enough about the local reflexive control of upper esophageal sphincter function to target pharmacotherapy for extraesophageal complications of gastroesophageal reflux disease?

A.M. Drewes (Aalborg)

The reflective control of the upper esophageal sphincter in the explanation of extraesophageal symptoms

The upper esophageal sphincter (UES) is a high pressure zone that is composed of muscle, cartilage and aponeuroses rather than just a simple ring of muscle. The zone is between 2 and 4 cm and the main muscles are the inferior pharyngeal constrictor, cricopharyngeus and the most proximal part of the esophagus. Cricopharyngeus is the most important muscle (*Figure 1*). For more detailed information the reader is referred to [1].

Normally the UES allows food to pass into the esophagus and allows reflux during belging and vomiting. The EUS pressure also decreases during sleep and in the elderly, and it has been discussed that the EUS under some circumstances may play a role in gastroesophageal reflux disease (GERD). However, the importance of the UES in GERD etiology remains controversial. Intraesophageal acid seems to increase the pressure in the UES [2]. On the other hand there is no correlation between episodes of reflux and UES activity [3] (*Figure 2*).

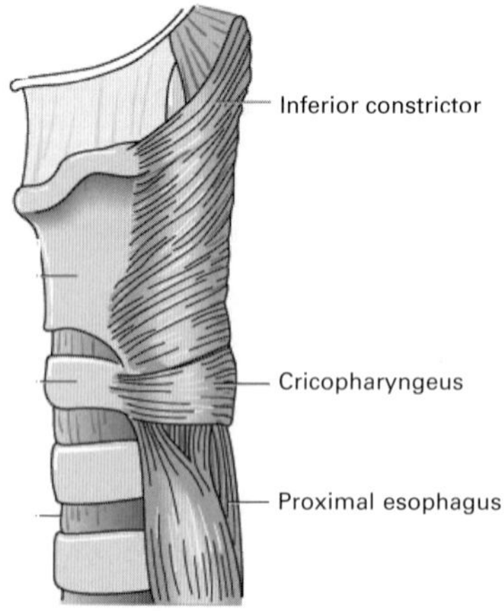

Figure 1. The upper esophageal sphincter is comprised of three adjacent muscles as illustrated together with cartilage and connective tissue.

One of the problems in understanding of UES functions may relate to the previous methods used to characterize the sphincter. First the sensors tend to move during swallowing and second there is axial asymmetry within the high-pressure zone. This complicates the interpretation of ordinary manometry. High-resolution manometry has the possibility to enhance the spatial resolution, and this method was used to obtain normative values in a series of 75 healthy volunteers [4]. Such data may in the future be used to characterize the UES in clinical manometric studies.

No matter to what extend the EUS projects against acid reflux there is no doubt that incompetence of the lower sphincter allowing large refluxates to pass into the esophagus is of major importance. Such refluxate has the possibility to enter the pharynx and contribute to extraesophageal symptoms such as asthma, chronic cough, globus, hoarseness, laryngitis, etc. For further information the reader is referred to e.g., [5]. However, many

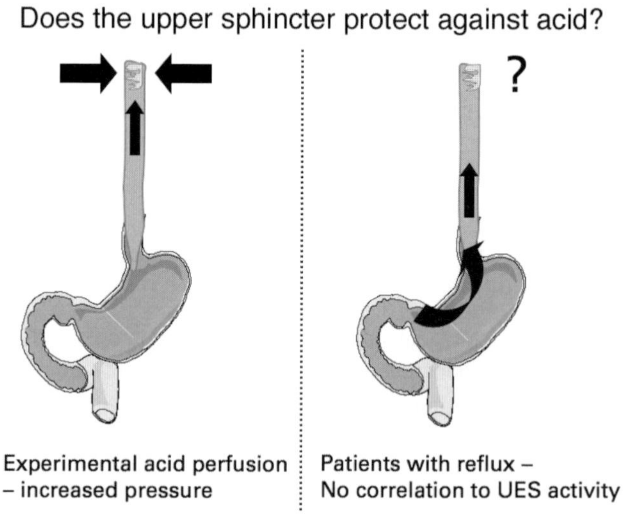

Figure 2. The controversial finding in experimental studies (left) where the pressure in the UES increases during intra-esophageal acid perfusion, whereas in the clinic (right) there is no correlation between episodes of reflux and UES activity.

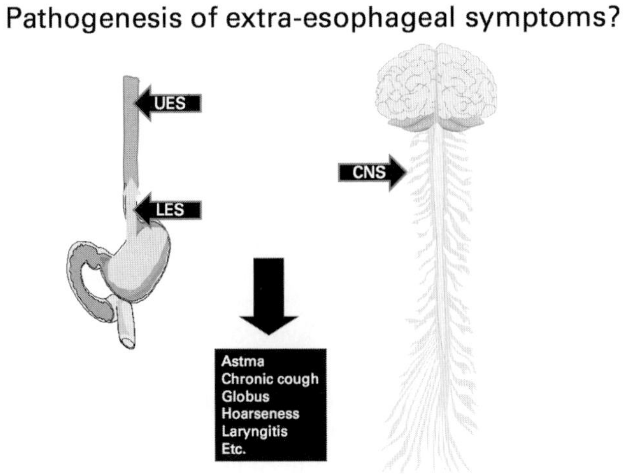

Figure 3. The pathogenetic mechanisms for extra-esophageal symptoms may be related to incompetence of the lower esophageal sphincter, incompetence of the upper esophageal sphincter and central hyperexcitability and viscero-visceral reflexes. Most likely combinations of these factors are often present.

patients continue to have symptoms despite sufficient medical or surgical treatment of the reflux, and in such patients hyperexcitability of the central nervous system and viscero-visceral reflex mechanisms may be of importance (*Figure 3*).

Viscero-visceral mechanisms in the explanation of extraesophageal symptoms

The mechanisms responsible for viscero-somatic convergence resulting in referred pain referral to somatic structures like the skin and muscle are not known in detail. Several theories have been suggested and for further information the reader is referred to [6]. However, schematically convergence between visceral and somatic structures on the same second order neuron in the spinal cord (or on neurons at higher levels in the neuraxis) is a plausible but simplified explanation (*Figure 4*). Hence, firing in the second order neuron causes the brain to "believe" that the somatic structures are suffering. This mislabeling can be explained by the fact that the brain is more used to encode spinal activation as being

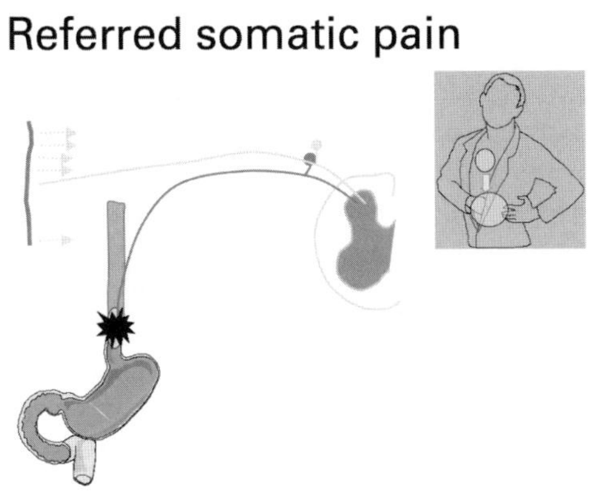

Figure 4. Referred pathways may be activated by impulses converging from esophageal pathways to central neurons also receiving somatic input. The activity in these central neurons may be interpreted by the patient as somatic pain in e.g., the abdomen.

somatic, as this is much more prevalent and important leading to e.g. withdrawal reflexes which protects the body against harmful stimulation.

Although viscero-somatic symptoms are well recognized in the clinic, hyperalgesia of one viscus may manifests clinically due to an inflammation or excess stimulation of another viscus [7]. This phenomenon termed viscero-visceral hyperalgesia is usually explained by partially overlapping innervation and extensive neuronal convergence of the different viscera. Viscero-visceral hyperalgesia is a complex form of hypersensitivity, which is likely to be explained by more than one mechanism. Since this phenomenon takes place preferentially between visceral organs which share, at least in part, their central projection, it is plausible that phenomena of central sensitization play an important role [8]. The concept of viscero-visceral hyperalgesia is shown in *Figure 5.* There is substantial experimental evidence documenting this phenomenon. In animal experiments, Garrison *et al.* [9] demonstrated that spinal neurons in the cat receiving input from the distal esophagus also received convergent input from the thoracic wall and the heart. In the same study, turpentine-induced inflammation of the distal esophagus resulted in a decreased threshold of the spinal neurons to esophageal distension. Evidence that the N-methyl-D-aspartate (NMDA) receptors play an important role in mediating this central neural hyperexitability exists [7].

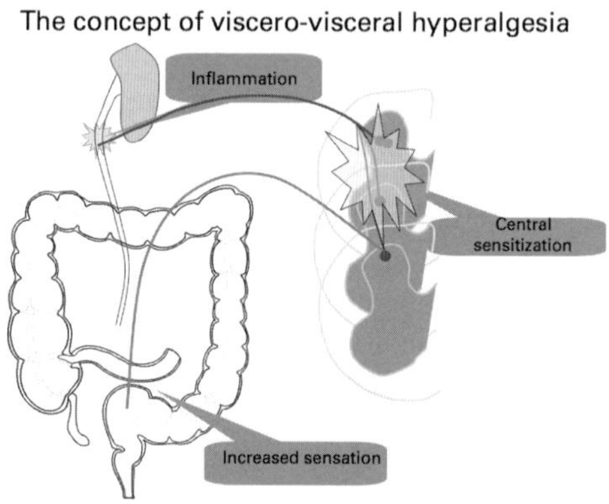

Figure 5. The concept of viscero-visceral hyperalgesia. A disease (or experimental stimulation) of the ureter may evoke hyperexcitability of neurons in the central nervous system. As visceral afferents innervate the spinal cord in a much more diffuse and widespread way as compared to somatic nerves the hyperexcitability may involve several segments. Hence, the input from other viscera such as the colon may also be amplified resulting in increased sensation in the remote organ.

Recently, human experimental studies supporting the role of viscero-visceral hyperalgesia in the clinic have also been conducted. Thus, acidification of the distal esophagus resulted in hyperalgesia in the proximal esophagus, and duodenal acidification has shown to induce esophageal hypersensitivity [10-12]. Recently we showed that acidification of the esophagus may involve widespread changes in the perception of pain from remote organs such as the rectum [13]. The evoked changes may not only be spinal as there is recent evidence from human studies that acidification of the esophagus with acid induce plastic changes in the cortical processing of pain evoked in the esophagus [14]. The above mentioned activation of NMDA receptors was also confirmed in a human study where acidification of the distal esophagus was performed prior to administration of the NMDA receptor antagonist ketamine. Hence, ketamine prevented the development of acid-induced hypersensitivity to electrical stimulation of the proximal esophagus [15]. The ability to model human viscero-visceral hyperalgesia under controlled experimental studies provides a unique approach in future exploration of pathophysiology and pharmacological interventions in patients with visceral hypersensitivity due to central sensitization.

The widespread visceral hypersensitivity in functional gastrointestinal disorders (irritable bowel syndrome, functional dyspepsia, etc.) may be at least partly due to this mechanism [16-18]. As an example a marked reduction in colonic perception thresholds and alternation in the viscerosomatic referral pattern were seen in patients with irritable bowel syndrome after lipid administration in the duodenum [19].

Viscero-visceral hyperalgesia may explain the epidemiological findings in several clinical conditions with organic diseases such as an increased number of anginal attacks in patients with gallbladder calcinosis, and increased number of colics in dysmenorrheic patients with urinary calculosis [7] (*Figure 6*). Evidence for viscero-visceral hyperalgesia has also been provided in experimental studies of organic diseases, e.g., in patients with GERD where increased sensitivity to gastric distension was shown [20]. Therefore the frequent airway symptoms in GERD may not only be related to direct aspiration of the gastric refluxate, but vasovagal reflex mechanisms evoked by acid related hyperalgesia may also be important [5]. Experimental tests can support this suspicion [21-23] although their usefulness in the individual patient still awaits further documentation.

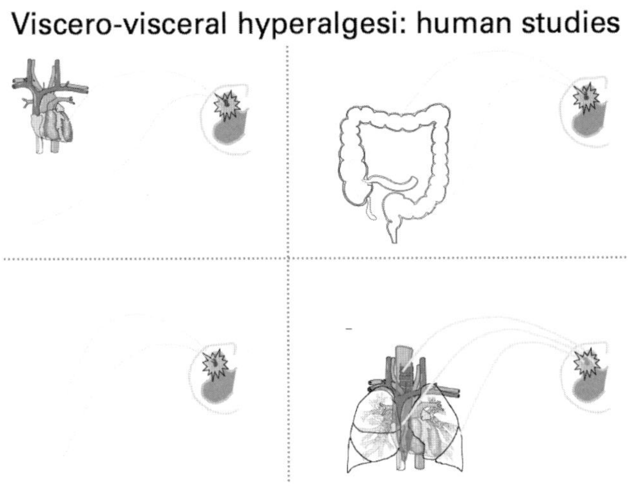

Figure 6. Schematic illustration human epidemiologic and experimental studies where evidence for viscero-visceral hyperalgesia have been demonstrated.

Treatment of extraesophageal symptoms

The treatment of extraesophageal symptoms rely on the prevalent mechanisms (*Figure 7*). In many patients where acid reflux is the dominant symptom proton pump inhibitors (PPI) are sufficient. H_2-blockers either alone or in combination with PPI are often preferable when there is evidence for night-time reflux. Some patients may need prokinetics or drugs improving sphincter and barrier function. However, many patients respond poorly to this treatment and in such cases viscero-visceral hyperalgesia should be considered. In these patients analgesics targeted at reducing central hyperexcitability may be a treatment option

Extra-esophageal symptoms ~
1. Sphincter incompetence
2. Viscero-visceral hyperalgesia
3. Central neuroplastic reorganization

↓

1. PPI ± H_2 blockers
2. Drugs improving LES (& UES)
3. Drugs improving barrier function
4. Prokinetics
5. Drugs against central hyperexcitability

Figure 7. Treatment of extra-esophageal symptoms depends on which mechanism is thought to be dominating. For details see text.

than acid inhibition. Whether simple analgesics such as paracetamol and weak opioids are preferred to more complex drugs such as ion-channel inhibitors and 5HT antagonists having many effects on the pain system still await further studies.

References

1. Singh S, Hamdy S. The upper oesophageal sphincter. Neurogastroenterol Mot 2005;17:3-12.
2. Andreollo NA, Thompson DG, Kendall GP, Earlam RJ. Functional relationships between cricopharyngeal sphincter and oesophageal body in response to graded intraluminal distension. Gut 1988;29:161-6.
3. Jacob P, Kahrilas PJ, Herzon G. Proximal esophageal pH-metry in patients with "reflux laryngitis". Gastroenterol 1991;100:305-10.
4. Ghosh SK, Pandolfino JE, Zhang Q, Jarosz A, Kahrilas PJ. Deglutitive upper esophageal sphincter relaxation: a study of 75 volunteer subjects using solid-state high-resolution manometry. Am J Physiol Gastrointest Liver Physiol 2006;291:G525-31.
5. Fass R, Achem SR, Harding S, Mittal RK, Quigley E. Review article: supra-oesophageal manifestations of gastro-oesophageal reflux disease and the role of night-time gastro-oesophageal reflux. Aliment Pharmacol Ther 2004;20:26-38.
6. Arendt-Nielsen L, Laursen RJ, Drewes AM. Referred pain as an indicator for neural plasticity. Prog Brain Res 2000;129:343-56.
7. Giamberardino MA. Recent and forgotten aspects of visceral pain. Eur J Pain 1999;3:77-92.
8. Qin C, Malykhina AP, Akbarali HI, Foreman RD. Cross-organ sensitization of lumbosacral spinal neurons receiving urinary bladder input in rats with inflamed colon. Gastroenterology 2005;129:1967-78.
9. Garrison DW, Chandler MJ, Foreman RD. Viscerosomatic convergence onto feline spinal neurons from esophagus, heart and somatic fields; effects of inflammation. Pain 1992;49:373-82.
10. Sarkar S, Aziz Q, Woolf CJ, Hobson AR, Thompson DG. Contribution of central sensitisation to the development of non-cardiac chest pain. Lancet 2000;356:1154-9.
11. Sarkar S, Hobson AR, Furlong PL, Woolf CJ, Thompson DG, Aziz Q. Central neural mechanisms mediating human visceral hypersensitivity. Am J Physiol Gastrointest Liver Physiol 2001;281:G1196-202.
12. Hobson AR, Aziz Q. Brain imaging and functional gastrointestinal disorders: Has it helped our understanding? Gut 2004;53:1198-206.
13. Frokjaer JB, Liao D, Bergmann A, et al. Three-dimensional biomechanical properties of the human rectum evaluated with magnetic resonance imaging. Neurogastroenterol Motil 2005;17:531-40.
14. Sami SA, Rössel P, Dimcevski G, et al. Cortical changes to experimental sensitization of the human esophagus. Neuroscience 2006;140:269-79.
15. Willert RP, Woolf CJ, Hobson AR, Delaney C, Thompson DG, Aziz Q. The development and maintenance of human visceral pain hypersensitivity is dependent on the N-methyl-D-aspartate receptor. Gastroenterology 2004;126:683-92.
16. Sanger GJ. Hypersensitivity and hyperreactivity in the irritable bowel syndrome: an opportunity for drug discovery. Dig Dis 1999;17:90-9.
17. Mertz H, Fullerton S, Naliboff B, Mayer EA. Symptoms and visceral perception in severe functional and organic dyspepsia. Gut 1998;42:814-22.
18. Munakata J, Naliboff B, Harraf F, et al. Repetitive sigmoid stimulation induces rectal hyperalgesia in patients with irritable bowel syndrome. Gastroenterology 1997;112:55-63.

19. Simren M, Abrahamsson H, Bjornsson ES. An exaggerated sensory component of the gastrocolonic response in patients with irritable bowel syndrome. Gut 2001;48:20-7.
20. Penagini R, Hebbard G, Horowitz M, et al. Motor function of the proximal stomach and visceral perception in gastro-oesophageal reflux disease. Gut 1998;42:251-7.
21. Drewes AM, Pedersen J, Reddy H, et al. Central sensitisation in patients with non-cardiac chest pain: A clinical experimental study. Scand J Gastroenterol 2006;41:1-10.
22. Drewes AM, Reddy H, Pedersen J, Funch-Jensen P, Gregersen G, Arendt-Nielsen L. Multimodal pain stimulations in patients with grade B oesophagitis. Gut 2006;55:926-32.
23. Reddy H, Staahl C, Arendt-Nielsen L, Gregersen H, Drewes AM, Funch-Jensen P. Sensory and biomechanical properties of the oesophagus in non-erosive reflux disease. Scand J Gastroenterol 2007;42:432-40.

What are the anatomical elements contributing to the structure of the upper esophageal sphincter?

R. Goyal (Boston)

The upper esophageal sphincter (UES) is the name given to a sphincter like area that is located between the esophagus and the pharynx. It is distinguished from the pharynx above and the esophagus below by the fact that it keeps the lumen closed at rest. The lumen opens and forcefully closes intermittently to allow passage of contents during various physiologic events such as swallowing. The functional behavior of the UES can be recorded by intraluminal pressure recording which shows a zone of high pressure called the upper high pressure zone (UHPZ) separating the pharyngeal and the esophageal pressures. Although presence of a functional UES or the UHPZ at the pharyngoesophageal junction is easily demonstrated, the anatomic components which constitute the UES or the UHPZ have been a subject of ongoing controversy.

Anatomy of the pharyngoesophageal junction area

The pharyngoesophageal junction areas that require consideration in relation to the UHPZ are the lower hypopharynx (part of the pharynx or laryngopharynx below the laryngeal opening into the pharynx) and the uppermost part of the cervical esophagus [1].

The anterior wall of the lower hypopharynx is an approximately 3.25 cm-high rigid structure. In adults, it is constituted by the arytenoid cartilage and the inter-arytenoid muscles (approximately 0.75 cm high) and posterior surface of the cricoid cartilage (approximately 2.5 cm high). The lower part of the pyriform sinuses, or the recesses on either side of the posteriorly bulging cricoid cartilage, are parts of the lower hypopharynx.

The posterior wall of the hypopharynx is entirely fibro-muscular in nature. The muscles that are present in the posterior wall of the hypopharynx are cricopharyngeus and thyropharyngeus. Anatomically, cricopharyngeus muscle refers to pharyngeal muscle connected to the cricoid catrilage. The cricopharyngeus muscle has been divided into the pars obliqua and the pars fundiformis. Fibers of the pars obliqua extends obliquely upwards to insert into the posterior midline pharyngeal raphe where they are joined by the fibers of the pars obliqua from the other side. Thyropharyngeus muscle is present superior to the pars obliqua fibers. Fibers of pars obliqua and the thyropharyngeus together constitute the inferior pharyngeal constrictor muscle. The lowermost fibers of the inferior pharyngeal constrictor are relevant to the discussion of the role of this muscle in UHPZ.

Fibers of the pars fundiformis extend horizontally around the posterior circumference of the hypopharynx to attach to the cricoid cartilage on the other side. The overall thickness of the pars fundiformis is around 0.7 cm. Posteriorly, the fibers of pars obliqua above and pars fundiformis below leave a triangular area of sparse muscle fibers called Killian's dehiscence (the site for formation of Zenker's diverticulum). Radiologists and clinicians usually refer only to the pars fundiformis of the cricopharyngeus muscle as the cricopharyngeus muscle (this terminology will be used in this commentary).

The cervical esophagus begins below the cricoid cartilage and is constituted by esophageal outer longitudinal and inner circular muscle fibers. The longitudinal muscle in the uppermost part of the esophagus is tendinous that is attached to the cricoid cartilage. The esophageal longitudinal muscle fibers arise from these tendons and fan out as they descend down dorsally to provide a complete covering of the posterior wall of esophagus by the longitudinal muscle. This arrangement of fibers leaves a V-shaped gap between and above them (Laimer's triangle) that is devoid of longitudinal muscle. Anteriorly also, this area of the esophagus is devoid of longitudinal muscle. The inner circular muscle appears to be similar to the circular muscle in the rest of the esophagus.

Radiological observations of the pharyngoesophageal area

Plain X-rays in the lateral projection show that the pharyngeal air column ends at the upper border of the hypopharynx and the airless segment end at the lower border of the cricoid cartilage. Because Valsalva maneuver causes reflex contraction of the cricopharyngeus muscle, during Valsalva maneuver impression of the contracted cricopharyngeus muscle can be seen in the area corresponding to the lower 1/4th of the cricoid cartilage. The esophagus below the cricopharyngeus muscle and the lower border of the cricoid cartilage is also identified as a well distended segment.

In this region, barium studies may show abnormalities such as Zanker's diverticulum and the dilated pyriform sinuses due pharyngeal muscle paralysis. In cricopharyngeus bar a prominent cricopharyngeus is seen in the posterior pharyngeal wall in the region of the lower 1/4th of the cricoid cartilage.

Thus, there is complete agreement between the anatomic and radiologic findings that:

- lower hypopharynx is around 3.2 cm high and is defined by the height of the cricoid cartilage and the arytenoids;
- cricopharyngeus muscle is present in the lower 1/4th of the cricoid cartilage;
- cervical esophagus starts just distal to the distal end of the cricoid cartilage and the cricopharyngeus (anatomic pars fundiformis);
- opening of the Zenker's diverticulum and the pyriform sinuses are present in the region of the hypopharynx.

Manometric observations of the pharyngoesophageal area

Manometric studies identify a 3-4 cm UHPZ between the atmospheric pressures in the pharynx and sub-atmospheric pressures in the esophagus. However, they do not identify what anatomic structures and muscles constitute the UHPZ.

Simultaneous cineradiographic and manometric studies

In order to identify the anatomic structures that contribute to the UHPZ, simultaneous cine-radiographic and manometric studies have been performed in human subjects. One of the reliably identifiable markers, on X-rays, in this area is position of the vocal cords. In the lateral projection, level of the vocal cords is marked by laryngeal air column. The vocal cords correspond to the upper border of the cricoid cartilage. The cricoid cartilage can also be identified in its entirety when it is calcified. The muscle contributing to the UHPZ can be deduced by the known location and the dimensions of the muscles.

Results of three simultaneous cine-radiographic and manometric studies are summarized in *Figure 1* [2-4]. These results show that most of the UHPZ corresponds with the anatomical and radiological lower hypopharynx that is located behind the cricoid and arytenoid cartilages. The peak of the UHPZ is present in the middle of the region of the cricoid cartilage [5]. Most surprisingly, the cricopharyngeus muscle was localized below the peak of the HPZ. Moreover, the cervical esophagus did not appear to contribute to the UHPZ. The above observations are not consistent with the generally held belief that the

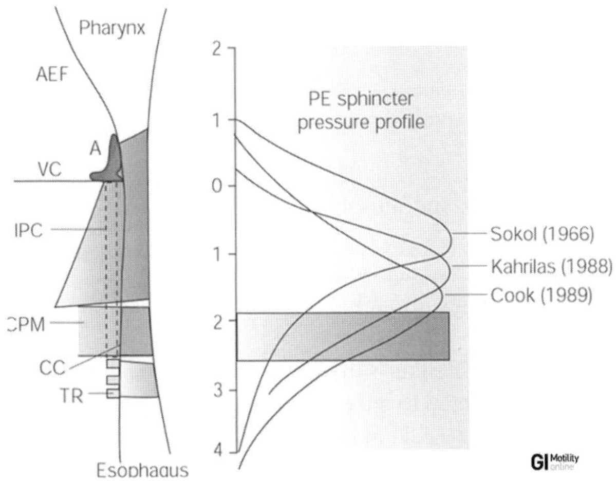

Figure 1. Anatomic correlates of the human upper high pressure zone. An important anatomic landmark in the pharyngo-esophageal segment is the vocal cords, which mark the junction of the arytenoids and the cricoid cartilage. Level of the vocal cords can be recognized by the air level in the laryngotracheal area. The bottom of the pharyngeal air column is a variable landmark and is present around the upper posterior part of the arytenoid cartilages. When calcified, entire cricoid cartilage may be visualized. The thyropharyngeus muscle and the oblique fibers of the crico-pharyngeus muscle constitute the inferior pharyngeal constrictor muscle. The horizontal fibers of the cricopharyngeus muscle (referred to as the cricopharyngeus muscle) is 0.7 cm wide and is present at the level of the lower 1/4 of the cricoid cartilage. Note that the peaks of none of these reported studies correspond with the level of the cricopharyngeus muscle (shown as the hatched area).
AEF: aryepiglottic fold; CC: cricoid cartilage; CPM: cricopharyngeus muscle; ESO: esophagus; IPC: inferior pharyngeal constrictor; TR: tracheal ring; VC: vocal cord; A: arytenoid.
(Original source: [5,6]).

cricopharyngeus is the main muscle of the UHPZ and therefore must form the peak of the UHPZ and that the uppermost part of the cervical esophagus contributes to the lower part of the UHPZ.

Other studies

Other studies using simultaneous high resolution manometry and imaging studies of the UHPZ and electrical recordings of the precisely identified muscles are needed to fully resolve this important issue. Studies of the electrical and mechanical behavior of the muscles in this area in experimental animals may also provide some supportive evidence for further testing in humans. Specifically remaining questions are:
- does cricopharyngeus muscle constitute peak of HPZ?
- does cervical esophagus contribute to the UHPZ?

As regard the first point, it has been argued [6] that the pressure of the UHPZ may peak in the region of the inferior pharyngeal constrictor because of its higher passive forces and low compliance. Therefore, although the peak HPZ corresponds with the location of the inferior pharyngeal constrictor, cricopharyngeus may be the most active muscle in the UES. It is possible that the head position used in these studies did not fully activate the cricopharyngeus resulting in lower pressures in the region of the cricopharyngeus. It is certainly possible that profile of the UHPZ may change with isolated activation of the cricopharyngeus. One study has reported that the peak UHPZ corresponds with level of the cricopharyngeus muscle [7]. Further studies to test this interesting suggestion are needed. As regards the contribution of the cervical esophagus to the UHPZ, evidence to support this view is scanty. Further studies to resolve this issue will also be rewarding. Use of recent, advanced imaging techniques and high resolution manometry will, no doubt, fully resolve these controversies in the future.

Why is accurate determination of the muscles responsible for upper high pressure zone important?

A full understanding of the anatomic landmark and muscles responsible for the UHPZ are important for several reasons:
- if the UHPZ is all above the cervical esophagus and is located entirely in the hypopharynx, then it should be more appropriately considered as pharyngeal or hypopharyngeal sphincter;
- if the UHPZ is entirely hypopharyngeal, then Zenker's diverticulum that opens just above the cricopharyngeus muscle should be considered to have opening within the UHPZ of the upper sphincter and this relationship may play a role in understanding the pathogenesis of Zenker's diverticulum.

References

1. Williams P, Warwick R. Gray's anatomy, 36th ed. Edinburgh: Churchill Livingstone, 1980:1308-13.
2. Sokol EM, Heitman P, Wolf BS, Cohen BR. Simultaneous cineradiographic and manometric study of the larynx, hypopharynx, and cervical esophagus. Gastroenterology 1966;51:960–74.
3. Kahrilas P, Dodds W, Dent J, Logeman J. Upper esophageal sphincter function during deglutition. Gastroenterology 1988;95:52-62.

4. Cook IJ, Dodds W, Dantas R, et al. Opening mechanisms of of the human UES. Am J Physiol 1989;257:G748-59.
5. Goyal RK, Martin SB, Shapiro J, Spechler, SJ. The role of cricopharyngeus muscle in pharyngoesophageal disorders. Dysphagia 1993;8:253-8.
6. Lang IM. Upper esophageal sphincter. GI Motility online, www.GIMotilityonline.com doi:10.1038/gimo12, 2006.
7. Nilsson ME, Isberg A, Schiratzki H. The location of the upper oesophageal sphincter and its behaviour during bolus propagation — a simultaneous cineradiographic and manometric investigation. Clin Otolaryngol Allied Sci 1989;14:61-5.

What is the significance of a cricopharyngeal bar and is it synonymous with upper esophagealsphincter achalasia?

R.O. Dantas, R.A. Cassiani (São Paulo)

Cricopharyngeal bar may be seen in the posterior wall of the hypopharynx as a smooth rounded indentation visible on lateral radiographs of barium swallows at the level of the 5th or 6th cervical vertebral body. Videoradiographic studies report a prevalence of 5-11%, with dysphagia being associated with bar in only 15% of the cases [1].

This radiological finding was considered as consequence of spasm of the cricopharyngeus or complete or incomplete failure of the cricopharyngeal relaxation [2], and was often called "cricopharyngeal achalasia" [3]. However, more recent studies have shown that there is no problem with cricopharyngeal relaxation and that the find is not consequence of cricopharyngeal achalasia [4-6], with no enough data to support the adequation of the terms spasm or achalasia to explain the finding. Manometrically normal relaxation of the cricopharyngeus has been commonly seen in patients with a permanent cricopharyngeal bar. For swallows of a 10 ml bolus of liquid barium the duration of upper esophageal sphincter (UES) relaxation was 0.56 ± 0.04 seconds for healthy volunteers and 0.54 ± 0.07 seconds for patients with cricopharyngeal bar [4].

Cricopharyngeal bar cause a problem in the UES opening [4], but causes dysphagia in the minority of patients [5]. When a patient with cricopharyngeal bar has dysphagia another explanation for the symptom should be evaluated. Often esophageal or pharyngeal dysfunction is the dominant mechanism of the dysphagia [5].

The reason why the cricopharyngeal bar do not cause dysphagia in most of the patients may be the normal UES flow seen in these patients. The UES sagittal diameter, UES transverse diameter and UES area are reduced when compared to normal subjects, but the UES flow is the same of normal subjects. With swallows of a 10 ml bolus of liquid barium the duration of UES opening (flow duration) was 0.58 ± 0.02 seconds for healthy volunteers and 0.61 ± 0.03 seconds for patients with cricopharyngeal bar [4]. The most important functional difference from the normal subjects is the significant increase in the upstream intrabolus pressure, which should sustain the normal flow [4]. These results are similar to that seen in patients with Zenker's diverticulum [6,7].

A recent study found a cricopharyngeal protrusion on the posterior hypopharyngeal wall in 29% of human cadavers of people who were over 60 years old [8]. The cricopharyngeal was completely relaxed although it had an anatomical protrusion, showing that the failure to relax is not the cause of the cricopharyngeal protrusion [8]. This cricopharyngeal protrusion is seen only in the elderly [9].

The antero-posterior UES opening and hyoid bone and thyroid cartilage anterior excursion are reduced in the elderly compared with young, what are associated with increased intrabolus pressure, suggesting an higher pharyngeal outflow resistance in the elderly compared to the young [10,11]. These results are similar to that found in patients with cricopharyngeal bar [4], suggesting that the cricopharyngeal bar is related to the aging process. However, the cricopharyngeal bar may be seen in subjects younger than 50 years [4]. The opening of the UES in elderly patients with cricopharyngeal bar is significantly reduced when compared with elderly patients without cricopharyngeal bar [12], so the aging process is not the single explanation of the UES alteration. Histologic examination of the cricopharyngeal muscle of patients with cricopharyngeal bar showed muscle fiber degeneration, interstitial fibrosis and inflammatory myopathy [5,8]. These alterations may cause a reduced compliance, or stretchability, of the relaxed UES [4].

In summary, cricopharyngeal bar is not synonymous of achalasia, cause dysphagia in some but not all patients, cause a reduction in UES opening, has a normal flow through the UES and an increase in the upstream intrabolus pressure.

References

1. Cook IJ. Cricopharyngeal function and dysfunction. Dysphagia 1993;8:244-51.
2. Palmer ED. Disorders of the cricopharyngeus muscle: a review. Gastroenterology 1976;71:510-9.
3. Leonard JR, Smith H. Cricopharyngeal achalasia. Ann Otol Rhinol Laryngol 1970;79:907-11.
4. Dantas RO, Cook IJ, Dodds WJ, Kern MK, Lang IM, Brasseur JG. Biomechanics of cricopharyngeal bars. Gastroenterology 1990;99:1269-74.
5. Cook IJ. Disorders causing oropharyngeal dysphagia. In: Castell DO,Richter JE, eds. The Esophagus, fourth edition. Philadelphia: Lippincott Williams & Wilkins, 2004:196-220.
6. Singh S, Hamdy S. The upper esophageal sphincter. Neurogastroenterol Motil 2005;17(Suppl 1): 3-12.
7. Cook IJ, Gabb M, Panagopoulos V, et al. Pharyngeal (Zenker's) diverticulum is a disorder of upper esophageal sphincter opening. Gastroenterology 1992;103:1229-35.
8. Leaper M, Zhang M, Dawes PJD. An anatomical protrusion exists on the posterior hypopharyngeal wall in some elderly cadavers. Dysphagia 2005;20:8-14.
9. Xu S, Tu L, Wang Q, Zhang M. Is the anatomical protrusion on the posterior hypopharyngeal wall associated with cadavers of only the elderly? Dysphagia 2006;21:163-6.
10. Kern M, Bardan E, Arndorfer R, Hofmann C, Ren J, Shaker R. Comparison of upper esophageal sphincter opening in healthy asymptomatic young and elderly volunteers. Ann Otol Rhinol Laryngol 1999;108:982-9.
11. Bammer T, Salassa JR, Klingler PJ. Comparison of methods for determining cricopharyngeal intrabolus pressure in normal patients as possible indicator for cricopharyngeal myotomy. Otolaryngol Head Neck Surg 2002;127:299-308.
12. Leonard R, Kendall K, Mckenzie S. UES opening and cricopharyngeal bar in nondysphagic elderly and nonelderly adults. Dysphagia 2004;19:182-191.

Do we have valid and reliable means of quantifying severity of pharyngeal dysphagia? Move toward standardization

B. Martin-Harris (Charleston)

Measurement of swallowing impairment

There has been a dramatic proliferation of methods and technologies geared toward the evaluation of swallowing function. A recent *Medline* search (1966 - October Week 4, 2006) that included the key words relating to swallowing and measurement yielded over 8,700 citations of studies involving human participants and 772 review articles on the cross-matched topics. The reported measurement methods included in these reports range from measures of pressure, bolus clearance, penetration, aspiration, muscle activity, timing, sensation, bolus flow, and kinematics. The instrumental technologies include both direct and indirect visualization procedures such as the modified barium swallowing study (MBSS) or videofluoroscopic swallowing evaluation (VFE), undoubtedly the most widely and carefully studied of all the available methods, fiberoptic endoscopic evaluation of swallowing (FEES), fiberoptic endoscopic evaluation of swallowing with sensory testing (FEEST), manometry, manofluorography (MFG), multichannel intraluminal impedence testing (MII), ultrasonography, electromyography, and scintigraphy. Consistent with many areas of medical practice, technologic advances have often been introduced prior to the development of standardized, reliable, and valid measurement methods that permit not only the quantification of impairment, but also the establishment of the external validity of the measures. The MBSS is clearly the predominant technique chosen by speech-language pathologists (SLP) for assessment of oropharyngeal swallowing impairment according to the frequency of CPT and Medicare billing codes (i.e., average of 20,000 billing entries each year) [1]. FEES, the second most commonly applied instrumental technique for the assessment or oropharyngeal swallowing function, permits early and late direct visualization of the pharynx and larynx relative to the timing of the swallow, permits observations regarding pre- and post-swallowing dynamics, and allows for inferences to be made of swallowing function [2,3]. However, there are several limitations to this type of exam. Many of the critical physiologic components known to contribute to the synergy of a safe and efficient swallowing mechanism are obscured during this endoscopic exam [3]. The oral cavity cannot be viewed because of the pharyngeal position of the scope. Additionally, the dynamics of the pharynx, larynx, and cervical esophagus are obliterated at the very height of the swallow as the tip of the endoscope (and consequent reflected light) opposes structures during hyolaryngeal excursion [3]. FEES and MBSS, however, are considered highly complimentary evaluative tools, are often used in association with each other at various times in a dysphagic patient's clinical course, and should be selected based on the candidacy of the patient and the questions that the clinician seeks to answer. Based on the widespread utilization of the MBSS, the comprehensive scope of the examination, and the plethora of studies that have tested the clinical utility of the exam, the MBSS will be the focus of the remaining discussion regarding measurement standards. In fact, the MBSS is considered the closest instrument to a "gold standard" in the fields of speech-language pathology and radiology, has been rigorously tested for its utility to predict and effect immediate patient outcomes, but has not been adequately tested empirically for its clinical utility relative to long-term patient outcome [4-7].

The MBSS, a videofluoroscopic recording of swallowing function, permits the visualization of bolus flow in relation to structural movement over time [8]. This evaluation method is considered an optimal tool by many practicing SLPs because it permits the visualization of bolus flow in relation to structural movement throughout the upper aerodigestive tract in real time [8-14]. The MBSS also permits detection of the presence and timing of aspiration, i.e., entry of ingested material below the level of the true vocal folds into the trachea, and assists in identifying the physiologic and often treatable causes of the aspiration [8-15].

Swallowing physiology as a foundation for measurement

Swallowing is a complex physiologic event comprised of simultaneous and sequential contractions of muscles of the oral-facial region, pharynx, larynx, and esophagus. Descriptions of swallowing physiology were attempted well before the development of a sophisticated modality for viewing the rapid contractions and movements of the muscles and structures associated with swallowing. In 1813, Magendie was the first to separate swallowing into phases or stages representing the anatomic regions traversed by the "bolus," or ball of material, to be swallowed [16]. The rapid sequential and overlapping motions characterizing adult human swallowing behavior were better appreciated with the introduction of radiography, and especially video radiography. Recent studies have shown that when temporal onsets of swallowing measures are studied for their contributions to these phases, the correlations between the kinematic and bolus flow events are so tight, that the events form one single factor, oropharyngeal [17].

The onsets of the tested oropharyngeal swallow events did not segment into an oral and pharyngeal phase, inconsistent with the traditional phase description of the swallowing mechanism. Rather, the oropharyngeal events from the onset of oral bolus transport to hyoid return to rest were so closely correlated that they loaded onto one factor in the solution. This finding speaks to the overlap between the initiation of oral and pharyngeal components of swallowing and highlights the artificiality of separating the swallowing continuum into isolated phases… Rather, in keeping with the physiologic model of swallowing, the onsets commingled bolus flow with structural movement measures. The phase nomenclature appears to relate more to the regions of bolus passage instead of to the functional movement of structures. Clinicians are often misguided in their observations of swallowing function when primary attention is focused on bolus flow characteristics such as transit times and estimates of "residue" or "pooling" in preference to attending to the underlying physiologic component(s) of swallowing that cause the aberration in bolus flow. Recognition of the impaired physiologic component(s), in lieu of describing an "oral phase" or "pharyngeal phase" disorder, is essential for the application of the appropriate treatment strategies that effect improvement in the physiologic swallow component

In contrast to describing a disordered swallowing phase, swallowing clinicians should attempt to evaluate the known literature-based functional targets of swallowing impairment [17] (*Figure 1*). The meaning of the term, domain, in the field of topology is defined as a connected open set, and will be used in the remaining discussions of this paper to eliminate

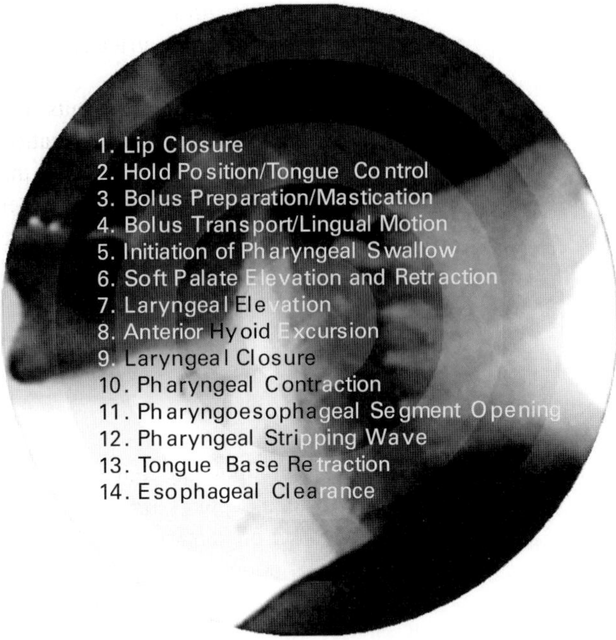
1. Lip Closure
2. Hold Position/Tongue Control
3. Bolus Preparation/Mastication
4. Bolus Transport/Lingual Motion
5. Initiation of Pharyngeal Swallow
6. Soft Palate Elevation and Retraction
7. Laryngeal Elevation
8. Anterior Hyoid Excursion
9. Laryngeal Closure
10. Pharyngeal Contraction
11. Pharyngoesophageal Segment Opening
12. Pharyngeal Stripping Wave
13. Tongue Base Retraction
14. Esophageal Clearance

Figure 1. Functional targets of swallowing impairment.

the arbitrary topographic limits connoted by the word phase [19]. The term, components, will represent the physiologic movement thought to contribute to the overall domain.

Regional domain: oral

Whereas the late oral and early pharyngeal components of swallowing are the most critical from a safety point of view, the oral preparatory and early oral transport aspects of swallow are the most aesthetically and psychologically important. During the oral preparatory stage of swallow, the bolus is manipulated by lingual motion, masticated (if necessary) and contained in the oral cavity by an anterior lip seal (component 1) and by lateral and posterior tongue to palatal contact. The tongue is the major mobile element of the oral phase of swallow and plays a complementary role in mastication during the oral preparatory phases. The tongue also plays a major role in bolus containment (component 2) and airway maintenance [20-23]. The back of the tongue assumes a slightly elevated position due to contraction of various muscle groups, and opposes an actively contracted soft palate that is drawn downward and forward. This glosso-palatine mechanism ensures that portions of the bolus do not fall prematurely over the base of the tongue [11,12]. The ingested material is mixed with saliva and tasted during mastication (component 3), a motion that is integrated into the oral swallowing process [20,21]. At the conclusion of the oral preparatory phase, when the ingested material is of adequate size and consistency for safe and efficient swallowing, it is collected and formed into a cohesive bolus on the center of the tongue and ready for lingual transport (component 4). If there are inefficiencies in the system, such as muscle weakness or sensory loss, residual material may remain in the oral cavity placing the patient at risk for inadequate nutrition/hydration or airway compromise.

Regional domain: pharyngeal

As the bolus is propelled through the oral cavity *via* upward and forward motion of the tongue, the head of the bolus reaches the region of the posterior oral cavity or oropharynx. When the sensory receptive fields in these areas are stimulated, the pharyngeal swallow is initiated (component 5) and respiration halts [19,20,23]. The pharyngeal swallow is characterized by five mechanical events that have been shown to overlap during synchronized video recordings of structural swallowing movements. These events function to protect the airway and clear the pharynx of ingested material and include:

- elevation and retraction of the soft palate (component 6);
- elevation (component 7) and anterior displacement (component 8) of the hyoid bone and larynx;
- laryngeal closure (component 9);
- pharyngeal contraction (component 10);
- opening of the pharyngoesophageal region (component 11) [8,10-13,24-31].

Contraction (e.g., stripping) of the pharyngeal constrictors (component 12) is coincident with the forceful retraction of the tongue (component 13) that applies strong positive pressure on the bolus tail assisting in pharyngeal clearance and prevention of pharyngeal residue [24,25,27,32]. Hyolaryngeal elevation and forward movement are intimately related and move as a functional unit. These critical motions, observed during the MBSS, appear to be physiologically linked to laryngeal closure (e.g., airway protection and aspiration prevention) and to opening and distension of the pharyngoesophageal segment (PES). Opening of the segment permits entry of the ingested material into the cervical esophageal region [24-31]. The traction placed on the cricoid cartilage during this brisk motion pulls this cartilage anteriorly and away from the posterior pharyngeal wall, opening the then compliant PES region [24-31]. This compliance is related to relaxation of the cricopharyngeal muscle, the primary muscular component of the segment [23,33]. As the larynx descends toward its rest position in the latter stages of pharyngeal swallowing, respiration is resumed and characterized by a small expiratory airflow in most adult human swallows [34-38].

Regional domain: esophageal

The mechanics of the esophageal body and lower esophageal sphincter (LES) are less complex and easier to study because of their slow speed relative to oropharyngeal swallow events. The bolus head enters the cervical esophageal region through the distended PES, continues through the esophagus and is propelled and cleared (component 14) *via* primary and secondary esophageal peristaltic muscle contractions [39,40]. These contractions continue until the bolus head and tail progress through the passively relaxed LES and advance into the stomach. There are a few behavioral interventions available to modify the contractile characteristics of the esophagus and improve esophageal clearance [8]. However, clinical evidence and preliminary research indicate that esophageal clearance in the upright position appears to have some functional impact on pharyngeal clearance and possibly airway protection [41]. Therefore, observations of esophageal clearance in the upright, eating and drinking position are made by clinicians during the MBSS exam in order to gain an impression of the potential impact of incomplete or slowed esophageal clearance on oropharyngeal swallowing function, on the potential for aspiration of residual esophageal contents, and on the nutritional status of the patient. Based on the wealth of information gained from the MBSS, clinicians also attempt to estimate the severity of the impairment(s) and make critical intake and diet texture recommendations, swallowing therapy recommendations, and predictions regarding the functional outcomes of the patient [8,10,14]. However, there remain no standardized, reliable, or valid tools for making such judgments. Furthermore, there is insufficient evidence that the observations of swallowing impairment made during the MBSS relate to the short-term or long-term outcomes of the patient [42]. There is a sense of urgency to pursue this knowledge in view of the recent demand for evidence-based practices in all aspects of behavioral medicine [42,43]. The urgency is also reflected in the fact that the incidence of aspiration pneumonia, an infectious disease frequently associated with disordered swallowing, high morbidity, and high mortality rates has reached epidemic proportions in the United States [44]. Results from an extensive review of the literature overseen by the Agency for Health Care Policy and Research adds to the compelling need for standardized MBSS assessment [4]. Whereas the report confirmed evidence that inclusion of a dysphagia management program resulted in decreased aspiration pneumonia rates in acute care patients with stroke, there was insufficient evidence to support that the MBSS or other instrumented exams further decreased pneumonia rates in stroke patients or any dysphagic patient population [42]. However, some evidence suggested that when patients with dysphagia aspirate on a MBSS exam, they have approximately 50% greater risk of developing aspiration pneumonia than patients with dysphagia who do not aspirate during the MBSS [4]. Thus, the investigators acknowledged that in addition to observed aspiration on MBSS, other factors including type and degree of swallowing impairment, cognitive status of the patient, and age may play equal or greater roles in causing pneumonia.

As clinicians treating potentially life-threatening swallowing disorders in elderly and medically fragile populations, we have a responsibility to identify and understand the effects and outcomes of our diagnostic and therapeutic practices for the patients we serve. "For clinicians and patients, outcomes research provides evidence about benefits, risks, and results of treatments so they can make more informed decisions" [43]. Until we develop evidence-based, standardized, diagnostic tools for measuring swallowing impairment during a MBSS exam and methods for training students and clinicians in the implementation of these tools, a clinical trial comparing one diagnostic (i.e. instrumented or non-instrumented) method to another in terms of patient outcome is clearly premature.

What is a gold standard?

By definition, a gold standard is a test by which all other tests are measured. Ideally, this test demonstrates 100% sensitivity and 100% specificity. The realistic state of affairs is that swallowing clinicians, like clinicians in most areas of clinical practice, will not ever achieve this ideal regardless of the rigor associated with the design and implementation of the optimally designed clinical trial. Even if the gold standard were not the desired aim, the state of affairs is that clinicians do not have a universally accepted terminology or a tool that has been empirically based, reliable, and valid for converting clinical information into a quantifiable metric for the diagnosis of swallowing impairment. Empirical evidence and standardization are lacking for the selection of the measured physiologic components, the types of measures that are employed, and categorization of functional swallowing components into regional domains. This lack of standardization in measurement methods across clinics and laboratories impedes our understanding of true functional results in studies that profess to document rehabilitative (swallowing therapy) and restorative (surgery and medications) effects of treatment, produces ambiguous reporting of outcomes, and hinders our understanding of what restorative and rehabilitative targets should be in order to impact the overall health and well-being of dysphagic patients.

Myths

Protocol (e.g., procedural standardization) alone makes a standardized examination

Clearly there is empirical evidence demonstrating the positive and negative effects of bolus textures, tasks, and interventions on immediate observations of swallowing function. The known variability in human subjects, regardless of the etiology of their swallowing impairment(s), precludes the development of one identical protocol for all dysphagic patients. However, the critical necessity for using materials and protocol methods that are standardized as much as possible to compare performance from one evaluating center to another (e.g., Protocol 201) has undoubtedly been established. In addition to the protocol, the measurements used to qualify or quantify clinical observations made during the MBSS must be standardized for meaningful comparison of results.

Standardization means clinically practical

Standardized methods of measurement may not be clinically practical. The logistic demands of clinical practice provide unfortunate, but necessary constraints on the time allotted to obtain and analyze evaluative measures. Discrete frame-by-frame analysis may not be practical and may not add to the clinical yield of the procedure. Further, the often wide range of variability of temporal measures displayed by individuals with normal swallowing function speaks to the notion that discrete temporal measures may not ideally capture the nature of the swallowing impairment. For example, it has been shown that the bolus flow and kinematic characteristics of oropharyngeal swallowing can be functionally grouped from visual observations of general temporal coordination and do not require the measurement of discrete event timings [37]. This methodology, if shown to have external validation, may be a desired method for semi-quantifying swallowing impairment in both clinical and research environments.

Reliability is a necessary and sufficient condition for validity

Because each of the physiological components is obtained from clinician judgment or interpretation of visualization of the bolus flow findings, it is necessary to estimate inter-rater (between rater) reliability and intra-rater (within rater) reliability. Inter-rater reliability assessment provides an indication of error attributable to raters (clinicians). It quantifies the extent to which different clinicians make the same clinical judgment about physiological swallowing impairment on a given patient. Inter-rater reliability assessment reflects on the "generality" of the ratings [45]. "Generality" is important in signifying that the obtained physiologic impairment ratings are not the idiosyncratic results of clinician's subjective interpretation of the bolus flow. Stated differently, one wants raters to be interchangeable. Ideally, one desires inter-rater reliability to be 1.0. If a test item, for example, cannot be reliably measured, its overall utility in the assessment of patients is nil. Further, reliability is primarily dependent on training the measurement task and on familiarity (or experience) with the impairment targeted for measurement. High intra-rater and inter-rater agreements on the desired measures does not necessitate validity. Measures must be validated regarding their relationship/correlation to each other (construct validity) and their relationship to external indicators of health status and quality of life (external validity).

Study designs that measure few dependent variables capture swallowing impairment

The fact is that unifactorial analyses often fail to capture the complexity of the swallowing impairment. In order to truly establish what swallowing measures (components) matter, one must test multiple relevant factors within one analysis to truly gain a picture of an impairment profile [46]. Such analyses, however, require large samples sizes and, depending on the study question, often require homogeneous patient populations. These studies are doable, however, the multifaceted, and medically complex nature of dysphagic patients demands increased implementation of such study designs to further our understanding of the variation in swallowing behavior that occurs with diseases or conditions, and that occur relative to our interventions. Clearly, one challenge is determining the parsimonious set of measures that contributes to true variation/aberration in swallowing function and their contribution to the outcome of the patient.

We have made tremendous strides in the clinical science of swallowing assessment over the past 30 years. This carefully controlled work has established a solid foundation for a new and evolving approach to the study of swallowing function. A comprehensive study is underway that is directed toward discovering the truths buried in these myths and aims to:
- create and test a tool measuring the functional components of swallowing observed on MBSS in a large cohort of dysphagic patients;
- quantify swallowing impairment based on physiology;
- empirically reduce measured components into a parsimonious, non-redundant, clinically relevant, and clinically practical set of measures that result in clinical action and relate to health status and quality of life patient outcomes.

Preliminary results are confirmatory regarding the hypothesized redundancy of several of the measures that we typically obtain during the MBSS, and that clinicians should be focusing restorative efforts toward the synergistic mechanism of swallowing, rather than isolated components alone [47]. If the current model under test fits the swallowing impairment model in patients with conditions and diseases, clinicians will be better able to predict swallowing outcomes and target treatments (surgical restoration and rehabilitation methods) to those components that make the most functional impact on the patient's ability to eat and that optimize health and quality of life.

Acknowledgments
The author wishes to acknowledge the continued contributions of the MUSC research team, particularly Martin Brodsky, Ph.D, at the MUSC Evelyn Trammell Institute for Voice and Swallowing and The Evelyn Trammell Voice and Swallowing Center at Saint Joseph's Hospital of Atlanta. The author's work cited in the manuscript was supported by the National Institute on Deafness and Other Communication Disorders (5 K23 DC005764-2) and the Mark and Evelyn Trammell Trust.

References

1. Personal communication from the Centers for Medicare & Medicaid Internal Data Systems: HCFA Customer Information System, Part B Extract Summary System, September 27, 2001.
2. Kidder TM, Langmore SE, Martin BJW. Indications and techniques of endoscopy in evaluation of cervical dysphagia: comparison with radiographic techniques. Dysphagia 1994;9(4):256-61.
3. Langmore S, Schatz K, Olson N. Fiberoptic endoscopic evaluation of swallowing safety: new procedure. Dysphagia 1988;2(4):216-9.
4. Sonies BC, Parent LJ, Morrish K, Baum BJ. Durational aspects of the oral-pharyngeal phase of swallow in normal adults. Dysphagia 1988;3:1-10.
5. Logemann JA, Pauloski BR, Rademaker A, et al. Impact of the diagnostic procedure on outcome measures of swallowing rehabilitation in head and neck cancer patients. Dysphagia 1992;7(4):179-86.
6. Teasell RW, McRae M, Heitzner J, Bhardwaj A, Finestone H. Frequency of videofluoroscopic modified barium swallow studies and pneumonia in stroke rehabilitation patients: a comparative study. Arch Phys Med Rehabilit 1999;80:294-8.
7. Aviv JE. Prospective, randomized outcome study of endoscopy versus modified barium swallow in patients with dysphagia. Laryngoscope 2000;110:563-74.
8. Logemann J.A. Manual for the videofluorographic study of swallowing, 2nd ed. Austin: ProEd, 1993.
9. Ramsey GH, Watson JS, Gramiak R, Weinberg SA. Cinefluorographic analysis of the mechanism of swallowing. Radiology 1955;64:498-518.
10. Logemann J.A. Evaluation and treatment of swallowing disorders. Austin: ProEd, 1998.
11. Dodds WJ, Logemann JA, Stewart ET. Physiology and radiology of normal oral and pharyngeal phases of swallowing. Am J Roentgenol 1990;154::953-63.
12. Dodds WJ, Stewart ET, Logemann JA. Radiologic assessment of abnormal oral and pharyngeal phases of swallowing. Am J Roentgenol 1990;154:965-74.
13. Jones B, Donner MW. Normal and abnormal swallowing: imaging in diagnosis and therapy. New York: Springer Verlag, 1991.
14. Martin-Harris B, Logemann J, McMahon S, Schleicher MA, Sandidge J. Clinical utility of the modified barium swallow. Dysphagia 2000;15(3):136-41.
15. Rosenbek JC, Robbins JA, Roecker EB, Coyle JL, Wood JL. A penetration-aspiration scale. Dysphagia 1996;11(2):93-8.
16. Magendie F. Mémoire sur l'usage de l'épiglotte dans la déglutition. Paris: Meguigon-Marvis, 1813.
17. Martin-Harris B, Michel Y, Castell DO. Physiologic model of oropharyngeal swallowing revisited. Otolaryngol Head Neck Surg 2005;133:234-40.
18. Insall, Matt and Weisstein, Eric W. "Connected Set." From MathWorld—A Wolfram Web Resource. http://mathworld.wolfram.com/ConnectedSet.html. Retrieved from the World Wide Web: November 8, 2006.
19. Storey AT. Interactions of alimentary and upper respiratory tract reflexes. In: Sessle B, Hannam A, eds. Mastication and swallowing: biological and clinical correlates. Toronto: University of Toronto Press, 1976:22-36.
20. Palmer JB, Rudin JH, Lara,G, Cromptom AW. Coordination of mastication and swallowing. Dysphagia 1992;7(4):187-200.
21. Kahrilas PJ, Lin S, Logemann JA, Ergun GA, Facchini F. Deglutitive tongue action: volume accommodation and bolus propulsion. Gastroenterology 1993;104(1):152-62.
22. Gilbert RJ, Daftary S, Campbell TA, Weisskoff RM. Patterns of lingual tissue deformation associated with bolus containment and propulsion during deglutition as determined by echo-planar MRI. J Magnet Res Imag 1998;8(3):554-60.
23. Yoshida T. Electromyographic and x-ray investigations of normal deglutition. Otologia (Fukuoka) 1979;25:824-82.
24. Atkinson M, Kramer P, Wyman S, Ingelfinger F. The dynamics of swallow. I. Normal pharyngeal mechanisms. J Clin Invest 1957;36:581-98.
25. Sokol EM, Heitmann P, Wolf BS, Cohen B. Simultaneous cineradiographic and manometric study of the pharynx, hypopharynx, and cervical esophagus. Gastroenterology 1966;51:960-74.
26. Kahrilas PJ, Dodds WJ, Dent J, Logemann JA, Shaker R. Upper esophageal sphincter function during deglutition. Gastroenterology 1988;95:52-62.
27. McConnel FMS, Cerenko D, Mendelsohn MS. Manofluorographic analysis of swallowing. Otolaryngol Clin N Am 1988;21:625-37.
28. Jacob P, Kahrilas PJ, Logemann J, Shah V, Ha T. Upper esophageal sphincter opening and modulation during swallowing. Gastroenterology 1989;97(6):1469-78.
29. Logemann J, Kahrilas PJ, Cheng J, et al. Closure mechanism of laryngeal vestibule during swallowing. Am J Physiol 1992;21(262):G338-G44.
30. Cook IJ, Dodds WJ, Dantas RO, et al. Timing of videofluoroscopic, manometric events, and bolus transit during the oral and pharyngeal phases of swallowing. Dysphagia 1989;4(1):8-15.
31. Ekberg O, Sigurjonsson S. Movement of the epiglottis during deglutition. Gastrointest Radiol 1982;7:101-7.
32. Pouderoux P, Kahrilas PJ. Deglutitive tongue force modulation by volition, volume, and viscosity in humans. Gastroenterology 1995;108(5):1418-26.

33. Ghosh SK, Pandolfino JE, Zhang Q, Jarosz A, Kahrilas PJ. Deglutitive upper esophageal sphincter relaxation: a study of 75 volunteer subjects using solid-state high-resolution manometry. Am J Physiol Gastrointest Liver Physiol 2006;291:G525-31.
34. Martin BJW. The influence of deglutition on respiration. Unpublished doctoral dissertation, Northwestern University, Evanston IL, 1991.
35. Martin-Harris B. Coordination of laryngeal dynamics and peripheral respiratory patterns: isolated and sequential swallows. Presentation at the Tenth Annual Meeting of the Dysphagia Research Society, Albuquerque, NM, 2001.
36. Martin-Harris B, Brodsky MB, Price CC, Michel Y, Walters B. Temporal coordination of laryngeal dynamics and breathing during swallowing: single liquid swallows. J Appl Physiol 2003;94:1735-43.
37. Martin-Harris B, Brodsky MB, Michel Y, Ford CL, Walters B, Heffner J. Breathing and swallowing dynamics across the adult lifespan. Arch Otolaryngol Head Neck Surg 2005;131:762-70.
38. Klahn MS, Perlman AL. Temporal and durational patterns associating respiration and swallowing. Dysphagia 1999;14(3):131-8.
39. Castell DA, Diederrich LL, Castell JA. Esophageal motility & pH testing, 3rd ed, Highlands Ranch, Colorado: Sandhill Scientific Inc., 2000.
40. Levine MS. Radiology of the esophagus. Philadelphia: W.B. Saunders Company, 1989.
41. Brenner MH, Curbow B, Legro MW. The proximal-distal continuum of multiple health outcome measures: the case of cataract surgery. Med Care 1995;33:AS236-44.
42. Agency for Health Care Policy and Research. Diagnosis and treatment of swallowing disorders (dysphagia) in acute-care stroke patients. Evidence Report/Technology Assessment, 1999, No.8 (AHCPR 99-E023/24).
43. Outcomes Research: FACT Sheet. Agency for Healthcare Research and Quality, 2000. (AHRQ Pub. No. 00-P011).
44. Baine WB, Yu W, Summe JP. Epidemiologic trends in the hospitalization of elderly medicare patients for pneumonia, 1991-1998. Am J Public Health 2001;91:1121-3.
45. Tinsley HEA, Weiss DJ. Interrater reliability and agreement of subjective judgments. J Counsel Psychol 1975;22(4):358-76.
46. Munro BH. Statistical methods for health care research, 4th ed. Philadelphia: Lippincott, 2001.
47. Martin-Harris B. Do we have valid and reliable means of quantifying severity of pharyngeal dysphagia? World Organization for Specialized Studies on Diseases of the Esophagus, OESO 2006; Avignon, France.

Is it possible to establish a protocol for video fluoroscopic evaluation of swallowing?

A.C. Wuttge-Hannig, C.E.M. Hannig (München)

The answer is: there is no universal protocol to perform a swallowing study [1-13].

However, certain rules can be established for a good examination.

The three "columns", which should be observed, are the choice of Contrast Medium, the type of documentation and the best examination procedure for the individual problem of the patient.

The first item, which should be answered is: why is it absolutely necessary to do a dynamic study of the swallowing process including the oral phase, the pharyngeal phase and the early esophageal phase including the whole esophagus and the esophagogastric junction (EGJ).

When we look at the physiology of the oro-, pharyngeal and esophageal transit times respectively we have to consider that five cranial nerves (nerve V, nerve VII, nerve IX, X and XII) are involved in the swallowing act and have to coordinate within the swallowing time the action of 26 cervical muscle groups. The transit time from the oral cavity to the pharynx is only 0.2 sec, the pharyngeal transit time is about 0.5 sec and the whole time of transit from oral cavity to esophagus is 0.7 sec. The pharyngeal constrictors lead to a bolus velocity in the cervical esophagus up to 70 cm/sec and the pressure generation during the pharyngeal contractions is between 300 and 500 mmHg [14,15].

The epidemiologic data and the great socio-medical importance of those studies is highlightened by an article from Ekberg *et al.* [16]. The main information we can get from this article is the fact, that 35-40% of the elderly population in nursing-homes suffer from chronic aspiration and most of them die of it without having got a proper examination. Often the nurses are not even aware of the fact of aspiration. Logeman [17] stresses that 7-8% of patients suffering from cerebral ischemia die within the very first year from aspiration pneumonia. These facts may sufficiently underline the great importance of swallowing studies especially in neurologic patients. Also elderly patients, who mainly suffer from several types of neurologic or mixed neurologic and gastrointestinal diseases need this work-up. Although the examination is not very expensive, it is not as much performed as it would be needed by the upper mentioned reasons.

The cause of this is the lack of expertise within the diagnostic radiologists and also the nursing persons and to some part also to a lack of experienced speech- and language-pathologists. The drammatic rise of 1200% of publications in this field for the future is quite promising.

Why is it not possible to establish a mixed protocol for any patient being referred for dynamic study ?

The reason for this is, that every patient shows up with a very different quality of complaints like dysphagia, odynophagia, aphagia, globus sensation, hoarseness, laryngitis posterior, heartburn, chest pain or other disturbances.

So is it absolutely necessary to tailor the examination to the patients complaints [9] and to use the adequate consistency and to imitate the situation and the position which provocates the complaint. This necessity may be underlined by the fact, that about 40% of our patients suffered from gastroenterologic diseases, 35% of the patients of neurologic diseases; but there was a overlapping group with as well neurologic and gastroenterologic underlying disease in 25%.

Material and methods

The only commun rules we can give for the different groups of illnesses, which might permit to choose an adequate protocol consists in the consideration of the the main three columns.

The first column consists in the choice of the radiologic technique

Up to now videofluoroscopy at a frame rate of 25 frames/sec with reduced radiation by a pulsing fluoroscopy-system allows a registration of the swallowing act and frame by frame analysis. With or without this pulsing sequences videofluoroscopy works at a very low dose and can also be used for young persons, children or even babies. A disadvantage of the videodocumentation is the fact that it cannot be implicated in a modern PACS system for archivation, thus not allowing an immediate access from every part of the interdisciplinary swallowing rehabilitation group.

In the last years we sometimes also use a technique of dynamic digital imaging with a frame rate of 8-30 frames/sec, which shows an excellent special resolution and also allows a much better frame-by-frame analysis; but it has a slightly higher radiation dose. The main positive aspect is the possibility to implicate the system into PACS of the hospital. A second advantage is the modern fluoroscopy with modern multi functionally devices with a flat detector, which allows digital registration of up to 30 frames/sec from the pulsed fluoroscopy signal. This technique is called dynamic fluorograbbing. The spacial resolution is no as good as in DSI but clearly better than a normal videodocumentation.

The age of the patient and the clinical question are decisive if high speed digital recording or if dynamic fluorograbbing is used.

Most of our 15,000 patients studied since 1982 were examinated either by cineradiography or by videofluoroscopy. Only in the last year the use of dynamic digital recording/dynamic fluorograbbing was possible.

Of course, it is possible to adapt the velocity of frames to the anatomic structure which has to be studied. So we start the examination of the oral cavity and the pharynx with velocity of about 15-30 frames going down to 8 frames in region of the upper esophagus and 4 frames in the region of mid-esophagus and the EGJ.

The second column is the contrast medium

The tailoring of the examination includes changes of consistency of the applicated bolus as well as the volume. The adaption of the rheology ranges from liquid to semisolid, solid or crumbly. The constract medium used normally is BaSO4, or a Tenner's solution in not-aspirating patients. Especially Tenner's-Barium solution gives a very good mucosal coating [18]. It can be completed by Barium paste, thickened contrast material or a mixture of contrast medium with normal food like yoghurt, bread or thickened liquids. In neurologic impaired patients a water-soluble, possibly iso-osmolar contrast medium should be used. Iotrolan or Gastromiro®, but absolutely not Gastrografin®, can be applied. It is possible to adapt the liquid jodine contrast medium to different rheology. A higher stress for solid-food-dysphagia is our marsh mellow consisting of a 1.4 cm sphere which is made of a gelatine basis added with fruit flavour and of course barium for giving the contrast [7,19,20]. The most difficult consistency to swallow is a mixed consistency like crackers or salad in liquid contrast medium because the sensoric system of mouth has to be very sensible in the oral bolus preparation of a mixed rheology.

• Cave

In any case of suspected aspiration it is absolutely dangerous to apply a water soluble hyper osmolar contrast medium like Gastrografin® (mecluminamidotricloat) or Telebrix Gastro® (mecluminioexithalmat). Because of the about seven times higher osmolarity to serum the aspiration of the very liquid substances easily leads to penetration to the alveolar part of the lung leading to a sudden alveolar and interstitiell fluid instream into lung causing an edema. Also the chemotoxic induced release of a histamin from the mastcells can additionally cause a bronchospasm. Sometimes it is is quite useful before starting the study and after having performed history-taking to give to the patient a waterswallow to look at the swallowing performance and to estimate his risk of aspiration.

A central attention must be given to the pharyngoesophageal interactions. Therefore a swallowing examination consists in the evaluation of the oral, the pharyngeal and the pharyngo-laryngeal and the esophageal phase. In *Figure 1* the pharyngoesophageal interactions are demonstrated.

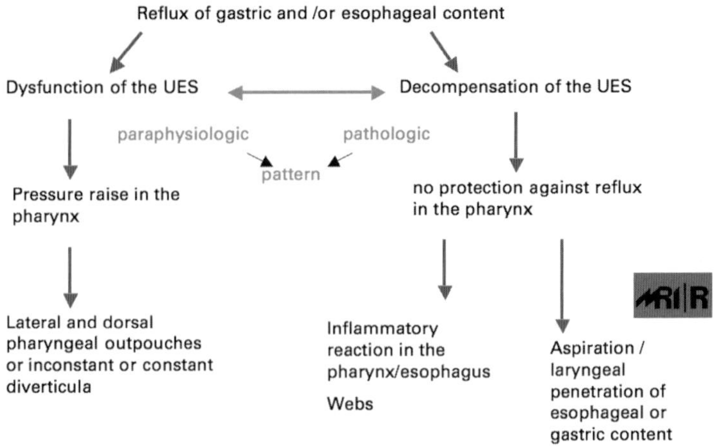

Figure 1. Dysfunction of the UES.

The third column consists in the examination performance or how to begin a study

Since different swallowing disorders are visible only in special positions, it is very important to begin with the most valuable position. Since aspiration and other handicaps of the patient do not permit more projections the best one for the suspected problem has to be performed at first.

Figure 2 shows the different approaches of projection and contrast medium in the different suspected areas of disease. Semisolid iodine means a mixture of iotrolan with for example bread.

These considerations are based on our experience of pharyngolaryngoesophageal interactions with is shown in *Figure 3*.

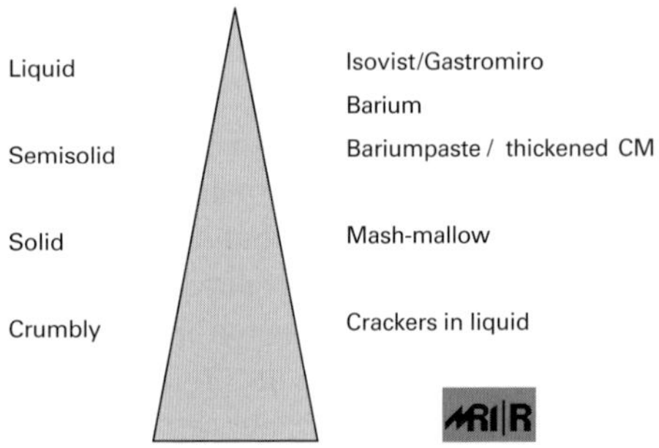

Figure 2. Examination tailored to patient's complaints

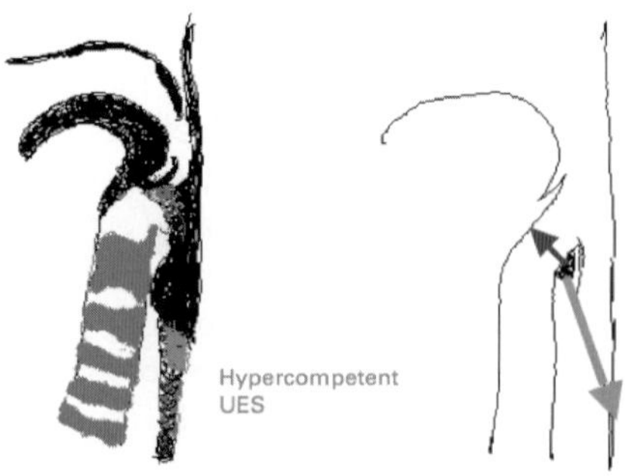

Figure 3. Laryngeal involvement indirectly caused by GER. In these cases there is a hypercompetent UES due to reflux, hindering the gastric content to enter into the pharynx. Since the UES is a sphincter sling fixed at the cricoid cartilage, its hypercompetence hinders the laryngeal closure. Therefore the approximation of the arythenoids against the basis of the epiglottis is delayed or failing.

In the case of otherwise normal findings in patients with suspected laryngeal dysfunctions and aspirations we always perform of the so called stress drinking. It consists in drinking at least half a cup of diluted barium ($BaSO_4$ in 20 g%). The patient is asked in lateral position to empty the cup as quick as possible and this drinking is documented with videofluoroscopy. The depth of penetration into the larynx of the bolus in stress drinking has a positive correlation with the grade of UES-dysfunction and indirectly with the amount of reflux in distance to the LES.

In conclusion the dynamic imaging of the swallowing act helps, if performed well adapted to the complaints of the patient, to recognize early functional disorders and helps to start earlier rehabilitative therapy; this reduces the costs of hospital and health system. An efficient individual therapy planning has to be based on the tailored examination mentioned above.

References

1. Donner MW. Radiology in swallowing disorders In: Heuck FHW, Donner MW, eds. Radiology today, 2nd ed. Springer Verlag, 1983.
2. Donner MW, Gayler BW, Beck TJ. Cineradiography of the gastrointestinal tract. In: Alimentary tract radiology. Moshby Corp, 1983.
3. Bosma JF, Donner MW. Physiology of the pharynx. Otolaryngology 1980;2:332-45.
4. Bosma JF, Donner MW, Tanaka E, Robertson D, Anatomy of the pharynx, pertinent to swallowing. Dysphagia 1986;1:23-33.
5. Curtis DJ, Cruess DF, Dachman AH. Normal erect swallowing normal function and incidence of variations. Invest Radiol 1985;20,5:717-25.
6. Groher M. Dysphagia – Diagnosis and management, 2nd ed. Boston, London, Oxford, Singapore, Sydney, Toronto, Wellington: Butterworth-Heinemann, 1992.
7. Hannig C. Radiologische Funktionsdiagnostik des Pharynx und des Ösophagus. Berlin Heidelberg: Springer-Verlag, 1995.
8. Hannig C, Wuttge-Hannig A. Erkrankungen des Ösophagus. In: Freyschmidt J, Feuerbach ST, eds. Handbuch diagnostische Radiologie. Springerverlag, 2007:28-139.
9. Jones B, Donner MW. Normal and abnormal swallowing-imaging in diagnosis and therapy. New York: Springer Verlag, 1991.
10. Wuttge-Hannig A, Beer A, Gebhardt A, Hellerhoff P, Wuttge R, Hannig C. Alternative methods for the diagnostic of deglutition. In: Schindler O, Ruoppolo G, Schindler A, eds. Deglutologia. Omega Edizioni, 2001.
11. Wuttge-Hannig A, Hannig C. The post-operative pharynx and larynx. In: Ekberg O, ed. Radiology of the pharynx and the esophagus. Heidelberg, New York: Springer Verlag, 2004:85-97.
12. Wuttge-Hannig A, Hannig C. Evaluation of the swallowing reflex in stress drinking in videofluoroscopy – Is it a tool for the measurement of pharyngeal dysfunction in reflux disease? Eur Radiol 2004;14(2):210-1.
13. Wuttge-Hannig A, Hannig C. Radiologische Funktionsdiagnostik von Schluckstörungen bei neurologischen Krankheitsbildern und bei therapierten onkologischen Kopf-Hals-Erkrankungen. In: Bartolome G, Schröter-Morasch H, eds. Schluckstörungen in Dysphagie, Elsevier 2006, 4th.ed.
14. Dodds WJ , Hogan WJ, Lynden SB, Stewart ET, Stef JJ, Arndorfer RC. Quantitation of pharyngeal motor function in normal human subjects. J Appl Physiol 1975;39:692-6.
15. Kennedy JG, Kent RD. Physiological substrates of normal deglutition. Dysphagia 1988;3:24-38.
16. Ekberg O, Hamdy S, Woisard V, Wuttge-Hannig A, Ortega P. Social and psychological burden of dysphagia : its impact on diagnosis and treatment. Dys Spring 2002;17(2):139-46.
17. Logemann JA. Swallowing physiology and pathophysiology. Otolaryngol Clin N Am 1988;21,4:613-23.
18. Tenner R. Verbesserte Detailerkennbarkeit bei der Doppelkontrastuntersuchung des Magens durch neue Kontrastmittelmischung. Röntgen-Blätter 1984;37:13-5.
19. Hannig C, Wuttge-Hannig A, Daschner H, Baum ST, Günthner ST. Bariumsulfat - Gelatinekugeln zur Diagnostik spezieller pharyngo-ösophagealer Fragestellungen. Röntgenpraxis1989;43:15-9.
20. Hannig C, Wuttge-Hannig A, Hörmann M, Herrmann IF. Kinematographische Untersuchung des Pathomechanismus der Aspirationspneumonie. Fortschr Röntgenstr 1989;150,3:260-7.

What can we expect from high resolution manometry?

G. Hebbard (Melbourne)

In order to consider what we can expect from high resolution manometry (HRM) we need to consider a number of related questions:
- what is HRM?
- what benefits will it provide?
- how will HRM help us to understand esophageal function/dysfunction and manage patients?

What is high resolution manometry?

At present there is no forma definition of what constitutes HRM. Resolution may be enhanced in space (more closely spaced recording points), time (higher sampling rates) or pressure (more accurate recording techniques); however at present the term would generally be accepted to relate to high spatial resolution. The techniques that underlie HRM have been leveraged from developments in manometric assembly design and construction, as well as computerised data acquisition, which not only facilitates acquisition, but also allows the data to be represented in novel forms.

A "functional" definition of HRM is that it provides a sampling of all mechanically significant pressure events within the lumen of a segment of gut. The recording requirements for this will vary with the region being studied and may include radial as well as longitudinal spatial resolution and electrical/mechanical stability of pressure transducers, as well as dynamic characteristics of the recording system relating to sampling frequency, rise rates, digitisation steps, etc.

HRM is not technology dependent and may be achieved using water perfused or solid state systems. The first recordings were made using HRM by Clouse (who used the term topographic manometry to describe the use of HRM with spatiotemporal display of the data) in the esophagus [1]. HRM with STA has since also been used in the pharynx, stomach, small intestine and anorectum [2-5].

HRM is an enabling technology for spatiotemporal analysis in which the structure of pressure events is depicted in three dimensions, with pressure plotted against both time and position in the gut. The use of the computer to display the HRM data in sophisticated forms is logical as interpretation of multiple line plots is difficult, and there is no reason why the computer should remain an "electronic chart recorder" as many early computerised recording systems could justifiably be described. The human eye is attuned to images and recognition of visual pattern and presentation of data in a visual form is efficient and intuitive. If we are to display the data using these methods however, we will be interpolating data between measured points, so it is vital that we have a sampling of all mechanically significant events, otherwise the interpolation becomes misleading.

What benefits can high resolution manometry provide?

We need to recognise that using "standard" manometric techniques, we are taking a very limited sample of pressures involved in the movement of gut contents and potentially missing mechanically significant events or being misled by movement of structures such as the lower esophageal sphincter (LES) or diaphragm. Ideally, in order to understand the mechanics of the transit of fluids and solids in the gut, we would like to know the three dimensional array of pressures and associated fluid movements, however this is not achievable at present (outside of computer simulation). Nevertheless, closely spaced recording points will allow an improved sampling of the relevant pressures, and improved accuracy in pressure measurement will allow better assessment of the relatively small pressure gradients that are likely to be important in the flow of fluids in the gut.

The use of closely spaced recording points allows improved definition of pressures created by anatomical structures whilst preserving positional tolerance (i.e. tolerance for a change in relative position of the manometric catheter and segment of gut). This is most dramatically seen at the LES where these issues were first identified. The sleeve was initially validated against an array of sideholes and HRM has recently been revalidated against the sleeve! [6]. The use of an array of sensors is in fact superior to the use of the sleeve at the LES as it allows definition of the esophageal and diaphragmatic components of the LES and monitoring of how these change with time. The "descent" of the diaphragm can be appreciated and even small hiatus hernia can be defined. The evanescent nature of hiatus hernia can be appreciated over a period of observation and as the "top" and "bottom" of the hernia open and close [7]. In some cases, the lower end of the LES can be seen allowing an assessment of esophageal length and shortening (*Figure 1*).

Closely spaced recording points will allow accurate assessment of pressure gradients allowing direct measurement of the pressures associated with movement of gastrointestinal (GI) contents [8-10]. These pressure gradients are related to the resistance of the segment of gut, such that a higher pressure gradient indicates a higher resistance to flow.

The continuous sampling of pressures from all sites allows prolonged accurate recordings from an entire segment of gut, even in an ambulatory setting. This allows the evaluation of longer term temporal patterns and more thorough investigation of the pressure correlates of intermittent symptoms eg regurgitation or chest pain (*Figure 1*).

Further insights will be obtained by integration of pressure information obtained at HRM with other techniques of measurement eg bolus position (by fluoroscopy or impedance), pH, neuromuscular activity, position/mechanical characteristics of the wall of gut. This will allow the correlation of pressure events with events detected on those studies.

From a technical point of view, HRM makes it easier to perform studies. The probe can be placed and left in that position for the entire study. Incorrect positioning or displacement during the study is appreciated earlier and is more obvious because of the increased spatial resolution. This not only reduce chances of probe misplacement or displacement during a study, but makes studies more reliable. Problems with single recording channels are more obvious because of the interpolation and spatiotemporal representation and this will increase the recognition of technical problems, HRM is also more tolerant of technical problems in a single sensor as information is still gathered from the surrounding sensors. This makes studies easier and faster to perform and more tolerable for patients.

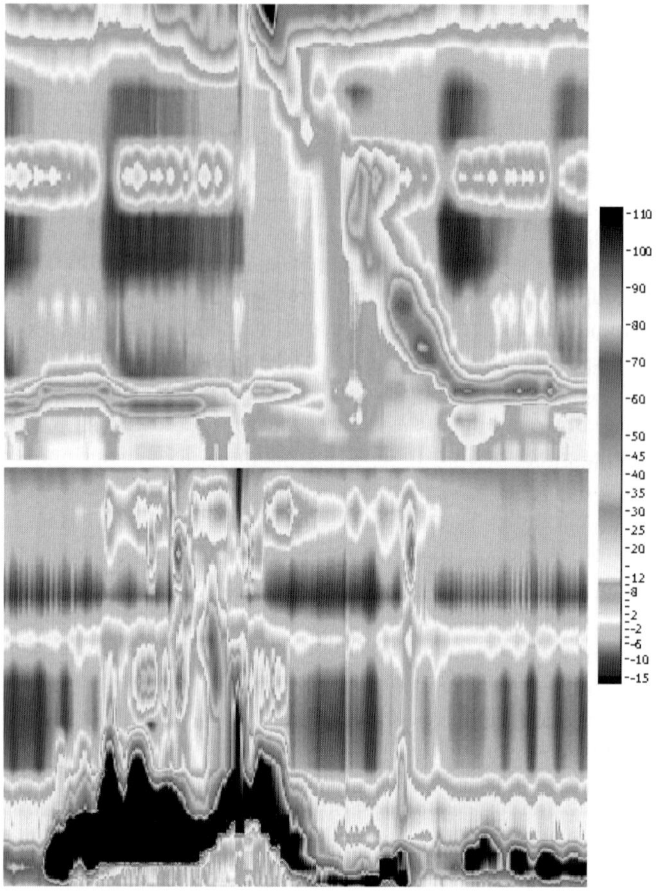

Figure 1. HRM from a patient with chest pain. The stationary study is shown in the top panel (normal). An ambulatory HRM study was done and the data in the bottom panel was collected during a period of chest discomfort. Note the increase in pressure in the LES, uncoordinated contractions in the body of the esophagus and esophageal shortening indicating longitudinal muscle contraction. (See page XV for colour figure).

How will high resolution manometry help us to understand esophageal function/dysfunction and manage patients?

Using the data from HRM and the processing and display power of computers, information can be presented in novel ways as, if we can be confident that we are not "missing" mechanically significant events it be comes legitimate to interpolate between recording points and represent these pressures as a three dimensional graph of pressure against both time and position along the GI tract (the spatiotemporal or topographic plot). Use of spatiotemporal representations allows better appreciation of the structure of pressure waves and makes the information more accessible to non-experts and patients.

The ability of HRM to provide improved spatial resolution in mobile areas such as the LES whilst maintaining position tolerance will allow insights into mechanisms of reflux and dysphagia. For example, compared to the sleeve the extra information obtained using HRM at the diaphragm allows definition of position of the diaphragm and an appreciation of the evanescent nature of small hiatus hernia [7], and subtle abnormalities such as the problems induced by poor coordination between the upper and lower components of the pressure wave can be detected [11].

The ability to measure pressure gradients along the manometric catheter allows assessment of the forces associated with the movement of fluids within the GI tract in both physiological and pathophysiological situations [8,10,12-14], and new computational methods can be developed to deal with these complex datasets to improve our understanding of the physiology of the esophagus [15]. We can expect this improved understanding of physiology and of the functional significance of subtle motor abnormalities to improve our understanding of symptoms and the classification of motility disorders

Will HRM help experts to diagnose "barn door" achalasia? Probably not. However even experts will be assisted in the "difficult" cases where increased resolution and the spatiotemporal representation of pressure allows them to appreciate subtle abnormalities that they had not noticed using standard data collection methods.

A study showed that in a series of studies in an established manometry laboratory HRM led to a more accurate diagnosis compared to conventional manometry [11]. The combination of HRM with methods that allow assessment of bolus position is a particularly powerful technique in the investigation of difficult cases of dysphagia.

For non-experts the changes are likely to be more obvious, increasing the chances of correct diagnosis in routine cases. It is likely that accuracy and technical quality of manometry will increase because of improved position tolerance of the manometric catheter and reduced susceptibility to the effects of movement of the esophagus or surrounding structures with respect to the catheter (i.e. pseudorelaxation due to esophageal shortening). Representation of data as a spatiotemporal plot is more attuned to ability of human brain to recognise and recall patterns in images, which is likely to improve diagnostic accuracy in routine use; however this has not been formally tested. Improved methods of data presentation and understanding of conditions will make motility studies more accessible and allow improved communication with colleagues and patients, who anecdotally find spatiotemporal representation more easily understood than conventional line plots.

The ability of HRM to record all of the mechanically relevant pressures over an entire study prolonged recordings of entire segment of gut for example during a post-prandial study allows us to evaluate unusual symptoms such as chest pain, post-prandial regurgitation or belching (*Figure 1*).

References

1. Clouse RE, Staiano A, Alrakawi A, Haroian L. Application of topographical methods to clinical esophageal manometry. Am J Gastroenterol 2000;95(10):2720-30.
2. Andrews JM, O'Donovan DG, Hebbard GS, Malbert CH, Doran SM, Dent J. Human duodenal phase III migrating motor complex activity is predominantly antegrade, as revealed by high-resolution manometry and colour pressure plots. Neurogastroenterol Motil 2002;14(4):331-8.
3. Williams RB, Pal A, Brasseur JG, Cook IJ. Space-time pressure structure of pharyngo-esophageal segment during swallowing. Am J Physiol Gastrointest Liver Physiol 2001;281(5):G1290-300.
4. Faas H, Hebbard GS, Feinle C, et al. Pressure-geometry relationship in the antroduodenal region in humans. Am J Physiol Gastrointest Liver Physiol 2001;281(5):G1214-20.
5. Indireshkumar K, Brasseur JG, Faas H, et al. Relative contributions of "pressure pump" and "peristaltic pump" to gastric emptying. Am J Physiol Gastrointest Liver Physiol. 2000;278(4):G604-16.
6. Bredenoord AJ, Weusten BL, Timmer R, Smout AJ. Sleeve sensor versus high-resolution manometry for the detection of transient lower esophageal sphincter relaxations. Am J Physiol Gastrointest Liver Physiol 2005;288(6):G1190-4.
7. Bredenoord AJ, Weusten BL, Timmer R, Smout AJ. Intermittent spatial separation of diaphragm and lower esophageal sphincter favors acidic and weakly acidic reflux. Gastroenterology 2006;130(2):334-40.

8. Scheffer RC, Samsom M, Hebbard GS, Gooszen HG. Effects of partial (Belsey Mark IV) and complete (Nissen) fundoplication on proximal gastric function and esophagogastric junction dynamics. Am J Gastroenterol 2006;101(3):479-87.
9. Pandolfino JE, Ghosh SK, Zhang Q, Jarosz A, Shah N, Kahrilas PJ. Quantifying EGJ morphology and relaxation with high-resolution manometry: a study of 75 asymptomatic volunteers. Am J Physiol Gastrointest Liver Physiol 2006;290(5):G1033-40.
10. Pandolfino JE, El-Serag HB, Zhang Q, Shah N, Ghosh SK, Kahrilas PJ. Obesity: a challenge to esophagogastric junction integrity. Gastroenterology 2006;130(3):639-49.
11. Fox M, Hebbard G, Janiak P, et al. High-resolution manometry predicts the success of oesophageal bolus transport and identifies clinically important abnormalities not detected by conventional manometry. Neurogastroenterol Motil 2004t;16(5):533-42.
12. Ghosh SK, Pandolfino JE, Zhang Q, Jarosz A, Shah N, Kahrilas PJ. Quantifying esophageal peristalsis with high-resolution manometry: a study of 75 asymptomatic volunteers. Am J Physiol Gastrointest Liver Physiol 2006;290(5):G988-97.
13. Ghosh SK, Pandolfino JE, Zhang Q, Jarosz A, Kahrilas PJ. Deglutitive upper esophageal sphincter relaxation: a study of 75 volunteer subjects using solid-state high-resolution manometry. Am J Physiol Gastrointest Liver Physiol 2006;291(3):G525-31.
14. Scheffer RC, Samsom M, Haverkamp A, Oors J, Hebbard GS, Gooszen HG. Impaired bolus transit across the esophagogastric junction in postfundoplication dysphagia. Am J Gastroenterol 2005;100(8):1677-84.
15. Ghosh SK, Janiak P, Schwizer W, Hebbard GS, Brasseur JG. Physiology of the esophageal pressure transition zone: separate contraction waves above and below. Am J Physiol Gastrointest Liver Physiol 2006;290(3):G568-76.

Can activation of peripheral sensory nerves be exploited to treat oropharyngeal dysphagia?

I.J. Cook (Sydney)

Oropharyngeal dysphagia following stroke carries a high morbidity, mortality, and cost. Stroke is the third leading cause of death in industrialized countries. Dysphagia occurs acutely in up to 90% of stroke patients [1,2]. Whilst the majority recovers spontaneously, dysphagia persist beyond 6 months in up to 40% [3]. The cost implications are significant because the resulting complications significantly increase institutionalisation and hospital readmission rates following stroke [4]. Any therapy that can be shown to improve the swallow, accelerate recovery and rehabilitation could be expected to reduce mortality and health costs. Current therapies for post-stroke pharyngeal dysphagia rely on dietary modification and modification of swallow technique; both therapeutic avenues with questionable efficacy. There are only two published randomised controlled trials evaluating any therapy for oropharyngeal dysphagia; one concluding benefit from dietary modification alone [5], the other inconclusive on the efficacy of swallow therapy [6]. A therapy capable of hastening recovery and prompting an effective swallow would represent a major advance. Could afferent pathways stimulation represent a novel approach to such therapy?

Central control of swallowing and the importance of afferent input

The pharyngeal swallow motor pattern is orchestrated by the medullary central pattern generator (CPG) comprised of two groups of neurons:

- the dorsal swallowing group adjacent to the nucleus tractus solitarius (NTS), responsible for generation and timing of the swallowing sequence;
- the ventral swallowing group located ventrolaterally, responsible for switching and distributing the signals to motor nuclei.

The CPG receives input both from the cerebral cortex and sensory inputs from the periphery (*Figure 1 and 2*). Cortical stimulation, either by direct electrical stimulation in animals [7] or by transcranial magnetic stimulation (TMS) in animals [8] and humans [9] can elicit a swallow *via* polysynaptic projections from cortex to the medulla. Cortical stimulation by TMS, reproducibly evokes EMG responses in the mylohyoid, pharynx and proximal esophagus [7,10]. TMS has been exploited to demonstrate that pharyngeal musculature is discretely and somatotopically represented on the motor and promoter cortex of both hemispheres but displays interhemispheric asymmetry [10]. This cortical dominance determines which patients with cortical stroke will get dysphagia while the

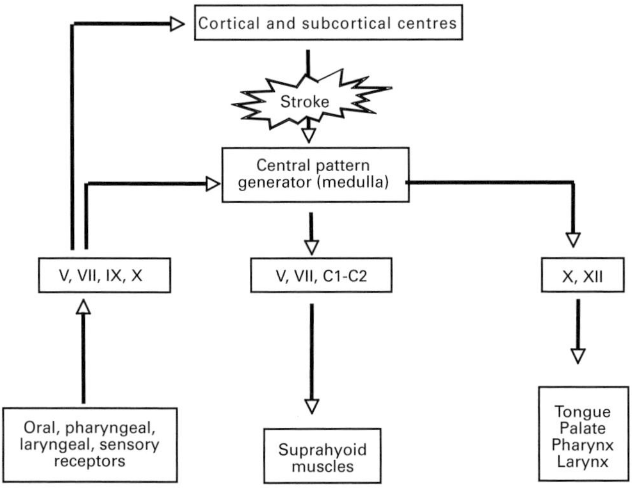

Figure 1. Schema of central neural control of the pharyngeal swallow (see text).

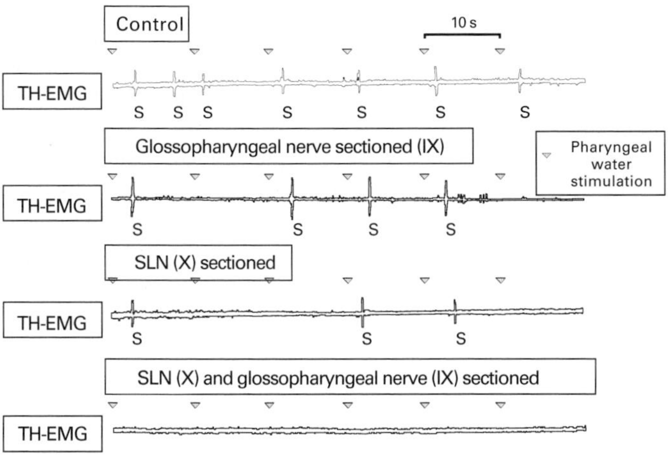

Figure 2. Electromyographic findings (thyrohyoid muscle) indicating swallow responses to peripheral afferent nerve stimulation. Note that sectioning the glossopharyngeal nerve reduces swallow frequency, but less markedly than does sectioning the internal branch of the superior laryngeal nerve (SLN). However sectioning both nerves abolishes the swallow.

degree of plasticity demonstrated by the unaffected hemisphere predicts swallow recovery in these patients [11]. This phenomenon of plasticity in the unaffected hemisphere is a potential therapeutic target to hasten recovery (see below).

Afferent input, relayed through the NTS in the dorsal medulla, is mandatory before normal voluntary swallowing can be initiated. For example, it is impossible to initiate the normal swallow voluntarily in the absence of bolus or saliva in the oropharynx. Liquid and pressure stimuli to the oropharynx and hypopharynx can induce or modulate a pharyngeal swallow response (V, IX & X nerves). Electrical stimulation of the V and IX nerves are a much less reliable means of stimulating the swallow, particularly in the sheep, although such stimulation does induce short latency potentials in the NTS [12]. The normal swallow cannot be dependent upon these response because of their inconsistency. However, V & IX nerve activity probably serves a role in facilitating the swallow response to concurrent simulation *via* the superior laryngeal nerve and sectioning of IX nerve, blocks the swallow response initiated by SLN stimulation [13]. In contrast, direct electrical stimulation of the internal branch of the superior laryngeal nerve (ISLN) alone was shown 50 years ago to be very effective at initiating the highly specific swallow sequence in the anaesthetized dog [14,15] and subsequently in the decerebrate sheep, rabbits and cats [16,17]. In the human it appears that intact SLN afferent traffic is important in generating an effective and safe volitional swallow. Blockade of the ISLN by transcutaneous infiltration into the paraglottic compartment with bupivacaine results in effortful swallowing and laryngeal penetration of liquids in humans [18].

Evidence that central or peripheral stimulation might be exploited therapeutically in the human

The available data raise two important questions likely to be relevant to therapy in cortical stroke because the peripheral connections; *via* the NTS to the medullary CPG are intact in this condition:

- **can acute peripheral afferent nerve stimulation (V, IX, X) [18-45] facilitate a functional swallow?**
- **can chronic afferent nerve stimulation hasten recovery of swallowing, perhaps by enhancing cortical plasticity of the unaffected hemisphers?**

In the dog vigorous transcranial magnetic stimulation (TMS) can initiate the entire swallow response [8]. Unfortunately stimuli of this intensity can cause seizures in the human. However, low intensity TMS can activate measurable responses in pharyngeal and esophageal musculature and these pharyngeal motor responses can be studied in the context of prior or concurrent afferent nerve stimulation to assess whether peripheral afferent stimulation might facilitate corticofugal pathways to the pharynx. Indeed, Hamdy *et al.* showed that prior stimulation of trigeminal or vagal nerves (utilizing TMS coils focused over supraorbital branch of V and over the vagal trunk in the neck respectively) facilitated cortical swallowing motor pathways as demonstrated by higher amplitude and shorter latency of EMG response in the pharyngeal muscles [46]. A study of 16 stroke patients showed that pharyngeal electrical stimulation caused videofluroscopically identifiable changes in the swallowing parameters such as pharyngeal transit time, swallowing response time and the aspiration score [47]. These observations, together with the wealth of animal data above, would indicate the likelihood of being able to facilitate the pharyngeal swallow by appropriately timed combinations of stimuli to trigeminal, GP and SLN and that stimulus parameters (train length, duration and frequency) are likely to determine the magnitude of the response.

As mentioned, recovery of swallowing following unilateral hemispheric stroke correlates with the phenomenon of plasticity in the unaffected hemisphere [11]. Short term stimulation of pharyngeal afferents transiently increases the cortical representation of pharyngeal muscles in the dominant hemisphere in healthy controls and in the non-affected hemisphere in dysphagic stroke patients [11]. In the clinical setting, tactile and thermal stimulation to the faucial pillars was explored. Although such stimulation improved swallow triggering and mean pharyngeal transit time in 23 of 25 patients, this approach is ineffectual as the effect is very transient [48,49]. Subsequently, animal studies on plasticity indicate that temporary changes in the sensory input or motor output can produce persistent changes in the organisation of sensory and motor areas of the cerebral cortex [44]. These findings support the hypothesis that chronic afferent stimulation may accelerate cortical plasticity and hasten recovery. In the healthy human, 10 minutes of pharyngeal electrical stimulation (5 Hz) induces both enhanced pharyngeal EMG responses and an increase in the size of cortical representation capable of inducing a swallow *via* TMS with that response persisting for an hour after the stimulus [50]. Furthermore, it is promising that such stimulation has been shown to induce in the short term, improvements swallow function in the stroke patient and that the increase in total hemispheric excitability correlated significantly with aspiration scores and temporal swallow measures demonstrated radiographically [47]. It remains to be tested whether such changes translate to hastened recovery in the stroke patient. This will require a prospective randomized clinical trial to determine the clinical utility of the technique.

Conclusions

The plausibility of these hypotheses has been demonstrated in animal models and to some extent by indirect inference from human studies. However, despite strong evidence for a crucial and fairly direct role of superior laryngeal nerve (X) stimulation in initiation of swallowing in various animals, this phenomenon is yet to be confirmed in humans. The most likely therapeutic application of peripheral nerve stimulation lies in its probable ability to influence central plasticity and perhaps thereby hasten swallow recovery after cortical stroke. Proof of this concept will require carefully designed, prospective randomised controlled trials combined with assessment of cortical and corticobulbar function as well as objective measures of swallow recovery.

References

1. Kidd D, Lawson J, Nesbitt R, MacMahon J. Aspiration in acute stroke: a clinical study with videofluoroscopy. Q J Med 1993;86:825-9.
2. Nilsson H, Ekberg O, Olsson R, Hindfelt B. Dysphagia in stroke: a prospective study of quantitative aspects of swallowing in dysphagic patients. Dysphagia 1998;13:32-8.
3. Hamdy S, Rothwell JC. Gut feelings about recovery after stroke: the organization and reorganization of human swallowing motor cortex. Trends Neurosci 1998;21:278-82.
4. Smithard DG, O'Neill PA, Park C, et alF. Complications and outcome after acute stroke: does dysphagia matter? Stroke 1996;27:1200-4 (published erratum appears in Stroke 1998;29(7):1480-1).

5. Groher ME. Bolus management and aspiration pneumonia in patients with pseudobulbar dysphagia. Dysphagia 1987;1:215-6.
6. DePippo KL, Holas MA, Reding MJ, Mandel FS, Lesser ML. Dysphagia therapy following stroke: a controlled trial. Neurology 1994;44:1655-60.
7. Jean A, Car A. Inputs to the swallowing medullary neurones from the peripheral afferent fibers and the swallowing cortical area. Brain Res 1979;178:567-72.
8. Valdez D, Salapatek A, Niznik G, Linden R, Diamant N. Swallowing and upper esophageal sphincter contraction with transcranial magnetic-induced electrical stimulation. Am J Physiol 1993;264:G213-9.
9. Aziz Q, Rothwell JC, Barlow J, et al. Esophageal myoelectric responses to magnetic stimulation of the human cortex and the extracranial vagus nerve. Am J Physiol 1994;30:G827-35.
10. Hamdy S, Aziz Q, Rothwell JC, et al. The cortical topography of human swallowing musculature in health and disease. Nat Med 1996;2:1217-24.
11. Hamdy S, Aziz Q, Rothwell JC, et al. Recovery of swallowing after dysphagic stroke relates to functional reorganization in the intact motor cortex. Gastroenterology 1998;115:1104-12.
12. Ciampini G, Jean A. Role of glossopharyngeal and trigeminal afferents in the initiation and propagation of swallowing. I Glossopharyngeal afferents. J Physiol (Paris) 1980;76(1):49-60.
13. Sinclair W. Role of the pharyngeal plexus in initiation of swallowing. Am J Physiol 1971;221:1260-3.
14. Doty RW, Bosma JF. An electromyographic analysis of reflex deglutition. J Neurophysiol 1956;19:44-60.
15. Doty R. Influence of stimulus pattern on reflex deglutition. Am J Physiol 1951;66:142-51.
16. Jean A. Brain stem control of swallowing: neuronal network and cellular mechanisms. Physiol Rev 2001;81:929-69.
17. Miller A. Deglutition. Physiol Rev 1982;62:129-84.
18. Jafari S, Prince RA, Kim DY, Paydarfar D. Sensory regulation of swallowing and airway protection: a role for internal superior laryngeal nerve in humans. J Physiol 2003;550:287-304.
19. Ambalavanar R, Tanaka Y, Selbie WS, Ludlow CL. Neuronal activation in the medulla oblongata during selective elicitation of the laryngeal adductor response. J Neurophysiol 2004;92:2920-32.
20. Ashida C, Kojima A, Kobashi M, Koga T. Oro-pharyngeal chemoreceptor activation induces gastric motor response in healthy volunteer subjects. J Smooth Muscle Res 2004;40:211-7.
21. Barkmeier JM, Bielamowicz S, Takeda N, Ludlow CL. Modulation of laryngeal responses to superior laryngeal nerve stimulation by volitional swallowing in awake humans. J Neurophysiol 2000;83:1264-72.
22. Beyak MJ, Collman PI, Valdez DT, Xue S, Diamant NE. Superior laryngeal nerve stimulation in the cat: effect on oropharyngeal swallowing, oesophageal motility and lower oesophageal sphincter activity. Neurogastroenterol Motil 1997;9:117-27.
23. Diamant N. Normal esophageal physiology. In: Cohen S, Soloway R, eds. Diseases of the esophagus. Volume 1. New York: Churchill Livingstone, 1982:1-34.
24. Ezure K, Oku Y, Tanaka I. Location and axonal projection of one type of swallowing interneurons in cat medulla. Brain Res 1993;632:216-24.
25. Goyal RK, Padmanabhan R, Sang Q. Neural circuits in swallowing and abdominal vagal afferent-mediated lower esophageal sphincter relaxation. Am J Med 2001;111:95S-105S.
26. Hammond CS, Davenport PW, HUtchinson A, Otto RA. Motor innervation of the cricopharyngeus muscle by the recurrent laryngeal nerve. J Appl Physiol 1997;83:89-94.
27. Harada H, Takakusaki K, Kita S, Matsuda M, Nonaka S, Sakamoto T. Effects of injecting GABAergic agents into the medullary reticular formation upon swallowing induced by the superior laryngeal nerve stimulation in decerebrate cats. Neurosci Res 2005;51:395-404.
28. Jafari S, Prince RA, Kim DY, Paydarfar D. Sensory regulation of swallowing and airway protection: a role for the internal superior laryngeal nerve in humans. J Physiol 2003;550:287-304.
29. Kajii Y, Shingai T, Kitagawa J, et al. Sour taste stimulation facilitates reflex swallowing from the pharynx and larynx in the rat. Physiol Behav 2002;77:321-5.
30. Kitagawa J, Shingai T, Takahashi Y, Yamada Y. Pharyngeal branch of the glossopharyngeal nerve plays a major role in reflex swallowing from the pharynx. Am J Physiol Reg Int Compar Physiol 2002;282.
31. Kobler JB, Datta S, Goyal RK, Benecchi EJ. Innervation of the larynx, pharynx, and upper esophageal sphincter of the rat. J Compar Neurol 1994;349:129-47.
32. Lamkadem M, Zoungrana OR, Amri M, Car A, Roman C. Stimulation of the chewing area of the cerebral cortex induces inhibitory effects upon swallowing in sheep. Brain Res 1999;832:97-111.
33. Lang IM, Medda BK, Ren J, Shaker R. Characterization and mechanisms of the pharyngoesophageal inhibitory reflex. Am J Physiol 1998;275.
34. Ootani S, Umezaki T, Shin T, Murata Y. Convergence of afferents from the SLN and GPN in cat medullary swallowing neurons. Brain Res Bull 1995;37:397-404.
35. Paterson WG. Alteration of swallowing and oesophageal peristalsis by different initiators of deglutition. Neurogastroenterol Motil 1999;11:63-7.
36. Reynolds R, Effer G, Bendeck M. The upper esophageal sphincter in the cat: the role of central innervation assessed by transient vagal blockade. Can J Physiol Pharmacol 1987;65:96-9.
37. Saito Y, Ezure K, Tanaka I. Intracellular activity of superior laryngeal nerve motoneurons during fictive swallowing in decerebrate rats. Brain Res 2002;956:262-7.

38. Sinclair W. Initiation of reflex swallowing from the naso- and oropharynx. Am J Physiol 1970;218:956-9.
39. Sugimoto T, Umezaki T, Takagi S, Narikawa K, Shin T. Crossing inputs of the superior laryngeal nerve afferents to medullary swallowing-related neurons in the cat. Neurosci Res 1998;30:235-45.
40. Sumi T. Some properties of cortically evoked swallowing and chewing in rabbits. Brain Res 1969;15:107-20.
41. Takagi M, Noda T, Yamada Y. Comparison of SLN-evoked swallows during rest and chewing in the freely behaving rabbit. Brain Res 2002;956:74-80.
42. Umezaki T, Matsuse T, Shin T. Medullary swallowing-related neurons in the anesthetized cat. Neuroreport 1998;9:1793-8.
43. Venker-van Haagen AJ, Van den Brom WE, Hellebrekers LJ. Effect of superior laryngeal nerve transection on pharyngeal muscle contraction timing and sequence of activity during eating and stimulation of the nucleus solitarius in dogs. Brain Res Bulle 1999;49:393-400.
44. Wang X, Merzenich MM, Sameshima K, Jenkins WM. Remodelling of hand representation in adult cortex determined by timing of tactile stimulation. Nature 1995;378:71-5.
45. Zoungrana OR, Lamkadem M, Amri M, Car A, Roman C. Effects of lingual nerve afferents on swallowing in sheep. Exp Brain Res 2000;132:500-9.
46. Hamdy S, Aziz Q, Rothwell JC, Hobson A, Barlow J, Thompson DG. Cranial nerve modulation of human cortical swallowing motor pathways. Am J Physiol 1997;272:G802-8.
47. Fraser C, Power M, Hamdy S, et al. Driving plasticity in human adult motor cortex is associated with improved motor function after brain injury. Neuron 2002;34:831-40.
48. Lazzara G, Lazarus C, Logemann JA. Impact of thermal stimulation on the triggering of the swallow reflex. Dysphagia 1986;1:73-7.
49. Rosenbek JC, Robbins J, Fishback B, Levine RL. Effects of thermal application on dysphagia after stroke. J Speech Hear Res 1991;34:1257-68.
50. Hamdy S, Rothwell JC, Aziz Q, Singh KD, Thompson DG. Long-term reorganization of human motor cortex driven by short-term sensory stimulation. Nat Neurosci 1998;1:64-8.

Imaging techniques in the diagnosis of diseases of the foregut

What is the role of radiology in the detection and evaluation of esophageal stenosis, diverticula and hiatal hernia

F.I. Habib, L. Candeloro (Rome)

Stenosis

Esophageal strictures, either benign or malignant are cause of dysphagia. The most common benign stricture in the lower third of the esophagus is due to gastroesophageal reflux disease (GERD); other causes are scleroderma and sequelae of nasogastric intubation. Upper and middle esophageal strictures may be due to mediastinal irradiation, ingestion of caustic substances, congenital esophageal stenosis. The diagnostic evaluation or these patients often begins with a barium examination. Barium swallow is always indicated in patients with recurrent strictures. On the hand radiology is useful whenever location, diameter and length of the structuring lesion are relevant for management. Barium swallow is more sensitive than endoscopy for detection of relatively open strictures, that are

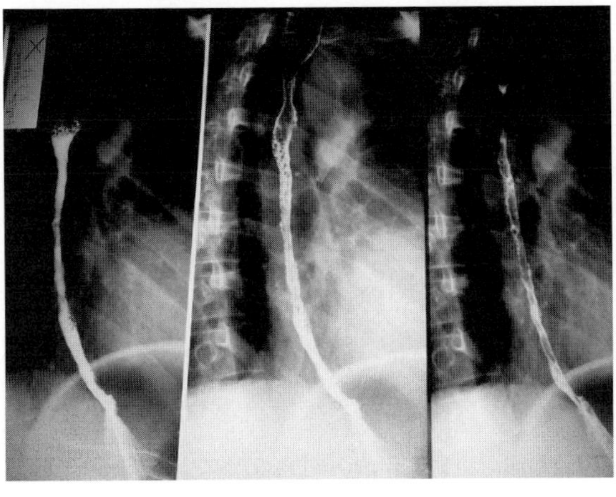

Figure 1. Extremely long stricture due to ingestion of caustic substance.

> 10 mm in diameter. When an esophageal stenosis is detected at barium examination, the underlying cause is usually suggested by the clinical history, the appearance and location of the stricture and the presence of other associated radiographic findings [1,2]. Radiological findings can help direct further endoscopic evaluation and intervention depending on the localization, size, complexity of the lesion, as well as the presence of associated abnormalities that may impact the type of therapeutic modality employed. If barium swallow raises the suspicion of malignancy, it may be necessary to perform a diagnostic endoscopy prior any intervention to determine the extent and type of the tumor [3]. Endoscopic ultrasound can analyze the individual esophageal layers and accurately define the depth of tumor penetration [4,5] with the technical limitation of the inability of the instrument to pass through an incompletely obstructing esophageal cancer. Computed tomography is useful for evaluating the presence or the absence of aortic or tracheo-bronchial invasion, with the only limitation of the inability to gauge the depth of the invasion [6]. A recent study by Ito *et al.* [7] stressed the usefulness of digital radiography in detecting and evaluating stenosis, particularly of middle esophagus, measuring the percentage of esophageal stenosis (PES). PES increases in proportion to tumor infiltration, when compared to histology, and these authors found that PES is a good index for differentiating T1a, T1b and T2 tumors.

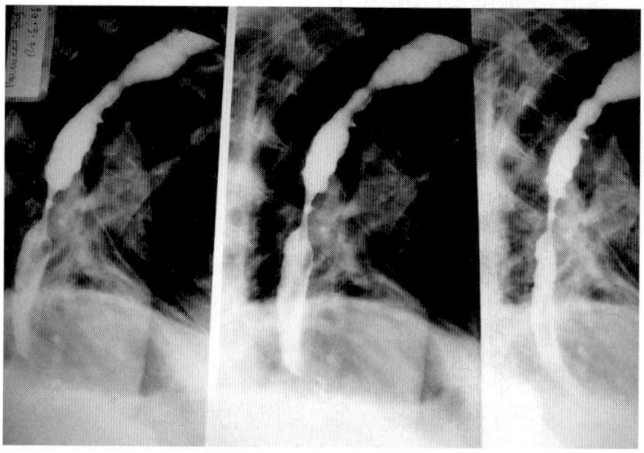

Figure 2. Malignant stricture of the middle esophagus with abrupt proximal and distal margins.

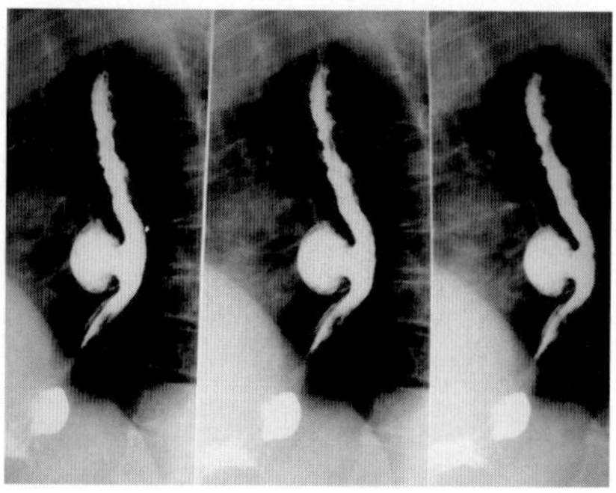

Figure 3. Mid esophageal diverticulum with wide-mouth, located near the tracheal bifurcation, associated with non peristaltic esophageal contractions.

Esophageal diverticula

Diverticula are out pouching of one or more layers of the esophageal wall and are distinct in true and false, or intramural depending from the number of layers involved: all in the true, mucosa and submucosa in the false and just mucosa in the intramural. Esophageal body diverticula are divided also in traction parabronchial diverticula and epiphrenic diverticula. The first are believed to be caused by fibrosis secondary to mediastinal inflammation due to tuberculosis or fungal infections but that can be associated with esophageal motility abnormalities such as achalasia and diffuse esophageal spasm [8,9]. Epiphrenic diverticula are located in the distal 10 cm of the esophagus, are false diverticula, associated with esophageal motility disorders or long-standing strictures [10]. Intramural diverticulosis may be segmental or diffuse in the esophagus, usually associated with chronic inflammation, stasis or distal obstruction [11].

Midthoracic and epiphrenic diverticula are usually asymptomatic, discovered during investigations for symptoms like dysphagia or regurgitation. Radiological evaluation for esophageal diverticula include barium swallow and computer tomography scan, the latter is helpful in defining the adjacent anatomic structures of traction diverticula in the mediastinum.

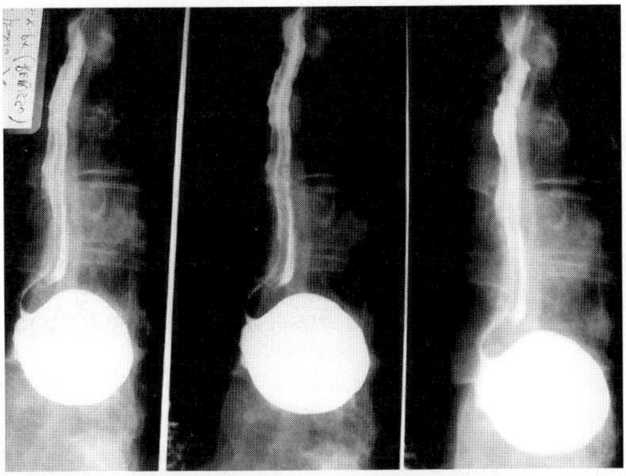

Figure 4. Epiphrenic diverticulum, large round pouch, associated with non-coordinated opening of the cardias.

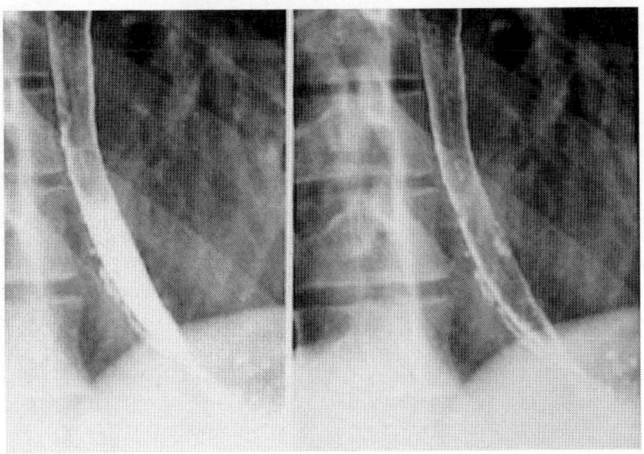

Figure 5. Intramural pseudodiverticulosis in a young man, 42 years old, complaining of dysphagia for solids.

Hiatal hernia

Hiatal hernia is the upward displacement of the stomach through the diaphragm into the thoracic cavity. There are two types of hiatal hernia: sliding and paraesophageal. In the sliding hernia a portion of the proximal stomach herniates through a wide hiatal opening because of a circumferential laxity of the crural diaphragm and phrenoesophageal membrane. Most sliding hernias are asymptomatic, except for the propensity to develop reflux disease. The cardias, at rest, lies just below the esophageal hiatus; during swallowing it moves through the hiatus upwards for a short distance into the chest; when the bolus arrives in the stomach the cardias returns to its resting position below the diaphragm. Failure of the cardias to return to its resting position is indicative of hiatal hernia. When a sliding hernia enlarges more than 3 cm its presence is obvious, because gastric folds are visible, traversing the diaphragm either during swallow and at rest. The paraesophageal hernia is less common than the sliding hernia and its main clinical significance lies in its potential for obstructive or ischemic complication. It results from a localized defect of the phrenoesophageal membrane, with the gastroesophageal junction (GEJ) fixed in its original position. It is the gastric fundus that herniates, some times all the stomach herniates in the chest with its greater curvature rolling up in an ogano-axial volvolus [12].

A sliding hiatal hernia may impair antireflux barriers at the GEJ and promote gastro-esophageal reflux. This can occur in many ways including the incompetence of the lower esophageal sphincter, caused by its dislocation to the chest from the abdomen. Hiatal hernia is highly prevalent in patients with esophagitis and Barrett's esophagus [13,14], and patients with hiatal hernia seem to

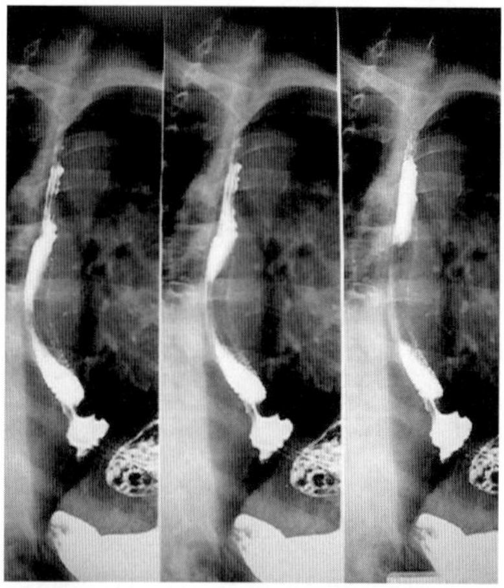

Figure 6. Small sliding hernia, about 3 cm.

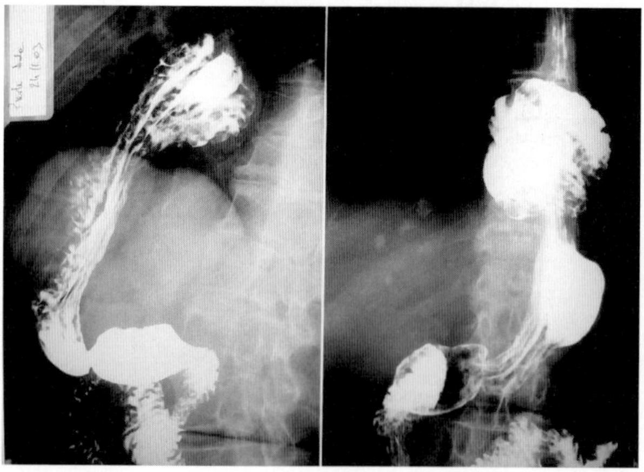

Figure 7. Large sliding hernia, about 8 cm of the proximal stomach is in the thoracic cavity.

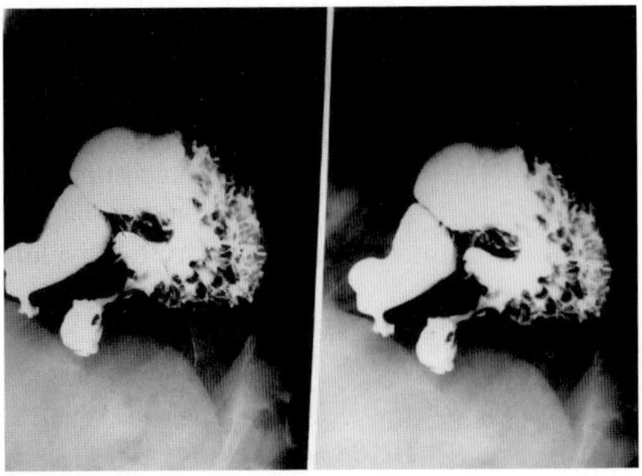

Figure 8. Paraesophageal hernia with organo-axial volvolus of the herniated stomach.

complain of more severe heartburn and regurgitation than those without, even in absence of esophagitis [15]. Most studies are hampered by the diagnostic criteria, endoscopic rather than radiological, used in the definition of hiatal hernia. Lack of standardization regarding the degree of air insufflation and difficulty in recognizing anatomical landmarks account for the less accurate findings obtained at endoscopy in diagnosing and measuring hiatal hernia. A recent study [16] in which attention was focused on the diagnosis of hiatal hernia by means of fluoroscopy, radiology confirmed the presence of a hiatal hernia, diagnosed at endoscopy in 23 patients, only in 65%, and detected a hiatal hernia in one patient with negative endoscopy, showing high sensitivity but lack of specificity of the endoscopic criteria.

References

1. Luedtke P, Levine MS, Rubesin SE, Weinstein DS, Laufer I. Radiologic diagnosis of benign esophageal strictures: a pattern approach. Radiographics 2003;23:897-909.
2. Gupta S, Levine MS, Rubesin SE, Katzka DA, Laufer I. Usefulness of barium studies for differentiating benign and malignant strictures of the esophagus. Am J Roentgenol 2003;180:737-44.
3. O'Connor JB, Richter JE. Esophageal strictures In: Castell DO, Richter JE eds. The esophagus, 3rd ed. Philadelphia: Lippincott Williams & Wilkins, 1999:473-83 .
4. Yoshikane H, Tsukamoto Y, Niwa Y, et al. Superficial esophageal carcinoa evaluation by endoscopic ultrasonography Am J Gastroenterol 1994;89:702-7.
5. Shinkai M, Niwa Y, Arisawa T, Ohmiya N, Goto H, Hayakawa T. Evaluation of prognosis of squamous cell carcinoma of the esophagus by endoscopic ultrasonography Gut 2000;47:120-5.
6. Wakelin SJ, Deans C, Crofts TJ, Allan PL, Plevris JN, Paterson-Brown S. A comparison of computerized tomography, laparoscopic ultrasound and endoscopic ultrasound in the preoperative staging of esophagogastric carcinoma. Eur J Radiol 2002;41:161-7.
7. Ito B, Niwo Y, Ando N et al. Diagnosis of the depth of invasion of esophageal carcinoma using digital radiography Eur J Radiol 2005;54:377-83.
8. Dodds WJ, Steff JJ, Hogan WJ, Hoke SE, Stewart ET, Arndorfer RC. Radial distribution of esophageal peristalsic pressure in normal subjects and patients with esophageal diverticulum. Gastroenterology 1975;69:584-90.
9. Kaye MD. Esophageal motor dysfuntion in patients with diverticula of the mid thoracic esophagus. Thorax 1974;29:666-72.
10. Hurwitz AL, Way LW, Haddad JK. Epiphrenic diverticulum in association with unusual motility disturbance: report of surgical correction. Gastroenterology 1975;68:795-8.
11. Hammon JWJr, Rice RP, Postlethwait RW, Young WG Jr. Esophageal intramural diverticulosis: a clinical and pathological survey. Ann Thorac Surg 1974;17:260-7.
12. Kahrilas PJ, Pandolfino JE. Hiatus hernia. In: Castell DO, Richter JE, eds. The esophagus, 4th ed. Philadelphia: Lippincott Williams & Wilkins, 2004;389-407.
13. Jones MP, Sloan SS, Rabine JC, Ebert CC, Huang CT, Kahrilas PJ. Hernia size is the dominant determinant of esophagitis presence and severity in gastroesophageal relux disease. Am J Gastroenterol 2001;96:1711-17.

14. Avidan B, Sonnenberg A, Schnell TG, Chejfec G, Metz A, Sontag SI. Hiatal hernia size, Barrett's length, and severity of acid reflux are all risk factors for esophageal adenocarcinoma. Am J Gastroenterol 2002;97:1930-6.
15. Petersen H, Johannessen T, Sandvik AK, et al. Relationship between endoscopic hiatus hernia and gastroesophageal reflux symptoms. Scand J Gastroenterol 1991;26:921-6.
16. Emerenziani S, Habib FI, Ribolsi M, et al. Effect of hiatal hernia on proximal esophageal acid clearance in gastro-esophageal reflux disease patients. Aliment Pharmacol Ther 2006;23:751-7.

The value of esophageal capsule endoscopy in detection of esophageal mucosal abnormalities

R. Eliakim (Haifa)

Gastroesophageal reflux disease (GERD) and its complications are a common health care problem. GERD is the second most common diagnosis and cause for outpatient visits in the USA [1].

Barrett's esophagus is a premalignant condition that occurs in up to 15% of patients with chronic GERD and may lead to adenocarcinoma of the esophagus, the second fasted growing cancer in the Western world [2]. The risk of esophageal adenocarcinoma in patients with Barrett's esophagus is approximately 0.4% per patient year and some guidelines recommend endoscopic screening for Barrett's esophagus in patients with chronic GERD [3].

Many millions worldwide suffer from cirrhosis of the liver. Bleeding from esophageal varices, a complication of portal hypertension in cirrhotic patients carries a mortality rate of at least 20% with each bleeding episode. National guidelines of few societies recommend screening endoscopy for esophageal varices in 1-3 years intervals depending on the presence or absence of varices [2]. The application of esophageal capsule endoscopy (ECE) has been considered and suggested in these three conditions, as it is a noninvasive procedure requiring no sedation, that could prove more patient friendly and increase adherance to guidelines.

Esophageal capsule endoscopy

ECE (PillCam ESO, Given Imaging, Yoqneam, Israel) is a dual-camera wireless capsule endoscope (11 x 27 mm) that obtains 14 images per second, which are transmitted to a recorder and then downloaded to a working station for interpretation (*Figure 1*).

Procedure

The swallowing procedure for ECE was built to increase visualization of the esophagus by increasing both esophageal transit time and number of esophageal frames seen per second. In the original description, after 2-3 hours of fasting, the patient ingests 100 ml of water to clear the esophagus from saliva. Then after the patient swallows the capsule in the supine

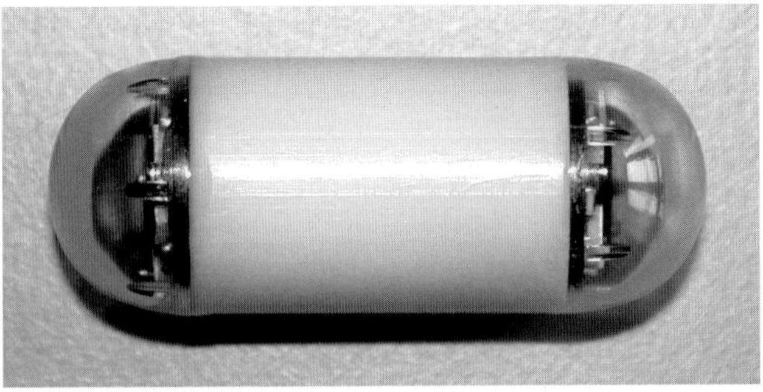

Figure 1. The PillCam ESO wireless capsule endoscope.

position with 10 ml of water and remains in that position for 2 minutes. He is then passively raised to 30 degrees for another 2 minutes, 60 degrees for another minute and then drinks some water in the sitting position [4]. This ingestion procedure was then used in bigger studies. The original esophageal capsule used 4 frames per second. The new capsule captures 14 frames per second. Due to deviations from the recommended ingestion protocol and inconvenience of supine capsule ingestion, a new simple ingestion protocol was developed that would be both easier to follow and improve gastroesophageal junction visualization [5]. The subject is positioned lying in the right lateral decubitus position with their head on a pillow. The patient swallows the capsule with a single sip (15 ml) from an Ingestion Cup (~300 ml cup filled with water, with cover, and a flexible straw), placed on the bed, close to the subject's mouth. After ingestion of the capsule while remaining lying on the right side, the subject is asked to drink additional sips of water for 7 minutes, one sip (~15 ml) every ~30 seconds. Then the subject is asked to sit upright and drink an additional sip of water.

Results

Since the first feasibility study has been published, bigger studies comparing ECE to conventional endoscopy in the diagnosis of esophagitis, Barrett's esophagus and esophageal varices were published [6-11].

Barrett's esophagus

The test characteristics of ECE for the diagnosis of Barrett's esophagus are shown in *Table I*. Over 200 patients were examined in these studies using the old ingestion procedure, in either multicenter [6], or single center studies [7,9]. Some studies used the 4 frames per second capsule and others the 14 frames per second capsule. The results suggest that ECE is an accurate method for diagnosis of suspected Barrett's esophagus with good sensitivity, specificity and negative predictive value (NPV). ECE can be used as a screening tool to detect Barrett's, possibly increasing the amount of subjects adhering to guidelines, followed by endoscopy with biopsies in those with positive findings. This strategy will eliminate the need for endoscopy in patients with negative findings. Larger multicenter studies using the new ingestion protocol and 14 frames per second capsule are needed to confirm these results.

Table I. Test characteristics of ECE reported in various trials for the diagnosis of Barrett's esophagus in patients with chronic heartburn.

	Sensitivity	Specificity	PPV	NPV
Eliakim [6] (multicenter)	97	99	97	99
Lin [9]	67	84	56	89
Koslowsky [7] (4 fps)	75	NR	NR	NR
Koslowsky [7] (14 fps)	1000	100	100	100
Sharma [10]	73	86	86	74

Esophagitis

ECE has very good test characteristics for the diagnosis of esophagitis in patients with chronic heartburn symptoms, when compared with traditional endoscopy with sensitivity of 89%, specificity 99% positive predictive value (PPV) of 97% and NPV 94% [4,6].

Since symptoms are enough and there is no need for endoscopy to diagnose reflux disease, this procedure should be reserved for the evaluation of patients with chronic reflux symptoms suspected to have GERD related complications.

Esophageal varices

Detection of esophageal varices is a third potential use for ECE. Active endoscopic screening and treatment of large varices is indicated by the European and American societies. Using ECE might be more attractive for screening of such patients as no sedation is needed.

Two pilot studies were recently published comparing ECE to conventional endoscopy in the detection of varices and portal gastropathy [8,11]. The 3 center 32 patients study [8], showed an overall diagnostic concordance of 97% for varices and 91% for portal gastropathy, while the 21 patients French study found an overall concordance of 84% [11]. ECE correctly indicated the need for primary prophylaxis in 100% of patients.

A multicenter international trial is ongoing to verify and expand these findings.

Conclusions

ECE shows promising results in the screening of patients with chronic reflux symptoms (for Barrett's) and in chronic liver disease (for varices).

References

1. Russo M, Wei J, Thiny M, et al. Digestive and liver statistics 2004. Gastroenterology 2004;126:1448-53.
2. Sharma VK, Eliakim R, Sharma P, Faigel D. ICCE consensus for esophageal capsule endoscopy. Endoscopy 2005;37:1060-4.
3. Sampliner RE. Practice parameters committee of the American College of Gastroenterology. Updated guidelines for the diagnosis, surveillance, and therapy of Barrett's esophagus. Am J Gastroenterol 2002;97:1888-95.
4. Eliakim R, Yassin K, Shlomi I, et al. A novel diagnostic tool for detecting esophageal pathology: the PillCam esophageal video capsule. Aliment Pharmacol Ther 2004;20:1083-9.

5. Gralnek IM, Rabinovitz R, Afik D, Eliakim R. A simplified ingestion procedure for esophageal capsule endoscopy: initial evaluation in healthy volunteers. Endoscopy 2006;38:213-8.
6. Eliakim R, Sharma VK, Yassin K, et al. A prospective study of the diagnostic accuracy of the Given esophageal capsule endoscopy versus conventional endoscopy in patients with chronic gastroesophageal reflux diseases. J Clin Gastroenterol 2005;39:572-8.
7. Koslowsky B, Jacob H, Eliakim R, Adler SN. PillCam ESO in esophageal studies -Improved diagnostic yield of 14 frames per second (FPS) compared with 4 FPS. Endoscopy 2006;38:27-30.
8. Eisen G, Eliakim R, Zaman A, et al. The accuracy of PillCam ESO capsule endoscopy versus conventional upper endoscopy for the diagnosis of esophageal varices. A prospective three-center pilot study. Endoscopy 2006;38:31-5.
9. Lin O, Schembre D, Kozarek R. Blinded comparison of esophageal capsule endoscopy versus conventional endoscopy for the diagnosis of Barrett's esophagus in patients with chronic gastroesophageal reflux disease. Gastrointest Endosc 2006;9396:761A.
10. Sharma P, Rastogi A, Esquivel R, et al. accuracy of wireless capsule endoscopy for the detection of Barrett's esophagus. Gastroenterology 2006;130:S1812.
11. Lapalus MG, Dumortier J, Fumex F, et al. Esophageal capsule endoscopy versus esophagogastroduodenoscopy for evaluation of portal hypertension: a prospective comparative study of performance and tolerance. Endoscopy 2006;38:36-41.

What can be expected from 3D dimensional endoscopic ultrasonography in staging of esophageal cancer?

M. Abu-Suboh Abadia, J. Dot Bach, J. Armengol-Miro
(Barcelona)

During the last decade three dimensional ultrasound images have been very popular within ultrasound diagnosis. Ten years ago we regarded 3D ultrasonography (US) as a troublesome, as there was a large quantity of volume data to achieve the reconstruction. Nowadays the rapid progress of computing technology makes able a real-time 3D US image.

Endoscopic ultrasonography (EUS) for gastrointestinal (GI) diseases was first developed in 1980. Since then, the scope of its applications has gradually expanded. In 1990 Hashimoto *et al.* first reported the use of a hand-made prototype system for three dimensional EUS. In 1994, Olympus developed the first commercially available 3D EUS processor. Now, advanced systems make possible to produce a three dimensional display of tumors and to estimate the volume of lesions.

The system for 3D-EUS consists in a 3D image processor, an ultrasound unit, a 3D probe driving unit and a 3D scanning ultrasound probe. The ultrasound probe is automatically moved inside the sheath by the driving unit, and 3D information is obtained from around the probe by mechanical spiral scanning.

The main indications for three dimensional studies are:

- volume calculation (tumors, cysts, stomach and gallbladder);
- evaluation of the vascular architecture;
- support of interventional ultrasonography;
- support of EUS, miniprobes, endorectal ultrasound and laparoscopic US.

Three dimensional EUS offers a new perspective into anatomy and pathology allowing to visualize at the same time the surface and the interior of a lesion and provides better resolution than other techniques for 3D images of GI lesions, allowing more accurate volume calculations.

But we still got some problems to solve regarding to this technique. Imaging of the esophagus is difficult because movement due to cardiac pulsation and respiration disturbs linear EUS imaging, especially in the middle esophagus. Is difficult to control probes in stenotic lesions. We need usually 30 seconds no scan, and it's too much time for the esophagus because the water is loosed in the stomach in this time of period. Lesions of more than 40 mm are difficult to visualize as a whole lineal image in a single scan and the probes have a poor penetration (about 3 cm).

The main applications of EUS in esophageal cancer are the initial staging and the re-staging after neoadjuvant therapy. The first staging of the tumor (T staging) and the nodal involvement (N staging) are important because the outcome of esophageal cancer is strongly associated with the stage, and an accurate clinical staging is critical for selecting an appropriate treatment option, and reducing unnecessary tests and treatments.

If we take a look at the algorithm of the *Figure 1*, we can see that after performing a CT scan and a PET scan if distant metastases are not demonstrated, a more accurate locoregional staging should be obtained by EUS with or without fine needle aspiration.

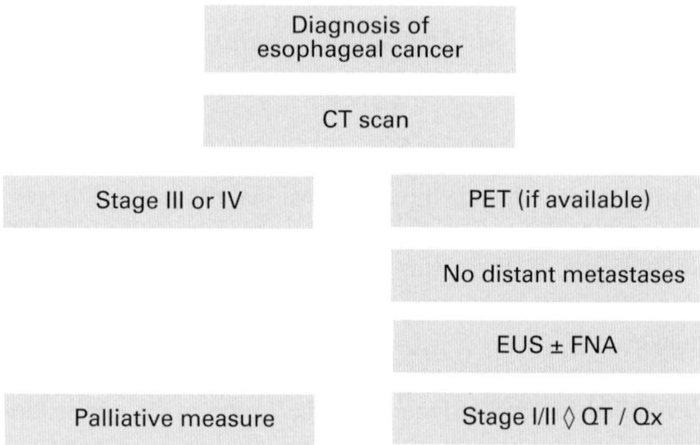

Figure 1. Algorithm for the staging of esophageal cancer (modified from Jones B. AGA Institute Postgraduate Course, 2006).
QT: chemotherapy,
Qx: surgery.

The CT scan is the most commonly used staging procedure for its availability, its capacity in ruling out distant mestastasic disease and the changes in treatment course that would occur if it demonstrates metatastases. PET scan uses 18-fluorodeoxyglucose for the detection of nodal or distant metastases. It's not accurate for the assessment of locoregional disease but it's useful for distant metastases especially for the detection of stage IV.

For the initial staging EUS is useful in determining the depth of tumor invasion (T stage) and the nodal involvement (N stage). A metaanalysis of 27 trials shows a T staging accuracy of 89%. The use of EUS produces an icrease in diagnosis of stage III and IV avoiding unnecessary surgery.

The graphic in *Figure 2* compares the accuracy of EUS and CT scan for T staging, and we can see that EUS is superior to CT scan and this superiority is for each T stage.

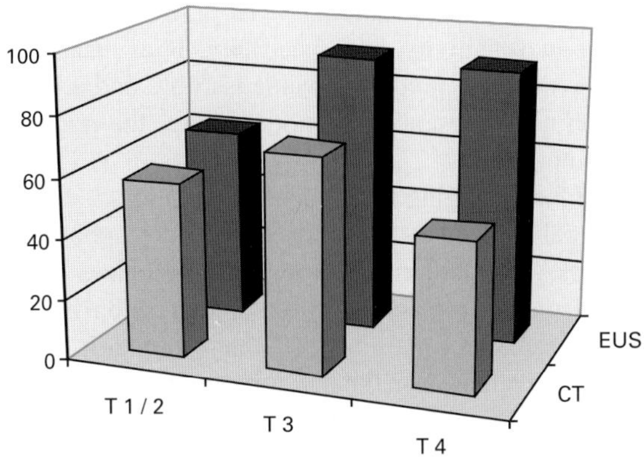

Figure 2.

Standard EUS working at frequencies between 7.5 and 12 MHz has an accuracy of 80% (50-90%) compared with pathologic staging. These instruments are able to visualize the esophageal wall as a five layered structure. But the distinction of subgroups of T1 can be problematic, and this distinction is especially important if we consider a nonsurgical therapy as endoscopic mucosal resection (EMR) or photo-dynamic therapy (PDT). For this purpose high frequency catheters are available that work at frequencies between 20-30 MHz. It provides a more detailed visualization permitting the delineation of nine layers in the esophageal wall. It permits the determination of the tumor extension into the muscularis mucosa with an accuracy as high as 84% (compared with histology). But high frequency catheters have some problems as its limited depth of penetration into the surrounding tissues (about 3 cm), and the difficulty to obtain an adequate acoustic coupling with the esophageal wall.

Three dimensional EUS (working at frequencies between 12 and 20MHz) uses a surface rendering method that can provide both, a surface image and a cross-sectional US image and it could be useful for the assessment of superficial tumors before to EMR or PDT. There are no prospective studies comparing 3D-EUS with EUS or other techniques for T staging of esophageal cancer. But results in the assessment of early gastric carcinoma invasion and rectal cancer invasions are promising.

The other item of the initial staging is the assessment of nodal involvement, and it's specially important because in esophageal cancer, metastases occur early and often. A tumor limited to the mucosa (T1m) has a prevalence of nodal metastases of 5%, but if the tumor involves the submcosa, the prevalence of nodal metastases if of 25%, for a T2 the prevalence is between 40-50% and 80% for T3 and T4.

For nodal staging EUS has a sensitivity of 71% with an specificity of 79% that may increase adding EUS-FNA of celiac and mesenteric nodes. In the *Table I*, we compare the sensitivity, specificity and accuracy of CT scan, EUS and EUS-FNA for nodal staging.

Classic endosonographic criteria for malignancy in lymph nodes are the following features: round, hypoechoic with sharp border and with a size of more than 5 mm. When all four suspicious features are present in a visualized lymph node, there is chance of 80-100 % of metastatic involvement, but only 25% of malignant nodes will have all of these features. Is for that reason that there are new proposed EUS criteria for improving nodal staging, and these new criteria are: the presence of more than 5 lymph

Table I.

	Sensitivity	Specificity	Accuracy
CT	29%	89%	51%
EUS	71%	79%	74%
EUS-FNA	83%	93%	87%

nodes, the presence of any celiac lymph node and the presence of a T3 or T4. The use of these new criteria produces an increasing in sensitivity and specificity: if a visualized lymph node presents one or less features the negative predictive value is 100% and a FNA is not needed. By the other hand if a lymph node presents 6 or more features the positive predictive value is 100% and a FNA is not needed.

Three dimensional EUS is not so useful for N staging for its poor penetration.

The other utility of EUS in esophageal cancer is the assessment of response to chemotherapy. Willis *et al.* reported that cross-sectional measurement of tumor sizes using two dimensional EUS is a reliable clinical method of assessing tumor regression before surgery, but assuming, occasionally, a significant error margin in volume estimation.

The treatment response ideally needs to be evaluated on the basis of tumor cells number and/or tumor volume. Three dimensional EUS has demonstrated its utility for the tumor volume measurement, and to assess the shrinkage after chemotherapy.

Summarizing, three dimensional EUS offers a new perspective into anatomy and pathology, allowing more accurate assessment of longitudinal invasion, and more accurate volume calculations, but there're still technical problems to be solved. It may be helpful for the assessment of superficial esophageal lesions and tumor shrinkage after neoadjuvant therapy. We should guess, that in the near future, 3D EUS image to be a useful modality for diagnosis and interventional method but further prospective studies are needed.

Bibliography

1. Dittler HJ, Bollschweiler E, Siewert JR. [What is the value of endosonography in the preoperative staging of esophageal carcinoma?]. Dtsch med Wochenschr 1991;116:561.
2. Flamen P, Lerut A, Van cutsem E et al. Utilitity of positron emisión tomography for the staging of patients with potentialy operable esophageal carcinoma. J Clin Oncol 2000; 18:3202.
3. Harewood GC, Kumar KS. Assessment of Clinical Impact of Endoscopic Ultrasound on Esophageal Cancer. J Gastroenterol Hepatol, 2004, 19(4):433-9
4. Murata Y, Suzuki S, Hashimoto H. Endoscopio ultrasonography of the upper gastrointestinal tract. Surg Endosc 1988;2:180.
5. Rosch T. Endosonographic staging of esophageal cancer: a review of literature result. Gastrointest Endosc Clin N Am. 1995;5;537.
6. Sabet EA, Okay T. Minamoto T, Mai M, Sawabu N. Three-dimensional endoscopic ultrasonography for the assessment of early gastrc carcinoma invasion : Could it provide diagnostic innovations?. Digestive Endoscopy, 2002;14:53-60
7. Tio TL, Coene PP, den Hartog Jager FC, Tytgat GN. Preoperative TNM classification of esophageal carcinoma by endosonography. Hepatogastroenterology 1990;37:376.
8. Tokiyama H, Yanai H, Nakamura H, Takeo Y. et al. Three-dimensional endoscopic ultrasonography of lesions of the upper gastrointestinal tract using a radial-linear switchable thin ultrasound probe. Journal of Gastroenterology and Hepatology, 1999;14(12):1212-8
9. Vazquez-Sequeiros E, Wiersema MJ, Clain JE, Norton ID, Levy MJ, Romero Y, Salomao D, Dierkhising R, Zinsmeister AR. Impact of lymph node staging of therapy of esophageal carcinoma. Gastroenterology 2003;125(6):1626-35
10. Vilgrain V, Mompoint D, Palazzo L, et al. Staging of esophageal carcinoma : comparison of results with endoscopic sonography and CT. Am J Roentenol 1990;115:277.
11. Watanabe M, Kida M, Yamada Y, Saigenky K. Measuring Tumor Volume with three dimensinal endoscopic ultrasonography: and explerimental and clinical study. Endoscopy, 2004, 36(11):976-81
12. Wiersema MJ, Wiersema LM, High resolution 25-megahertz ultrasonography of the gastrointestinal wall: histologic correlates. Gastrointestinal Endosc. 1993;39:499-504.
13. Yoshino J, Nakazawa S, Inui K, Katoh Y, Wakabayshi T, Okushima T, Kobayashi T, Watanabe S. Surface-rendering Imaging of Gastrointestinal lesions by three dimensional endoscopic ultrasonography.

Is videofluoroscopy the best technique for evaluation of dysphagia?

P. Pokieser, M. Scharitzer (Vienna)

Dysphagia means a sensation of mechanical difficulty during movement of food through the mouth, the pharynx or the esophagus. The underlying causes of dysphagia are numerous along the whole pathway of the upper gastrointestinal (GI) tract including impaired swallowing due to oral, pharyngeal or upper esophageal structural abnormalities or motor dysfunction. Dental problems, neurological diseases, tumors of the oral cavity, the larynx, pharynx or esophagus, motility disorders and reflux disease, benign morphologic diseases of the GI tract, like webs, rings, strictures and diverticula may lead to swallowing problems. This wide spectrum of pathologic conditions explains the need of a multidisciplinary diagnostic approach. Videofluoroscopy of deglutition is established to evaluate the whole swallowing tract additional to endoscopy, manometry and pH monitoring in a complementary and not competitive collaboration. There is no best test but a best team approach for the multidisciplinary evaluation of dysphagia. The purpose of this article is to discuss the strengths and weaknesses of videofluoroscopy in different clinical settings.

Strengths of videofluoroscopy

Videofluoroscopy investigates the entire swallowing tract

The examination includes all areas of action, involved in swallowing. The film documents with 25 frames per second the oral intake and the bolus formation on the back of the tongue and the voluntary initiation of the automatic pharyngeal swallow. The strong movement of the back of the tongue, separation and closure of the nasopharynx by the soft palate, rapid movements of the epiglottis, hyoid and larynx are recorded. Further, laryngeal closure, complete opening of the upper esophageal sphincter (UES), esophageal transport and opening of the lower esophageal sphincter (LES) are included, the transport through stomach and duodenum represent the final observations of a complete study [1,2].

The radiologic report can be structured into comments about function and morphology of the Seven Functional Units [2] (*Figure 1*):

- oral cavity and tongue: deficient bolus formation and transport, weakness of the tongue, structural deficit or mass;
- soft palate: deficient closure of the oral cavity or nasopharynx, nasal regurgitation, structural deficit or mass;
- epiglottis: insufficient tilt, asymmetric movement, structural deficit or mass;
- hyoid and larynx: lax movement, aspiration or penetration – pre- intra- post-deglutitive –, structural deficit or mass;
- pharyngeal constrictors: late or absent initiation of the involuntary swallow, pharyngeal weakness – bilateral-unilateral, diverticulum, structural deficit or mass;

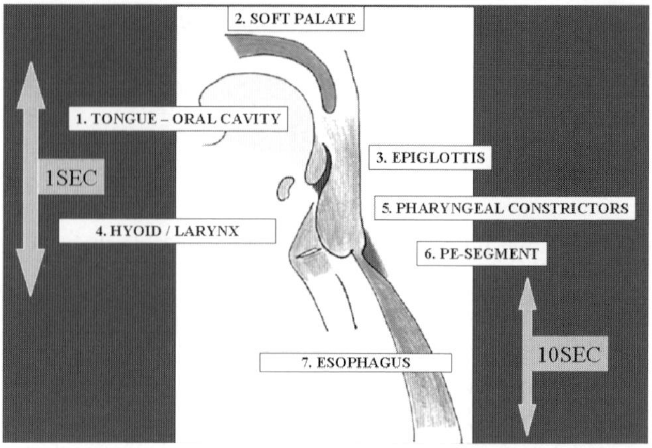

Figure 1. This graph demonstrates the seven functional units of swallowing, providing a practical structure for analysis and radiologic reports of videofluoroscopy studies. In the majority of dyphagic patients, analysis of the entire swallowing tract with videofluoroscopy is indicated.

- UES: late or incomplete opening, gaping, diverticulum, stenosis, structural deficit or mass;
- esophagus, LES, stomach, duodenum: delay of esophageal transport, non propulsive esophageal contractions, stenosis, diverticulum, hernia, lax esophagogastric junction (broadening, funnel shaped cardia, obtuse angle of His), gastric stasis, gastric or duodenal ulcers, erosions, structural deficit or mass.

Dysphagic patients may suffer from multiple causes of dysphagia, for example a neuromuscular compromise of the pharyngeal swallow, combined with an esophageal stenosis. Videofluoroscopy as the first test can detect both, giving valuable information for planning detailed diagnostic work up and therapy. Videofluoroscopy bridges the diagnostic demands of oropharyngolaryngeal and esophago-gastroduodenal clinical settings.

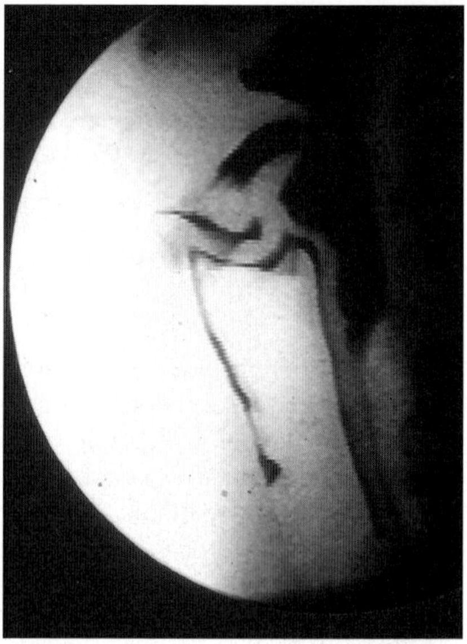

Figure 2. During aspiration, the inner larynx contracts and the endolaryngeal surface is visualised by aspirated contrast material, a typical document of dynamic radiologic pathophysiology.

Videofluoroscopy investigates function and morphology

Videofluoroscopy combines visualisation of bolus transport with documentation of movements of anatomical structures. The latter modify their appearance during action, which turns the radiographic anatomy into radiographic physiology. Pathologic structures, like diverticula, webs, rings or other types of stenoses show their pathophysiologic mechanism only during action. Typically Schatzki's ring or Zenker's diverticulum show the compromise of the GI-tract only during bolus passage for splits of a second only [3-5] (*Figure 3*).

Videofluoroscopy can evaluate the esophagus distal to a stenosis

Videofluoroscopy can investigate the pharynx and the esophagus distally to a stenosis, which cannot be passed by the endoscope [2] (*Figure 4*). Furthermore static radiographic images often fail to depict esophageal stenoses of the upper third, where narrowings are often visible for only about 0.1-0.3 seconds.

Videofluoroscopy can visualise the transport of different materials

Routinely, high density barium suspension is used. Thinned with water, the consistency can be lowered to detect aspiration with a deficient laryngeal closure. Isoosmolar contrast material is given to individuals, who are at high suspicion of aspiration or suffer from a reduced lung function. Liquid barium bolus may fail to detect mild esophageal narrowing

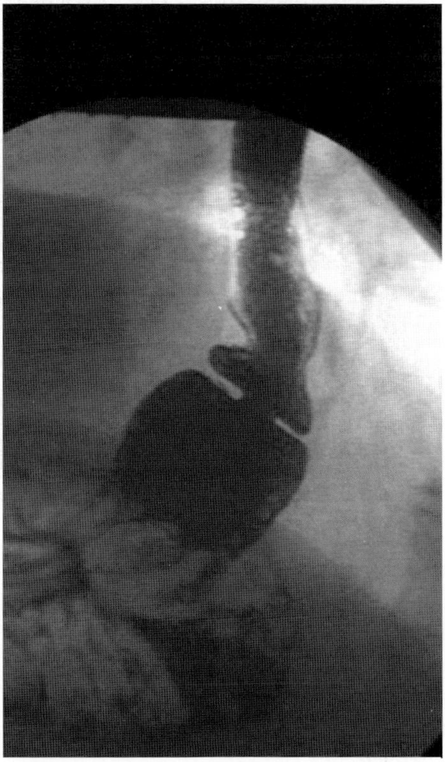

Figure 3. Schatzki's ring: videofluoroscopy can estimate the extent of narrowing during bolus passage, when the maximal width of the stenosis is visible. Endoscopy can be performed more easily with the videofluoroscopic information, especially when dilatation of the ring is considered.

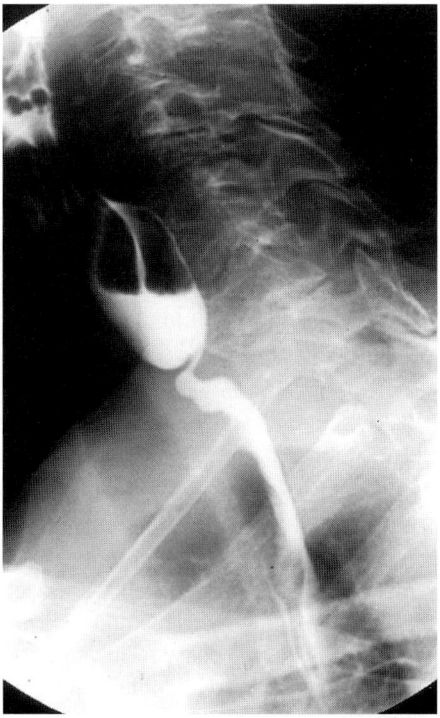

Figure 4. Dynamic imaging depicts high grade benign stenosis, caused by a ventral web at the level of the upper esophageal sphincter. The endoscope could not pass over the narrowing.

and will not reproduce symptoms in many patients with dysphagia. Barium paste is thick like tooth paste and helps to detect for example pharyngeal weakness. With a 13-14 mm placebo tablette, the width of a stenosis can be measured accurately [2] (*Figure 5*).

Monitoring the transport of the tablette by videofluoroscopy, parallel the patient can be asked to tell, if symptoms occure or not. An impaction of a tablette at the level of a Schatzki's ring often is not recognised by the patient. In turn the tablette may provoke symptoms instead of a normal width of the esophagus. This might be valuable information for further work up with endoscopy, manometry or pH monitoring.

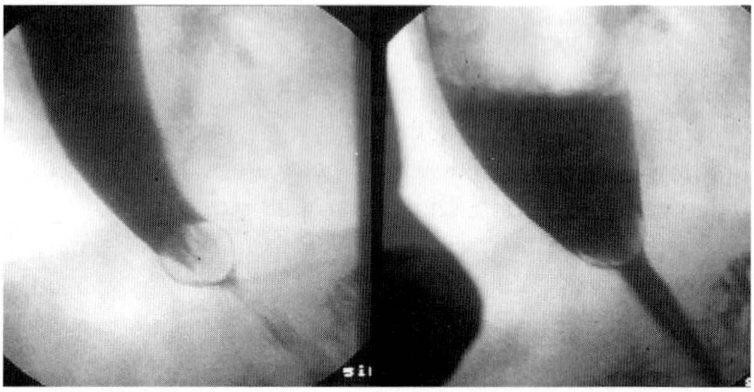

Figure 5. In this patient, 4 months after fundoplication, a placebo tablette gets stuck at the level of a narrowed fundoplication. The known diameter of the tablette helps to approximate the width of the stenosis.

Weaknesses of videofluoroscopy

Videofluoroscopy cannot exclude malignancy

Weakness of radiography to detect small malignancies is well known and endoscopy is the method of choice, if evaluation of the mucosa is of diagnostic interest. Therefore, any stenosis, detected by videofluoroscopy should undergo endoscopy. Videofluoroscopy is helpful in patients with high grade malignant stenosis near the UES, where endoscopy is difficult to perform [1,2].

Videofluoroscopy causes radiation exposure

Depending on the clinical situation, the screening time of videofluoroscopy ranges from 20-200 sec [1,2,8], and for a typical videofluoroscopic examination a dose-area product between 0.2-0.4 mSv are reported [6,7]. The radiation doses compare adequate with the effective doses associated with other common radiological upper GI studies and therefore radiation disadvantage is well within acceptable limits. Without any radiation, magneetic resonance imaging (MRI) is under development for clinical evaluation of deglutition. But dynamic MRI of the pharyngeal and esophageal phase of swallowing remains an interesting tool of clinical research, an interesting imaging option for clinical use in future.

Videofluoroscopy has a low availability

To obtain expertise in videofluoroscopy, even trained radiologists need a lot of training. Acceptance to integrate videofluoroscopy into the repertoire of radiological departments is rising, but still the availability of videofluoroscopy is low [1,2,8].

Videofluoroscopy evaluation depends mostly on the skill and interest of the radiologist performing the exam

The clinical interpretation of videofluoroscopic images depends on subjective judgements and interreader variability varies according to the rater's experience and quality of image. Highest levels of agreement are obtained, if interdisciplinary discussions are possible, especially in complicated cases [9]. A standardization of interpretation of videofluoroscopic assessment (7 functional units) is an attempt to provide a checklist of possible findings to facilitate the recognition and correct valuation of radiographic signs.

Conclusion

Videofluoroscopy provides a descriptive overview of function and morphology of the entire swallowing tract. Videofluoroscopy is complementary to endoscopy, pH- monotoring and manometry. There is no best test for evaluation of dysphagia, but the best choreography of tests is provided by our ability to cooperate among different disciplines.

References

1. Jones B, Donner M. Examination of the patient with dysphagia. Radiology 1988;167:319-26.
2. Ekberg O, Pokieser P. Radiologic evaluation of the dysphagic patient. Eur Radiol 1997;7:1285-95.
3. Schatzki R, Gary JE. Dysphagia due to a diaphragm-like localized narrowing in the lower esophagus ("lower esophageal ring"). Am J Roentgenol 1953;70:911-23.
4. Schima W, Schober E, Stacher G, et al. Association of midoesophageal diverticula with oesophageal motor disorders. Videofluoroscopy and manometry. Acta Radiol 1997;38:108-14.
5. Scharitzer M, Pokieser P, Schober E, et al. Morphological findings in dynamic swallowing studies of symptomatic patients. Eur Radiol 2002;12(5):1139-44.
6. Zammit-Maempel I, Chapple CL, Leslie P. Radiation dose in videofluoroscopic swallow studies. Dysphagia 2007;22(1):13-5.
7. Wright RE, Boyd CS, Workman A. Radiation doses to patients during pharyngeal videofluoroscopy. Dysphagia 1998;13(2):113-5.
8. Eisenhuber E, Schima W, Stadler A, et al. Evaluation of swallowing disorders with videofluoroscopy in Austria: a survey. Eur J Radiol 2005;53(1):120-4.
9. Scott A, Sci A, Perry A, et al. A study of interrater reliability when using videofluoroscopy as an assessment of swallowing. Dysphagia 1998;13:223-7.

Bolus transit and dysphagia: what can be expected from combined manometric and videofluoroscopic study of swallow?

P. Clavé (Mataró)

Dysphagia is a symptom that refers to difficulty with or discomfort during the progression of the alimentary bolus from the mouth to the stomach. From an anatomical standpoint dysphagia may result from oropharyngeal or esophageal dysfunction and from a pathophysiological standpoint from structure-related or functional causes. The prevalence of **oropharyngeal functional dysphagia** is very high: it affects more than 30% of patients who have had a cerebrovascular accident, 52%-82% of patient's with Parkinson's disease, it is the first symptom for 60% of patients with amyotrophic lateral sclerosis (ALS), it affects up to 44% of patients with multiple sclerosis, up to 84% of patients with Alzheimer's disease, and more than 60% of older institutionalized patients [1-4]. The severity of oropharyngeal dysphagia varies from moderate difficulty to complete inability to swallow and may give rise to two groups of clinically relevant complications:

- a decrease in the efficacy of deglutition leading to malnutrition and/or dehydration in up to 25%-75% of patients;
- a decrease in deglutition safety, leading to choking and tracheobronchial aspiration which result in pneumonia in 50% of cases, with an associated mortality of up to 50% [1,2].

The current state of the art of oropharyngeal dysphagia management aims at identifying early patients at risk for dysphagia, assessing alterations in the biomechanical events of oropharyngeal swallow response, and attempting to prevent and treat potential complications of dysphagia such as aspiration pneumonia and malnutrition [5].

Dysphagia may result from a wide range of structural alterations that impair bolus progression, the most common being esophageal and ENT tumors, neck osteophytes, postsurgical esophageal stenosis, and Zenker's diverticulum [2]. Dysphagia may also be a side effect in patients with head and neck cancers undergoing radiotherapy. Most hospitals are fully equipped to diagnose and treat structural causes of dysphagia. However, oropharyngeal dysphagia is more frequently a functional disorder of deglutition affecting bolus propulsion and oropharyngeal configuration and caused by systemic or neurological diseases, or associated with aging [2,3]. In many hospitals there is a big discrepancy between the high prevalence, morbidity, mortality and costs caused by nutritional and respiratory complications of functional oropharyngeal dysphagia and the low level of human and material resources dedicated to dysphagic patients. Diagnosis and management of oropharyngeal dysphagia requires a multidisciplinary approach. A dysphagia multidisciplinary team should include several professional domains: nurses, speech-swallow therapists, gastroenterologists, ENT specialists, neurologists, surgeons, rehabilitation physicians, dietitians, radiologists, geriatricians, etc. The goals of a multidisciplinary dysphagia team include:

- early identification of patients with dysphagia;
- diagnosis of any medical or surgical etiology for dysphagia that may respond to specific treatment, the exclusion of ENT and esophageal tumors, and gastroesophageal reflux and its complications;
- characterization of specific biomechanical events responsible for functional dysphagia in each patient;
- the design of therapeutic strategies to provide the patient with safe and effective deglutition, or the provision of an alternative route to oral feeding based on objective and reproducible data [2,5].

Videofluoroscopy (VFS) is the gold standard to study the oral and pharyngeal mechanisms of dysphagia [1,2,7,8]. VFS is a dynamic exploration that evaluates the safety and efficacy of deglutition, characterizes the alterations of deglutition in terms of videofluoroscopic signs, allows accurate measurement of the oropharyngeal swallow response and helps to select and assess specific therapeutic strategies. Technical requirements for clinical VFS are an X-ray tube with fluoroscopy and a videotape recorder; and there are computed-assisted methods of analysis of images allowing quantitative temporal and spatial measurements [5,6,9]. Main observations during VFS are done in the lateral plane while swallowing 3-20 mL boluses of three viscosities: liquid, nectar and pudding. Viscosity can be defined as the measure of a fluid's resistance to flow, a concept similar to friction, and is measured in the International System of Units as Pascal seconds. Thin liquids have a viscosity from 1-20 mPas, nectar fluids have 250-300 mPas and pudding fluids 3,500-4,000 mPas [6]. We keep the patient at a minimal risk for aspiration by starting the study with low volumes and thick consistencies, introducing liquids and high volumes as tolerated [2,5-7]. VFS signs measuring efficacy of deglutition include apraxia of swallow, reduced range of tongue control and weak bolus propulsion, oral residue, pharyngeal residue, nasopharyngeal regurgitation and impaired upper esophageal sphincter (UES) opening [5-7]. Residue in the mouth, the vallecula, or the pyriform sinus is found in up to 50% of patients with neurogenic dysphagia. In contrast, impaired UES opening is found in less than 15% of these patients [6].

Videofluoroscopic signs measuring swallowing safety are reduced glossopalatal seal, laryngeal penetration (bolus reaches the laryngeal vestibule) or aspiration (bolus enters the airway). VFS can determine whether aspiration occurs before, during or after the swallow response. Predeglutitive aspirations are caused by impaired glossopalatal seal. Aspirations during swallow responses are caused by a delay in triggering the pharyngeal swallow or impaired deglutitive airway protection (laryngeal elevation, epiglottic descent, and closure of vocal folds). Post-swallow aspiration is caused by an ineffective pharyngeal clearance. Pre- and post-deglutitive aspirations occur in less than 10% of patients with neurogenic dysphagia. In contrast, up to 40% of our patients with neurogenic dysphagia showed aspirations during pharyngeal phase of swallow response, one-third without cough (silent aspirations) [3-6].

In biomechanical terms, the oropharyngeal swallow response consists of the temporal arrangement of oropharyngeal structures from a respiratory to a digestive pathway, the transfer of the bolus from the mouth to the esophagus, and the recuperation of the respiratory configuration [10]. Configuration of the oropharynx during swallow response is defined by opening (O) or closing (C) events occurring at the glossopalatal junction (GPJ), velopharyngeal junction (VPJ), laryngeal vestibule (LV), and UES that can be measured during videofluoroscopic studies (*Figure 1*). Healthy subjects presented a short swallow response (GPJO-LVO < 740 ms), fast laryngeal vestibule closure (LVC < 160 ms) and fast UES opening (UESO < 220 ms) [6]. In contrast, we found the swallow response severely impaired in patients with neurogenic dysphagia and also in older people [3-6]. Overall duration of oropharyngeal swallow response (OSR) in these patients was significantly longer than in healthy subjects due to delay in the early phase of oropharyngeal reconfiguration from a respiratory to a digestive pathway. We found prolonged intervals to LVC and UESO are the key abnormalities of swallow response leading to unsafe deglutition and aspiration in neurological patients, doubling that of healthy subjects (*Figure 2*) [6]. Transfer of the bolus from the mouth through the pharynx to the esophagus is mainly caused by the squeezing action of the tongue against the palate providing driving forces to propel swallowed material across the UES with minimal resistance [12]. The pharyngeal contraction facilitates pharyngeal clearance [13]. We assessed bolus propulsion forces by measuring the bolus velocity and translational kinetic energy in milli-Joules (mJ) of the bolus prior to entering the UES. Healthy subjects presented high bolus velocity

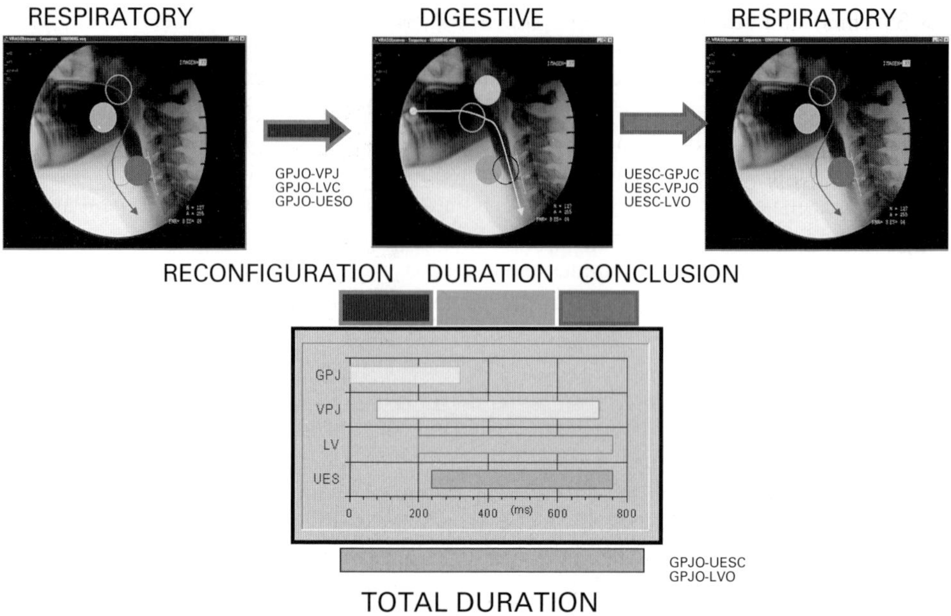

Figure 1. Configuration of the oropharynx during swallow response. Each phase of the response (reconfiguration, duration and conclusion) is defined by opening (O) or closing (C) events occurring at the glossopalatal junction (GPJ), velopharyngeal junction (VPJ), laryngeal vestibule (LV), and upper esophageal sphincter (UES). (See page XVI for colour figure).

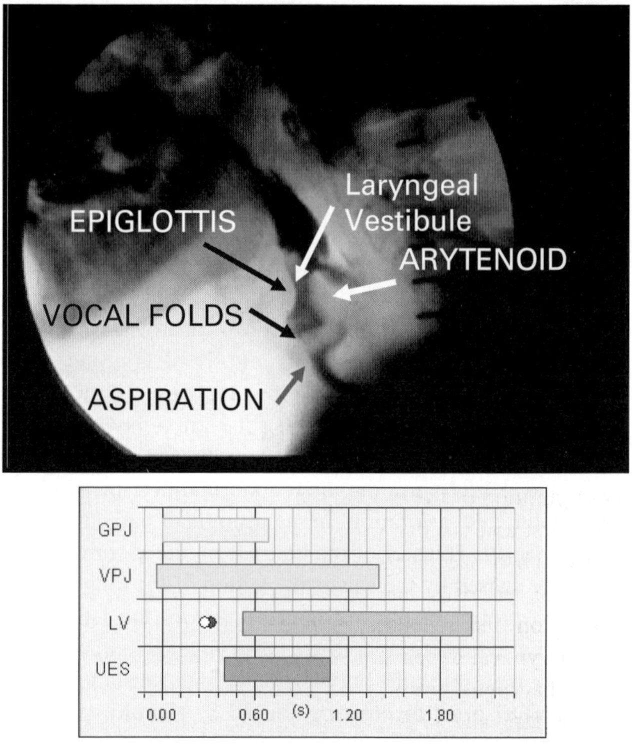

Figure 2. Swallow response in a patient with neurogenic dysphagia and aspiration during swallow. Diagram at the bottom of each tracing depicts timing of swallow response showing severe delay in LVC and UESO. White dots represent timing of laryngeal penetration and the red point, time of aspiration. (See page XVI for colour figure).

(> 35 cm/s) and strong bolus propulsion forces (> 0.33 mJ). In contrast, neurological patients showed slow bolus velocity (< 22 cm/s) and weak bolus propulsion forces (< 0.20 mJ) causing post swallow residue [6]. We also found that older people with oropharyngeal dysphagia presented even more impaired tongue propulsion forces (< 0.14 mJ) and slower bolus velocity (< 10 cms/s) [3].

Mechanisms of UES opening: the four main mechanisms that participate in UES opening are:

- the interruption of vagal input to the cricopharyngeal muscle allowing muscular relaxation;
- the anterior traction on the sphincter caused by contraction of hyoid muscles;
- the intrabolus propulsion forces caused by tongue thrust;
- the compliance of the sphincter allowing complete relaxation, low residual pressures and no resistance during swallowing (*Figure 3*) [14].

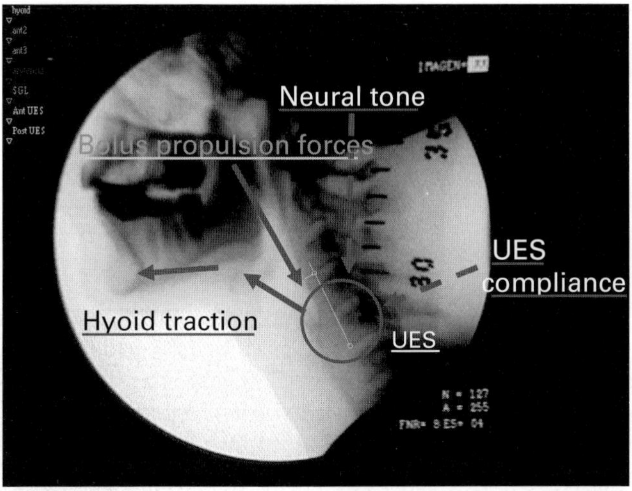

Figure 3. Mechanisms of UES opening. Timing of swallow response, the extent of hyoid motion and UES opening and bolus propulsion forces can be assessed during videofluoroscopic studies. UES relaxation and compliance is assessed by pharyngo-esophageal manometry. (See page XVII for colour figure).

The integrity of swallow response, the extent of hyoid motion and UES opening and bolus propulsion can be assessed during videofluoroscopic studies. UES relaxation and compliance is assessed by pharyngoesophageal manometry [8,15]. We perform manometric studies using perfusion techniques and a trans-nasal probe with a 6 cm sleeve or with five side holes 1 cm apart to straddle the UES, simultaneously monitoring surface EMG of the hyoid muscles. Initially, we did manometric and VFS studies simultaneously. However, the presence of the manometric probe altered the accuracy of the measurement of the configuration of the oropharynx and also the extent of hyoid motion. Now we conduct the VFS first and use the X-ray facility to locate the manometric probe at the end of the VFS study. Then we perform the manometric study, using the same bolus characteristics (volume, viscosity and density) that we used in theVFS studies. Failure of manometric relaxation and reduced sphincter compliance are uncommon findings in patients with oropharyngeal dysphagia and cause a steep rise in residual (nadir) sphincter pressure and hypopharyngeal pressure as bolus volume increases [15] (*Figure 4*). By combining the manometric and VFS findings we can define three main patterns of reduced UES opening:

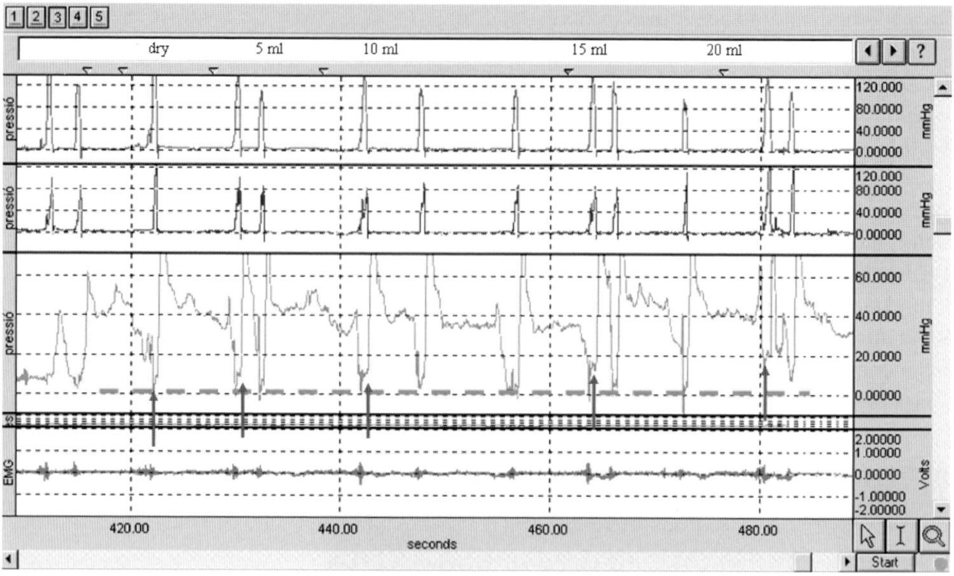

Figure 4. Pharyngeoesophageal manometry with surface EMG of hyoid muscles. Representative tracing in a patient with a Zenker diverticulum showing reduced sphincter compliance. Note that residual pressure is normal during dry swallows and that fibrosis of the sphincter causes increased resistance and increased residual (nadir) pressures with increased bolus volume. Note that nadir UES pressure is over 20 mmHg during 20 mL swallows. (See page XVII for colour figure).

- impaired UES caused by low bolus propulsion is observed in up to 15% patients with neurodegenerative diseases and characterized by delayed swallow response, short hyoid motion, weak bolus propulsion, and normal manometric relaxation [2,8]. Many of these patients also presented reduced safety of deglutition. Treatment includes increasing the viscosity and reducing the volume of the bolus, improving hyoid motion, tongue thrust and airway protection by rehabilitation procedures that should be provided by experienced swallow-therapists and include changes in head posture, heightened sensory input, and active swallow maneuvers, and probably in the future electrical stimulation of hyoid muscles and pharmacological modulation of swallow response;
- impaired neural UES relaxation observed in spastic neurological diseases such as Parkinson disease or brain injury is characterized by delayed or absent swallow response, short hyoid motion, weak bolus propulsion, and reduced or even absent neuromuscular relaxation and reduced sphincter compliance on manometry [2,8,15]. Treatment must combine treatment of neurogenic dysphagia and improvment of neuromuscular relaxation of the sphincter. Efficacy of cricopharyngeal myotomy in patients with impaired swallow response is fair to poor and injection of botox in the sphincter could be a therapeutic alternative for these patients;
- impaired UES opening in patients with Zenker's diverticulum or isolated cricopharyngeal bars show normal swallow response, wide hyoid motion, strong bolus propulsion and reduced sphincter compliance caused by sphincter fibrosis [2,8,15]. Treatment of this group of patient is surgical and combines cricopharyngeal myotomy and resection of the diverticulum. Results in patients with preserved swallow response are excellent.

Summary and conclusions

To the question: what can be expected from combined manometric and videofluoroscopic studies of swallow? We can answer: manometry and VFS are complementary methods to study the pathophysiology and select the treatment of patients with oropharyngeal dysphagia:

VFS can assess the signs of safety and efficacy of deglutition, the timing of swallow response and the mechanisms of aspiration, the extent of hyoid motion and UES opening and the strength of bolus propulsion forces.

Manometry can assess the UES compliance and hypopharyngeal pressure, and the mechanism of incomplete UES opening.

Identification of functional oropharyngeal dysphagia as a major neurological and geriatric syndrome will induce many changes in the provision of medical and social services in the near future. Education of health professionals in the diagnosis and treatment of dysphagia and its complications, early diagnosis, development of specific complementary explorations in the clinical setting, improvement in dietary strategies to avoid aspirations and malnutrition, and research into its pathophysiology are the cornerstones to allow maximal recovery potential for patients with functional oropharyngeal dysphagia.

References

1. Cook IJ, Kahrilas PJ. AGA technical review on management of oropharyngeal dysphagia. Gastroenterology 1999;116:455-78.
2. Clave P, Terre R, de Kraa M, Serra M. Approaching oropharyngeal dysphagia. Rev Esp Enferm Dig 2004;96:119-31.
3. Clavé P, Verdaguer A, Arreola V. Oral-pharyngeal dysphagia in the elderly. Med Clin (Barc) 2005;124(19):742-8.
4. Terre-Boliart R, Orient F, Bernabeu M, Clavé-Civit P. Oropharyngeal dysphagia in patients with multiple sclerosis. Rev Neurol 2004;39(8):707-10.
5. Clavé P, Almirall J, Esteve M, Verdaguer A, Berenguer J, Serra-Prat M. Dysphagia – a team approach to prevent and treat complications. Campden Publishing Ltd. Hospital Healthcare Europe 2005/2006. N5-N8, 2005.
6. Clavé P, de Kraa M, Arreola V, et al. The effect of bolus viscosity on swallowing function in neurogenic dysphagia. Aliment Pharmacol Ther 2006;24:1385-94.
7. Clavé P. A picture is worth a thousand words: Videofluoroscopic diagnosis of oropharyngeal dysphagia. Nutr Matt 2001;3:1-2.
8. Clavé P. Métodos de estudio de la neurofisiología de la deglución y de la disfagia orofaríngea. Rev Esp Enferm Dig 2004;96(Supl. II):47-9.
9. Logemann JA, Kahrilas PJ, Begelman J, Dodds WJ, Pauloski BR. Interactive computer program for biomechanical analysis of videoradiographic studies of swallowing. AJR Am J Roentgenol 1989;153:277-80.
10. Kahrilas PJ, Lin SZ, Chen J, et al. Oropharyngeal accommodation to swallow volume. Gastroenterology 1996;111:297-306.
11. Kahrilas PJ, Lin S, Rademaker AW, Logemann JA. Impaired deglutitive airway protection: a videofluoroscopic analysis of severity and mechanism. Gastroenterology 1997;113:1457-64.
12. Nicosia MA, Robbins JA. The fluid mechanics of bolus ejection from the oral cavity. J Biomech 2001;34:1537-44.
13. Kahrilas PJ, Logemann JA, Lin S, et al. Pharyngeal clearance during swallowing: a combined manometric and videofluoroscopic study. Gastroenterology 1992;103:128-36.
14. Cook IJ, Dodds WJ, Dantas RO, Massey B. Opening mechanisms of the upper esophageal sphincter. Am J Physiol (Gastrointestinal. Liver Physiol) 1989;20:G747-59.
15. Williams RBH, Wallace KL, Ali GA, Cook IJ. Biomechanics of failed deglutitive upper esophageal sphincter relaxation in neurogenic dysphagia. Am J Physiol (Gastrointestinal. Liver Physiol) 2002;283:G16-26.

What is the predictive role of the degree of esophageal emptying by timed barium swallows of patients with achalasia?

E.-H. Metman, L. Picon, L. Negreanu (Tours)

Barium swallow has long been used to diagnose achalasia. The classic radiological finding associated with achalasia is the "bird's beak" appearance of the distal esophagus. Other radiological findings include an air-fluid level or a tortuous, sigmoid esophagus (especially in long-standing achalasia).

No current treatment restores the normal peristalsis of the esophagus. The endoscopic (pneumatic dilation and botulinum toxin injection) and surgical methods have as end points the symptom relief and the achievement of esophageal emptying through reduction of the lower esophageal sphincter (LES) functional obstruction.

The success rate of the Rigiflex pneumatic dilations vary from 50% to 93% [1]. This variability was attributed to technical differences, although the data in the litterature are conflicting. The decision to stop therapy is usually based on symptomatic relief. The "clinical approach" assumes that symptomatic improvement is associated with physiologic improvement which is not always the case. Eckardt *et al.* compared a detailed score of clinical symptoms before and after treatment and observed that symptomatic improvement may not accurately reflect optimal or complete esophageal emptying [2].

The timed barium esophagogram (TBE) was firstly used by Oliveira et al. in 23 achalasia patients studied retrospectively before and after pneumatic dilation or Clostridium botulinum toxin injection [3]. The method was a further development of the barium swallow, introducing functional and dynamic dimensions to the assessment. In their original paper the authors stated that their purpose was "to define a simple, noninvasive, and widely available barium technique that could serve as an objective measure of esophageal baseline and post-therapy emptying in achalasia patients".

Other advantages of the TBE pointed out by Oliveira's work are: it is a diagnostic modality that could be used outside the tertiary centers, or when manometry is not available and also as a diagnostic tool which offers acceptable accuracy before the use of more advanced and more costly technology.

Their original technique was to obtain upright frontal spot films of the esophagus at 1, 2 and 5 minutes after ingestion of 100-200 ml of low-density (45% weight in volume) barium sulfate (volume of barium determined by patient tolerance). The degree of esophageal emptying was calculated by comparing 1 and 5 minutes spot films by height or area (height x width).

The authors concluded that timed barium swallow was a simple and reproducible technique and that both qualitative assessment and estimated that change in area based on height-times-width measurements of the barium column was an accurate methods of estimating esophageal emptying [3].

After the initial description, the method (or its variants) was used in treated and non treated achalasia patients.

Two studies by Vaezi *et al.* discussed the predictive value of the esophageal emptying on TBE before and after treatment of achalasia patients.

In the first study [4] there was a 73% concordance between the degree of symptom improvement and degree of esophageal emptying by barium esophagogram (results of 53 pneumatic dilatations in 37 achalasia patients). The patients reporting only slight symptom improvement (< 50%) showed almost always (17/19 patients, 89%) a poor

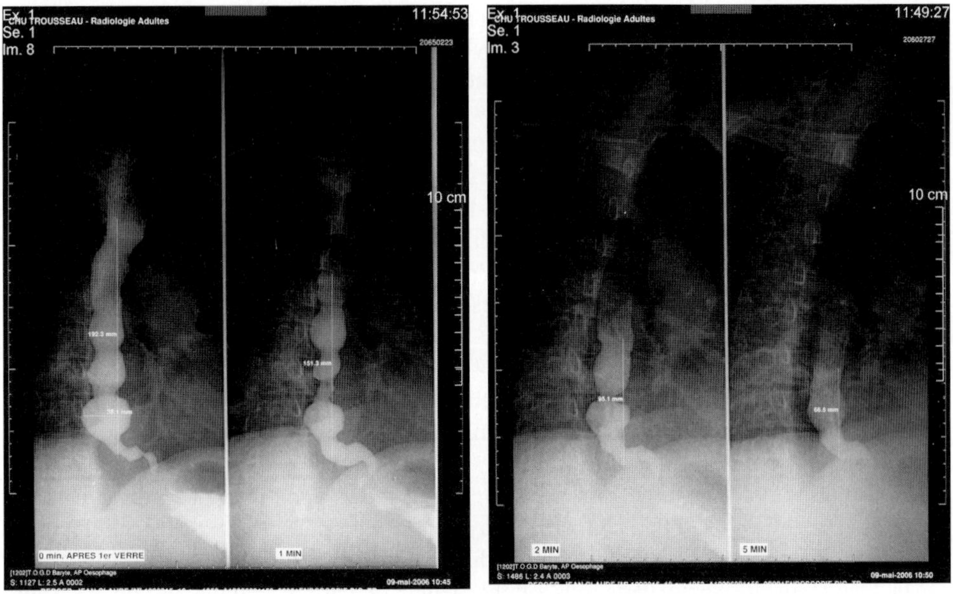

Figure 1.

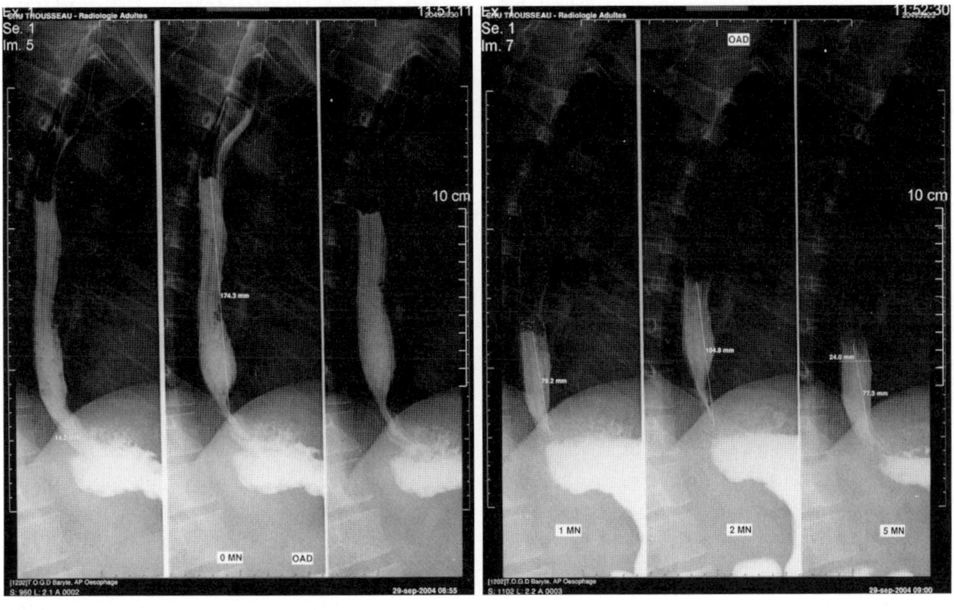

Figure 2.

esophageal emptying on TBE. The study also showed that up to 30% of dilated patients still had poor esophageal emptying of barium (< 50%) although they reported 90-100% symptom improvement [4].

Starting from the hypothesis that the group of patients with poor esophageal emptying would have an earlier relapse of their symptoms when followed long term, the same team conducted a new study [5]. A comparison between the patients with poor esophageal emptying (discordant group) with the patients whose symptom resolution correlated with marked improvement in esophageal emptying (concordant group) was realized. The primary end point was to determine if the timed barium esophagogram is a better predictor of long term treatment success (mean follow up of 6 years) after therapy than symptom assessment alone. The results confirmed the predictive value of the TBE emptying: 77% of the patients from the concordant group were still in symptomatic remission while this was the case in none of the discordant group. In fact, (90%) patients with discordant findings failed therapy within one year of pneumatic dilations while the failure rate was constant and slow for the concordant group. Furthermore, patients in the concordant group available for follow up continued to have complete esophageal emptying as well as long term symptomatic remission [5].

The TBE can be considered a predictor of poor long term outcome if patients continue to have post pneumatic dilation retained barium. Based on the TBE results a closer follow up and a more aggressive further therapy might be offered to these patients in order to ensure long term remission.

However in a recent study from Sweden, which shows good inter observer evaluation of the parameters of the TBE, comparing day to day variations, the esophageal emptying appeared not so accurate for the evaluation due to poor reproductibility [6].

In fact there are some variations of the height of barium column during the same examination at time 0 and also at time 1 and 2 minutes in our experience (*Figures 1 and 2*).

There is a need for standardization of the technique, and definition of the best criteria:

- pre-therapy 1 minute height predictive of immediate or late results of therapy for Vela *et al.* [7];
- percentage change in volume between 1 and 5 minutes after treatment was predictive for Montazeri *et al.* [8];
- pre- and post-therapeutic barium height at five minutes was predictive of results for Vaezi *et al.* [5].

Esophageal manometry is probably the best technique for the evaluation of the response after pneumatic dilation but because of cost and lack of availability in many centers, post-procedure manometry is not currently offered to all patients. The development of a method that could objectively evaluate the therapy results seemed natural and the results of the TBE are convincing. A good correlation between post therapy reduction in LES pressure and barium column height was shown in achalasia patients undergoing pneumatic dilation by the same team of Vaezi *et al.* [7], so this is another argument for the use of TBE in the patient's response to therapy evaluation.

References

1. D'Alteroche L, Metman EH. Traitement endoscopique et instrumental des troubles moteurs de l'œsophage. In :Boyer J, Ponchon T, eds. Endoscopie digestive interventionelle. Paris : Doin, 2002:55-66.
2. Eckardt VF, Aignherr C, Bernhard G. Predictors of outcome in patients with achalasia treated by pneumatic dilation. Gastroenterology 1992;103:1732-8.

3. de Oliviera JMA, Birgisson S, Doinoff C, et al. Timed barium swallow: a simple technique for evaluating esophageal emptying in patients with achalasia. Am J Radiol 1997;169:473-9.
4. Vaezi MF, Baker ME, Richter JE. Assessment of esophageal emptying post-pneumatic dilation: use of the timed barium esophagogram. Am J Gastroenterol 1999;94:1802-7.
5. Vaezi MF, Baker ME, Achkar E, Richter JE. Timed barium esophagogram: better predictor of long term success after pneumatic dilation in achalasia than symptom assessment. Gut 2002;50:765-70.
6. Kostic S, Andersson M, Hellström M, Lönroth H, Lundell L. Timed barium esophagogram in the assessment of patients with achalasia: reproducibility and observer variation. Dis Esophagus 2005;18:96-103.
7. Vela MF, Richter JE, Khandwala F, et al. The long-term efficacy of pneumatic dilatation and heller myotomy for the treatment of achalasia. Clin Gastroenterol Hepatol 2006;4:580-7.
8. Montazeri G, Nouri N, Estakhri A, et al. Lower oesophageal sphincter pressure and timed barium oesophagogram: two objective parameters in the non-invasive assessment of primary achalasia. Aliment Pharmacol Ther 2005;22:261-5.
9. Vaezi MF, Richter JE, Wilcox CM, et al. Botulinum toxin versus pneumatic dilation in the treatment of achalasia: a randomized trial. Gut 1999;44:231-9.

What are the current indications of radiology in patients with gastroesophageal reflux disease?

F.I. Habib (Rome)

Only 26% of subjects, proven to have pathological gastroesophageal reflux (GER) at 24-hour pH probe monitoring, were positive at the radiological examination for unprovoked spontaneous reflux [1]. Nevertheless radiology is important in GER disease (GERD) patients to recognize morphological changes due to acid reflux, changes in esophageal motor activity such as non peristaltic contractions with proximal escape, delayed clearing due to failure of secondary peristalsis and the presence and size of a hiatus hernia. It has been shown that GERD patients, particularly those presenting hiatal hernia, are characterized by a more compliant esophagogastric junction that could facilitate the flow of larger volumes of refluxate. The relationship between proximal aced exposure and volume of refluxate has been investigated by Orr *et al.* by perfusing 1 and 3ml of acid in the distal esophagus in healthy volunteers: higher volumes were associated with higher proximal migration [2].

During fluoroscopic examination GER may occur spontaneously, more frequently when the patient is lying on his right hand side, or during provocative maneuvers, such Valsalva maneuver or water siphon test, that enhance its occurrence [3,4].

References

1. Thompson JK, Koehler RE, Richter JE. Detection of gastroesophageal reflux: value of barium studies compared with 24-hr pH monitoring. Am J Roentgenol 1994;162:621-6.
2. Orr WC, Elsenbruch S, Harnish MJ, Johnson LF. Proximal migration of esophageal acid perfusions during walking and sleep. Am J Gastroenterol 2000;95:37-42.
3. Sellar RJ, DeCaestecker JS, Heading RC. Barium radiology: a sensitive test for gastro-esophageal reflux. Clin Radiol 1987;38:303-7.
4. Thompson JK, Koehler RE, Richter JE. Detection of gastroesophageal reflux: value of barium studies compared with 24-h pH monitoring. Am J Roentgenol 1994;162: 621-6.

Are there specific indications for esophageal scintigraphy in gastroesophageal reflux disease?

K.G. Chaudhuri, J.K. Chaudhuri, D.N. Chaudhuri, S. Fink, T.K. Chaudhuri, T.K. Chaudhuri (San Antonio)

Gastroesophageal reflux disease (GERD) is a common disease, with an estimated 18.6 million cases per year in the United States alone and 27.5 million patients treated worldwide between 1994 and 1999. Although the majority of patients with GERD do not have erosive disease which limits the value of endoscopy and barium swallows , esophageal pH monitoring and esophageal manometry are fortunately not so limited, and have gained increasing importance in diagnosing GERD [1]. Associated respiratory disease includes asthma, chronic cough, laryngitis, and aspiration pneumonia due to gastropulmonary aspiration (GPA). The latter was present in 18% of one series of patients with respiratory symptoms due to GERD [2]. We herein review the current status of esophageal scintigraphy in making the diagnosis of GPA.

Materials and methods

The procedure of esophagobronchial scintigraphy for the diagnosis of GPA is the end-point of the procedure for the diagnosis of GERD. The scintigraphic test for GER culminates into the scintigraphic test for GPA. Therefore, the scintigraphic procedure for studying GPA is the same as the scintigraphic procedure for studying GER.

The procedure begins with the patient (child or adult) in a recumbent position after an overnight fast. A total radiopharmaceutical (Tc-99m-Sulfur Colloid) dose of 100 microcuries for a child and 1.0 millicurie for an adult is given, uniformly mixed in a meal of formula for a child and egg sandwich and milk for an adult. A smalll amount of non-reactive liquid is given at the end of the radioactive feeding to clear the esophagus. Infants should be burped after feeding.

Imaging begins as soon as possible after feeding. The subject lies supine under a gamma camera and sequential images of the stomach and esophagus are recorded every minute for 60 minutes to detect any GER. Thereafter, the adult subject (not children) lies in the Trendelenburg position with occasional external compression of the abdomen. A couple of hours later, a single anterior static scintigraphic image of the stomach and esophagus was obtained to detect GER, and all four views of the lungs were obtained to detect GPA. These images may be repeated during the next 24 hours with particular attention to the 24-hour images.

Results

The diagnosis of GPA is made based upon the presence of tracer activity within the lung fields, provided that surface contamination has been ruled out.

GPA tends to occur during sleep, when esophageal peristalsis and possible protective reflex contraction of the upper esophageal sphincter is most likely to be suppressed.

Because of this, some diagnosticians administer the radioactive meal in the evening, and image the lungs the next morning after the patient has a night of uninterrupted sleep. This morning-after test provides greater sensitivity of the test.

Summary

Esophageal scintigraphy can quantitate the rates of emptying and reflux in all esophageal segments simultaneously and correlation with esophageal manometry data has been reported at 95% and 96% [3].

Gastric aspiration causes a chemical burn which can cause a severe inflammatory reaction in the respiratory tract. However, many patients have "silent aspiration" manifested solely by arterial desaturation with radiologic evidence of aspiration [4]. We suggest that the scintigraphy is worthy of wide application in patients with GERD who have unexplained cough or dyspnea, particularly in the presence of unexplained pulmonary pathology. An example of this would be a patient with GERD and idiopathic pulmonary fibrosis. In such a case, positive esophageal/pulmonary scintigraphy would suggest a very rigorous long-term regimen of gastric acid suppression.

References

1. Napierkowski J, Wong RK. Extraesophageal manifestations of GERD. Am J Med Sci 2003;326:285-99.
2. Roca R, Rosztoczy A, Izbeki F, et al. Prevalence of respiratory symptoms and disease associated with gastroesophageal reflux disease. Digestion 2005;71:92-6.
3. Mariani G, Barreca M, Bellini M, et al. Radionuclide gastroesophageal motor studies. J Nucl Med 2004;45:1004-28.
4. Marik PE. Aspiration pneumonitis and aspiration pneumonia. N Engl J Med 2001;344:665-71.

What is the role of esophageal intraluminal impedance in the evaluation of patients with gastroesophageal reflux with persistent symptoms on proton pump inhibitor?

D. Pohl, R. Tutuian (Zurich)

Multichannel intraluminal impedance (MII) is a technique that has recently been made applicable to research and clinical practice [1]. By measuring changes in electrical resistance to alternating current (i.e. impedance) within the esophagus this method can detect the presence of liquids and gas within the esophagus independent on the H^+ concentration [2]. Measuring impedance changes at multiple levels it can detect not only the presence of fluids at various levels in the esophagus but it can also determine direction of bolus movement. Hereby MII can distinguish between swallows and gastroesophageal reflux (GER) of liquid, gas or mixed composition.

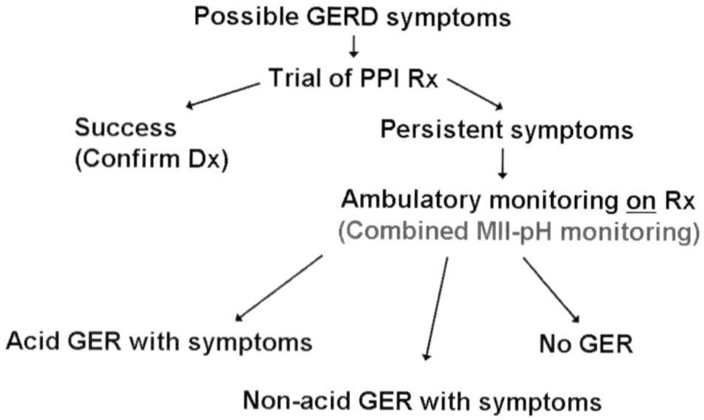

Figure 1. Role of combined MII-pH monitoring in the current GERD diagnostic algorithm.

Combined with pH, multichannel intraluminal impedance (i.e. combined MII-pH monitoring) provides the opportunity to detect all types of reflux episodes independent of their pH [3]. This is an important development as the wide use of proton pump inhibitor (PPI) trials as first diagnostic step in patients suspected of having GER disease (GERD) led to a shift in the patient population referred for reflux monitoring. In our experience the largest proportion of patients referred for reflux monitoring are those with symptoms not responding to PPI therapy [4]. Both patient and referring physician are interested if the persistent symptoms are or not due to ongoing reflux.

Persistent symptoms on proton pump inhibitor therapy

Soon after the introduction in clinical practice (i.e. in Europe mid 1980ies and USA end 1980ies) PPI's have been recognized to be very potent suppressants of gastric acid production [5]. Pre-clinical studies documented irreversible acid suppression in virtually all cultured parietal cells leading many to believe that treatment with once daily PPI inhibits the entire gastric acid production [6]. Studies in human volunteers and patients documented the excellent gastric acid control but also documented that in some individuals a residual gastric acid production remains [7]. Reasons for this residual acid production include the fact that not all parietal cells are activated at once (i.e. during the period when plasma PPI concentrations are in the therapeutic range) and that new proton pumps are generated and parietal cells are constantly replaced in *in vivo* situations.

Despite these considerations PPIs remain the main medical treatment in patients with GERD. Large multicenter studies documented the ability of once daily PPI to heal erosive esophagitis lesions in up to 90% of patients within 8 weeks of therapy [8]. The same study found though that symptomatic response is not as good as healing rates. The analysis of patient diaries revealed that approximate 65-70% achieved complete symptom resolution within one month implying that 30-35% of patients on once daily PPI therapy have persistent symptoms.

In patients with persistent symptoms on PPI therapy possible mechanisms of symptoms include:

- persistent acid GER due to insufficiently high dosed PPIs;
- persistent non-acid GER (i.e. PPI control the intragastric acidity but patients continue to reflux liquids with a pH above;
- symptoms not associated with reflux (i.e. symptoms due to causes other than reflux).

Combined multichannel intraluminal impedance-pH monitoring in patients with persistent symptoms on proton pump inhibitor therapy

Combined MII-pH monitoring is performed similar to conventional pH monitoring. Impedance rings can be mounted on pH catheter without changing the dimension of the catheter, making this examination, from the patient perspective, no different than catheter-based pH monitoring. Impedance rings are arranged such that bolus presence data is recorded 3, 5, 7, 9, 15 and 17 cm above the lower esophageal sphincter (LES) while the pH sensor remains at the traditionally 5 cm above the LES location.

During combined MII-pH monitoring reflux episodes are identified by changes in intraluminal impedance (i.e. rapid decline in impedance to at least 50% of esophageal baseline in at least two distal channels progressing over time from distal to proximal) and information from the pH sensor is used to classify episodes as acid or non-acid based on the concomitant changes in pH. Reflux episodes are considered to be acid if the lowest pH value recorded at the time of an impedance detected reflux episode is below 4.0. Conversely reflux episodes are considered to be non-acid if the lowers pH value remains above 4.0. Recognizing that from the chemist's point of view solutions with a pH between 4.0 and 7.0 are should be considered acidic a recent consensus proposed separating non-acid reflux episodes into weakly acidic (i.e. nadir pH between 4.0 and 7.0) and weakly alkaline (i.e. nadir pH above 7.0) [3]. While some authors have embraced the more exact nomenclature, others prefer using the term non-acid reflux in order to underscore the difference between these reflux episodes and the acid reflux episodes identified by conventional pH-metry. The main point is though that both terms (non-acid and weakly acidic) refer to the same reflux episodes (i.e. reflux episodes with a pH above 4).

Given the new challenges raised by patients with persistent symptoms on acid suppressive therapy as discussed above and the availability of the technology to detect reflux episodes independently of the acid concentration Mainie *et al.* investigated the frequency of the three mechanisms (i.e. ongoing acid reflux, non-acid reflux or no reflux associated with symptoms) in a group of 168 patients with persistent GERD symptoms on PPI bid ± H2RA qhs [9]. Out of the 144 patients who reported symptoms during the monitoring period 16 (11%) had a positive symptom index (SI) [10] for acid reflux, 53 (37%) a positive SI for non-acid reflux and 75 (52%) patients had no association between symptoms and GER. A positive symptom association with non-acid reflux was more common ($p < 0.05$) in patients with typical reflux symptoms (42%) than in patients with atypical symptoms (22%). Similar results were recently reported by Zerbib *et al.* in 71 patients with persistent symptom on PPI therapy [11]. During ambulatory impedance-pH monitoring, a positive symptom association probability (SAP) [12] was noticed in 22/60 (36%) who recorded symptoms during the monitoring period. Furthermore 19/22 patients had a positive SAP for non-acid reflux.

Clinical relevance of the combined impedance-pH findings

To date there are few data on the clinical relevance of results of combined impedance-pH monitoring. In a small, uncontrolled study Mainie *et al.* reported on the surgical outcome in a group of 19 patients who underwent laparoscopic Nissen fundoplication following combined impedance-pH monitoring on PPI therapy [13]. In 14 (73%) patients impedance-pH monitoring documented a positive SI for non-acid reflux and in 4 (21%) a positive SI for acid reflux. At a mean follow-up of 14 months (range 7-25 months) after surgery, 16/17 patients with a positive SI pre-operatively asymptomatic or markedly improved. Although these data need to be confirmed by larger, controlled studies these first outcome data suggests that symptomatic non-acid reflux is clinically relevant.

Conversely one should not underestimate the clinical value of negative results during impedance-pH monitoring (i.e. documentation of no symptom association with reflux). Prior to the introduction of impedance-pH monitoring a normal distal esophageal acid exposure on PPI therapy did not exclude the possibility of symptoms being associated with non-acid reflux. A negative combined impedance-pH monitoring offers additional confidence that symptoms reported on PPI therapy are not due to GER.

Conclusions

Combined multichannel intraluminal impedance and pH (MII-pH) monitoring allows detection of GER episodes regardless of the acidity of the refluxate. In approximately 35-45% of patients with persistent reflux symptoms on acid suppressive therapy MII-pH monitoring documents a positive symptom association with ongoing non-acid or persistent acid reflux. Documenting a positive symptom association with non-acid reflux has clinical consequences as some of these patients might be good candidates for anti-reflux surgery. Based on these we conclude that combined MII-pH monitoring is currently the gold standard to clarify the relationship between symptoms and reflux in patients with persistent symptoms on PPI therapy.

References

1. Tutuian R, Vela MF, Shay SS, Castell DO. Multichannel Intraluminal Impedance (MII) in esophageal function testing and gastroesophageal reflux monitoring. J Clin Gastroenterol 2003;37:206-15.
2. Silny J. Intraluminal multiple electric impedance procedure for measurement of gastrointestinal motility. J Gastrointest Motil 1991;3:151-62.
3. Sifrim D, Castell D, Dent J, Kahrilas PJ. Gastro-oesophageal reflux monitoring: review and consensus report on detection and definitions of acid, non-acid, and gas reflux. Gut 2004;53:1024-31.
4. Tutuian R. How PPIs have altered the GERD treatment landscape. Drug Benefit Trends 2004;16(8):408-25.
5. DeVault KR. Overview of medical therapy for gastroesophageal reflux disease. Gastroenterol Clin North Am 1999;28:831-46.
6. Richardson P, Hawkey CJ, Stack WA. Proton pump inhibitors. Pharmacology and rationale for use in gastrointestinal disorders. Drugs 1998;56:307-35.
7. Peghini PL, Katz PO, Bracy NA, et al. Nocturnal recovery of gastric acid secretion with twice-daily dosing of proton pump inhibitors. Am J Gastroenterol 1998;93:763-7.
8. Castell DO, Kahrilas PJ, Richter JE, et al. Esomeprazole (40 mg) compared with lansoprazole (30 mg) in the treatment of erosive esophagitis. Am J Gastroenterol 2002;97:575-83.
9. Mainie I, Tutuian R, Shay S, Vela M, Zhang X, Sifrim D, Castell DO. Acid and non-acid reflux in patients with persistent symptoms despite acid suppressive therapy. A multicenter study using combined ambulatory impedance- pH monitoring Gut 2006;55:1398-402.
10. Wiener GJ, Richter JE, Copper JB, Wu WC, Castell DO. The symptom index: a clinically important parameter of ambulatory 24-hour esophageal pH monitoring. Am J Gastroenterol 1988;83:358-61.
11. Zerbib F, Roman S, Ropert A, et al. Esophageal pH-impedance monitoring and symptom analysis in GERD: a study in patients off and on therapy. Am J Gastroenterol 2006;101:1956-63.
12. Weusten BL, Roelofs JM, Akkermans LM, Van Berge-Henegouwen GP, Smout AJ. The symptom-association probability: an improved method for symptom analysis of 24-hour esophageal pH data. Gastroenterology 1994;107:1741-5.
13. Mainie I, Tutuian R, Agrawal A, Adams D, Castell DO. Combined multichannel intraluminal impedance-pH monitoring identifies patients with persistent reflux symptoms on acid suppressive therapy who benefit from a laparoscopic Nissen fundoplication. Br J Surg 2006;93:1483-7.

Can intraluminal impedance measurement be used as a screening test for Barrett's esophagus?

F. Fornari, D. Sifrim (Leuven)

Impedance is the average electrical resistance between two adjacent electrodes. By positioning a catheter containing several paired electrodes into the esophagus is possible to measure impedance values during resting conditions, as well as during episodes of intraluminal flow related to swallows or gastroesophageal reflux (GER) [1,2]. Basal values of intraesophageal impedance depend on the cross-sectional area and electrical conductivity of the medium around the impedance electrodes. Initial experience with impedance-pH studies in patients with GER disease (GERD) suggested differences in the baseline impedance related with the presence of esophageal mucosa damage, particularly Barrett's esophagus. As shown in *Table I*, impedance pull-through of the lower esophageal sphincter (LES) and distal esophagus has found significantly reduced impedance values in patients with erosive esophagitis and Barrett's esophagus compared to healthy volunteers. In addition, the columnar lined esophageal mucosa had significantly lower impedance values than squamous mucosa, and the length of Barrett's mucosa determined by impedance correlated significantly ($r = 0.66$, $P < 0.05$) with that determined endoscopically [3].

Table I. Impedance values of the gastric fundus, lower esophageal sphincter (LES) and distal esophagus (columnar and squamous epithelium) in normal subjects and patients with erosive esophagitis or Barrett's esophagus.

	Fundus	LES	Distal esophagus	
			Columnar	Squamous
Normal (n =14)	471 (377-566)	1,877 (1,555-4,844)	–	2,227 (1,950-3,880)
Esophagitis (n = 9)	499 (373-624)	1,249 (837-2,181)*	–	2,158 (1,787-2,604)
Barrett (n = 12)	492 (373-598)	640 (530-858)**	1,050 (825-1,358)***	2,045 (1,338-2,713)

*p < 0.05 *versus* normal; **p < 0.05 *versus* esophagitis; ***p < 0.05 *versus* squamous

Further studies confirmed the association between erosive esophagitis, including Barrett's esophagus, and low basal esophageal impedance values. From a large series of asymptomatic volunteers and GERD patients with different degrees of esophagitis, impedance monitoring of the distal esophagus (2cm-segment above LES) showed progressive lower impedance values with increasing severity of mucosal damage. Endoscopy negative GERD patients had lower impedance values but significant overlap with normal subjects. Distal impedance values higher than 2000Ω practically excluded severe esophagitis or Barrett's esophagus, with a negative predictive value of 96%.

Therefore, a simplified impedance measurement might be useful for screening strategies in patients with GERD [4].
The ability of impedance monitoring to exclude severe esophagitis and Barrett's esophagus can be partially explained by studies from Gonzalez-Correa *et al.*, in which tissue resistivity (impedance) was measured in different esophageal epitheliums, including inflamed and non-inflamed squamous and columnar epithelium, as well as in columnar dysplasia and adenocarcinoma. Squamous non-inflamed mucosa had an impedance value three- to four-fold greater than columnar non-inflamed mucosa. Within columnar mucosa, inflammation was associated with a small but nevertheless significant reduction in impedance values [5].

In the light of these evidences, impedance monitoring can be used to exclude the presence of columnar lined epithelium at the level of impedance sensors in the esophagus, particularly in patients with a lower probability of harbour severe reflux esophagitis or Barrett's metaplasia. When low basal impedance level is found during routine investigation for GERD, patients might benefit with endoscopic screening for Barrett's esophagus. Further studies are needed to define the best positioning of the impedance sensors in order to predict the absence of short columnar lined epithelium, keeping the accuracy for reflux detection.

References

1. Silny J. Intraluminal multiple electric impedance procedure for measurement of gastrointestinal motility. J Gastrointest Motil 1991;3:151-62.
2. Sifrim D, Silny J, Holloway RH, Janssens JJ. Patterns of gas and liquid reflux during transient lower oesophageal sphincter relaxation: a study using intraluminal electrical impedance. Gut 1999;44:47-54.
3. Sifrim D, Holloway R, Tack J, Silny J, Lerut A, Janssens J. Impedance patterns at the gastroesophageal junction and distal esophagus in patients with Barrett's esophagus. Gastroenterology 2000;118:2634.
4. Emerenziani S, Zhang X, Blondeau K, Sifrim D. Patients with severe esophagitis and Barret's esophagus have a distinctive low intraluminal impedance. A screening test? United European Gastroenterology Week 2004.
5. Gonzalez-Correa CA, Brown BH, Smallwood RH, Stephenson TJ, Stoddard CJ, Bardhan KD. Low frequency electrical bioimpedance for the detection of inflammation and dysplasia in Barrett's oesophagus. Physiol Meas 2003;24:291-6.

What is the role of radiology in patients with chest pain?

C.M.E. Hannig, A.C. Wuttge-Hannig (München)

The center of interest in radiologic examinations is he so called "non-cardiac-chest-pain", which is characterized by retrosternal pain without any evidence of electrocardiographic or coronary angiographic pathology. Also other reasons for chest-pain like neurogenic disorders or intercostal neuropathy has to be ruled out.

Aim of our study was to assess the value of dynamic radiologic recording of the pharyngoesophageal motility in the detection of esophageal motor dysfunction. In all patients with positive results these were correlated to 24-hour pH-monitoring and 24-hour manometry. In our interdisciplinary working group for Dysphagia in Munich since 1982 we have examined 11,663 patients with dysphagia. Seven hundred and eighty-three of them suffered from retrosternal pain. Cardiac reasons and other neurogenic causes had been ruled out before [1-5].

Material and methods

It is essential to perform a dynamic radiographic recording of the motion phenomena of the esophagus during deglutition and bolus passage. For this either videofluoroscopy or in the last time digital dynamic recording methods at a frame rate between 16-30 frames/sec were performed [6-8].

Because the better special and temporal resolution digital dynamic registration turned out to be superior to videofluoroscopy for the diagnostic work-up.

Results

In our patient population of 783 patients we found 83 with diffuse esophageal spasm, 102 suffering from vigorous achalasia and 140 with hypermotile achalasie. Three hundred and fifty-six patients showed evidence of gastroesophageal reflux disease (GERD) with reflux associated motor disturbances of the tubular esophagus. In 53 patients a nutcracker esophagus was detected by non radiologic inverstigations.

Diffuse esophageal spasm is defined as well by means of radiology as by means of manometry. It consists in motility disorders associated with repetitive only occasional attack-like simultaneous non propulsive contractions of the smooth muscle portion of the tubular esophagus. This entity is one of the typical reansons for non-cardiac-chest-pain. The pain is supposed to be caused ischemia in the area of the spastic muscle areas because the contractions keep the muscles away from blood supply.

The diagnosis can only be made in correlation to the clinical findings and the functional radiological pattern. Manometry, especially 24-hour manometry is the "gold-standard" for a definitive diagnosis. Since coronary spasm as well as diffuse esophageal spasm are sensitive to nitro-application and calcium antagonists like nifedipine, the pharmacologic characterisation is not possibile. There is a high number of patients falsely classificated as coronary patients. The fast ingestion of a cold liquid as well as a solid bolus can provoque diffuse esophageal spasm. Not rarely diffuse esophageal spasm is the reason for bolus impaction, the so-called "Steakhouse-Syndrom". We found a special form of diffuse esophageal spasm in cases of long-lasting disease. This is a form of spasm, which leads to a extreme hypertrophy of the smooth muscles of the esophagus and shows an radiologic appearance like a skrew-driver image. Specially in these patients a long distance botox-injection is indicated [1-3].

Vigorous achalasia is characterized by a not-existing or less-accentuated dilatation of the esophagus and presents also segmental non propulsive contractions of the smooth muscle portion of the esophagus. Generally simultaneous contractions scattered all over the esophagus in the sense of segmental contractions can be observed. Also in these cases the contractions are very strong and lead again to a reduced bloods supply to the esophagus, causing he typical "non-cardiac chest-pain". In difference to the diffuse esophageal spasm it consists in a deficiency of the lower esophageal sphincter (LES), which presents a failing or incomplete swallowing reflex-triggered opening function [3].

In the case of diffuse esophageal spasm in addition to the 24-hour pH-monitoring also endoscopy is necessary because a submucous located cancer of the cardia can imitate the same symptoms. Also a paraneoplastic origin of this disease is possible. Therapy again is based on nitroglycerin applications or calcium-antagonists and in the last time more and more to the use of botox. If conservative therapy fails, a myotomy of the LES has to be performed.

Chest-pain may also be caused by hypomotile achalsia. This is mainly due to the volume effect of the dilatated esophagus and the dysfunction of the cardia.

The role of GERD is underestimated as co-factor for non cardiac chest pain. The typical heartburn has only a diagnostic value of 50% in normal radiologic examinations. The observation of an reflux event has not to be over-estimated and its sensitivity is described in the litterature also in the range of 50%.

By dynamic recording it is possible to evaluate the reaction of the tubular esophagus on reflux events and in 35% we could observe a typical hypermotile reaction with associated chest pain. These finding of course have to be confirmed by endoscopy and pH-monitoring [3-5].

The diagnostic work-up of nutcracker esophagus

In nutcracker esophagus pressure amplitudes over 300 mmHg is the dominant finding in manometric records. It is sometimes impossible to diagnose this entity during a radiologic examination even if the patient is asked to swallow in a recumbent position and the peristasis is investigated. In a few patients a little spasm above the level of the bolus can be observed. The sensitivity of this finding is not to be estimated to be to high.

Results

In 3 of 83 cases od diffuse esophageal spasm dynamic radiology missed the diagnosis in comparison to the gold-standarts of 24-hour manometry. Three of 102 patients with vigorous achalasia were missed compared to the 24-hour manometry results. All forms of hypomotile or amotile achalasia were found als well during radiologic examinations as during manometry. GERD was missed in 45/356 patients, which means that the simultaneous 24-hour pH-recording and the the reflux aspiration showed a 12.7% higher incidence of disease.

In conclusion videofluoroscopy and now especially digital dynamic recording are non-invasive, medication independent, not time-consuming, in-expensive methods. In our patient population a all over accuracy of max 87.3%. We propose, that dynamic radiography should be performed as first step in any case of cardiac chest pain after a negative cardiologic examination.

References

1. Hannig C, Wuttge-Hannig A. Röntgendiagnostik von Motilitätsstörungen des Pharynx und Ösophagus. Leber Magen Darm1987;1:7-17.
2. Hannig C. Radiologische Funktionsdiagnostik des Pharynx und des Ösophagus. Berlin Heidelberg: Springer-Verlag, 1995.

3. Hannig C, Wuttge-Hannig A. Erkrankungen des Ösophagus. In: Freyschmidt J, Feuerbach S, eds. Handbuch diagnostische Radiologie. Springerverlag 2007:28-139.
4. Wuttge-Hannig A, Hannig C. Evaluation of the swallowing reflex in stress drinking in videofluoroscopy – Is it a tool for the measurement of pharyngeal dysfunction in reflux disease? Eur Radiol 2004;14(2):210-1.
5. Wuttge-Hannig A, Hannig C. The post-operative pharynx and larynx. In: Ekberg O, ed. Radiology of the pharynx and the esophagus. Heidelberg, New York: Springer Verlag 2004:85-97.
6. Dodds WJ, Harell GS. Motility disorders chapter. In: Margulies AR, Burhenne HJ, eds Alimentary tract roentgenology, Vol. 1. St. Louis: Mosby 1973.
7. Donner MW. Spezielle Röntgendiagnostik von Funktionstörungen der Speiseröhre. In: Siewert JR, Blum AL, Waldeck F, eds. Funktionsstörungen der Speiseröhre. Springer Verlag, 1976:80-100.
8. Donner MW, Saba GP, Martinez OR. Diffuse disorders of the esophagus: a practical approach, Semin Roentgenol 1981;XVI,3.

- Ekberg O. The symptomatic esophagus and GERD. Acta Radiol 2003;44(2):119-20.
- Groher M. Dysphagia – Diagnosis and management, 2nd ed. Boston London Oxford Singapore Sydney Toronto Wellington: Butterworth-Heinemann, 1992.
- Tenner R. Verbesserte Detailerkennbarkeit bei der Doppelkontrastuntersuchung des Magens durch neue Kontrastmittelmischung. Röntgen-Blätter 1984;37:13-5.

Is there a reliable correlation between the radiographic and manometric findings for diagnosing esophageal motor disorders?

K.R. DeVault (Jacksonville)

When a cardiac etiology has been excluded in a patient with chest pain, the attention appropriately turns to the esophagus. Gastroesophageal reflux disease is a common etiology that will often respond to control of acid with a proton pump inhibitor. Esophageal motility disorders (EMD) are other potential causes of chest pain. Traditionally, EMD are defined by their peristaltic patterns on esophageal manometry, but some information can be obtained from radiographic testing. In fact, in carefully performed research studies, the correlation between peristalsis as measured by manometry and video barium studies is quite good [1]. I will answer this question by first looking at the accuracy of radiology in the various manometrically defined EMD and then apply that information to the problem of noncardiac chest pain.

Achalasia

Achalasia is the prototypical EMD characterized by a incompletely relaxing, often hypertensive lower esophageal sphincter (LES) and lack of peristalsis in the body of the esophagus. In a study of 21 patients with a barium swallow considered classic for achalasia, 19 of 21 (90%) had a manometry that demonstrated achalasia [2]. The other two patients had significant esophageal dysmotility but were not felt to have achalasia by manometry. Barium testing is a reasonable test in patients suspected of having achalasia, but manometry is always required for confirmation and endoscopy is needed to exclude secondary achalasia due to a malignancy at the esophagogastric junction. Of the three tests (barium, manometry and endoscopy) the barium study is probably the least helpful and certainly the least mandatory [3].

Diffuse esophageal spasm

Diffuse esophageal spasm (DES) is manometrically characterized by a combination of simultaneous and peristaltic contractions in the body of the esophagus. Some patients may also have repetitive simultaneous contractions after swallowing. In a small study of 14 patients diagnosed with DES by radiology, 8 of 14 (57%) met the manometric criteria [4]. The other 6 all had either an incompletely relaxing LES or other nonspecific changes. Conversely, in a group of patients diagnosed with DES manometrically, 72% had an abnormality reported on barium, but only 28% had the classic "corkscrew" appearance [5]. Nellemann *et al.* were able to show that patients with normal clearance of both a liquid and solid bolus were highly predictive of a normal study [6]. Like other studies, their abnormal studies were likely to predict that the patient has a manometric disorder, but they did not reliably predict which specific disorder. Interestingly, a recent study using combined manometry and impedance testing found that 51% of DES patients had complete bolus transit [7]. Patients with chest pain were more likely to have complete bolus transit compared to those presenting with dysphagia.

Nutcracker esophagus

Nutcracker esophagus is a manometric condition that is common in chest pain patients and is characterized by higher than expected, yet normally propagated contractions in the body of the esophagus. Shortly after the disorder was first described, a study found that a video-barium study was normal in 55% of patients with nutcracker esophagus and nonspecifically abnormal in the remainder [8]. In Patti's study, barium studies were abnormal in 58% of patients with nutcracker esophagus, although no radiologist even suggested nutcracker esophagus as a diagnosis to explain the abnormalities they were seeing [5].

Nonspecific or disorders with ineffective esophageal motility

Most experts use the term ineffective esophageal motility (IEM) in place of the older term nonspecific esophageal motility disorders. A resent study performed video esophagus studies on 33 patients with IEM finding the studies to be normal in 45% and various abnormalities in the rest [9]. Patients with IEM can be segregated into those with normal and those with impaired bolus using impedance testing although the signficance of this segregation is not clear [10].

How does this apply to patients with chest pain?

From the above review, barium studies are rarely normal in specific disorders like achalasia, are usually abnormal in DES, but are either normal or have very nonspecific changes in most of the other esophageal motility disorders. Achalasia and DES are rare in chest pain. In a large series of patients undergoing manometry for chest pain, only 28% had any type of abnormal esophageal motility of those only 10% (< 3% of the total) had DES and 2% (< 1% of total) achalasia [11]. The actually diagnostic yield of barium studies in patients with chest pain is not well defined, but a study of 50 chest pain patients suggested that barium and endoscopy were both relatively unhelpful in this population [12]. These data certainly lead one to surmise that for this particular symptom (chest pain) radiology has a very low yield and therefore should not be recommended. On the other hand, barium studies are much more useful in patients presenting with dysphagia where the likelihood of a specific disorder is much higher [13].

References

1. Ott DJ, Chen YM, Hewson, et al. Esophageal motility: assessment with synchronous videotape fluoroscopy and manometry. Radiology 1989;173:419-22.
2. Amaravadi R, Levine MS, Rubesin SE, Laufer I, Redfern RO, Katzka DA. Achalasia with complete relaxation of lower esophageal sphincter: radiographic-manometric correlation. Radiology 2005;235(3):886-91.
3. Patient Care Committee, Society for Surgery of the Alimentary Tract. Esophageal achalasia. SSAT patient care guidelines. J Gastrointest Surg 2004;8(3):367-8.
4. Prabhakar A, Levine MS, Rubesin S, Laufer I, Katzka D. Relationship between diffuse esophageal spasm and lower esophageal sphincter dysfunction on barium studies and manometry in 14 patients. AJR Am J Roentgenol 2004;183(2):409-13.
5. Patti MG, Gorodner MV, Galvani C, et al. Spectrum of esophageal motility disorders: implications for diagnosis and treatment. Arch Surg 2005;140(5):442-9.
6. Nellemann H, Aksglaede K, Funch-Jensen P, Thommesen P. Bread and barium. Diagnostic value in patients with suspected primary esophageal motility disorders. Acta Radiol 2000;41(2):145-5.
7. Tutuian R, Mainie I, Agrawal A, Gideon RM, Katz PO, Castell DO. Symptom and function heterogenicity among patients with distal esophageal spasm: studies using combined impedance-manometry. Am J Gastroenterol 2006;101(3):464-9.
8. Chobanian SJ, Curtis DJ, Benjamin SB, Cattau EL Jr. Radiology of the nutcracker esophagus. J Clin Gastroenterol 1986;8:230-2.
9. Shakespear JS, Blom D, Huprich JE, Peters JH. Correlation of radiographic and manometric findings in patients with ineffective esophageal motility. Surg Endosc 2004;18(3):459-62.
10. Tutuian R, Castell DO. Clarification of the esophageal function defect in patients with manometric ineffective esophageal motility: studies using combined impedance-manometry. Clin Gastroenterol Hepatol 2004;2(3):230-6.
11. Katz PO, Dalton CB, Richter JE, Wu WC, Castell DO. Esophageal testing of patients with noncardiac chest pain or dysphagia. Results of three years' experience with 1161 patients. Ann Intern Med 1987;106(4):593-7.
12. de Caestecker JS, Blackwell JN, Brown J, Heading RC. The oesophagus as a cause of recurrent chest pain: which patients should be investigated and which tests should be used? Lancet 1985;2(8465):1143-6.
13. Fuller L, Huprich JE, Theisen J, et al. Abnormal esophageal body function: radiographic-manometric correlation. Am Surg 1999;65(10):911-4.

What can be expected from the four-electrode impedance planimetry in the evaluation of esophageal wall tension and sensitivity in patients with chest pain?

H. Gregersen (Aalborg)

Balloon (bag) distension is a commonly used technique for studying the physiology and mechanics of visceral organs, e.g. the mechanosensitive pathways. Impedance planimetry is a technique developed specifically for gastrointestinal distension studies

This article describes the bag distension technique impedance planimetry and several new modifications and applications of impedance planimetry.

Impedance planimetry

Impedance planimetry is a technique for the measurement of luminal cross-sectional area (CSA) during distension of hollow organs such as the esophagus. The term impedance planimetry was introduced in 1991 [1] and is a method to measure the area of a plane by the measurement of electrical impedance. Impedance planimetry utilizes a simple electrical principle based on Ohm's law. In brief excitation electrodes inside a catheter-mounted fluid-filled bag generates a constant electrical current field. Two detection electrodes placed between the excitation electrodes measures the electrical potential difference that is proportional to the CSA of the bag (*Figure 1*).

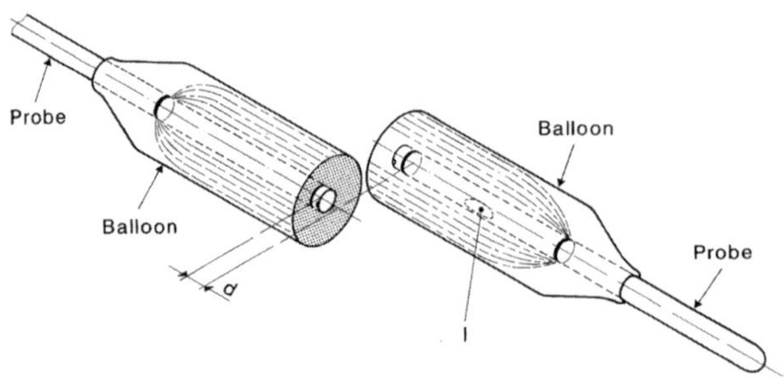

Figure 1. Sketch of a conventional impedance planimetric probe with one set of excitation electrodes and one set of detection electrodes for measurement of cross-sectional area in the middle of the balloon. d denotes the distance between the detection electrodes.

Impedance planimetry has been used in a large number of scientific and clinical studies, e.g. for diagnosing unexplained chest pain [2], systemic sclerosis [3-5], studying rectal function in patients with spinal lesions [6] and for evaluation of peristaltic reflex activity and tone [7-9].

Impedance planimetry is a distension technique that provides data on the size of the bag. CSA data can be used with concomitant pressure measurements to derive the wall tension and wall strain and the mechanical data can be related to sensory data. Impedance planimetry has obvious advantages over distension techniques based on volume measurements, i.e. in volume measurements the degree of wall stretch is not known due to possible elongation of the bag, and tone cannot be differentiated from phasic muscle contractions with most bag designs used to date.

Impedance planimetry was the basis for the first tensiometer for the gastrointestinal (GI) tract developed by Gregersen *et al.* [10] and has been used to evaluate GI smooth muscle function *in vivo* [7,11,12]. In recent years impedance planimetry has been further developed into new applications:

- the functional luminal imaging probe (FLIP);
- the multimodal pain stimulation probe;
- the axial force probe.

These new applications are outlined in more detail below

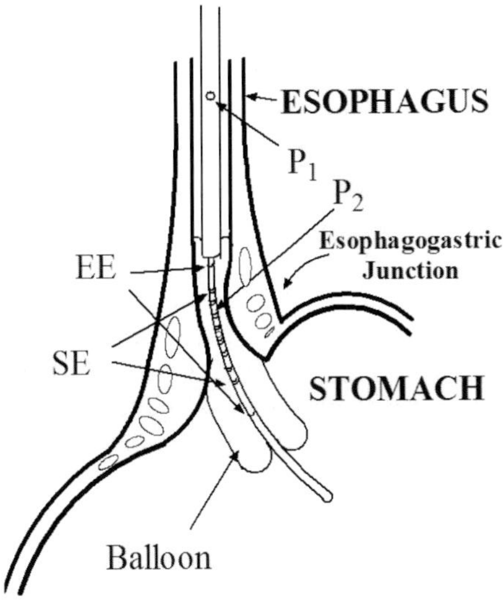

Figure 2. The functional luminal imaging probe with electrodes for eight measurements of cross-sectional area in the EGJ. P1 and P2 illustrate the sideholes for pressure measurements, EE are the two excitation electrodes and SE are the sensing electrodes. (Courtesy of Dr. McMahon).

New techniques based on impedance planimetry

Functional lumen imaging probe

The impedance planimetry technique has been used extensively to determine the CSA in hollow organs of the body and in particular in the GI organs [13-17]. Impedance planimetry has recently been further developed into multi-electrode systems for the purpose of measuring up to eight cross-sections inside a saline filled bag in the esophagogastric junction (EGJ) [18,19] (*Figure 2*). Until now, FLIP is the first technique to give a clear 3D outline of the geometric profile of the sphincter at various levels of distension [19] (*Figure 3*). Competence of the sphincter is better derived from geometry and pressure data gathered during distension than by measuring the pressure at fixed points. The closely spaced CSA measurement allow the reconstruction of the geometry and this in turn allows the generation of images which represent this part of the lumen of the GI tract when it is physiologically active. The EGJ is the barrier mechanism that prevents the refluxing of stomach contents into the esophagus. This closing off must be related to a narrowing of the lumen which can be represented by CSAs measured in this region. Hence, FLIP could represent a major step forward in the diagnosis, monitoring and evaluation of diseases such as gastroesophageal reflux disease (GERD) and achalasia.

Using CSA and pressure measurements the FLIP has the potential to provide new information on the biomechanical functioning of the EGJ in healthy volunteers and in patients with disorders such as GERD where an ineffective junction allows acid from the stomach to travel back up into the esophagus. The technique may have a role in assisting with drug therapy and surgical therapies for reflux.

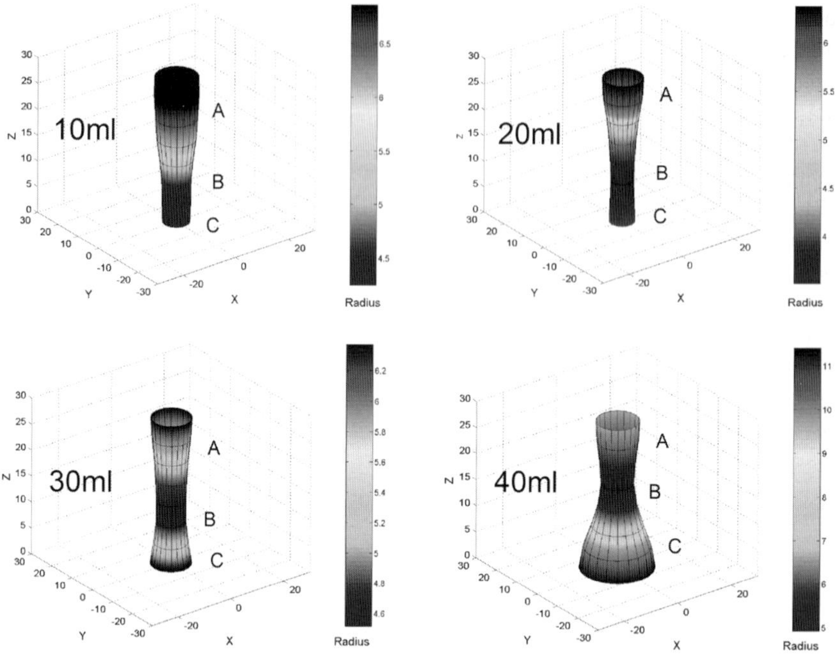

Figure 3. Three dimensional reconstruction of the geometry of the EGJ shown at bag fill volumes of 10 ml, 20 ml, 30 ml and 40 ml, respectively. The color represents radii (mm). In each case A represents the position in the luminal image of the ampulla of the esophagus, B represents the EGJ and C represents the point at which the esophagus enters the stomach. x, y and z are the three orthogonal directions (mm). (Courtesy of Dr. McMahon). (See page XVIII for colour figure).

Multimodal probe

As pain is a multidimensional perception it is obvious that the reaction to a single stimulus of a given modality can represent only a limited fraction of the entire pain experience. The possibility for combining different methods for stimulation and assessment will approximate the clinical situation where many different nerves and pathways are activated. Thus, the method will give a more comprehensive and differentiated information about the nociceptive system compared to stimuli using single or a few modalities [20]. For comprehensive experimental studies mimicking the clinical situation, a multimodal testing approach must therefore be used where the test battery will increase the probability for activation of a range of relevant nervous mechanisms. Such sophisticated methods will be able to select the best test procedures to explore different basic aspects of pain as well as pharmacological modulations. In the GI tract difficulties with access to the organs and technical limitations of the currently available models have until now made such a multimodal stimulation approach difficult.

Some authors have combined mechanical and electrical stimuli [21,22] or mechanical and chemical stimuli [23,24]. Drewes and Gregersen recently introduced several multimodal models with combined chemical, mechanical, electrical, cold and warmth stimuli to assess the sensation of the esophagus together with acid sensitization [14]. The model has currently been extended to stimulate the proximal esophagus, duodenum and rectum and have been used in to unravel the pain mechanisms in different patients and in drug research. Mechanical stimulation is achieved with impedance planimetric bag distension. Thermal stimulation is achieved by recirculating fluid inside the bag with concomitant measurement of temperature. Chemical and electrical stimulation is achieved be means of sideholes placed proximal to the bag and by electrodes on the outside of the bag. Sensitization with acid was added to the protocol to evoke hyperalgesia (*Figure 4*) [14,25-27].

The multimodal approach gives the possibility for a differentiated stimulation of receptors in the superficial and deep layers of the esophagus. The possibility for induction of hyperalgesia with e.g., acid perfusion and evoking central phenomena such as summation, allodynia and referred pain makes the model clinically relevant with respect to increase the knowledge of peripheral and central symptom mechanisms. The symptom assessment should ideally also be multimodal and for example include quantitative and qualitative sensation, assessment of referred pain and neurophysiologic measurements (for details see [26]).

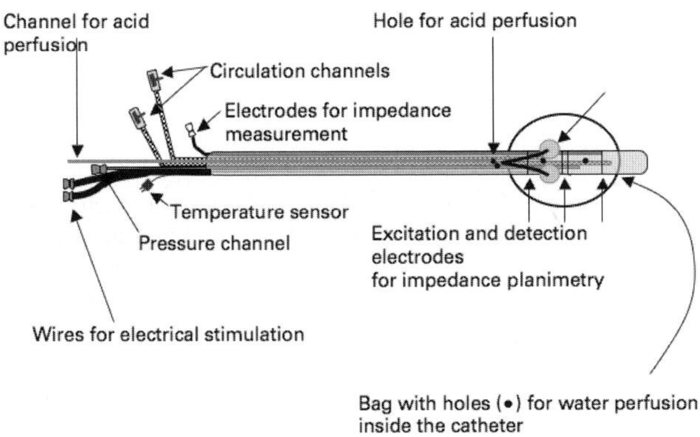

Figure 4. The probe assembly for multimodal pain stimulations. (Courtesy of Dr Asbjørn Drewes).

Axial force probe

The primary effect of esophageal peristalsis is to develop a force (flow) in the axial direction to pass the food into the stomach. The most common method to study esophageal peristalsis is manometry using low-compliance perfused catheters. However, manometry only measures the radial pressure which is an indirect measurement of the radial force but not the axial force. Videofluoroscopy is also used to visually assess esophageal contractility but it does not provide quantitative information on force in axial direction. Several attempts have been made to develop techniques to measure the axial force in the esophagus [28-32]. Despite promising initial results from these studies based on strain gauge technology, these methods have never been thoroughly tested or did not gain acceptance in clinical studies.

Electrical impedance technologies are becoming increasing popular in gastroenterology. The principle of impedance planimetry is to create an electric field between two excitation electrodes placed in a bag with conductive fluid. Two detection electrodes placed close to each other measure the CSA based on Ohm's law. Using this technique, the only variable is the CSA and the other parameters are constants implemented in the calibration. For the axial force probe we took advantage of our experience with impedance planimetry and modified the design to keep the CSA constant but allowed the distance between the detection electrodes to vary (Gravesen *et al.,* yet unpublished data).

The probe is custom made to measure axial force and pressure at different positions on the probe (*Figure 5*). A bag placed distal to the force transducer serves to provide a mechanical stimulus distal to the force transducer. The force measurement apparatus is located inside a channel with an inner diameter of 3.5 mm. Two pieces of catheters has mounted an excitation and detection electrode. These two catheter pieces are fixed to the channel, with a wire around the inner catheter, through the wall of the surrounding probe, and fixed to the outer probe in such way that the detection electrodes are close to each other when no axial force is applied (*Figure 5*). The channel for axial force measurement is filled with saline and voltage measurements are made between the detection electrodes inside the channel. Any axial force applied distal to the force section will elongate the probe and move the inner catheters apart, increasing the distance and the impedance between the detection electrodes.

Data obtained in humans volunteers shows that force depends on the amount of fluid in the distal bag and on the swallowed volume, whereas pressure is relatively insensitive to such changes (*Figure 6*). This clearly demonstrates the limitations of the manometric technique and the need for a more direct measure of the motility.

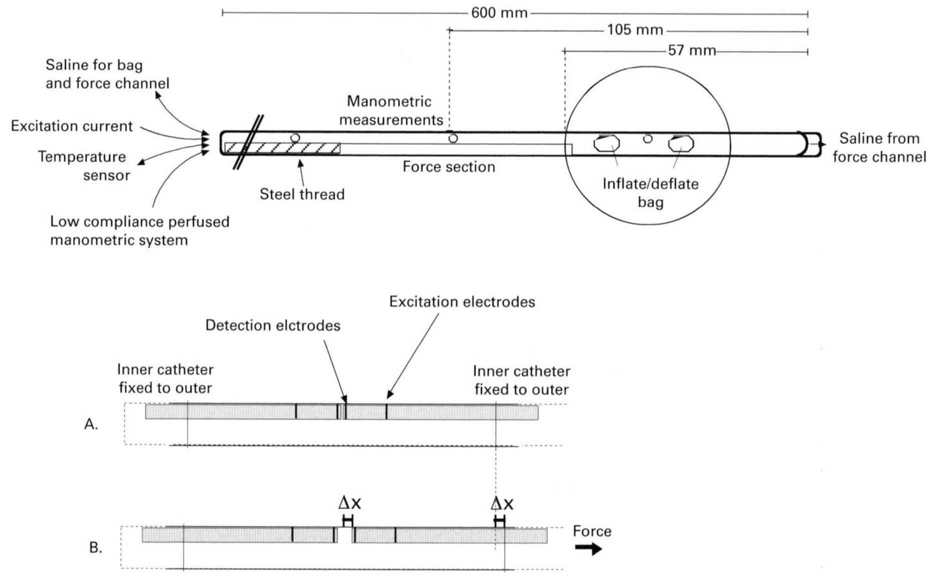

Figure 5. Top. Sketch of the force probe. The conductive saline was slowly perfused through the channel where the force was measured. The assembly enables measurement of pressure in the bag and force proximal to the bag. **Bottom.** Sketch of the axial force electrodes. The channel was filled with conductive saline and the excitation electrodes created an electric field. The impedance between the detection electrodes was measured and used for calibration. When force was applied, distal to the force section, the probe elongates and pulls the inner catheters apart and decreases the diameter. This increases the impedance which correlates with the axial force. (Modified from yet unpublished paper). (Courtesy of Flemming Gravesen).

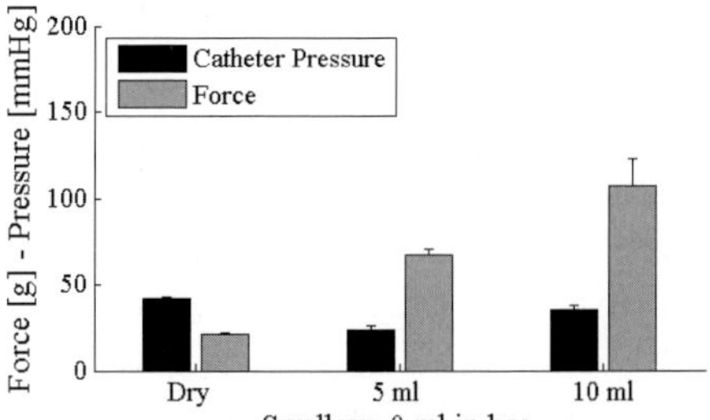

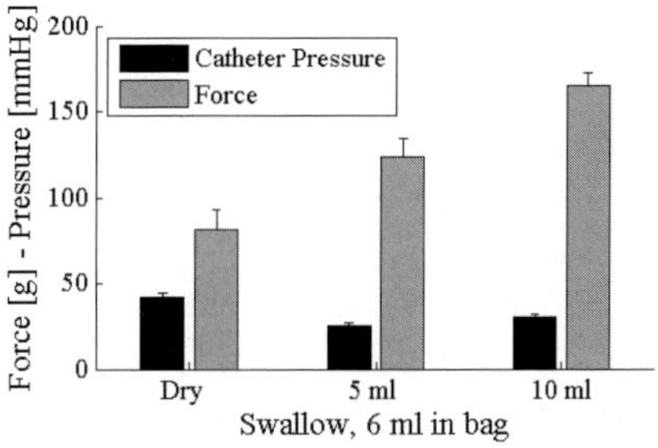

Figure 6. The peak pressure and peak force during dry, 5 ml and 10 ml swallows with the bag inflated with 0 ml (left) and 6 ml (right). The was a significant difference between pressure measurements and force measurements. (Modified from yet unpublished paper). (Courtesy of Flemming Gravesen).

Future perspectives with impedance planimetry

Distension techniques have been used for a long time in experimental and clinical studies of the GI tract. They have added significantly to our knowledge on GI physiology and pathophysiology. Impedance planimetry has proven to be a useful technique for obtaining data on wall tension, deformation and mechanosensory properties and it has now been further developed for new applications. These are especially useful for obtaining the geometric structure of the organ under study and for evaluation of the sensory function upon multimodal stimulation. It can be expected that these techniques will be further modified and made commercial within a short time frame.

References

1. Gregersen H, Djurhuus JC. Impedance planimetry: a new approach to biomechanical intestinal wall properties. Dig Dis Sci 1991;9:332-40.
2. Rao SS, Gregersen H, Hayek B, Summers RW, Christensen J. Unexplained chest pain: the hypersensitive, hyperreactive, and poorly compliant esophagus. Ann Intern Med 1996;124:950-8.
3. Pedersen J, Gao C, Egekvist H, et al. Pain and biomechanical responses to distention of the duodenum in patients with systemic sclerosis. Gastroenterology 2003;124:1230-9.
4. Villadsen GE, Storkholm JH, Hendel L, Vilstrup H, Gregersen H. Impedance planimetric characterisation of the eosophagus in systemic sclerosis patients with severe involvement of the oesophagus. Dig Dis Sci 1997;42:2317-26.
5. Villadsen GE, Storkholm JH, Zachariae H, Hendel L, Bendtsen F, Gregersen H. Esophageal pressure-cross-sectional area distributions and secondary peristalsis in relation to subclassification of systemic sclerosis. Neurogastroenterol Motil 2001;13:199-210.
6. Krogh K, Mosdal C, Gregersen H, Laurberg S. Rectal wall properties in patients with acute and chronic spinal cord lesions. Dis Colon Rectum 2002;45:641-9.
7. Gregersen H, Gilja OH, Hausken T, et al. Mechanical properties in the human gastric antrum using B-mode ultrasonography and antral distension. Am J Physiol 2002;283:G368-75.
8. Gregersen H, Christensen J. Gastrointestinal tone. Neurogastroenterol Motil 2000;12:501-8.
9. Gregersen H, Orvar K, Christensen J. Biomechanical wall properties and tone during phase I and phase II of the MMC. Am J Physiol 1992;263:G795-801.
10. Gregersen H, Barlow J, Thompson D. Development of a computer-controlled tensiometer for real-time measurements of tension in tubular organs. Neurogastroenterol.Motil 1999;11:109-18.
11. Gao C, Petersen P, Liu W, Arendt-Nielsen L, Drewes AM, Gregersen H. Sensory-motor responses to volume-controlled duodenal distension. Neurogastroenterol Motil 2002;14:365-74.
12. Gregersen H. Biomechanics of the gastrointestinal tract. Springer Verlag, 2002.
13. Gao C, Arendt-Nielsen L, Liu W, Petersen P, Drewes AM, Gregersen H. Sensory and biomechanical responses to ramp-controlled distension of the human duodenum. Am J Physiol 2003;284:G461-71.

14. Drewes AM, Gregersen H, Arendt-Nielsen L. Experimental pain in gastroenterology: a reappraisal of human studies. Scand J Gastroenterol 2003;38:1115-30.
15. Petersen P, Gao C, Arendt-Nielsen L, Gregersen H, Drewes AM. Pain intensity and biomechanical responses during ramp-controlled distension of the human rectum. Dig Dis Sci 2003;48:1310-6.
16. Drewes AM, Pedersen J, Liu W, Arendt-Nielsen L, Gregersen H. Controlled mechanical distension of the human oesophagus: sensory and biomechanical findings. Scand J Gastroenterol 2003;38:27-35.
17. Andersen IS, Gregersen H, Buntzen S, Djurhuus JC, Laurberg S. New probe for the measurement of dynamic changes in the rectum. Neurogastroenterol Motil 2004;16:99-105.
18. McMahon BP, Frokaer JB, Drewes AM, Gregersen H. A new measurement of oesophago-gastric junction competence. Neurogastroenterol Motil 2004;16:543-6.
19. McMahon B, Frokjaer J, Liao D, Kunwald P, Drewes A, Gregersen H. A new technique for evaluating sphincter function in visceral organs: application of the functional lumen imaging probe (FLIP) for the evaluation of the oesophago-gastric junction. Physiol Meas 2005;26:823-36.
20. Staahl C, Drewes AM. Experimental human pain models: a review of standardised methods for preclinical testing of analgesics. Basic Clin Pharmacol Toxicol 2004;95:97-111.
21. Hollerbach S, Hudoba P, Fitzpatrick D, Hunt R, Upton AR, Tougas G. Cortical evoked responses following esophageal balloon distension and electrical stimulation in healthy volunteers. Dig Dis Sci 1998;43:2558-66.
22. Mehta AJ, De Caestecker JS, Camm AJ, Northfield TC. Sensitization to painful distention and abnormal sensory perception in the esophagus. Gastroenterology 1995;108:311-9.
23. DeVault KR. Acid infusion does not affect intraesophageal balloon distention- induced sensory and pain thresholds. Am J Gastroenterol 1997;92:947-9.
24. Hu WH, Martin CJ, Talley NJ. Intraesophageal acid perfusion sensitizes the esophagus to mechanical distension: a Barostat study. Am J Gastroenterol 2000;95:2189-94.
25. Drewes AM, Schipper KP, Dimcevski G, et al. Multimodal induction and assessment of allodynia and hyperalgesia in the human oesophagus. Eur J Pain 2003;7:539-49.
26. Drewes AM, Gregersen H. Multimodal pain stimulation of the gastrointestinal tract. World J Gastroenterol 2006;12:2477-86.
27. Drewes AM, Reddy H, Staahl C, et al. Sensory-motor responses to mechanical stimulation of the esophagus after sensitization with acid. World J Gastroenterol 2005;11:4367-74.
28. Russell C, Bright N, Buthpitiya G, Alexander L, Walton C, Whelan G. Esophageal propulsive force and its relation to manometric pressure. Gut 1992;33:727-32.
29. Williams D, Thompson D, Heggie L, Bancewicz,J. Responses of the human esophagus to experimental intraluminal distension. Am J Physiol 1993;265:G196-203.
30. Williams D, Thompson D, Heggie L, Ohanrahan T, Bancewicz J. Esophageal clearance function following treatment of esophagitis. Gastroenterology 1994;106:108-16.
31. Williams D, Thompson D, Marples M, Heggie L, Ohanrahan T, Bancewicz, J. Diminished esophageal traction forces with swallowing in gastroesophageal reflux disease and in functional dysphagia. Gut 1994;35:165-71.
32. Winship D, Zboralske F. The esophageal propulsive force: esophageal response to acute obstruction. J Clin Invest 1967;46:1391-401.

What information can be expected from the neurophysiologic techniques (magnetoencephalography, positron emission tomography scan and functional magnetic resonance imaging) in the evaluation of patients with functional disorders of the esophagus?

A.R. Hobson (Harlow)

Brain imaging: techniques

Four main brain imaging techniques have been used to study esophageal sensory processing; positron emission tomography (PET), functional magnetic resonance imaging (fMRI), magnetoencephalography (MEG) and cortical evoked potentials (CEP) [1]. PET relies on the principle of detecting positron-emitting radionuclides that are intravenously injected into a subject positioned so that the head is placed in a specialized detection system. The most commonly used radionuclide used in gastrointestinal (GI) research is ^{15}O, which is prepared as $H_2{}^{15}O$ labelled water. This approach is used to create perfusion images that measure blood-flow to the brain. Cerebral blood-flow has been used a surrogate measure of brain activation as increases in regional cerebral blood-flow (rCBF) have been closely correlated to regional glucose consumption and more latterly with neuronal activity. These studies have predominantly utilised block design paradigms that compare images taken during active task periods and rest periods [2-4].

Using a similar study design, fMRI produces images of active brain regions by detecting indirect effects of neural activity on local blood-flow, volume and oxygen saturation, giving detailed information regarding the functional neuroanatomy of the brain. Together PET and fMRI have demonstrated that esophageal sensation and pain is processed in a multitude of cortical and sub-cortical regions including the primary somatosensory cortex (S1), secondary somatosensory cortex (S2), insula cortex (IC), anterior cingulate cortex (ACC), prefrontal cortex, thalamus and brainstem [5]. This network of brain activation is broadly similar to that seen in response to somatic pain with subtle differences possible reflecting psychophysiological differences in the perception of these two sensory modalities. For instance, esophageal pain has been described as more unpleasant than somatic pain elicited from the area of referral on the anterior chest wall, and may be attributed to some of the reported differences in activation of the limbic cortex [6].

One of the limitations of using metabolic brain imaging techniques to study esophageal sensory processing is that the recorded image is not specific to the experimental stimulus. That is, brain activity has been observed in response to and in anticipation of a given stimulus. In addition, the magnitude of activation is closely related to the novelty of the stimulus and the subject's emotional state [7,8].

To overcome some of these limitations we can use CEP and MEG. Neurophysiologists have used CEP to study somatosensory, visual, auditory and pain pathways for many years and this technique involves the brief presentation of a sensory stimulus which is time and phase locked to the recording of the electroencephalogram (EEG) *via* surface electrodes placed on the scalp. The event-related signal is small in amplitude but occurs at the same moment in time following each stimulus, whilst the large amplitude background EEG occurs randomly. In order to extract the desired signal, repeated stimuli are given and the subsequent brain activity averaged. This reduces the unwanted, randomly occurring EEG whilst enhancing the event-related CEP. The resultant waveform represents the brain's response to a stimulus as it changes on a millisecond-by-millisecond basis.

CEP responses are reproducible and have been recorded in response to stimulation of many regions of the GI tract [9-11], and these responses reflect the known physiological characteristics of the afferents that innervate these regions. Importantly, the GI CEP response provides an objective correlate of perceived sensation, with the response increasing in amplitude whilst decreasing in latency, as the stimulation intensity increases (*Figure 1*) [9-11]. This ability to record objective neurophysiological measures which correspond directly to subjective pain ratings overcomes many of the limitations of previous studies of visceral hypersensitivity [12]. In addition, it has recently been shown that the CEP response to proximal esophageal stimulation is enhanced following distal esophageal acidification in a model of esophageal sensitisation, indicating that CEP enables us to detect changes in the sensitivity of the central GI pain pathway [13].

CEP also has several practical advantages over other brain imaging techniques. These include the fact that the equipment needed to perform these studies is inexpensive (< £ 10,000), available in most hospitals, and can be performed in individual patients as a routine clinical assessment. However, its major disadvantage is that whilst we know that CEP represents a summation of cortical activity related to specific stages in the cortical

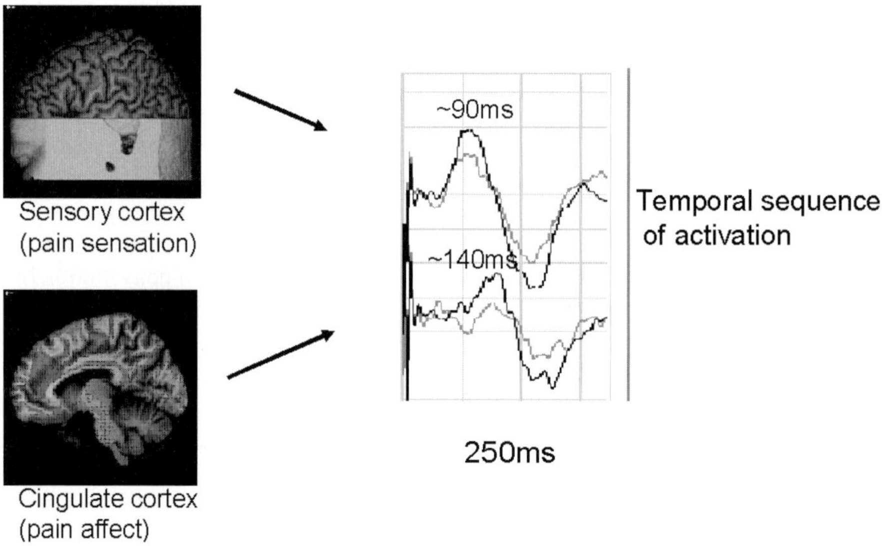

Figure 1. This figure shows the evoked field response recorded with MEG/SAM following painful and non-painful electrical stimulation of the esophagus. The top trace is recorded from a virtual electrode positioned in the lateral portion of the primary somatosensory cortex and the peak latency of this response is 90 ms. This corresponds to the P1 component of the EEP and is consistent with this regions role in the sensory discriminatory aspects of pain processing. The lower trace is recorded from a virtual electrode positioned in the perigenual cingulate cortex and the peak latency of this response is 140 ms. This later response is consistent with this regions involvement in affection/ cognitive processing of esophageal pain. (Figure reproduced with permission from [12]). (See page XVIII for colour figure).

processing of GI sensation and pain, the signal is distorted as it passes through the skull and scalp making localisation of the neural correlates of the response difficult.

MEG detects the minute magnetic fields generated by groups of active cortical neurons using highly sensitive sensors known as SQUIDS (super conducting quantum interference device). Unlike the electrical signal recorded with EP, which is distorted by all of the structures that lie between the cortical source and recording electrode, the magnetic field generated by an active group of cortical neurons passes through these structures unattenuated. The major advantage of using MEG therefore is that it has comparable spatial resolution to PET and fMRI in addition to millisecond temporal resolution, therefore pain related cortical activity can be imaged dynamically as it changes in real time. In addition, as the signal detected with MEG is the magnetic component of the electrical field recorded with CEP, it can be used to temporally correlate activity occurring within specific cortical regions with the scalp recorded CEP.

Using this approach it has been demonstrated that the earliest esophageal CEP component (P1), which occurs approximately 80-110 ms following esophageal stimulation, reflects activation of cortical regions involved in processing the sensory discriminatory aspects of esophageal pain (S1, S2 and posterior insula), whilst later components (N1, P2) are an amalgamation of cortical activity within regions that process both sensory discrimination and the affective/ ognitive components [14]. It is clear therefore that these later components represent secondary processing of esophageal sensation/pain (*Figure 1*).

In summary, functional brain imaging techniques have allowed us to determine the functional neuroanatomy of esophageal sensory processing, evaluate the effects of factors such as psychological modulation and esophageal injury and begun to identify specific neurophysiological abnormalities in patients with pain assumed to be esophageal in origin. Great progress has been made in this field and using a combination of these techniques in future clinical and research studies should help us to design and test the therapies of the future in this difficult to treat patient population with functional esophageal disorders.

References

1. Hobson AR, Aziz Q. Brain imaging and functional gastrointestinal disorders: has it helped our understanding? Gut 2004;53(8):1198-206.
2. Aziz Q, Andersson JL, Valind S, et al. Identification of human brain loci processing esophageal sensation using positron emission tomography. Gastroenterology 1997;113(1):50-9.
3. Aziz Q, Furlong PL, Barlow J, et al. Topographic mapping of cortical potentials evoked by distension of the human proximal and distal oesophagus. Electroencephalogr Clin Neurophysiol 1995;96(3):219-28.
4. Aziz Q, Thompson DG, Ng VW, et al. Cortical processing of human somatic and visceral sensation. J Neurosci 2000;20(7):2657-63.
5. Derbyshire SW. A systematic review of neuroimaging data during visceral stimulation. Am J Gastroenterol 2003;98(1):1.
6. Strigo IA, Duncan GH, Boivin M, Bushnell MC. Differentiation of visceral and cutaneous pain in the human brain. J Neurophysiol 2003;89(6):3294-303.
7. Phillips ML, Gregory LJ, Cullen S, et al. The effect of negative emotional context on neural and behavioural responses to oesophageal stimulation. Brain 2003;126:669-84.
8. Yaguez L, Coen S, Gregory LJ, et al. Brain response to visceral aversive conditioning: a functional magnetic resonance imaging study. Gastroenterology 2005;128(7):1819-29.
9. Hobday DI, Hobson AR, Sarkar S, Furlong PL, Thompson DG, Aziz Q. Cortical processing of human gut sensation: an evoked potential study. Am J Physiol Gastrointest Liver Physiol 2002;283(2):G335-9.
10. Hobson AR, Sarkar S, Furlong PL, Thompson DG, Aziz Q. A cortical evoked potential study of afferents mediating human esophageal sensation. Am J Physiol Gastrointest Liver Physiol 2000;279(1):G139-47.

11. Hollerbach S, Hudoba P, Fitzpatrick D, Hunt R, Upton AR, Tougas G. Cortical evoked responses following esophageal balloon distension and electrical stimulation in healthy volunteers. Dig Dis Sci 1998;43(11):2558-66.
12. Hobson AR, Aziz Q. Brain processing of esophageal sensation in health and disease. Gastroenterol Clin North Am 2004;33(1):69-91.
13. Sarkar S, Hobson AR, Furlong PL, Woolf CJ, Thompson DG, Aziz Q. Central neural mechanisms mediating human visceral hypersensitivity. Am J Physiol Gastrointest Liver Physiol 2001;281(5):G1196-202.
14. Hobson AR, Furlong PL, Worthen SF, Hillebrand A, Barnes GR, Singh KD, Aziz Q. Real-time imaging of human cortical activity evoked by painful esophageal stimulation. Gastroenterology 2005;128(3):610-9.

How can we use cortical evoked potentials to distinguish patients with esophageal hypersensitivity?

A.R. Hobson (Harlow)

Patients presenting with symptoms of chest pain in the absence of cardiac disease have presented clinicians with a diagnostic enigma for well over a century [1]. Synonyms such as, irritable heart and non-cardiac chest pain (NCCP), have been used to describe this condition, however these descriptive labels contribute little insight into the aetiology of patient's symptoms.

Esophageal hypersensitivity is prevalent in the NCCP population with studies demonstrating that approximately 50% of patients report pain at lower stimulation levels when compared to controls [2]. Recent studies which have attempted to explore mechanisms of esophageal hypersensitivity have provided complimentary evidence to support the fact that modulation of peripheral, central (spinal) and/or psychological factors can lead to a reduction in esophageal pain thresholds [3,4]. Whilst these studies have proved valuable in our understanding of the potential mechanisms of esophageal hypersensitivity, they also serve to highlight the dilemma faced by researchers working in this area.

This dilemma begins with the fact that current techniques employed to evaluate esophageal sensation rely predominantly on subjective reporting of pain ratings, a method proven to be susceptible to response bias and incapable of objectively dissociating between the potential candidate mechanisms of visceral hypersensitivity [5]. Cortical neural activity can be recorded objectively in real-time using two methods, magnetoencephalography (MEG) and electroencephalography (EEG) [5]. We have recently demonstrated that when MEG and EEG are recorded in response to repetitive esophageal stimulation then highly reproducible esophageal evoked potentials (EEP) can be recorded [6]. EEP represent the sequence of voltage changes within the brain that occur following an esophageal stimulus. Each component of the EEP relates to a specific step in the processing of esophageal sensory information [7,8].

We have previously demonstrated that EEP can be used to determine the neurophysiological characteristics of esophageal afferent pathways, detect changes in the sensitivity of these afferents following experimental acidification and using MEG we have identified the cortical neural correlates of each EEP component [6-9]. These studies have shown that EEP is a robust method which provides objective, stimulus specific neural measures of esophageal afferent pathway sensitivity.

The relevance of these findings to esophageal pain comes from a recent paper in which EEP responses were examined in a cohort of non-cardiac chest pain patients. In this study, 32 patients presented in clinic with symptoms of angina-like chest pain in the absence of any cardiac abnormality (as tested by exercise ECG and coronary angiography). All had a previous trial of proton pump inhibitors which did not alleviate symptoms and there was no evidence of motor abnormalities or gastroesophageal reflux on physiological testing. Esophageal balloon distension and electrical stimulation revealed evidence of esophageal hypersensitivity using the method of ascending limits technique. An electrical stimulation intensity which was 75% of the difference between the subjects sensory and pain thresholds was then used to elicit EEP. These data showed that NCCP patients with esophageal hypersensitivity could be separated into two distinct groups [10].

Figure 1 shows the esophageal CEP responses in selected patients from both sub-groups and demonstrates that these seemingly identical patients have drastically different neurophysiological profiles. Patients in panel A demonstrate visceral hypersensitivity to esophageal stimulation in addition to short latency large amplitude CEP responses. This is the same type of response seen in the acid model of esophageal sensitisation and is consistent with this patient having sensitisation of their gastrointestinal (GI) afferent pathways.

In contrast, patients in panel B, whilst still demonstrating visceral hypersensitivity, have long latency early CEP components, indicating that the afferent signal arriving at the cortex is not exaggerated, yet the late responses, which reflect affective processing, are enhanced when compared to normal. This profile is consistent with a second proposed sub-group of NCCP, those that are hypervigilant of visceral sensations. In summary, this paper demonstrated that patients with NCCP, can be sub-classified on the basis of sensory responsiveness and neurophysiological profiles.

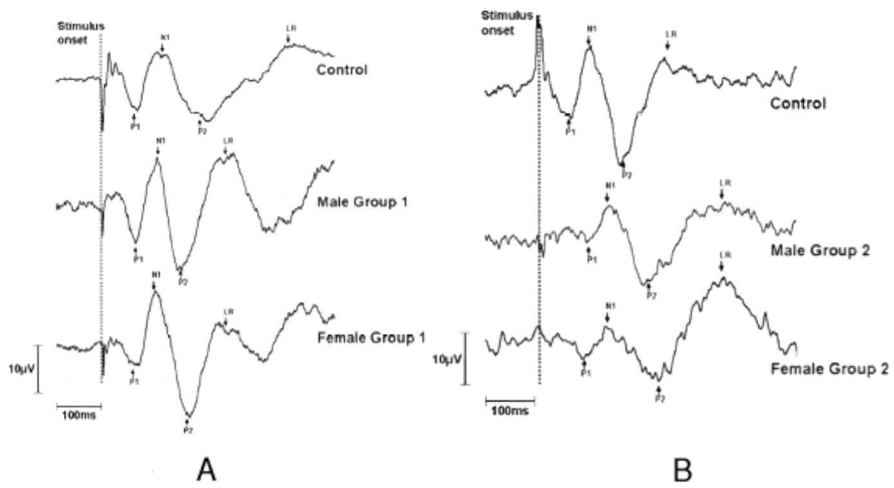

Figure 1. Shows representative EEP responses in NCCP patients. Panel A shows EEP consistent with enhanced afferent pathway sensitivity as equivalent response is seen to normal despite using reduced sensory input to elicit the response. Panel B shows EEP consistent with enhanced psychological (hypervigilance) processing of esophageal afferent information as early components are attenuated whilst later cognitive components are enhanced. (Reproduced with permission of [10]).

In summary, whilst these preliminary observations hold promise, they require confirmation in a larger cohort of patients. However, if this approach is successful then it may allow us to identify specific abnormalities within the central nervous system processing of GI sensation in individual patients, allowing us to objectively differentiate between those with sensitised GI afferents from those that are hypervigilant to GI sensations. The ability to differentiate between these two groups has obvious advantages when deciding to treat them with drugs that maybe anti-hyperalgesic in contrast to analgesic.

References

1. Achem SR, DeVault KR. Unexplained chest pain at the turn of the century. Am J Gastroenterol 1999;94(1):5-8.
2. Hobson AR, Aziz Q. Brain processing of esophageal sensation in health and disease. Gastroenterol Clin North Am 2004;33(1):69-91.
3. Phillips ML, Gregory LJ, Cullen S, et al. The effect of negative emotional context on neural and behavioural responses to oesophageal stimulation. Brain 2003;126:669-84.
4. Sarkar S, Aziz Q, Woolf CJ, Hobson AR, Thompson DG. Contribution of central sensitisation to the development of non-cardiac chest pain. Lancet 2000;356(9236):1154-9.
5. Hobson AR, Aziz Q. Brain imaging and functional gastrointestinal disorders: has it helped our understanding? Gut 2004;53(8):1198-206.
6. Hobson AR, Furlong PL, Worthen SF, et al. Real-time imaging of human cortical activity evoked by painful esophageal stimulation. Gastroenterology 2005;128(3):610-9.
7. Hobson AR, Sarkar S, Furlong PL, Thompson DG, Aziz Q. A cortical evoked potential study of afferents mediating human esophageal sensation. Am J Physiol Gastrointest Liver Physiol 2000;279(1):G139-47.
8. Hollerbach S, May A, Kamath MV, Shine G, Upton AR, Tougas G. Objective assessment of cognitive factors involved in visceral perception by using event-related cerebral evoked responses to esophageal target stimulation in man. Dig Dis Sci 2001;46(4):790-801.
9. Sarkar S, Hobson AR, Furlong PL, Woolf CJ, Thompson DG, Aziz Q. Central neural mechanisms mediating human visceral hypersensitivity. Am J Physiol Gastrointest Liver Physiol 2001;281(5):G1196-202.
10. Hobson AR, Furlong PL, Sarkar S, et al. Neurophysiologic assessment of esophageal sensory processing in noncardiac chest pain. Gastroenterology 2006;130(1):80-8.

Pathopysiology and controversies in gastroesophageal reflux disease

What is the prevalence of gastroesophageal reflux disease in Asian countries?

T.K. Cheung, B.C.Y. Wong (Hong Kong)

The reported population prevalence of gastroesophageal reflux disease (GERD) in eastern Asia ranged from 2.5% to 6.7% for at least weekly symptoms of heartburn and/or acid regurgitation [1-5]. Typical GERD symptoms are consistently less common among the general populations of Asia than those in the West which have a prevalence of around 20% for weekly reflux symptoms [6-11]. No reliable data are available on the prevalence of esophagitis in the general population [12]. In case studies the prevalence of reflux esophagitis ranged from 3.4% to 16.3% [13-15]. However, these are likely to overestimate the true prevalence.

A large study in Hong Kong in patients undergoing routine or emergency upper endoscopy (n = 16,606) showed that 3.8% of the patients had esophagitis demonstrated by endosocpy and the majority (94%) had Los Angeles Classification grade A or B esophagitis and only 14 patients (0.08%) had esophageal stricture [13]. A large Japanese study reported esophagitis in 16.3% of patients visiting a hospital for routine physical examinations (n = 6,010) and 87% had mild esophagitis [14]. Lee *et al.* examined 7,015 patients coming for self-paid check-up and 3.4% of patients found to have esophagitis in which 98.3% were classified as mild esophagitis [15]. In summary, the prevalence of reflux esophagitis appears to be lower in Asian population and the disease spectrum is milder in Asians.

Prevalence of Barrett's varies between different countries. In a study of multi-ethnic Malaysian population, Barrett's esophagus was reported in 1.6% of those undergoing elective endoscopy for upper abdominal or reflux complaints [16]. A much lower prevalence was found in southern Chinese patients undergoing upper endoscopy, of whom only 0.06% were found (n = 22,628) [13]. More data are required to determine the true prevalence of Barrett's esophagus in Asians.

Rosaida *et al.* have shown that in a prospective study, 65.5% of their patients had non erosive reflux disease (NERD) [17]. In another study from Hong Kong, it was found that 46.7% (215 of 460 subjects) of patients with typical reflux symptoms had no endoscopic evidence of esophagitis [18]. In a study from Singapore [19], patients with NERD were significantly younger, more likely to have minor psychiatric morbidity and were less likely to respond to proton pump inhibitors (PPI) when compared with patients with erosive esophagitis.

The prevalence of GERD in Asia may be increasing [12,20]. In a 1999 re-survey of a cohort of community residents in Singapore who were interviewed in an earlier study in 1994, Lim *et al.* reported a more than 6 fold increase in the reporting of reflux symptoms, from a prevalence of 1.6% to a prevalence of 9.9% [21]. In a 1-year follow-up study in Hong Kong, Wong *et al.* reported an increase in the annual, monthly and weekly prevalence of GERD from 29.8%, 8.9% and 2.5% to 34.1%, 10.1% and 2.7%, respectively [1,2].

Why is the incidence of adenocarcinoma of the esophagus and gastric cardia increasing?

There has been a rise in the incidence of adneocarcinoma of the gastric cardia and esophagus in the United States [22] and Western Europe [23]. In Japan, adenocarcinoma of the esophagus is still rare, although there has been an increase in the annual death rate from 3.7 (1960) to 6.9 (1995) per 100,000 population. Two large prospective studies on the geographic prevalence of Barrett's esophagus in Japan, the Sendai Barrett's Esophagus Study (S-BEST) and the Far East Study (FEST), have recently investigated the epidemiology of Barrett's esophagus. Results from both studies showed that overall prevalence of the condition is lower than in the West: 0.9-1.2% in Japan compared with 1-4% in Europe and 5-12% in USA. Similar to the situation in the West, the condition was shown to be most prevalent in elderly male patients and least prevalent in patients with *Helicobacter pylori.* In contrast, the incidence of esophageal adenocarcinoma and gastric cardia carcinoma *versus* esophageal squamous cell carcinoma and gastric noncardia adenocarcinoma did not increase over a 15-year period (1981-1995) in a Taiwan study [24]. Another study from Korea also show that the ratio of esophageal adenocarcinoma compared to squamous cell carinoma has not increased among patients with esophageal carcinoma over a 30-year period (1970-1999) [25].

The strongest risk factor for esophageal adenocarcinoma is Barrett's esophagus. Patients with Barrett's esophagus have a 50- to 100-fold increased risk of developing adenocarcinoma compared with the general population [26] and it is an acquired condition secondary to longstanding GERD [27]. The risk of developing adenocarcinoma in patients with Barrett's esophagus has been estimated to be 0.5% per year [28]. Patients with recurrent symptoms of reflux has also been found to have increased risk of esophageal adenocarcinoma [29,30]. However, there is no data supporting a rising incidence of GERD in the USA or Europe. The incidence of GERD is increasing in Asian countries but baseline prevalence is still very low [12,20].

It has been suggested that the increasing prevalence of obesity in the Western world may explain the rising trends in incidences of adenocarcinoma of the esophagus and gastric cardia [31]. A recently published meta-analysis showed a positive association between body mass index (BMI) and risk of adenocarcinoma of the esophagus and possibly of the gastric cardia [32]. A recent published cohort study carried out at the Netherlands showed that the relative risks (RRs) (95% CI's) of esophageal adenocarcinoma were 1.40 (0.95-2.04) and 3.96 (2.27-6.88) for overweight (BMI 25.0-29.9 kg/m2) and obese subjects (BMI $\geq$ 30.0 kg/m$_2$), respectively, compared to subjects with normal weight (BMI 20.0-

24.9 kg/m$_2$). For gastric cardia adenocarcinoma, the RRs were 1.32 (0.94-1.85) and 2.73 (1.56-4.79) [33]. Central obesity can lead to a higher intra-abdominal pressure which may result in increase incidence of gastroesophageal reflux. Frequent reflux of gastric acid or bile may result in the formation of Barrett's esophagus which is thought to the premalignant lesion for the development of esophageal adenocarcinoma.

The eradication and the decreasing rate of *H. pylori* infection has also been proposed to be another possible reason for this trend. In a population-based case control study in Swden, *H. pylori* seropositivity was associated with a reduced risk for esophageal adenocarcinoa with an odds ratio (OR) of 0.3 (95% CI = 0.2-0.6) but not with esophageal squamous cell carcinoma (OR = 1.1) or gastric cardia adenocarcinoma (OR = 0.9) [34]. On the other hand, gastric atrophy was found to be associated with an increased risk for gastric cardia adenocarcinoma (OR = 4.5, 95% CI = 2.5-7.8) [34].

Other risk factors that have been associated with esophageal adenocarcinoma and gastric cardia cancers include lower esophageal sphincter relaxing drugs [35], tobacco smoking [29,36] and the low intake of fruit and vegetables [37]. Studies have shown a reduced risk of developing esophageal cancers in cohorts using non-steroidal anti-inflammatory drugs [35,38]. None of these appeared to contribute significantly to the increasing incidence of adenocarcinoma of the esophagus and gastric cardia.

References

1. Wong WM, Lai KC, Lam KF, et al. Prevalence, clinical spectrum and health care utilization of gastro-oesophageal reflux disease in a Chinese population: a population-based study. Aliment Pharmacol Ther 2003;18:595-604.
2. Wong WM, Lai KC, Lam KF, et al. Onset and disappearance of reflux symptoms in a Chinese population: a 1-year follow-up study. Aliment Pharmacol Ther 2004;20:803-12.
3. Wang JH, Luo JY, Dong L, Gong J, Tong M. Epidemiology of gastroesophageal reflux disease: a general population-based study in Xi'an of Northwest China. World J Gastroenterol 2004;10:1647-51.
4. Fujiwara Y, Higuchi K, Watanabe Y, et al. Prevalence of gastroesophageal reflux disease and gastroesophageal reflux disease symptoms in Japan. J Gastroenterol Hepatol 2005;20:26-9.
5. Watanabe Y, Fujiwara Y, Shiba M, et al. Cigarette smoking and alcohol consumption associated with gastro-oesophageal reflux disease in Japanese men. Scand J Gastroenterol 2003;38:807-11.
6. Locke GR 3rd, Talley NJ, Fett SL, Zinsmeister AR, Melton LJ 3rd. Prevalence and clinical spectrum of gastroesophageal reflux: a population-based study in Olmsted County, Minnesota. Gastroenterology 1997;112:1448-56.
7. Agreus L, Svardsudd K, Talley NJ, Jones MP, Tibblin G. Natural history of gastroesophageal reflux disease and functional abdominal disorders: a population-based study. Am J Gastroenterol 2001;96:2905-14.
8. Haque M, Wyeth JW, Stace NH, Talley NJ, Green R. Prevalence, severity and associated features of gastro-oesophageal reflux and dyspepsia: a population-based study. N Z Med J 2000;113:178-81.
9. Frank L, Kleinman L, Ganoczy D, et al. Upper gastrointestinal symptoms in North America: prevalence and relationship to healthcare utilization and quality of life. Dig Dis Sci 2000;45:809-18.
10. Kennedy T, Jones R. The prevalence of gastro-oesophageal reflux symptoms in a UK population and the consultation behaviour of patients with these symptoms. Aliment Pharmacol Ther 2000;14:1589-94.
11. Sandler RS, Everhart JE, Donowitz M, et al. The burden of selected digestive diseases in the United States. Gastroenterology 2002;122:1500-11.
12. Wong BC, Kinoshita Y. Systematic review on epidemiology of gastroesophageal reflux disease in Asia. Clin Gastroenterol Hepatol 2006;4:398-407.
13. Wong WM, Lam SK, Hui WM, et al. Long-term prospective follow-up of endoscopic oesophagitis in southern Chinese—prevalence and spectrum of the disease. Aliment Pharmacol Ther 2002;16:2037-42.
14. Furukawa N, Iwakiri R, Koyama T, et al. Proportion of reflux esophagitis in 6010 Japanese adults: prospective evaluation by endoscopy. J Gastroenterol 1999;34:441-4.
15. Lee SJ, Song CW, Jeen YT, et al. Prevalence of endoscopic reflux esophagitis among Koreans. J Gastroenterol Hepatol 2001;16:373-6.
16. Rajendra S, Kutty K, Karim N. Ethnic differences in the prevalence of endoscopic esophagitis and Barrett's esophagus: the long and short of it all. Dig Dis Sci 2004;49:237-42.
17. Rosaida MS, Goh KL. Gastro-oesophageal reflux disease, reflux oesophagitis and non-erosive reflux disease in a multiracial Asian population: a prospective, endoscopy based study. Eur J Gastroenterol Hepatol 2004;16:495-501.

18. Wu JC, Chan FK, Ching JY, Leung WK, Lee YT, Sung JJ. Empirical treatment based on "typical" reflux symptoms is inappropriate in a population with a high prevalence of Helicobacter pylori infection. Gastrointest Endosc 2002;55:461-5.
19. Ang TL, Fock KM, Ng TM, Teo EK, Chua TS, Tan J. A comparison of the clinical, demographic and psychiatric profiles among patients with erosive and non-erosive reflux disease in a multi-ethnic Asian country. World J Gastroenterol 2005;11:3558-61.
20. Ho KY, Cheung TK, Wong BC. Gastroesophageal reflux disease in Asian countries: Disorder of nature or nurture? J Gastroenterol Hepatol 2006;21:1362-5.
21. Lim SL, Goh WT, Lee JM, Ng TP, Ho KY. Changing prevalence of gastroesophageal reflux with changing time: longitudinal study in an Asian population. J Gastroenterol Hepatol 2005;20:995-1001.
22. Pohl H, Welch HG. The role of overdiagnosis and reclassification in the marked increase of esophageal adenocarcinoma incidence. J Natl Cancer Inst 2005;97:142-6.
23. Botterweck AA, Schouten LJ, Volovics A, Dorant E, van Den Brandt PA. Trends in incidence of adenocarcinoma of the oesophagus and gastric cardia in ten European countries. Int J Epidemiol 2000;29:645-54.
24. Chang SS, Lu CL, Chao JY, et al. Unchanging trend of adenocarcinoma of the esophagus and gastric cardia in Taiwan: a 15-year experience in a single center. Dig Dis Sci 2002;47:735-40.
25. Son JI, Park HJ, Song KS, et al. A single center's 30 years' experience of esophageal adenocarcinoma. Korean J Intern Med 2001;16:250-3.
26. Cameron AJ, Lomboy CT, Pera M, Carpenter HA. Adenocarcinoma of the esophagogastric junction and Barrett's esophagus. Gastroenterology 1995;109:1541-6.
27. Schuchert MJ, Luketich JD. Barrett's esophagus-emerging concepts and controversies. J Surg Oncol 2007;95:185-9.
28. Shaheen NJ, Crosby MA, Bozymski EM, Sandler RS. Is there publication bias in the reporting of cancer risk in Barrett's esophagus? Gastroenterology 2000;119:333-8.
29. Lagergren J. Adenocarcinoma of oesophagus: what exactly is the size of the problem and who is at risk? Gut 2005;54 Suppl 1:i1-5.
30. Lagergren J, Bergstrom R, Lindgren A, Nyren O. Symptomatic gastroesophageal reflux as a risk factor for esophageal adenocarcinoma. N Engl J Med 1999;340:825-31.
31. Calle EE, Kaaks R. Overweight, obesity and cancer: epidemiological evidence and proposed mechanisms. Nat Rev Cancer 2004;4:579-91.
32. Kubo A, Corley DA. Body mass index and adenocarcinomas of the esophagus or gastric cardia: a systematic review and meta-analysis. Cancer Epidemiol Biomarkers Prev 2006;15:872-8.
33. Merry AH, Schouten LJ, Goldbohm RA, van den Brandt PA. Body Mass Index, height and risk of adenocarcinoma of the oesophagus and gastric cardia: a prospective cohort study. Gut 2007.
34. Ye W, Held M, Lagergren J, et al. Helicobacter pylori infection and gastric atrophy: risk of adenocarcinoma and squamous-cell carcinoma of the esophagus and adenocarcinoma of the gastric cardia. J Natl Cancer Inst 2004;96:388-96.
35. Ranka S, Gee JM, Johnson IT, Skinner J, Hart AR, Rhodes M. Non-steroidal anti-inflammatory drugs, lower oesophageal sphincter-relaxing drugs and oesophageal cancer. A case-control study. Digestion 2006;74:109-15.
36. Wu AH, Wan P, Bernstein L. A multiethnic population-based study of smoking, alcohol and body size and risk of adenocarcinomas of the stomach and esophagus (United States). Cancer Causes Control 2001;12:721-32.
37. Terry P, Lagergren J, Hansen H, Wolk A, Nyren O. Fruit and vegetable consumption in the prevention of oesophageal and cardia cancers. Eur J Cancer Prev 2001;10:365-9.
38. Anderson LA, Johnston BT, Watson RG, et al. Nonsteroidal anti-inflammatory drugs and the esophageal inflammation-metaplasia-adenocarcinoma sequence. Cancer Res 2006;66:4975-82.

Pathogenesis of eosinophilic esophagitis

K. Mönkemüller, H. Neumann, P. Malfertheiner (Magdeburg)

Eosinophilic esophagitis (EE) is a chronic inflammatory disease of the esophagus, characterized by a T_H2-type allergic inflammatory response [1,2]. This type of inflammatory response is also seen in allergic diseases such as asthma or atopic dermatitis, which are also present in 50-70% of patients with EE or their relatives [3-6]. The pathophysiologic mechanisms of EE are not well understood but recently major advances in the understanding of this condition have been achieved [7-18]. Knowledge of the pathophysiology of eosinophilic esophagitis is essential to better understand this disease and to develop appropriate treatment options. Currently, the mainstay of medical therapy are either topical or systemic corticosteroids. Additional therapies included leukotriene receptor antagonists (e.g. montelukast) und IL-5 blockers (e.g. mepolizumab) [17-22]. Elimination diets, avoiding the presumed allergen have also shown promising results [16,23].

Pathophysiology

The exact pathogenesis of EE is unknown. The main pathophysiological disturbances in EE are eosinophilic and mast cell infiltration of the esophageal mucosa and derangements in the T helper cell 2 (T_H2) type immune responses [2,10,12-15]. We will briefly address these pathophysiologic mechanisms.

Infiltration of the esophagus with eosinophils, mast cells and lymphocytes

In contrast to the other segments of the gastrointestinal (GI) tract, there no eosinophils present in the normal esophageal mucosa [1,2]. Therefore, a major research question in the study of EE is to understand the mechanisms of eosinophils infiltration and perpetuation in the esophagus. There are various other esophageal diseases associated with eosinophilic infiltration such as parasitic infestations, gastroesophageal reflux disease and autoimmune diseases [1,2,24,26]. However, in EE there is strong data showing that the infiltration of eosinophils in EE through occurs through unique mechanisms [6,7]. The infiltration of eosinophils and mast cells is clearly associated with histological changes such as increased basal layer cell thickness [27]. Thus, it is important to differentiate EE from the above mentioned entities. In addition to eosinophils there are other inflammatory cells present in EE. These include polymorphonuclear leucocytes, various subsets of T-lymphocytes and mast cells [9]. This demonstrates that cellular components of the T_H2-type reaction are present in EE and these elements result in an allergic inflammatory response [2,9]. Clinical and experimental data documenting the role of eosinophils in EE show that the eosinophilic inflammation and infiltration acutely resolves with the use of systemic or topic corticosteroids [17,19]. The possible mechanisms of corticosteroids upon eosinophilic inflammation include induction of apoptosis, down-regulation of chemotactic factors, and inhibition of proinflammatory mediators [2].

Atopic or allergic response

An allergic response has been strongly implicated in the pathogenesis of EE [2,3,9]. The published data support a immune mediated response to exogenous allergens. This is supported by epidemiological and clinical evidence showing that many patients with EE (50%-80%) have seasonal variations in their symptoms and/or coexistent atopic condition such as asthma, atopic dermatitis and/or allergic rhinitis [1,2,6-19,25,26]. Laboratory data confirm this allergic predisposition as the IgE level and eotaxin are also frequently elevated in EE [2,7,13,27]. Additionally, there are various studies documenting allergic responses to either orally or nasally ingested allergens, as well as improvement following removal of the causative (allergen-containing) foods [11,12,16,23].

A recent experiment in mice showed that the eosinophilic infiltration of the esophagus was induced by inhalation of antigens, whereas the intragastric application of the same antigens did not result in eosinophilic infiltration of the esophagus [12]. Additional support for a role of inhaled antigens in the pathogenesis of EE comes from clinical studies and epidemiologic data showing a correlation of asthma and EE, with a corresponding sensitivity to aeroallergens [13-15]. However, there are data demonstrating that orally ingested allergens can also result in EE, especially in children [14]. Furthermore, exclusion diets have also shown to be beneficial in EE [16,23].

Despite these contrasting data, it is clear that EE is not an immediate allergic condition but occurs as a late phase reaction associated with T helper cell (T_H2)-type immune responses. Molecular studies have confirmed the presence of elevated levels of eosinophil-active T_H2 cytokines such as IL-4 and IL-5 in patients with EE [2,13,15]. The late phase reaction is caused by the induced synthesis and release of mediators such as leukotrienes and cytokines from the activated mast cells, which in turn recruit eosinophils and T_H2 lymphocytes to the site of inflammation. If the antigen stimulus persists it stimulates allergen-specific T_H2 cells, which in turn promote eosinophilia, release of IL-4 and IL-5 and further IgE production.

In the mouse model it could be demonstrated that IL-5 plays a central role in the induction of eosinophilic infiltration [8]. Whereas IL-5 induced eosinophilic trafficking into the esophagus and small intestine of wild-type mice, this was not the case in IL-5 deficient mice (i.e. these mice are resistant to develop EE) [8]. In this study it was also shown that eotaxin was also essential for eosinophil recruitment. In the absence of eotaxin, trafficking of eosinophils decreased 15-fold [8]. *In vitro* studies using human tissue of patients with EE showed that the mucosa is infiltrated with IL-5 secreting cells and that the squamous epithelial cells also secrete massive amounts of TNF-alpha [9,10]. These findings have important clinical implications as various therapies currently employed to treat EE target IL-5 and leukotrienes [20,22].

In another study involving mice, intratracheal administration of IL-13 lead to esophageal inflammation through IL-5, eotaxin and STAT-6 pathways [15]. IL-13 is produced by eosinophils and is also a T_H2-mediated cytokine. It has inflammatory and profibrotic capabilities which result in bronchial hyperreactivity. Intratracheal instillation of IL-13 also induces EE [2,8]. IL-13 shares signal transduction with IL-4. IL-4 regulates trafficking of eosinophils, attracts these into the tissue and promote their adhesion to endothelial surfaces.

In summary, the published data demonstrate an intimate connection between the development of eosinophilic inflammation in the esophagus as a result of external allergic triggers and intrinsic T_H2 cytokines, supporting an allergic pathogenesis of EE. IL-5 appears to be essential for eosinophil recruitment, differentiation and activation. Current therapies aim to decrease the eosinophilic infiltration by blocking the inflammatory pathways. These medications include topical or oral steroids, leukotriene antagonists (e.g. montelukast) and IL-5 receptors (mepoluzimab) [17-23]. However, it is still not known whether the late or permanent complications of EE can be prevented by the use of anti-inflammatory agents. Therefore, more studies into the pathophysiology of EE and clinical long-term follow-up data are needed.

References

1. Straumann A, Spichtin HP, Bernoulli R, et al. Idiopathic eosinophilic esophagitis: a frequently overlooked disease with typical clinical aspects and discrete endoscopic findings. Schweiz Med Wochenschr 1994;124:1419-29.
2. Furuta GT, Liacouras C, Collins MH, et al. Eosinophilic esophagitis in children and adults: a systematic review and consensus recommendations for diagnosis and treatment. Gastroenterology 2007;133:1342-63.
3. Straumann A, Spichtin HP, Grize L, et al. Natural history of primary eosinophilic esophagitis: a follow up of 30 patients for up to 11.5 years. Gastroenterology 2003;125:1660-9.
4. Attwood SE, Smyrk TC, DeMeester TR, et al. Esophageal eosinophilia with dysphagia, a distinct clinicopathologic syndrome. Dig Dis Sci 1993;38:109-16.
5. Kato M, Kephart GM, Talley NJ, et al. Eosinophil infiltration and degranulation in normal human tissue. Anat Rec 1998;252:418-25.
6. Steiner SJ, Gupta SK, Croffie JM, et al. Correlation between number of eosinophils and acid reflux index on same day esophageal biopsy and 24 hour esophageal pH monitoring. Am J Gastroenterol 2004;99:801-5.
7. Rosen R, Furuta GT. The role of non acid reflux in patients with eosinophilic esophagitis. A study using multi-channel intraluminal impedance. J Pediatr Gastroenterol Nutr 2005;41:42.
8. Mishra A, Hogan SP, Brandt EB, et al. IL-5 promotes eosinophil trafficking to the esophagus. J Immunol 2002;168:2464-9.
9. Straumann A, Bauer M, Fischer B, et al. Idiopathic eosinophilic esophagitis is associated with a Th2 type allergic inflammatory response. J Allergy Clin Immunol 2001;108:954-61.
10. Gupta SK, Fitzgerald JF, Kondratyuk T, et al. Cytokine expression in normal and inflamed esophageal mucosa: a study into the pathogenesis of allergic eosinophilic esophagitis. J Pediatr Gastroenterol Nutr 2006;42:22-6.
11. Mishra A, Rothenberg ME. Intratracheal IL 13 induces eosinophilic esophagitis by an IL 5, eotaxin–1 and STAT 6 - dependent mechanisms. Gastroenterology 2003;125:1419-27.
12. Mishra A, Hogan SP, Brandt EB, Rothenberg ME. An etiological role for aeroallergens and eosinophils in experimental esophagitis. J Clin Invest 2001;107:83-90.
13. Simon D, Marti HP, Heer P, Simon HU, Braathen LR, Straumann A. Eosinophilic esophagitis is frequently associated with IgE-mediated allergic airway diseases. J Allergy Clin Immunol 2005;115:1090-2.
14. Spergel JM, Beausoleil JL, Mascarenhas M, et al. The use of skin prick tests and patch tests to identify causative foods in eosinophilic esophagitis. J Allergy Clin Immunol 2002;109:363-8.
15. Furuta GT. Eosinophils in the esophagus: acid is not the only cause. J Pediatr Gastroenterol Nutr 1998;26:468-71.
16. Kagalwalla AF, Sentongo TA, Ritz S, et al. Effect of six-food elimination diet on clinical and histologic outcomes in eosinophilic esophagitis. Clin Gastroenterol Hepatol 2006;4:1097-102.
17. Arora A, Yamazaki K. Eosinophilic esophagitis: asthma of the esophagus? Clin Gastroenterol Hepatol 2004;2:523-30.
18. Attwood SE, Lewis CJ, Bronder CS, et al. Eosinophilic oesophagitis: a novel treatment using Montelukast. Gut 2003;52:181-5.
19. Arora AS, Perrault J, Smyrk TC. Topical corticosteroid treatment of dysphagia due to eosinophilic esophagitis. Topical corticosteroid treatment of dysphagia due to eosinophilic esophagitis in adults. Mayo Clin Proc 2003;78:830-5.
20. Stein ML, Collins MH, Villanueva JM, et al. Anti-IL-5 (mepolizumab) therapy for eosinophilic esophagitis. J Allergy Clin Immunol 2006;118:1312-9.
21. Teitelbaum JE, Fox VL, Twarog FJ, et al. Eosinophilic esophagitis in children: Immunopathological analysis and response to fluticasone propionate. Gastroenterology 2002;122:1216-25.
22. Straumann A, Conus S, Kita H, et al. Mepolizumab, a humanized monoclonal antibody to IL-5, for severe eosinophilic esophagitis in adults: a randomized, placebo-controlled double-blind trial. Gastroenterology 2007;132:P-90.
23. Markowitz JE, Spregel JM, Ruchelli F, et al. Elemental diet is an effective treatment for eosinophilic esophagitis in children and adolescents. Am J Gastroenterol 2003;98:777-82.
24. Furuta GT, Straumann A. Review article: the pathogenesis and management of eosinophilic oesophagitis. Aliment Pharmacol Ther 2006;24:173-82.
25. Müller-Stöver I, Richter J, Häussinger D. Infection with Gnathostoma spinigerum as a cause of eosinophilic oesophagitis. Dtsch Med Wochenschr 2004;129:1973-5.
26. Arnim U, Mönkemüller K, Malfertheiner P, Straumann A. Eosinophilic esophagitis - pathogenesis, clinical presentation and therapeutic management. Z Gastroenterol 2007;45:1257-63.
27. Blanchard C, Mingler MK, Vicario M, et al. IL-13 involvement in eosinophilic esophagitis: transcriptome analysis and reversibility with glucocorticoids. J Allergy Clin Immunol 2007;120:1292-300.

Eosinophilic esophagitis in adults

A. Straumann (Olten)

Eos is the name of the ancient Greek goddess of dawn. The term eosinophil was coined in 1879 by Paul Ehrlich to describe the bright red color – resembling dawn – exhibited by the characteristic cytoplasmic granules of these particular leukocytes. Eosinophilic esophagitis (EE) is a "young" disorder. Almost all relevant features of EE are insights gleaned within the past few years. The recognition of this disorder introduced the dawn of a new and exiting era of eosinophil research in gastroenterology. This review focuses on six relevant aspects of this chronic esophageal inflammatory disorder.

Definition: eosinophilic esophagitis a clearly defined entity or an omnium-gatherum of eosinophilic-inflammatory responses?

In 1993 and 1994, three authors independently described the clinical picture of EE using several series of patients [1-3], prompting this disorder's acceptance as a distinct entity in the adult as well as in the pediatric population [4-7]. The last few years have brought significant advances in understanding the pathogenesis of EE and up until now, clinical characteristics, endoscopical manifestations, immunopathogenic mechanisms, fundamental epidemiological data, natural course as well as therapeutic options of this esophageal disease have been properly elucidated [8,9]. Today, EE is clearly defined as a clinico-pathological disorder characterized by upper intestinal symptoms in combination with a dense esophageal eosinophilia, both of which persisting despite prolonged treatment with proton pump inhibitors. In addition, eosinophilic inflammation is absent in the stomach, small intestine and colon [9].

Epidemiology: eosinophilic esophagitis a rare curiosity or a substantial disease?

EE was originally considered rare, but is now increasingly recognized. Whether this increased recognition stemmed from an enhanced awareness or to a real increase in the incidence was long unclear. Some demographic data existed for pediatric patients [10], but none for adults. Thus, in order to obtain relevant demographic data, we analyzed our prospectively conducted database that enrolls confirmed EE patients from a demographically stable catchment area [11]. Throughout our 16-year observation period, an average annual incidence of 1.438 cases per 100,000 inhabitants was noted with a marked increase in newly-diagnosed cases during the last years. Based on the documented chronicity of EE, the steady incidence resulted in a constantly-increasing prevalence. Given the stability of the demographic and recording conditions, it is very likely that this remarkable trend reflects a real increase in EE and not just enhanced awareness. These data, confirmed by several other recently published studies [12,13], indicate that EE, once believed to be an extremely rare anomaly, occurs at a considerable frequency and may soon reach that of chronic inflammatory bowel diseases.

Clinical presentation: can we clinically suspect a patient with eosinophilic esophagitis?

EE is a predominantly male disease found in almost all age groups, but symptomatic episodes usually first peak in early childhood, and then again between the ages of 20-40 years. The primary symptom of EE in adult patients is dysphagia for solids sometimes leading to long-lasting episodes of food impaction. Almost half of the patients suffers additionally under non-swallowing-related retrosternal pain. Unfortunately, standard laboratory analyses are not contributory to establishing the diagnosis of EE. However, in most series, somewhat more than half of the patients had abnormalities in their peripheral blood [1,3]. In general, the increase is mild and almost never exceeds an absolute value of 1,500 cells/mm^3 [14]. Additonally, between 70 to 92% of EE patients have elevated serum IgE levels [3,6]. Taken together, EE patients present with a typical history of dysphagia, but with almost no conclusive findings in the physical examination or in the routine laboratory anaylses.

Endoscopic features: what can the endoscopist expect in a patient with eosinophilic esophagitis?

Unfortunately, the endoscopic signs of EE are often unremarkable, misleading or even absent. To date, at least 12 different endoscopic signs – e.g. as white exudates, solitary rings, corrugated rings giving the esophagus a trachea-like aspect, red furrows, strictures, lack of visible abnormalities – have been reported. We attempted a more precise characterization of this confusing picture [15]. In a group of 30 adult EE patients, we found that all presented with endoscopic abnormalities of the esophageal mucosa. However, only half of the patients had alterations that would clearly indicate the existence of an esophageal disorder. Furthermore, all but one patient presented a random combination of up to five different signs. EE therefore evokes a patchwork of different endoscopic signs rather than a single, characteristic picture. This heterogeneity, together with the usually discreet expression of the endoscopic signs, hinders the endoscopic recognition of EE and may likewise contribute to its underdiagnosis.

Natural course: what happens over time in a patient with eosinophilic esophagitis?

It is likely that EE is a chronic disorder. However, neither EE natural course nor information regarding potential long-term risks had been known. With the intent of defining the long-term course, we prospectively followed thirty adult patients with previously confirmed EE over a mean of 7.2 years [16]. All patients survived the study period in good health and stable nutritional state. Dysphagia persisted in almost all patients, exerting a major negative effect on socioprofessional activities on one patient and a minor impact on 15 individuals. The eosinophilic infiltration persisted in all patients, but the number of the tissue dwelling eosinophils spontaneously decreased over time. The inflammatory process evoked fibrosis of the esophageal lamina propria but did not spread to the stomach or duodenum. No case evolved to an eosinophilic gastroenteritis. Summarized, it is documented that EE is a primary chronic disease definitely restricted to the esophagus that leads to persistent dysphagia and an esophageal remodeling, but does not impact the nutritional state. To date, no malignant potential has been associated with this disease. Nevertheless, the disease has a relevant negative impact on the quality of live.

Therapeutic management: when should treat and how can we treat a patient with eosinophilic esophagitis?

Fortunately, only a minority of the adult patients with EE present with such severe disturbances that therapy is warranted. Nevertheless, we do not yet know whether consistent long-term therapy in patients having only minimal or absent symptoms could prevent eventual stricture formation. At this stage, treatment can be recommended only for symptomatic patients. But once diagnosed, EE management still remains largely controversial. Standard recommendations for EE-induced dysphagia in adult patients include systemic [17] or topical corticosteroids [18-20], leukotriene antagonists [21] and dilation [1]. Recently, beneficial effects of mepolizumab, a humanized antibody against IL-5, have been reported in two studies with various hypereosinophilic disorders, including one patient with EE [22,23]. All these treatment studies are limited to openlabeled clinical trials or even anecdotal case reports. Based on these investigations, we propose that a prudent course for managing symptomatic EE patients could be outlined as follows (*Figure 1*). If endoscopy detects neither visible stenosis nor significant resistance, first line therapy should be medical treatment with topical corticosteroids. Patients presenting with a visible stenosis and/or significant resistance during endoscopy, refractory to a course of topical corticosteroids, should be treated with dilation. Patients experiencing severe dysphagia, refractory to topical corticosteroids, may be treated with systemic corticosteroids or mepolizumab. Nevertheless, additional studies are still needed in order to evaluate the efficacy and safety of these various therapeutic approaches.

Outlook

During the last ten years, an enormous research effort in pediatric and adult EE has been undertaken and as a result, several pathogenic aspects of EE are now recognized and defined. Despite these advances, many questions remain:

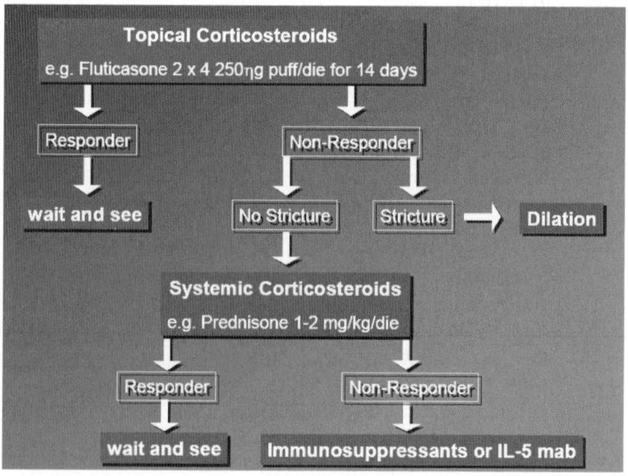

Figure 1. Therapeutic management of eosinophilic esophagitis in adults (2006).

- are we faced with an exploding increase in the EE prevalence?
- is EE definitely a benign disorder or are EE patients at risk for developing a malignant condition later on?
- what is responsible for the striking male dominance?
- do children with EE outgrow their disease?
- what are the best therapeutic strategies for EE?
- in order to prevent esophageal fibrosis and remodeling, should we treat the chronic inflammatory process in any case, independently of the presence of symptoms?

All these unsolved questions will stimulate and fuel the ongoing.

References

1. Attwood SE, Smyrk TC, Demeester TR, Jones JB. Esophageal eosinophilia with dysphagia. A distinct clinicopathologic syndrome. Dig Dis Sci 1993;38:109-16.
2. Vitellas KM, Bennett WF, Bova JG, Johnston JC, Caldwell JH, Mayle JE. Idiopathic eosinophilic esophagitis. Radiology 1993;186:789-93.
3. Straumann A, Spichtin HP, Bernoulli R, Loosli J, Voegtlin J. Idiopathic eosinophilic esophagitis: a frequently overlooked disease with typical clinical aspects and discrete endoscopic findings. Schweiz Med Wochenschr 1994;124:1419-29.
4. Kelly KJ, Lazenby AJ, Rowe PC, Yardley JH, Perman JA, Sampson HA. Eosinophilic esophagitis attributet to gastroesophageal reflux: improvement with an amino acid-based formula. Gastroenterology 1995;109:1503-12.
5. Walsh SV, Antonioli DA, Goldman H, et al. Allergic esophagitis in children: a clinicopathological entity. Am J Surg Pathol 1999;23:390-6.
6. Orenstein SR, Shalaby TH, DiLorenzo C, Putnam PE, Sigurdsson L, Kocoshis SA. The spectrum of pediatric eosinophilic esophagitis beyond infancy: a clinical series of 30 children. Am J Gastroenterol 2000;95:1422-30.
7. Spergel JM, Beausoleil JL, Mascarenhas M, Liacouras CA. The use of skin prick tests and patch tests to identify causative foods in eosinophilic esophagitis. J Allergy Clin Immunol 2002;109:363-8.
8. Arora AS, Yamazaki K. Eosinophilic esophagitis: asthma of the esophagus? Clin Gastroenterol Hepatol 2004;2:523-30.
9. Furuta GT, Straumann A. The pathogenesis and management of eosinophilic esophagitis. Aliment Pharmacol Ther 2006;24:173-82.
10. Noel RJ, Putnam PE, Rothenberg ME. Eosinophilic esophagitis. N Engl J Med 2004;351:940-1.
11. Straumann A. Simon HU. Eosinophilic esophagitis: escalating epidemiology? J Allergy Clin Immunol 2005;115:418-9.
12. Desai TK, Stecevic V, Chang CH, Goldstein NS, Badiazdegan K, Furuta GT. Association of eosinophilic inflammation with esophageal food impaction in adults. Gastrointest Endosc 2005;61:795-801.
13. Ronkainen J, Talley NJ, Aro P, et al. Prevalence of eosinophilia and eosinophilic esophagitis in adults in the community: a random population based study (Kalixana). Gastroenterology 2006;130 :575.
14. Rothenberg ME. Eosinophilic Gastrointestinal Disorders (EGID) J Allergy Clin Immun 2004;113:11-28.
15. Straumann A, Spichtin HP, Bucher KA, Simon HU, Beglinger C. Eosinophilic esophagitis: red on microscopy, white on endoscopy. Digestion 2004;70:109-16.
16. Straumann A, Spichtin HP, Grize L, Bucher KA, Beglinger C, Simon HU. Natural history of primary eosinophilic esophagitis: a follow-up of 30 adult patients for up to 11.5 years. Gastroenterology 2003;125:1660-9.
17. Liacouras CA, Wenner WJ, Brown K, Ruchelli E. Primary eosinophilic esophagitis in children: successful treatment with oral corticosteroids. J Pediatr Gastroenterol Nutr 1998;26:380-5.
18. Faubion WA, Perrault J, Burgart LJ, Zein NN, Clawson ML, Freese DK. Treatment of eosinophilic esophagitis with inhaled corticosteroids. J Pediatr Gastroenterol Nutr 1998;27:90-3.
19. Teitelbaum JE, Fox VL, Twarog FJ, et al. Eosinophilic esophagitis in children: Immunopathological analysis and response to fluticasone propionate. Gastroenterology 2002;122:1216-25.
20. Arora AS, Perrault J, Smyrk TC. Topical corticosteroid treatment of dysphagia due to eosinophilic esophagitis in adults. Mayo Clin Proc 2003;78:830-5.
21. Attwood SE, Lewis CJ, Bronder CS, Morris CD, Armstrong GR, Whittam J. Eosinophilic oesophagitis: a novel treatment using Montelukast. Gut 2003;52:181-5.
22. Garrett JK, Jameson SC, Thomson B, et al. Anti-interleukin-5 (mepolizumab) therapy for hypereosinophilic syndromes. J Allerg Clin Immun 2004;113:115.
23. Plötz SG, Simon HU, Darsow U, et al. Use of an anti-interleukin-5 antibody in the hypereosinophilic syndrome with eosinophilic dermatitis. N Engl J Med 2003;349:2334-9.

What is the distribution of values for post-prandial and nocturnal gastric acidity in gastroesophageal reflux disease with erosive esophagitis and no esophagitis?

S. Emerenziani, M. Cicala (Roma)

The reasons for the question

Although, of the gastric contents, acid reflux has recently been confirmed to play a major role in determining both symptoms and mucosal injuries in gastroesophageal reflux disease (GERD), little attention has been focused on gastric acidity in the pathophysiology of the erosive *versus* non-erosive disease (NERD). In the presence, and at the time, of failure of the antireflux barrier, esophageal reflux characteristics will reflect those of the content immediately below the gastroesophageal junction and, indeed, a significant direct relationship between gastric acidity (as assessed by pH probe at 10 cm below the lower esophageal sphincter – LES) and esophageal acid exposure, as well as between intragastric acid suppression and esophageal acid control, have been clearly shown.

In the early 90's, attempts to demonstrate increased gastric acid secretion in GERD led, in two large series, to conflicting results: in one study [1], Hirschowitz, matching the control group, found that erosive GERD was not associated with gastric acid or pepsin hypersecretion and that the severity of esophagitis was not related to the acid secretion rate while, in another study [2], gastric basal acid output was increased in 19% of heartburn patients and in 28% of esophagitis patients.

Recent studies have shown that NERD patients represent the vast majority (up to 75%) of the GERD population [3,4] Compared to esophagitis patients, NERD patients, presenting an overall reduced esophageal acid exposure, should achieve better symptomatic relief following proton pump inhibitor (PPI) treatment, at the same doses. Several clinical trials have actually shown the opposite [5,6], thus leading to various hypotheses being advanced, among which a possible gastric hyperacidity or a reduced acid suppression in NERD.

From acid secretion to integrated acidity studies

Several studies have since been focused on the gastric integrated acidity, derived from ambulatory 24-hour pH studies, which is less invasive and more physiological than the nasogastric aspiration technique and provides indirect assessment of gastric acid secretion. Gastric integrated acidity results not only from acid secretion but also from the buffering capacity of meals, rate of gastric emptying, saliva swallowed, non acid secretions and retrograde flow from the duodenum. Moreover, a direct correlation has been found between gastric acid secretion and post-prandial gastric integrated acidity in healthy subjects and in GERD patients [7].

In a study carried out in GERD patients, not stratified in terms of endoscopic findings, the post-prandial gastric integrated acidity, as well as the meal-stimulated gastric acid secretion were significantly higher than those in controls. However, no difference was found between GERD patients and controls as far as concerns gastric integrated acidity either during the nocturnal or the entire 24-hour recording time. These results do not support the hypothesis of a "global" gastric hyperacidity in GERD patients. In that same study, a significant correlation between esophageal and post-prandial gastric integrated acidity was found only in GERD patients [8].

A retrospective study on a very large series of GERD patients focused on the role of post-prandial esophageal integrated acidity in GERD pathogenesis: patients were stratified into GERD and non-GERD patients according to the 24-hour pH profile (esophageal pH < 4 for more than 4.2% of the total recording time = GERD). Since a direct relationship was found between gastric post-prandial integrated acidity and percentage of time below 4, as expected GERD patients demonstrated a greater post-prandial esophageal integrated acidity compared to those with physiological acid exposure. Only among patients with pathological reflux, did patients with symptoms show a greater post-prandial esophageal integrated acidity than those not reporting symptoms, during the test. However, the correlation between the symptom association probability (SAP) index and post-prandial esophageal integrated acidity was poor [9].

Erosive and non-erosive disease

Very few studies have assessed the relationship between esophageal and gastric acidity in GERD patients according to the presence/absence of erosive disease.

Gardner *et al.* investigating the relationship between gastric and esophageal integrated acidity at baseline and during treatment with PPI observed that these parameters did not differ between erosive and non-erosive patients. However, the mathematical analysis of esophageal acidity in relation to the accompanying value of gastric acidity showed that the higher gastric integrated acidity correlated with pathological esophageal acidity only in patients with erosive esophagitis (ROC curves were used). Furthermore, the authors examined the pharmacodynamic effects of PPI on post-prandial and nocturnal gastric acidity and their association with pathological esophageal acidity. At baseline, post-prandial and nocturnal gastric integrated acidity were not significantly different between patients with erosive and non-erosive disease. During PPI treatment, post-prandial gastric integrated acidity was predictive of pathological *versus* normal esophageal acidity in patients with erosive esophagitis, but not in NERD patients, thus suggesting that normalization of esophageal acidity requires a greater decrease in the post-prandial integrated gastric acidity in NERD disease. Thus, the less efficient pharmacological control of post-prandial gastric acidity in NERD patients, would account for the reduced symptomatic response to PPI in these patients [10]. Only 8 NERD patients were studied and the daily time was assessed as being equivalent to the post-prandial period. GERD was defined on the basis of the pH profile, all enrolled patients presenting a clearly pathological esophageal acid exposure (pH < 4 for more than 10% of the recording time).

Savarino *et al.* [11] assessed the 24-hour intragastric acidity in a large study population comprising NERD and esophagitis patients as well as normal subjects. The simple finding of the mean 24-hour gastric pH profile of the controls was comparable to those of NERD and esophagitis patients during the entire study, including also the night- and daytime periods, thus suggesting that mechanisms other than acid hypersecretion would account for the reduced response to PPI in NERD. Although a less sophisticated assessment of gastric acidity was used, i.e., the mean gastric pH, patients were enrolled on the basis of symptoms (both typical and atypical), thus including, for the first time, patients with physiological esophageal acid exposure. Furthermore, patients with a history of duodenal ulcer disease were excluded and the presence of *Helicobacter pylori* and of gastric atrophy were evaluated.

The analysis of the frequency of the different gastric pH values was further assessed by Gardner *et al.* using the database from the previous study in GERD patients, selected on the basis of a pathological esophageal acid exposure. The new analysis employed in this study was able to reveal differences between GERD patients and controls not only in the distribution of post-prandial gastric pH values, as already found by means of IA values, but also in the distribution throughout the entire 24-hour and nocturnal period. Compared to controls, as shown in *Figure 1*, patients more frequently presented pH values below 2.5 but fewer values above 3.5 over the 24 hours, a similar but more significant difference during the post-prandial (from 9.00 to 22.00) period and more values within the pH range of 2-6 in the nocturnal period. Findings were not stratified for presence/absence of erosive disease and, as pointed out by the authors, the analysis did not take into account gastric pH changes over time [12].

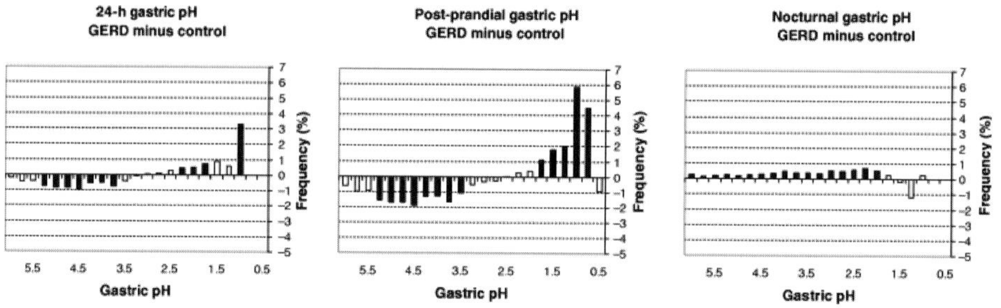

Figure 1. Histogram of difference in values for pH from 24-hour gastric pH recordings. Results are mean values of 26 control subjects and 26 GERD subjects. Each bin is 0.25 pH units. Values were calculated as the mean for GERD subjects minus the corresponding mean value for controls. Post-prandial pH was recorded from 09:00 to 22:00 hours and nocturnal pH from 22:00 to 09:00 hours. Closed symbols are significantly different ($P < 0.01$) by unpaired t-test comparing logarithm of frequencies. (From Gardner [12] with permission).

An unsolved question

Certain aspects should be considered when approaching NERD pathogenesis. In the selection of patients, attention should be paid to the possibility of mucosal healing by previous treatment: Case history of patients (in terms of previous endoscopy and therapy) and adequate washout are crucial. Several studies have demonstrated that about 50% of NERD patients present a physiological 24-hour pH profile, and, indeed, the lowest response to PPI treatment is observed in this subgroup. Therefore, studies aimed at clarifying the reasons for poor PPI response should focus on NERD not presenting with pathological esophageal pH. In healthy subjects and GERD patients, most gastroesophageal reflux events do occur in the post-prandial period, thus suggesting a relationship between the volume and the characteristics of the gastric contents and the likelihood of reflux.

Integrated acidity does not provide information on volume. Recent MR studies have shown that, contrary to the traditional theory of rapid and complete homogenization of the meal, gastric contents appear to be poorly mixed. Long after ingestion, the meal remains heterogeneous, with gastric secretion scarcely penetrating the center of the food bolus [13,14]. Future studies, on the influence of gastric acidity on GERD pathogenesis should take this evidence into consideration and should attempt to assess the gastric acidity not only at 10 cm below the LES, since a single value might not be representative of the regional variation in gastric acidity.

It is also important, when assessing gastric acidity, to take into account the numerous factors affecting gastric physiology and, hence, the interpretation of pH recording studies [15] (*Table I*). Of these factors, some may account for the differences observed in the above-mentioned studies.

Table I. Factors affecting the results of gastric pH recordings. (From Armstrong [15] with permission).

Inter-individual variability	Baseline, off therapy On therapy
Duration of previous therapy	
Subject's health status	Healthy Peptic ulcer disease or GERD Systemic illness (e.g. intensive care unit patient)
Helicobacter pylori status	
Feeding status	Fasted Regular food Enteral/parenteral nutrition
Position of pH electrode in the stomach	Body Antrum
Type of pH electrode	Glass Antimony Ion-sensitive field effect transistor (ISFET)

References

1. Hirschowitz BI. A critical analysis, with appropriate controls, of gastric acid and pepsin secretion in clinical esophagitis. Gastroenterology 1991;101:1149-58.
2. Collen MJ, Johnson DA, Sheridan MJ. Basal acid output and gastric acid hypersecretion in gastroesophageal reflux disease. Correlation with ranitidine therapy. Dig Dis Sci 1994;39(2):410-7.
3. Fass R, Fennerty B, Vakil N. Nonerosive reflux disease-current concepts and dilemmas. Am J Gastroenterol 2001;96:303-14.
4. Quigley EMM, Di Baise JK. Non-erosive reflux disease: the real problem in gastro-oesophageal reflux disease. Digest Liver Dis 2001;33:523-7.
5. Dean BB, Gano ADJ, Knight K, Ofman JJ, Fass R. Effectiveness of proton pump inhibitors in nonerosive reflux disease. Clin Gastroenterol Hepatol 2004;2:656-64.
6. Armstrong D, Talley NJ, Lauritsen K, et al. The role of acid suppression in patients with endoscopy-negative reflux disease: the effect of treatment with esomeprazole or omeprazole. Aliment Pharmacol Ther 2004;20:413-21.
7. Gardner JD, Ciociola AA, Robinson M. Measurement of meal-stimulated gastric acid secretion by in vivo gastric autotitration. J Appl Physiol 2002;92(2):427-34.

8. Gardner JD, Sloan S, Miner PB, Robinson M. Meal-stimulated gastric acid secretion and integrated gastric acidity in gastro-oesophageal reflux disease. Aliment Pharmacol Ther 2003;1;17:945-53.
9. Shih GL, Brensinger CM, Katzka DA, Metz DC. Postprandial oesophageal integrated acidity is a reliable predictor of gastro-oesophageal reflux disease. Aliment Pharmacol Ther 2005;15;21(12):1475-82.
10. Gardner JD, Gallo-Torres H, Sloan S, Robinson M, Miner PB. The basis for the decreased response to proton pump inhibitors in gastro-oesophageal reflux disease patients without erosive oesophagitis. Aliment Pharmacol Ther 2003;18(9):891-905.
11. Zentilin P, Dulbecco P, Bilardi C, et al. Circadian pattern of intragastric acidity in patients with non-erosive reflux disease (NERD). Aliment Pharmacol Ther 2003;17(3):353-9.
12. Gardner JD, Sloan S, Robinson M, Miner PB Jr. Frequency analyses of gastric pH in control and gastro-oesophageal reflux disease subjects treated with a proton-pump inhibitor. Aliment Pharmacol Ther 2004;20(11-12):1381-6.
13. Marciani L, Gowland PA, Spiller RC, et al. Effect of meal viscosity and nutrients on satiety, intragastric dilution, and emptying assessed by MRI. Am J Physiol Gastrointest Liver Physiol 2001;280(6):G1227-33.
14. Emerenziani S, Sifrim D. Gastroesophageal reflux and gastric emptying, revisited. Curr Gastroenterol Rep 2005;7(3):190-5.
15. Armstrong D. Gastric pH- the most relevant predictor of benefit in reflux disease? Aliment Pharmacol Ther 2004;20:19-26.

In patients with heartburn, can a correlation with esophageal acid perfusion be demonstrated?

R.C. Orlando (Chapel Hill)

Esophageal acid perfusion when performed in the clinical context is commonly referred to as the Bernstein test. The Bernstein test was devised over 40 years ago as a tool for the diagnosis of gastroesophageal reflux disease (GERD) in subjects with non-cardiac chest pain [1,2]. While the actual performance of the test over time has undergone a variety of iterations, its essentials remain the same. That is, it involves the nasal passage and fixation of a catheter system whose perfusion port is localized to mid-esophagus, some 5-cm above the lower esophageal sphincter. By means of the port, the distal esophagus is perfused alternately, and without the subject's knowledge, with 0.1N HCl (pH ~ 1.1) or isotonic saline (pH ~ 6.5). In the absence of symptoms, acid perfusion is continued for up to 30 minutes. The Bernstein test is considered "positive" (+) and diagnostic of GERD, if acid, but not saline, elicits heartburn or chest pain consistent with the clinical complaint; and the test is considered "negative" if neither acid nor saline elicit symptoms similar to the clinical complaint [3].

The principles forming the basis of the Bernstein test are fundamentally sound and based on the accepted premise that "heartburn" in GERD results from contact of the (distal) esophagus with refluxed gastric (hydrochloric) acid. Notably, and less well-appreciated is that for heartburn to occur the refluxed gastric acid must contact a (previously) "damaged" esophageal epithelium. Consequently, symptoms are invoked during the Bernstein test in GERD when luminal acid diffuses across a damaged esophageal epithelium in sufficient quantities to activate chemosensitive nociceptors within the organ. Activation of the nociceptors in turn provide the signal to the central nervous system (CNS) for the conscious perception of heartburn [4] (*Figure 1*). In contrast to those with GERD, healthy subjects

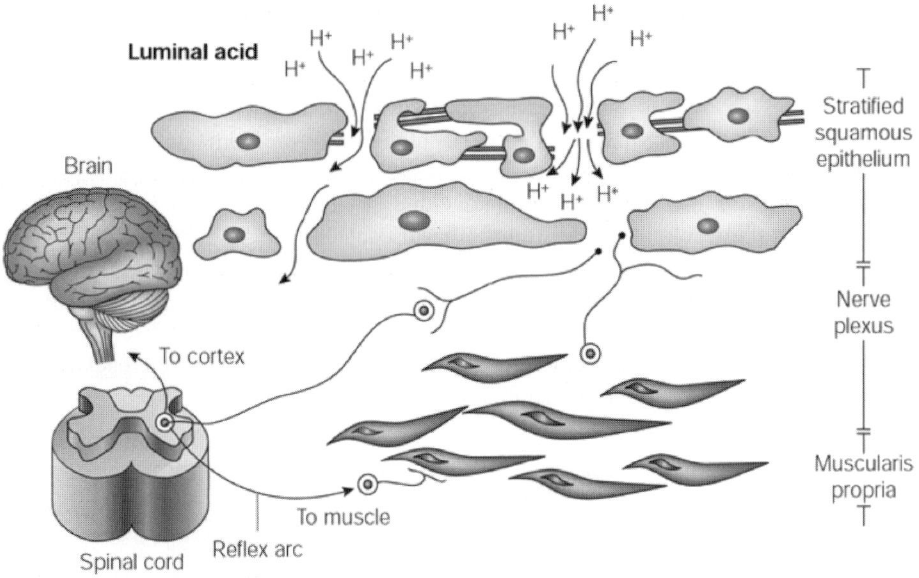

Figure 1. The presence of abnormal tissue resistance – demonstrated by defects within the intercellular junctional complex between cells of the surface layers of esophageal (stratified squamous) epithelium – is shown to enable the ready diffusion of refluxed gastric acid (H^+) into the intercellular space. Within this space, it encounters and activates chemosensitive nociceptors whose signals are transmitted *via* the spinal cord to the brain for symptom (heartburn) perception. Activation of the same nociceptors are also capable of initiating a short reflex arc to esophageal (longitudinal) smooth muscle as means of precipitating a sustained esophageal contraction. (Modified and reprinted with permission from [4]).

have no symptoms during the Bernstein test – this because the healthy epithelium limits the backdiffusion of acid into the tissue and so minimizes the rate and degree of nociceptor activation. Experimental evidence consistent with these concepts has been provided by monitoring CNS activity by functional magnetic resonance imaging during esophageal acid perfusion in both healthy and GERD subjects. The results showed that while esophageal acid perfusion triggers a signal to the same areas of CNS, the CNS signals in those with GERD were more rapid in onset and of greater magnitude than those in healthy subjects; and these differences are presumed to account for the fact that GERD subjects experienced "heartburn" during acid perfusion while healthy subjects remained symptom-free [5]. Currently there are two schools of thought relating to the means by which luminal acid produces the conscious symptom response in GERD. One suggests that the CNS events are the direct result of acid-activation of chemosensitive nociceptors within the esophageal wall [4]; the other suggests that acid-activation of the chemosensitive nociceptors first transmits the signal to the esophageal (longitudinal) musculature and that contraction of the (longitudinal) smooth muscle elicits the CNS signal for a symptom response [6]. Additional experiments are required to resolve this issue.

On endoscopy the reflux-damaged esophagus has two common forms: erosive esophagitis in which erosions are grossly evident and non-erosive reflux disease (NERD) in which the esophagus appears grossly normal [7]. Yet, despite the gross appearance, the esophageal epithelium in NERD is not "normal" – with significant abnormalities being reported on esophageal biopsy. Historically, using suction biopsy, the most sensitive and specific markers of NERD were reported to be basal cell hyperplasia and elongation of the rete pegs [8]. More recently, another lesion known as "dilated intercellular spaces" in esophageal squamous epithelium has been recognized on both light and electron microscopy as indicative of both erosive and non-erosive forms of GERD [8-13] (*Figure 2*). Further the lesion was shown to correlate with the symptom of heartburn in GERD and to resolve with the resolution of heartburn after a course of therapy with a proton pump inhibitor [14]. In addition, the lesion is present in GERD subjects irrespective of whether they had normal or abnormal acid contact time on 24-hour pH monitoring [9]. Experimental animal models of NERD also demonstrate that tissues containing dilated intercellular spaces are highly permeable and consequently that they can account for the backdiffusion of luminal acid into the tissue responsible for heartburn [15].

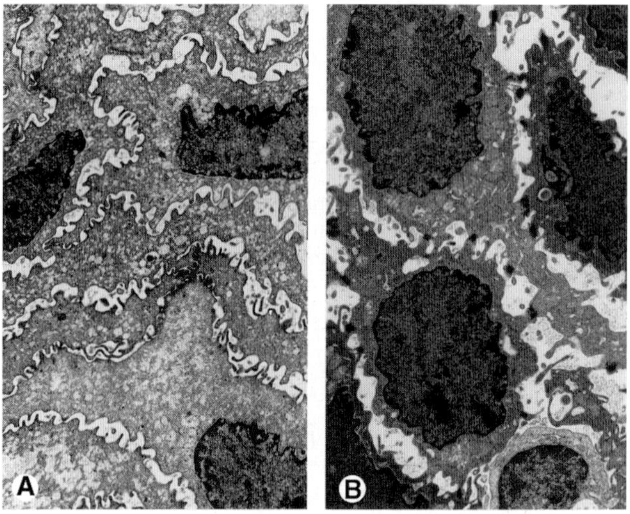

Figure 2. Transmission electron micrographs showing the differences in size of the intercellular spaces for normal (A) and non-erosive acid-damaged (B) esophageal epithelia. X9000 (Reprinted with permission from [4]).

The question posed above asks whether a correlation can be demonstrated between esophageal acid perfusion and "heartburn" – and the answer to this is that it depends – as it should – on whether the symptom of "heartburn" is the result of (active) GERD or not. Consequently, for accuracy, the question can be rephrased to ask whether a correlation can be demonstrated between esophageal acid perfusion and the "heartburn" of GERD? The reason for this is clear since many patients with self-described "heartburn" use the term indiscriminately to reflect other symptoms, e.g. belching and nausea, and others are labeled clinically as having the "heartburn" of GERD based solely on the presence of substernal (burning) pain, the latter symptom alone not pathognomonic of GERD since it occurs with other esophageal and non-esophageal conditions, e.g. esophageal motility disorders, cholelithiasis and panic attacks. The answer then to the question of whether a correlation can be demonstrated between esophageal acid perfusion and "heartburn" is affirmative when the "heartburn" results from GERD – though the correlation varies considerably among studies. Typically, specificity is high with values in one review ranging from 50% to 100% (average 86%) and sensitivity somewhat lower ranging from 42% to 100% (average 77%) [3]. Such variations are not surprising given differences in technique and patient populations selected for study. Moreover, a false negative test result will occur in GERD if acid suppression therapy is empirically initiated and esophageal healing occurs prior to study [16].

In summary, the Bernstein (esophageal acid perfusion) test correlates well with the symptom of heartburn when the symptom reflects a disease such as GERD that produces a damaged acid-permeable (distal) esophagus. And it doesn't correlate with symptoms mimicking "heartburn" when that symptom reflects the presence of other (esophageal or non-esophageal) disease unassociated with a damaged, acid-permeable, distal esophagus.

References

1. Bernstein LM, Baker LA. A clinical test for esophagitis. Gastroenterology 1958;34:760-81.
2. Bernstein LM, Fruin RD, Pacini R. Differentiation of esophageal pain from angina pectoris: role of the esophageal acid perfusion test. Medicine (Baltimore) 1962;41:143-62.
3. Richter JE. Provocative tests in esophageal diseases. In: Scarpignato C, Galmiche JP, eds. Functional investigation in esophageal disease. Frontiers of gastrointerstinal research. Basel: Karger, 1994;22:188-208.
4. Barlow WJ, Orlando RC. The pathogenesis of heartburn in nonerosive reflux disease: a unifying hypothesis. Gastroenterology 2005;128:771-8.
5. Kern M, Hofmann C, Hyde J, Shaker R. Characterization of the cerebral cortical representation of heartburn in GERD patients. Am J Physiol Gastrointest Liver Physiol 2004;286:G174-81.
6. Pehlivanov N, Liu J, Mittal RK. Sustained esophageal contraction: a motor correlate of heartburn symptom. Am J Physiol Gastrointest Liver Physiol 2001;281:G743-51.
7. Orlando RC. Reflux esophagitis. In: Yamada T, Alpers D, Owyang C, et al., eds. Textbook of gastroenterology. Philadelphia: JB Lippincott Williams & Wilkins, 1999:1235-63.
8. Calabrese C, Fabbri A, Bortolotti M, et al. Dilated intercellular spaces as a marker of oesophageal damage: comparative results in gastro-oesophageal reflux disease with or without bile reflux. Aliment Pharmacol Ther 2003;18:525-32.
9. Caviglia R, Ribolsi M, Maggiano N, et al. Dilated intercellular spaces of esophageal epithelium in nonerosive reflux disease patients with physiological esophageal acid exposure. Am J Gastroenterol 2005;100:543-8.
10. Ravelli AM, Villanacci V, Ruzzenenti N, et al. Dilated intercellular spaces: a major morphological feature of esophagitis. J Pediatr Gastroenterol Nutr 2006;42:510-5.
11. Solcia E, Villani L, Luinetti O, et al. Altered intercellular glycoconjugates and dilated intercellular spaces of esophageal epithelium in reflux disease. Virchows Arch 2000;436:207-16.
12. Tobey NA, Carson JL, Alkiek RA, Orlando RC. Dilated intercellular spaces: a morphological feature of acid reflux-damaged human esophageal epithelium. Gastroenterology 1996;111:1200-5.
13. Villanacci V, Grigolato PG, Cestari R, et al. Dilated intercellular spaces as markers of reflux disease: histology, semiquantitative score and morphometry upon light microscopy. Digestion 2001;64:1-8.
14. Calabrese C, Bortolotti M, Fabbri A, et al. Reversibility of GERD ultrastructural alterations and relief of symptoms after omeprazole treatment. Am J Gastroenterol 2005;100:537-42.
15. Tobey NA, Hosseini SS, Argote CM, Dobrucali AM, Awayda MS, Orlando RC. Dilated intercellular spaces and shunt permeability in nonerosive acid-damaged esophageal epithelium. Am J Gastroenterol 2004;99:13-22.
16. Massey BT. Wither the Bernstein test. Am J Gastroenterol 2004;99:416-20.

What are the causes of the antireflux effects of the Stretta procedure?

G. Triadafilopoulos (Stanford)

The Stretta procedure is an endoscopic therapy that delivers temperature-controlled radiofrequency energy to the muscle of the gastroesophageal junction (GEJ). The procedure significantly improves or eliminates gastroesophageal reflux disease (GERD) symptoms, improves patient quality of life and decreases medication use by increasing the antireflux barrier and significantly decreasing intraesophageal pH [1,2].

The 6 mm diameter Stretta catheter (Curon Medical Inc., Fremont, CA) contains a balloon/basket combination, which is adjustable by inflation to accommodate varying anatomy (6-30 mm outer diameter). After endoscopic positioning of the catheter and inflation of the balloon, the device deploys four nickel-titanium needle electrodes into the muscle of the GEJ and cardia. The Stretta generator delivers radiofrequency energy in an automated fashion under temperature and impedance control, using thermocouple monitoring while the power output is regulated by computer algorithm. Target tissue temperature is elevated and maintained at a predetermined level, while mucosal temperature is maintained a body temperature to prevent mucosal ulceration [3]. The end result of a Stretta session is the induction of several (> 50) linear burns within the muscle of the GEJ without associated mucosal scarring and stricture formation. Subsequent healing of these burns and collagen deposition within the muscle alters GEJ and cardia plasticity limits pathologic reflux without impairing esophageal clearance. The functional effect is noted within the ensuing 2 months and reaches a maximum 12 months after the procedure. Several potential mechanisms of action of Stretta have been proposed and investigated (*Table I*). They are broadly distinguished as mechanical, neurological, and placebo-induced.

Table I. Potential mechanisms of action of Stretta.

Mechanical	Lower esophageal sphincter pressure augmentation* Increased lower esophageal sphincter thickness* Gastric yield pressure increase* Improved gastric emptying*
Neurological	Decrease of transient lower esophageal relaxations* Sensory (vagal) denervation
Placebo effect	
*Associated with reduced esophageal acid exposure	

Mechanical effects of Stretta

Augmentation of the lower esophageal sphincter pressure profile

Stretta increases lower esophageal sphincter pressure (LESP) in porcine model of BoTox-induced LESP hypotension. In this model, BoTox was injected in the LES reducing the LESP. LESP was restored back to normal levels in Stretta-treated animals *versus* non-treated controls [4]. A modest increase of the post-prandial LESP 6 months after Stretta has also been found in 2 human trials [5,6].

Increased lower esophageal sphincter thickness

After Stretta, increased muscular wall thickness has been shown histopathologically in a canine model and endosonographically in a porcine model [7,8].

Gastric yield pressure increase

An increased gastric yield pressure (GYP) by 75% and LESP by 21% have been shown in a porcine model of reflux using BoTox injection followed by Stretta [4].

Improved gastric emptying

Stretta has been shown to accelerate gastric emptying. In one study with 17 patients, percentage gastric emptying at 90 minutes improved from 33 to 71%. It is postulated that the altered plasticity of the GEJ serves as a barrier to reflux, thus enhancing radionuclide clearance through the pylorus [9].

Neurological effects of Stretta

Decrease of transient lower esophageal relaxations

In a canine model, decreases in the transient lower esophageal sphincter relaxation (tLESR) frequency by 54% have been shown. In human Stretta studies incorporating 3-hour post-prandial esophageal manometry and pH monitoring after a standard meal (3,000 kJ, 55% fat) tLESR frequency was reduced by 25-70% [5,6].

Sensory (vagal) denervation

Early studies using Stretta in humans explored the possibility that radiofrequency ablation causes vagal injury at the level of the GEJ and cardia. DiBaise *et al.*, studied 8 patients before and after Stretta measuring pancreatic polypeptide levels in a standardized fashion, in which patients were asked to chew but not swallow toasted bacon and cheese sandwich. In such experiments, if pancreatic polypeptide (PP) levels are found below 25 pg/ml, vagal dysfunction is suggested. In this small group of patients, PP levels were 73.2 pg/ml before Stretta and fell to 54.4 pg/ml (NS) after the procedure, thus failing to support the hypothesis of vagal injury [5].

A recent report on 11 patients has claimed that Stretta causes distal esophageal desensitization [10]. In a modified Bernstein's test before and 6 months after Stretta, all patients had a positive Bernstein test before Stretta with a median time to report symptoms

(TRS) of 9 minutes; after the procedure, the median TRS was 17 minutes, significantly higher than the pre-procedural value. Such esophageal desensitization has been a theoretical concern since the initial Stretta US open-trial. In this trial, the percentage time with esophageal pH < 4.0 at 6-months after Stretta, albeit significantly reduced from 10.2% to 6.4% ($p \leq 0.0001$), did not normalize for all patients. This raised the possibility, for some, that ablation of the muscle of the GEJ desensitizes the esophagus, thus potentially masking symptoms of GERD. Therefore, critics of the procedure have proclaimed that Stretta maybe harmful to patients with GERD by allowing ongoing acid reflux after the procedure to cause distal esophageal mucosal damage without associated symptoms, even though no study has demonstrated worsened or silent esophagitis after Stretta.

To resolve this question, a recent *post hoc* study sought to determine if there was a correlation between the improvement in GERD outcomes and esophageal acid exposure after Stretta using the same data from the US open trial. If the effect of Stretta were due to reduced acid exposure, there would be a positive correlation between post-treatment control of GERD symptoms (GERD-HRQL and heartburn) and a reduced esophageal acid exposure, and a negative correlation between satisfaction and esophageal acid exposure. In contrast, if sensory denervation were responsible for the Stretta effect no such correlation would be found (*Figure 1*). The GERD-HRQL responder sub-group improved their median distal esophageal acid exposure time from a baseline of 10.4% to 4.3% ($p < 0.001$), while non-responders exhibited no change (10.9% to 7.7%, $p = 0.13$) (*Figure 2*). This evidence strongly suggests that the significant symptomatic improvement is due to a decrease in esophageal acid exposure and not due to desensitization of the esophageal body [11].

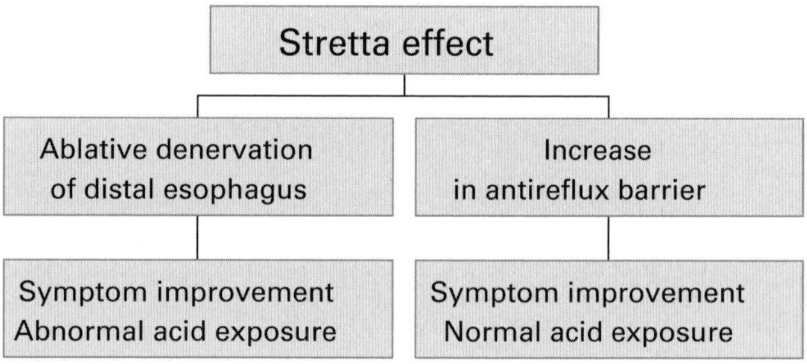

Figure 1. Two main interpretations that may explain the effect of Stretta.

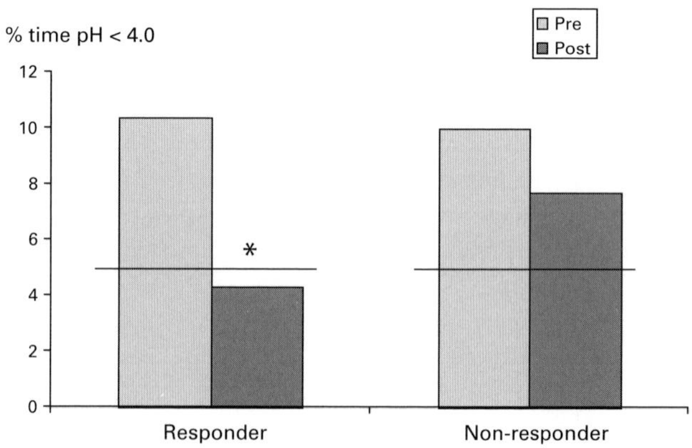

Figure 2. Distal esophageal acid exposure time (% time pH < 4.0) before and after Stretta, comparing responders and non-responders for GERD-HRQL outcome (*p < 0.05).

Placebo effect

The Stretta prospective, multicenter, sham-controlled, randomized trial enrolled 64 patients, 34 of whom were actively treated and 30 were sham-treated (balloon inflation only) with an option for Stretta at 6 months after the sham procedure. The primary endpoint of the trial was GERD symptom score improvement (GERD-HRQoL); secondary endpoints were general quality of life (SF-36), heartburn scores, acid exposure, and medication use (dose escalation). This trial showed a true benefit of Stretta over sham therapy, thereby making placebo effect an unlikely mechanism [12].

In conclusion, Stretta relieves GERD symptoms and quality of life, mostly by augmenting LESP and reducing the frequency of tLESRs which in turn decrease esophageal acid exposure and not by desensitizing the esophageal body. Nevertheless, the efforts for a better understanding on how the procedure works in GERD should be continued.

References

1. Triadafilopoulos G, DiBaise JK, Nostrant TT, et al. Radiofrequency energy delivery to the gastroesophageal junction for the treatment of GERD. Gastrointest Endosc 2001;53:407-15.
2. Triadafilopoulos G, Dibaise JK, Nostrant TT, et al. The Stretta procedure for the treatment of GERD: 6 and 12 month follow-up of the US open label trial. Gastrointest Endosc 2002;55:149-56.
3. Triadafilopoulos G. Stretta: an effective, minimally invasive treatment for gastroesophageal reflux disease. Am J Med 2003;115(3A):192S-200S.
4. Utley DS, Kim MS, Vierra MA, Triadafilopoulos G. Augmentation of lower esophageal sphincter pressure and gastric yield pressure after radiofrequency energy delivery to the gastro-esophageal junction: a porcine model. Gastrointest Endosc 2000;52(1):81-6.
5. DiBaise JK, Brand RE, Quigley EMM. Endoluminal delivery of radiofrequency energy to the gastroesophageal Junction in uncomplicated GERD: efficacy and potential mechanism of action. Am J Gastro 2002;97(4):833-42.
6. Tam WCE, Schoeman MN, Zhang Q, et al. Delivery of radiofrequency energy (RFe) to the lower oesophageal sphincter and gastric cardia inhibits transient lower oesophageal sphincter relaxations and gastro-oesophageal reflux in patients with reflux disease. Gut 2003;52:479-85.
7. Kim MS, Dent J, Holloway R, Utley DS. Radiofrequency energy delivery to the gastric cardia inhibits triggering of transient lower esophageal sphincter relaxation in a canine model. Gastrointest Endosc 2003;57:17-22.
8. Chang KJ, Utley DS. Endoscopic ultrasound (EUS) in vivo assessment of radiofrequency (RF) energy delivery to the gastroesophageal (GE) junction in a porcine model. Gastrointest Endosc 2001;53(5):AB 2001.
9. Noar M, Knight S, Bidlack D. Impaired gastric emptying in GERD patients improved after radiofrequency (RF) energy delivery to the gastroesophageal junction (Stretta procedure). Gastroenterology. 2002;122:A558.
10. Arts J, Van Olmen A, D'Haens G, et al. Radiofrequency delivery at the gastroesophageal junction in GERD improves acid exposure and symptoms and decreases esophageal sensitivity to acid infusion. AGA Plenary Session, DDW, 2003.
11. Triadafilopoulos G. Changes in symptom scores correlate with improvement in esophageal acid exposure after the Stretta procedure. Surg Endosc 2004;18:1038-44.

What is the value of intraluminal manometry?

M. Fox (Zurich)

The primary functions of the esophagus are to transport food and fluid from the mouth to the stomach and to prevent reflux of gastric contents. Although the underlying causes of gastroesophageal reflux disease (GERD) remain uncertain, the structure and function of the gastroesophageal junction (GEJ) is of key importance. In addition, esophageal dysfunction can exacerbate the condition by impairing the clearance of acid and other noxious substances (e.g. bile acid, pepsin) from the esophagus. The aim of esophageal manometry in this condition is to document and understand the physiological basis of GERD and to guide rational treatment. It is by these standards that the value of this investigation should be judged.

Patients with GERD present typically with heartburn and acid regurgitation; although dysphagia, chest pain, chronic cough and many other symptoms have been linked to the condition [1]. Conventional manometry can identify the occasional patient with major esophageal dysmotility (e.g. diffuse esophageal spasm, achalasia) that presents with "reflux symptoms"; however it is rare that such cases have no features suggesting the other diagnosis [2,3]. Rather in the majority of patients with reflux symptoms esophageal dysfunction as assessed by conventional manometry is not the major determinant of disease severity (i.e. acid exposure) [4,5], and basing therapeutic decisions (e.g. concerning anti-reflux surgery) on these findings has not been shown to improve outcomes [6,7]. Moreover even when dysmotility is present effective medical treatment is lacking. For these reasons guidelines do not recommend the routine use of manometry in GERD [8,9]. The likelihood that a patient with reflux symptoms be referred for physiologic measurement depends on the clinical history, examination, endoscopic findings and response to treatment. The presence of dysphagia, anaemia or weight loss demands endoscopic examination primarily to exclude malignancy. In the absence of "alarm findings" (or after endoscopy) a therapeutic trial of acid suppression using proton pump inhibitors (e.g.; omeprazole 20 mg b.d. for 2 weeks) is a reasonably accurate and cost-effective test to confirm the clinical diagnosis of GERD [8,10]. Even patients with atypical symptoms of GERD such as dysphagia and chronic cough often respond to acid suppression (although more prolonged high-dose treatment may be required). It is only when this approach has failed, and especially if surgical treatment of GERD is considered, that manometry in combination with ambulatory pH studies (± multi-channel intraluminal impedance – MII) is required to confirm the diagnosis [8,10].

At present conventional manometry with 4-8 pressure sensors including a sleeve sensor at the lower esophageal sphincter (LES) is the "reference standard" investigation of esophageal function. This technique defines esophageal dysfunction in terms of a few basic patterns: abnormal sphincter relaxation, esophageal spasm, hypertensive contractions, loss of tone and motility [11]. This classification is simple; however studies have shown that the esophageal function is complex comprising overlapping segments that contract in sequence to produce coordinated peristalsis and effective bolus transport (*Figure 1*) [12-14]. In addition research presented at OESO 2006 demonstrates that the GEJ has three distinct components (the intrinsic lower esophageal spincter – LES, the diaphragmatic crura plus the sling and clasp muscle fibres of the gastric cardia) that interact to form an effective

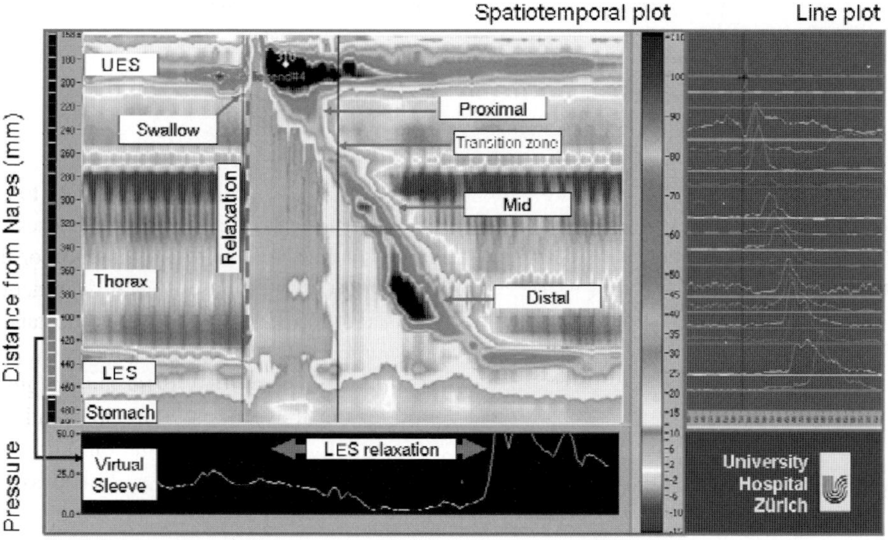

Figure 1. Normal water swallow as assessed by 32-channel, water perfused high resolution manometry (HRM). Time is on the x-axis and distance from the nares is on the y-axis. Each pressure is assigned a colour. The spatiotemporal plot presents the same information as the line plots; however the large volume of data is easier to appreciate in a single image than multiple line plots. Normal esophageal function is clearly demonstrated including the synchronous relaxation of the upper and lower esophageal sphincter on swallowing, and the increasing pressure and duration of the peristaltic wave as it passes distally. In addition subtle but functionally important pressure events are demonstrated. These include the transition zone (pressure trough) between the proximal and middle esophagus, the 'common cavity' pressure rise after the water swallow and the build up of intra-bolus pressure (the force that drives bolus transport) as peristalsis approaches the LES. (See page XIX for colour figure).

reflux barrier [15]. Indeed a high proportion of reflux events in patients with GERD occur during intermittent separations of the intrinsic and diaphragmatic components of the GEJ (*Figure 2*) [16]. These observations explain why pressure sensors spaced 4-6 cm apart cannot provide an adequate description of motor activity in the esophagus or the structure and function of the GEJ. It follows that conventional manometry cannot explain impaired esophageal clearance or the propensity to reflux in patients with GERD [14,16]. This is clinically relevant because esophageal symptoms and mucosal damage are more closely related to failed bolus transport and impaired clearance than measurements of esophageal motor activity by conventional manometry [17,18].

High-resolution manometry (HRM) is a new development in intraluminal pressure recording made possible by the development of miniaturised pressure sensors spaced at 1-2 cm intervals from the pharynx to the stomach. Data acquired by HRM can be analyzed and presented either as "line plots" or as a "spatiotemporal plot", a compact, visually intuitive display of esophageal function (*Figure 1*). HRM has practical advantages in everyday practice; in contrast to conventional manometry a pull-through is not required and shifts of position do not affect the reliability and reproducibility of pressure recordings [19]. Additionally HRM reveals the segmental character of esophageal peristalsis and the functional anatomy of the GEJ (*Figure 2*), a feature that facilitates the accurate placement

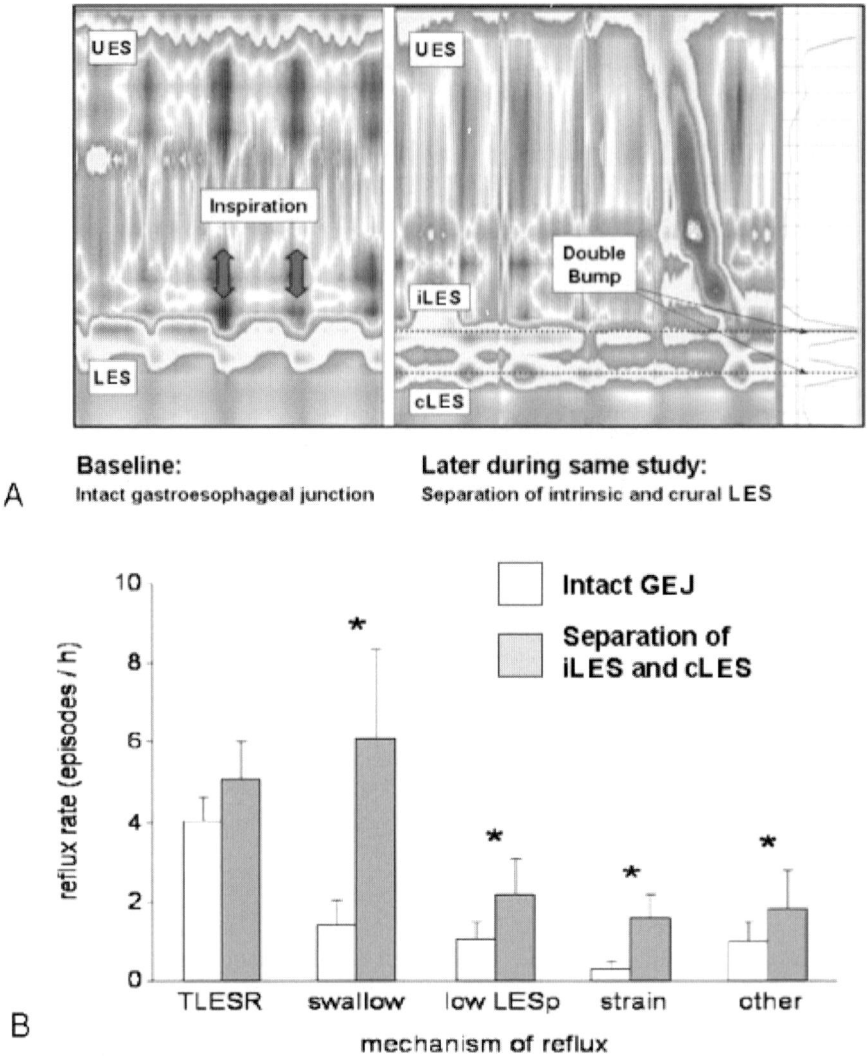

Figure 2. A. Contour plots of an individual patient at two points during a stationary HRM study. The left panel shows the gastroesophageal junction (GEJ) as a single high-pressure zone that rises and falls with respiration. The right panel shows spatial separation of the high-pressure zone into the intrinsic lower esophageal sphincter (iLES) and diaphragmatic crus (cLES) Partial relaxation of both components occurs during a dry swallow. The far right panel displays pressure measurements from the pharynx to the stomach at a single moment in time; "a virtual pull-through". Note the typical "double bump" indicating the presence of a small hiatus hernia (~3 cm). (See page XIX for colour figure). **B.** Reflux rate (episodes/hour) during periods of time when the GEJ is in the reduced (single pressure peak, open bars) and unreduced (double pressure peak, grey bars) hernia state. Significantly higher reflux rates were found during the unreduced state ($p \leq 0.05$). Transient LES relaxation was the most prevalent reflux mechanism during the reduced state; whereas the increase in reflux rate in the unreduced state is due to other reflux mechanisms ($p \leq 0.05$). (Reproduced from [16] with permission of the authors).

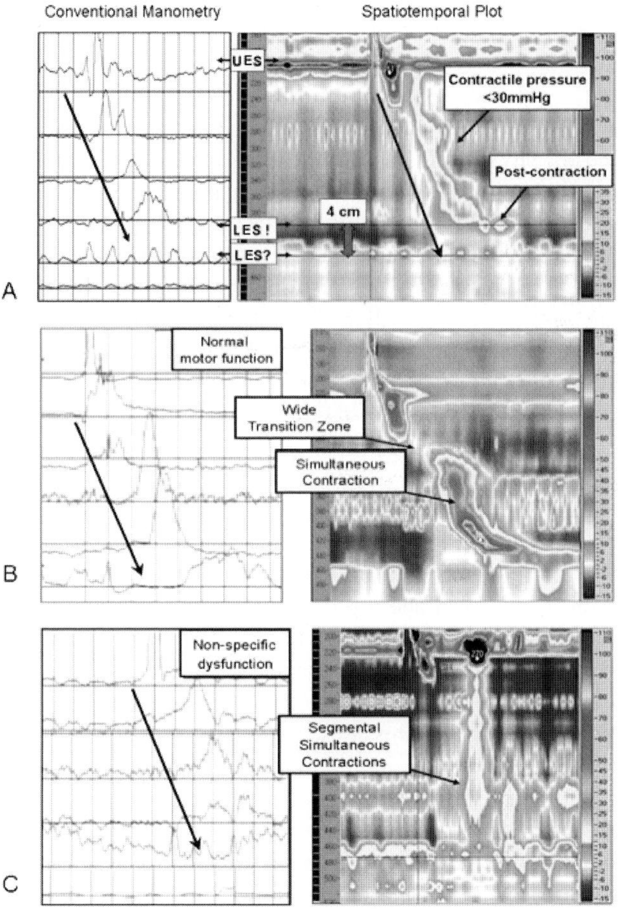

Figure 3. Three examples of conventional and high-resolution manometry in patients with reflux and/or regurgitation referred for physiological investigation. In each case conventional manometry was reported as "non-specific esophageal motor abnormality"; however HRM revealed distinct abnormalities of motor activity in each case with different effects on bolus transport. In the future HRM may guide specific management that addresses the underlying pathophysiology in such cases. **A.** This case illustrates two advantages of HRM. Firstly, the ease with which the appropriate position for pH studies can be found with HRM despite the presence of a large hiatus hernia and the absence of a high-pressure zone at the GEJ. Whereas it was not possible to locate the intrinsic LES by conventional manometry, HRM revealed the brief, weak LOS post-contraction. Secondly although this case would be labeled as "non-specific esophageal motor abnormality" or "ineffective esophageal function" on the basis of hypotensive contractile pressure, HRM reveals coordinated peristalsis from the UES to the LES indicating occlusive contraction and certainly consistent with bolus transport. **B.** Conventional manometry was essentially normal in this patient with longstanding dysphagia, chest pain and regurgitation; however HRM revealed focal abnormality of peristalsis with a wide proximal transition zone (pressure trough) and spasm in the mid-esophagus. Solid bolus escape was seen in this region on concurrent videofluoroscopy. **C.** Conventional manometry is not normal in this patient with "reflux symptoms", however the extent and nature of the motility disorder cannot be appreciated. The reason for this, clearly displayed by HRM, is that the esophageal spasm (simultaneous contraction) was not diffuse but segmental, occurring first in the mid- and then the distal-esophagus. LES function was normal and only mild reflux was present on pH studies (DeMeester score 21 (due to poor acid clearance)). Bolus escape and pendular movement of liquid barium was observed on concurrent videofluoroscopy. (Reproduced from [14]). (See page XX for colour figure).

of pH probes (*Figure 3A*) [20]. More fundamentally, HRM displays the pressure gradient during bolus transport, the force that directs the movement of food and fluid through the esophagus and across the GEJ [21,22]. As a result HRM increases the accuracy with which bolus transport can be predicted from manometry and identifies clinically important abnormalities not detected by conventional manometry [14,21]. In a clinical study of 212 consecutive patients referred for physiologic measurement HRM identified important esophageal dysfunction more accurately than conventional manometry (using final diagnosis at six month follow-up as the "gold standard") [20].

The value of HRM in GERD has not yet been studied; however its ability to distinguish between abnormalities of esophageal motor activity that disturb bolus transport from those that have no effect on function suggest that it will have a greater impact on clinical management than conventional manometry [14,20]. Patients with reflux symptoms rarely have major esophageal dysfunction but "non-specific motor disorders" are common [11]. Combining conventional manometry and MII clarifies the relevance of these findings for individual patients ("ineffective esophageal motility" is present if bolus transport is incomplete in > 30% swallows) [17], but this still does not describe the abnormal motor activity underlying impaired function. Most studies define esophageal dysmotility in GERD on the basis of contractile pressure < 30 mmHg; however studies with concurrent HRM and videofluoroscopy show that hypotensive contractions are consistent with normal function if peristaltic coordination is preserved and a positive pressure gradient from the proximal to the distal esophagus is maintained (*Figure 3A*). In contrast a wide "proximal transition zone" between the proximal and mid-distal esophagus and/or focal spasm in the smooth muscle esophagus (both difficult to detect with conventional manometry) can disrupt bolus transport despite normal contractile pressures (*Figure 3B, 3C*). It is intriguing to note that a wide "proximal transition zone" is more common in patients with reflux esophagitis than healthy controls and may impair esophageal clearance in this group [23]. In addition HRM provides a vivid demonstration of the dynamic interaction between the intrinsic and diaphragmatic components of the GEJ and it should be possible also to assess the contribution of the gastric cardia to the reflux barrier. Future studies will report on whether these measurements provide clinically relevant information that can be used to guide management. With the introduction of new, more effective prokinetics it may be that HRM can identify abnormalities in esophageal motor activity that respond to specific medications (e.g. nitrate donors, tegaserod) [24]. In patients that do not respond to medical therapy, it could be that the presence of esophageal dysmotility that impairs bolus transport (e.g. focal spasm) indicates the need for "partial" rather than "full" fundoplication, whereas other manometric abnormalities (e.g. hypotensive peristalsis) have no bearing on outcome and may resolve after surgery [6,7]. It can also be speculated that patients in whom the reflux barrier is unstable should be considered for antireflux surgery, whereas those with preserved GEJ anatomy should be treated with medications that suppress transient LES relaxation (e.g. baclofen).

In conclusion the value of conventional manometry in GERD is limited to the exclusion of major esophageal dysmotility and management decisions cannot based on its findings alone. Indeed in patients with reflux symptoms the main use of conventional manometry is only to guide catheter placement for pH ± MII studies. HRM is an important advance that provides detailed and objective information that can clarify the relationship between esophageal motor function, bolus transport and symptoms. This technology has improved our understanding of esophageal bolus transport and LES function. Although the value of HRM in GERD has yet to be established, there is a real possibility that improved understanding of the pathophysiology underlying reflux events and impaired esophageal clearance will guide rational treatment tailored to the needs of individual patients with reflux symptoms.

References

1. Fox M, Forgacs I. Gastro-oesophageal reflux disease. Br Med J 2006;332:88-93.
2. Costantini M, Crookes PF, Bremner RM, et al. Value of physiologic assessment of foregut symptoms in a surgical practice. Surgery 1993;114(4):780-7.
3. Tarkan D, Ergun G. Grand rounds in gastroenterology from Baylor College of Medicine - Dysphagia after laparoscopic fundoplication. Medscape Gastroenterol 2001;3(1).
4. Diener U, Patti MG, Molena D, Fisichella PM, Way LW. Esophageal dysmotility and gastroesophageal reflux disease. J Gastrointest Surg 2001;5(3):260-5.
5. DiBaise JK, Lof J, Quigley EM. Can symptoms predict esophageal motor function or acid exposure in gastroesophageal reflux disease? A comparison of esophageal manometric and twenty-four-hour pH parameters in typical and extraesophageal gastroesophageal reflux disease. J Clin Gastroenterol 2001;32(2):128-32.
6. Fibbe C, Layer P, Keller J, Strate U, Emmermann A, Zornig C. Esophageal motility in reflux disease before and after fundoplication: a prospective, randomized, clinical, and manometric study. Gastroenterology 2001;121(1):5-14.
7. Hakanson BS, Thor KB, Pope CE 2nd. Preoperative oesophageal motor activity does not predict postoperative dysphagia. Eur J Surg 2001;167(6):433-7.
8. NICE. (North of England Dyspepsia Guideline Development Group). Dyspepsia: managing dyspepsia in adults in primary care. National Institute of Clinical Excellance, London; 2004.
9. Pandolfino JE, Kahrilas PJ. American Gastroenterological Association medical position statement: clinical use of esophageal manometry. Gastroenterology 2005;128(1):207-8.
10. Talley N, Vakil N. Guidelines for the management of dyspepsia. Am J Gastroenterol 2005;100:2324-37.
11. Spechler SJ, Castell DO. Classification of oesophageal motility abnormalities. Gut 2001;49(1):145-51.
12. Clouse RE, Staiano A. Topography of the esophageal peristaltic pressure wave. Am J Physiol 1991;261:G677-84.
13. Li M, Brasseur JG, Dodds WJ. Analyses of normal and abnormal esophageal transport using computer simulations. Am J Physiol 1994;266:G525-43.
14. Fox M, Hebbard G, Janiak P, et al. High-resolution manometry predicts the success of oesophageal bolus transport and identifies clinically important abnormalities not detected by conventional manometry. Neurogastroenterol Motil 2004;16(5):533-42.
15. Brasseur JG, Ulerich R, Dai Q, Patel D, Soliman A, Miller LS. Pharmacological dissection of the gastro-oesophageal segment into three sphincteric components. J Physiol. 2007;580:961-75.
16. Bredenoord AJ, Weusten BL, Timmer R, Smout AJ. Intermittent spatial separation of diaphragm and lower esophageal sphincter favors acidic and weakly acidic reflux. Gastroenterology 2006;130(2):334-40.
17. Tutuian R, Castell DO. Combined multichannel intraluminal impedance and manometry clarifies esophageal function abnormalities: study in 350 patients. Am J Gastroenterol 2004;99(6):1011-9.
18. Bredenoord AJ, Weusten BL, Curvers WL, Timmer R, Smout AJ. Determinants of perception of heartburn and regurgitation. Gut 2006;55(3):313-8.
19. Nayar DS, Khandwala F, Achkar E, et al. Esophageal manometry: assessment of interpreter consistency. Clin Gastroenterol Hepatol 2005;3(3):218-24.
20. Clouse RE, Staiano A, Alrakawi A, Haroian L. Application of topographical methods to clinical esophageal manometry. Am J Gastroenterol 2000;95(10):2720-30.
21. Staiano A, Clouse RE. Detection of incomplete lower esophageal sphincter relaxation with conventional point-pressure sensors. Am J Gastroenterol 2001;96(12):3258-67.
22. Ghosh SK, Pandolfino JE, Zhang Q, Jarosz A, Shah N, Kahrilas PJ. Quantifying esophageal peristalsis with high-resolution manometry: a study of 75 asymptomatic volunteers. Am J Physiol Gastrointest Liver Physiol 2006;290(5):G988-97.
23. Janiak P, Ghosh S, Hebbard G, et al. Changes in upper esophageal motor function in reflux esophagitis defined by high resolution manometry. Gastroenterology 2001;DDW abstract.
24. Fox M, Fried M, Menne D, Stutz B, Schwizer W. The effect of tegaserod on esophageal function: a randomized controlled trial in healthy volunteers Aliment Pharmacol Ther 2006;24:1017-27.

Why does hiatal hernia rarely exist with achalasia?

V. Nilton Felix (São Paulo)

Fixation of the diaphragm to the lower end of the esophagus and to the cardia of the stomach is obtained by the diaphragmatic esophageal membrane that consists of elastic and fibrous tissue originating in the fascial coverings of the diaphragm, mostly from the abdominal side but partly from the thoracic side of the diaphragm.

This elastic and fibrous membrane has its origin lateral to the muscular ring of the hiatus, over which it passes, with slight attachments to fill the space between the inner margin of the muscle and the esophagus; it is inserted into the lower 2 or 3 centimeters of the esophagus and into the upper 1.5 to 2 centimeters of the stomach, in a fanlike manner.

The diaphragmatic esophageal membrane constitutes a flexible connection from the diaphragm to the esophagus and cardia, and permits some mobility during the act of swallowing and during respiratory movements. Its greatest strength is in its esophageal attachment, where it acts as an antagonist to the longitudinal muscle fibers of the esophagus, preventing these muscles from pulling the cardia through the hiatus.

The membrane with the circular and oblique muscle layers at the cardia can also play an important role in sphincteric action at the cardia by maintaining the normal angular anatomic relationship between the lower end of the esophagus and the stomach [1].

The normal peritoneal covering and attachments of the esophagus and cardia of the stomach, around the esophageal hiatus, are of great importance.

The abdominal portion of the esophagus is loosely covered with peritoneum on its anterior and left aspects. The uppermost part of the stomach is loosely covered below the esophagus for about 2 centimeters anteriorly and 3 centimeters posteriorly. The peritoneum then fuses with the serous covering of the gastric wall and the union of the two folds of peritoneum forms the gastrophrenic ligament, which fixes the cardiac end of the stomach to the diaphragm and continues to the left to form the phrenocolic ligament.

Beneath this loose peritoneal covering lie a triangular pad of fat and connective tissue and the attachments of the diaphragmatic esophageal membrane. This loose peritoneal attachment around the esophageal hiatus also permits flexible movement of the esophagus.

Sliding hernia is the most common variety of hiatal hernia and predisposing factors include increased elasticity, loss of tonicity of the diaphragmatic crura, dilatation of the esophageal hiatus and relaxation of gastroesophagodiaphragmatic ligaments because of constitutional weakness of connective tissue, obesity, multiple pregnancies, repeated vomits, chronic cough and the sucking action of the thoracic cavity in the presence of increased subdiaphragmatic pressure [2].

Reducible sliding hernias displace freely to either the thoracic or abdominal cavity depending on the respiratory phase, body position or degree of gastric filling, but, because of persistent abdominal pressure increase due professional activity, radical sportive practice or repeated great volume meals, sliding hernias become irreducible and subsequent esophageal shortening can occur.

The slow gastric emptying also is potentially capable to cause or increase hiatal hernia determining vomits or continuous pressure increase upwards through hiatal ring.

The entire hiatus is progressively incompetent, the cardiac end of the stomach protrudes above the diaphragm, the esophagus is elevated and is at the apex of the herniated portion of the cardia.

There is not a true hernial sac and may not be considered a true hernia and the diagnosis is best established by roentgenographic examination, including esophagoscopy to measure the length of the esophagus and to determine the possible presence of lesions associated with the hernia such as esophagitis and strictures.

Many of the hiatal hernias of elderly people probably result from incompetence of the hiatus, due to atrophy of this protective elastic membrane, that is sufficiently strong during the prime of life to protect the hiatal opening but, as atrophy of the elastic tissue associated with advancing years weakens the membrane, the stomach protrudes through the large hiatus to a position above the diaphragm.

In such cases, herniation probably would have occurred earlier in life if abnormal stress, such as trauma, respiratory difficulty or marked increase of intra-abdominal pressure had been applied.

During embryologic development the stomach descends behind the septum transversum. If its descent is delayed, the lumbar portion of the diaphragm will be imperfectly developed and the esophageal hiatus will form around the anlage of the stomach instead of around the lower part of the esophagus.

This will result in an abnormally large esophageal hiatus and in some instances in deficiency of its muscular ring and also abnormal attachments of the diaphragmatic esophageal membrane and the ligaments from the diaphragm to the stomach and spleen.

Acquired similar problem can be caused by traumatic or rheumatic vertebral column deformations.

Abnormal enlargement of the esophageal hiatus results in an abnormally wide space between the muscle ring and the walls of the esophagus – the more defective the hiatus, the more likely that herniation of the viscera will occur, because this abnormal relationship will permit much greater flexibility of the esophagus in the enlarged hiatus than is normal.

The esophagus rarely does not develop normally in length to reach the diaphragm and a portion of the cardiac end of the stomach remains in the thorax because of the congenitally short esophagus.

Marked variation found in the size of the hiatus during operative procedures, under normal conditions, reinforces considerable variation in its embryologic formation.

Achalasia has effects on both the muscles and nerves of the esophagus; however, the effects on the nerves are the most important. Early in achalasia, inflammation can be seen under the microscope in the muscle of the lower esophagus, especially around the nerves.

The patients have dysphagia, usually for liquids as well as solids that is not explained by fixed stenosis or inflammation in the esophagus. The barium swallow often, but not invariably, shows features suggestive of classic achalasia with a dilated esophagus that terminates in a beak-like narrowing caused by the dysfunctional lower esophageal sphincter (LES).

Classic achalasia is perhaps the best understood and best characterised esophageal motility disorder, in which there is degeneration of neurones in the wall of the esophagus [3,4]. The degenerative process appears to involve preferentially the nitric oxide producing inhibitory neurones that effect relaxation of esophageal smooth muscle [5,6].

The smooth muscle of the LES is normally tonically contracted at rest and relaxes when intramural neurones release their inhibitory neurotransmitters [7]. Loss of inhibitory innervation in the LES can cause basal sphincter pressures to rise and can interfere with normal relaxation.

Unlike the LES, the smooth muscle of the esophageal body does not exhibit resting tone and therefore loss of inhibitory neurones has little effect on resting pressure in the body of the esophagus. Inhibitory influences are necessary for normal peristalsis however and loss of inhibitory neurones can result in aperistalsis [8].

Certain recognized diseases can cause esophageal motor abnormalities similar or identical to those of primary achalasia. In Chagas disease seen in Central and South America, for example, esophageal infection with the protozoan parasite *Trypanosoma cruzi* can result in loss of intramural ganglion cells that causes aperistalsis and incomplete LES relaxation [9,10].

Symptoms are due primarily to the fact that swallow induced LES relaxation is inadequate either because it is incomplete in amplitude or too short in duration [10].

The clinical feature common to these atypical disorders is that affected patients have dysphagia which responds to treatments that decrease resting LES pressure (pneumatic dilation, Heller myotomy, botulinum toxin injection).

The manometric features proposed for a diagnosis of achalasia are: incomplete relaxation of the LES and aperistalsis in the body of the esophagus characterized either by simultaneous esophageal contractions.

Manometric features that are characteristic of achalasia but not required for the diagnosis include: elevated resting LES pressure and resting pressure in the esophageal body that exceeds resting pressure in the stomach.

This is supported too by a recent study that used high-frequency ultrasound probe catheter, concurrent manometry and ultrasound images of the esophagus, to demonstrate

Table I. Facts that explain why hiatal hernia rarely exists with achalasia.

Hiatal hernia (HH)	Achalasia (AC)	HH + AC in 3,600 patients Endoscopy = HH
Embryologic malformation of the hiatus	–	–
Acquired enlargement of the esophageal hiatus (traumatic, for example)	?	1
Elder patient	Younger patient	–
Weak hiatus	Strong hiatus	–
Obesity	Weight loss	–
Multiple pregnancies	?	1
Vomits	Regurgitations	–
Chronic cough	?	2
Increased subdiaphragmatic pressure (slow gastric emptying)	Reduced subdiaphragmatic pressure (slow esophageal emptying)	–
–	Acquired enlargement of the esophageal hiatus due to forced dilation of the cardia	3

that the LES and esophageal muscle thickness as well as esophageal muscle cross-sectional area are greater in patients with achalasia than in normal subjects [11].

A number of the patients operated upon for hiatal hernia have also had gastroduodenal ulcer, slow gastric emptying symptoms, cholecystic disease with vomits or obstructive carcinoma of the stomach.

Achalasia was rarely associated to hiatal hernia in our experience (3,600 patients with endoscopic diagnosis of hiatal hernia submitted to esophageal manometry): three patients submitted to repeated forceful dilation of the cardia, potentially capable to weak the connective tissue and the attachments of the diaphragmatic esophageal membrane, two elderly patients with chronic cough due to repeated pulmonary aspiration, one woman after multiple pregnancies and a man with traumatic column deformation (*Table I*).

In achalasia the patients are often young, have a strong hiatus seen at operative procedures, loose weight (do not present obesity) and do not have respiratory problems. The regurgitation, an almost passive phenomenon, does not force the hiatus and the slow esophageal emptying does not permit gastric distension.

Achalasia is a disease in which etiologic, physiopathologic and clinical events does not result predisposing mechanical efforts to hiatal hernia. On the contrary they could be considered antagonists to the sliding hernias through the hiatus, and could explain why hiatal hernia rarely exists with achalasia.

References

1. Harrington SW. Esophageal hiatus diaphragmatic hernia. Thoracic Surg 1938;8:127-48.
2. Hill LD, Tobias J, Morgan EH. Newer concepts of the pathophysiology of hiatal hernia and esophagitis. Am J Surg 1966;111:70-5.
3. Reynolds JC, Parkman HP. Achalasia. Gastroenterol Clin North Am 1989;18:223-55.
4. Goldblum JR, Whyte RI, Orringer MB. Achalasia. A morphologic study of 42 resected specimens. Am J Surg Pathol 1994;18:327-37.
5. Holloway RH, Dodds WJ, Helm JF. Integrity of cholinergic innervation to the lower esophageal sphincter in achalasia. Gastroenterology 1986;90:924-9.
6. Singaram C, Koch J, Gaumnitz EA. Nature of neuronal loss in human achalasia. Gastroenterology 1996;110:A259.
7. Saha HK, Sengupta JN, Goyal RK. Role of chloride ions in lower esophageal sphincter tone and relaxation. Am J Physiol 1992;263:115-26.
8. Yamato S, Spechler SJ, Goyal RK. Role of nitric oxide in esophageal peristalsis in the opossum. Gastroenterology 1992;103:197-204.
9. Spechler SJ. AGA technical review on treatment of patients with dysphagia caused by benign disorders of the distal esophagus. Gastroenterology 1999;117:233-54.
10. Felix VN, Cecconello I, Moraes Filho JPP, Pinotti WH. Achalasia: a prospective study comparing the results of dilatation and myotomy. Hepatogastroenterology 1998;45:97-108.
11. Mittal RK, Kassab G, Puckett JL, Liu J. Hypertrophy of the muscularis propria of the lower esophageal sphincter and the body of the esophagus in patients with primary motility disorders of the esophagus. Am J Gastroenterol 2003;98:1705-12.

What are the mechanisms of the association between *Helicobater pylori* infection and gastroesophageal reflux disease?

I. Sarosiek, M. Majewski, J. Sarosiek (Kansas City)

Direct impact of *Helicobacter pylori* on lower esophageal sphincter basal tone: Unlikely
Direct impact of *H. pylori* on transient lower esophageal sphincter relaxation: Unlikely
Direct impact of *H. pylori* on esophageal acid clearance: Unlikely
Direct impact of *H. pylori* on obesity epidemic: Unlikely

There is only very little evidence that *Helicobacter pylori* may have the potential for interaction with the quality of gastroesophageal refluxate (GER) as *H. pylori*-induced gastritis influences the acidity of gastric secretion, thus setting the stage for gastric disorders and indirectly only might mildly modify the esophageal mucosal inflammation related to GER.

The fact that the human esophageal mucosa is covered by the squamous epithelium lacking the skin-type of the keratin layer that is present in rodents, and the most aggressive neighborhood of the highly injurious acidic and peptic gastric milieu makes the contemplation of pathogenesis of GER disease (GERD) so challenging.

The integrity of the alimentary tract mucosa, and the esophageal mucosa in particular, depends upon an equilibrium between aggressive factors and protective mechanisms [1-10].

In patients with GERD, especially accompanied by endoscopic erosions, so called reflux esophagitis with Barrett's esophagus, the esophageal epithelium is under relentless challenge from acid and pepsin within the GER [1-3,7,11-14].

Since injurious components of the GER always act on the luminal aspect of the squamous epithelium, the mucus/buffer layer (0.095 μm thick) covering the mucosa represents a vanguard of mucosal defense, the so-called pre-epithelial barrier [6]. This mucus/buffer layer is continuously eroded by the luminal mechanical and chemical (acid/pepsin of GER) forces and restored due to continuous secretion from esophageal submucosal mucous glands as well as deposited freshly from swallowed salivary secretion [4,5,11,15,16]. Of note, as we have recently demonstrated for the first time in humans, both protective factors elaborated by salivary and esophageal submucosal mucous glands, especially bicarbonate and non-bicarbonate buffers, EGF, and TGFα are significantly augmented by stimulation of serotonin receptor $5HT_4$ [17].

We have published our finding that the content of mucin, the predominant and most protective component of mucus elaborated by esophageal submucosal mucous glands, in patients with reflux esophagitis is significantly impaired [18]. Furthermore, we have recently demonstrated for the first time in humans that healing of reflux esophagitis with rabeprazole (8 weeks of 20 mg QD) results in significant increase in the rate of secretion of esophageal mucin both in basal conditions (during mucosal exposure to initial saline) and during mucosal challenge with HCl/pepsin, mimicking the natural GER scenario ($P < 0.01$) (I. Sarosiek *et al. Am J Gastroenterol*, in submission).

This may indicate that an impairment in the protective qualities of the esophageal pre-epithelial barrier could be partly pre-existing and partly a secondary phenomenon related to severe inflammation of the esophageal mucosa and submucosal, narrowing the esophageal submucosal mucous glands ducts and their ability to secrete and deposit on the surface of the esophageal mucosa the freshly produced mucin.

In another novel, double-blind, placebo-controlled, cross-over designed study protocol we have demonstrated that administration of naproxen (500 mg BID) for 7 days results in significant decline of gastrin mucin production in basal conditions (by 39%, $P < 0.01$) and during stimulation with pentagastrin (by 49%, $P < 0.01$). Co-administration, however, of naproxen (500 mg BID) with rabeprazole (20 mg QD) resulted in significant restoration of an impairment in mucin production in pentagastrin-stimulated conditions (by 67%, $P = 0.003$) and in basal conditions (by 40%, $P = 0.05$) [19].

It is legitimate, therefore, to assume that the pharmacodynamic property of rabeprazole, augmenting mucin production, with or without co-administration of naproxen, within the esophageal and gastric mucous glands, may potentially benefit the upper gastrointestinal tract mucosal integrity [7].

Figure 1 shows the hypothetical overview of the various clinical scenarios in which the digestive power of the gastric milieu is encountering a strong or weak defense within the vanguard of protective potential within the esophageal pre-epithelial defense.

Considering the fact that any significant quantitative change in gastric juice acidity, which is always accompanied by proteolytic activity of pepsins, may negatively impact the existing equilibrium especially in patients with weaker mucosal protective mechanisms, one may anticipate that *H. pylori* may have some influence in some patients who respond to *H. pylori* antral gastritis by activating hyper secretion of acid leading to duodenal ulcer or body and/or pangastritis accompanied by hypochlorhydria.

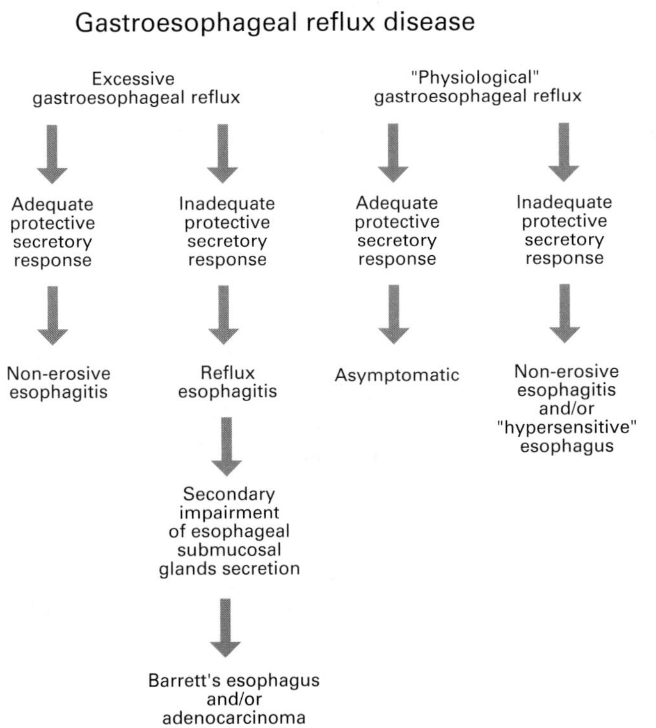

Figure 1. Hypothetical interrelationship between aggressive factors and protective mechanisms elaborated within salivary and esophageal submucosal mucous glands in pathogenesis of gastroesophageal reflux-related esophageal mucosal injury and complications [1,2,7, 17,18].

Furthermore, the prevalence of *H. pylori* colonization is continuously declining especially within industrialized nations, as increasing socio-economic status improves the hygiene of food preparation and storage. At the same time these nations are facing growing incidence of Barrett's esophagus and esophageal adenocarcinoma. But the real culprits of this coincidence are the epidemics of metabolic syndrome, overweight and obesity. A direct link between BMI and esophageal acid exposure in patients with GERD has been recently demonstrated. Speculation that declining *H. pylori* could be the factor in increasing incidence of Barrett's esophagus and AdCa, although tempting, should not be continued.

The other way to address the serendipity of these two phenomena is simply by eradication of *H. pylori* colonization among patients with GERD and assessment of severity of GER symptomatology before and after therapy with proton pump inhibitors (PPIs).

Recently, 690 patients from two similar randomized, placebo controlled trials of *H. pylori* eradication in non-ulcer dyspepsia were studied in Western population [20]. Symptoms were assessed during a 1-week run-in period, at 6 months and 12 months. Endoscopy was performed at baseline and at 3 months and 12 months to determine if esophagitis was present. As expected, antrum-predominant gastritis (55%) was more frequently found than corpus-predominant gastritis (6%). Erosive esophagitis developed in 7% of the eradicated group compared with 2% in the control group, but there was no significant difference after adjustment for any esophagitis present at baseline [20].

It seems that neither *H. pylori* infection nor its eradication causes GERD [21]. Furthermore, *H. pylori* eradication also does not impede antisecretory therapy with antisecretory drugs, especially PPIs [21].

Among patients treated with rabeprazole in clinical practice, *H. pylori* infection or its absence has no effect on the speed or degree of GERD symptom relief [22].

H. pylori induced duodenal ulcers frequently coincide with GERD, therefore it is plausible that the development of GERD following successful eradication of *H. pylori* represents the unmasking of an existing disorder rather than its *de novo* development [23].

In general, facing the GERD and *H. pylori* dilemma, regardless of patient diagnosis, the balance should be in favor of *H. pylori* eradication [24]. This is of great clinical importance in patients with body gastritis (*Figure 2*) who, if they are demonstrated by genotyping to

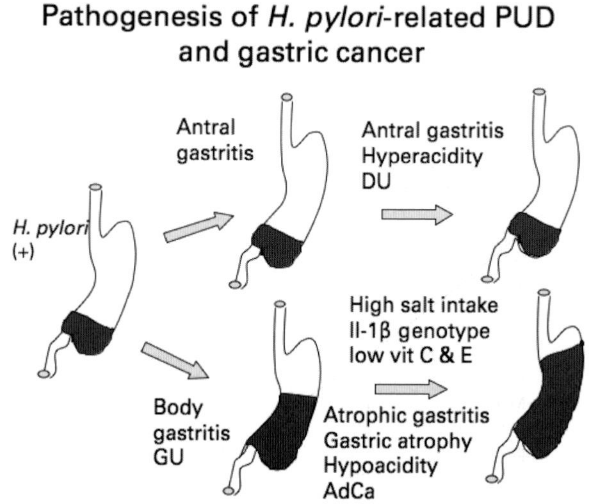

Figure 2. The inter-relationship between the type of *H. pylori*-induced gastritis and the development of clinical sequelae, thus setting the rationale for its eradication [25].

carry homozygous IL-1β511T proinflammatory allele, are more likely do develop gastric atrophy potentially setting the stage for subsequent development of gastric adenocarcinoma [8,21,25].

There is some degree of probability that if a clinical study based on a small sample size is conducted, patients with predominant antral gastritis may have slightly different final outcomes than patients with body gastritis. But this impact is too small to taken seriously into consideration during management of patients with GERD and/or *H. pylori* colonization.

The gastric outcome of *H. pylori* colonization should be taken most seriously and managed adequately by our state-of-the-art knowledge of *H. pylori* eradication.

In conclusion

A direct impact of *H. pylori* colonization on the motility of the esophageal body or LES is highly unlikely.

Some indirect impact on the quality of gastroesophageal refluxate, especially its acidity is plausible but its clinical relevance for the management of GERD symptoms and development of complications remains unproven.

References

1. Sarosiek J, McCallum RW. Mechanisms of esophageal mucosal defense. Best Pract Res Clin Gastroenterol 2000;14(5):701-17.
2. Sarosiek J, Jensen RT, Maton PN, et al. Salivary and gastric epidermal growth factor in patients with Zollinger-Ellison syndrome: its protective potential. Am J Gastroenterol 2000;95(5):1158-65.
3. Sarosiek J, Scheurich CJ, Marcinkiewicz M, McCallum RW. Enhancement of salivary esophagoprotection: rationale for a physiological approach to gastroesophageal reflux disease. Gastroenterology 1996;110(3):675-81.
4. Sarosiek J, McCallum RW. Do salivary organic components play a protective role in health and disease of the esophageal mucosa? Digestion 1995;56:32-7.
5. Sarosiek J, McCallum RW. What role do salivary inorganic components play in health and disease of the esophageal mucosa? Digestion 1995;56:24-31.
6. Sarosiek J, McCallum RW. What is the secretory potential of submucosal mucous glands within the human gullet in health and disease? Digestion 1995;56:15-23.
7. Namiot Z, Sarosiek J, Rourk RM, Hetzel DP, McCallum RW. Human esophageal secretion: mucosal response to luminal acid and pepsin. Gastroenterology 1994106(4):973-81;.
8. Sarosiek J, Marshall BJ, Peura DA, Hoffman S, Feng T, McCallum RW. Gastroduodenal mucus gel thickness in patients with Helicobacter pylori: a method for assessment of biopsy specimens. Am J Gastroenterol 1991;86(6):729-34.
9. Sarosiek J, Slomiany A, Slomiany BL. Evidence for weakening of gastric mucus integrity by Campylobacter pylori. Scand J Gastroenterol 1988;23(5):585-90.
10. Slomiany BL, Sarosiek J, Slomiany A. Gastric mucus and the mucosal barrier. Dig Dis 1987;5(3):125-45.
11. Marcinkiewicz M, Namiot Z, Edmunds MC, McCallum RW, Sarosiek J. Detrimental impact of acid and pepsin on the rate of luminal release of transforming growth factor alpha. Its potential pathogenetic role in the development of reflux esophagitis. J Clin Gastroenterol 1996;23(4):261-8.
12. Hirschowitz BI. A critical analysis, with appropriate controls, of gastric acid and pepsin secretion in clinical esophagitis. Gastroenterology 1991;101(5):1149-58.
13. Walker V, Taylor WH. Pepsin 1 secretion in chronic peptic ulceration. Gut 1980;21(9):766-71.
14. DeMeester TR, Johnson LF, Joseph GJ, Toscano MS, Hall AW, Skinner DB. Patterns of gastroesophageal reflux in health and disease. Ann Surg 1976;184(4):459-70.
15. Namiot Z, Yu ZJ, Piascik R, Hetzel DP, McCallum RW, Sarosiek J. Modulatory effect of esophageal intraluminal mechanical and chemical stressors on salivary prostaglandin E2 in humans. Am J Med Sci 1997;313(2):90-8.
16. Marcinkiewicz M, Sarosiek J, Edmunds M, Scheurich J, Weiss P, McCallum RW. Monophasic luminal release of prostaglandin E2 in patients with reflux esophagitis under the impact of acid and acid/pepsin solutions. Its potential pathogenetic significance. J Clin Gastroenterol 1995;21(4):268-74.

17. Majewski M, Jaworski T, Sarosiek I, et al. Significant enhancement of esophageal pre-epithelial defense by tegaserod: implications for an esophagoprotective effect. Clin Gastroenterol Hepatol 2007;5(4):430-8.
18. Namiot Z, Sarosiek J, Marcinkiewicz M, Edmunds MC, McCallum RW. Declined human esophageal mucin secretion in patients with severe reflux esophagitis. Dig Dis Sci 1994;39(12):2523-9.
19. Jaworski T, Sarosiek I, Sostarich S, et al. Restorative impact of rabeprazole on gastric mucus and mucin production impairment during naproxen administration: its potential clinical significance. Dig Dis Sci 2005;50(2):357-65.
20. Vakil N, Talley NJ, Stolte M, Sundin M, Junghard O, Bolling-Sternevald E. Patterns of gastritis and the effect of eradicating Helicobacter pylori on gastro-oesophageal reflux disease in Western patients with non-ulcer dyspepsia. Aliment Pharmacol Ther 2006;24(1):55-63.
21. Liu Y, Akiyama J, Graham DY. Current understandings of Helicobacter pylori, peptic ulcer and gastroesophageal reflux disease. Minerva Gastroenterol Dietol 2006;52(3):235-48.
23. Mc ND, Buckley M, O'Morain C. Helicobacter pylori-induced duodenal ulcer frequently coincides with gastro-esophageal reflux disease. Dig Liver Dis 2002;34(8):542-6.
24. Dent J. Review Article: is Helicobacter pylori relevant in the management of reflux disease? Aliment Pharmacol Ther 2001;15:16-21.
25. Ando T, El Omar EM, Goto Y, et al. Interleukin 1B proinflammatory genotypes protect against gastro-oesophageal reflux disease through induction of corpus atrophy. Gut 2006;55(2):158-64.

What is the role of *Helicobacter pylori* infection in the development of carditis?

R. Malekzadeh, S. Nasseri-Moghaddam (Tehran)

The process of carcinogenesis in the upper gastrointestinal (GI) tract is commonly believed to start with inflammation. Prolonged inflammation can potentially lead to atrophy and metaplasia, which in time may end up in dysplasia. Dysplasia is considered to be the precursor of cancer [1]. Where the "point of no return" lies in this transformation is not clear.

Over the past decades, the incidence of proximal gastric cancer has increased, while that of distal gastric cancer has decreased. This is mostly for the intestinal type gastric cancer [2,3]. Meanwhile the prevalence of gastroesophageal reflux disease (GERD) has increased substantially [4]. Carditis is commonly found on biopsies taken from the gastric cardia. Whether "carditis" is due to infection with *Helicobacter pylori* or a consequence of GERD is in dispute [5]. Hansen *et al.* have calculated the risk of developing cancer in different parts of the stomach in relation to *H. pylori* [6]. According to their data the risk is highest in the distal stomach (RR: 24, 95% CI: 2-∞ in the distal antrum, RR: 5.9, 95% CI: 2-17 in the proximal antrum) and lowest at the cardia (RR: 0.3, 95% CI: 0.1-0.6). In a meta-analysis, Forman *et al.* have nicely shown that non-cardia gastric cancer is related to *H. pylori*, while cardia cancers are not [7]. On the other hand, in a case-control study in Linxian, China, Limburg *et al.* have found that the OR for cardia cancer is 1.9 (95% CI: 1.1-3.2) for those infected with *H. pylori* [8]. In a well-designed population-based study form Sweden, Lagergren *et al.* have shown that the OR for carida cancer is 2 (95% CI: 1.4-2.9) in patients with GERD [9]. We argue that there are lines of evidence which support the link between *H. pylori* and inflammation at the cardia an that the issue may be different in the east and west.

Currently gastric cancer is the most common cancer in Iran. One of the hotspots for this cancer is "Ardabil" a province in the north-west of the country, along the western border of the Caspian littoral (*Figure 1*). The ASR for gastric cancer is 49.1 per 10^5 population among men and 25.4 per 10^5 population among females [10]. *Figure 2* compares the prevalence of gastric cancer in Ardabil with tha of other parts of the world. The "Digestive Disease Research Center, DDRC" of "Tehran University of Medical Sciences, TUMS" has established the "Aras Clinic" with collaboration of "Ardabil University of Medical Sciences", the "International Agency for Research on Cancer, IARC" and the "National Cancer Institute, NCI" for registering cases and providing care to gastric cancer patients of the area. Records from this clinic have revealed that the most common site for gastric cancer is the "cardia", comprising 25.3% of all gastric cancers with an ASR of 26.4 and 8.6 per 10^5 in males and females respectively [11]. Most of these cardia cancers occur on the right side (along the lesser curve aspect) of the stomach [12]. This may be explained by the "Maggenstrasse" theory which implies that the smooth muscle of the esophagus and upper stomach are arranged in a fashion that liquids travel along the right side of the cardia from the esophagus to the stomach [13]. Therefore, this area has the most contact with xenobiotics entering the GI tract, including potential carcinogens like N-nitroso compounds.

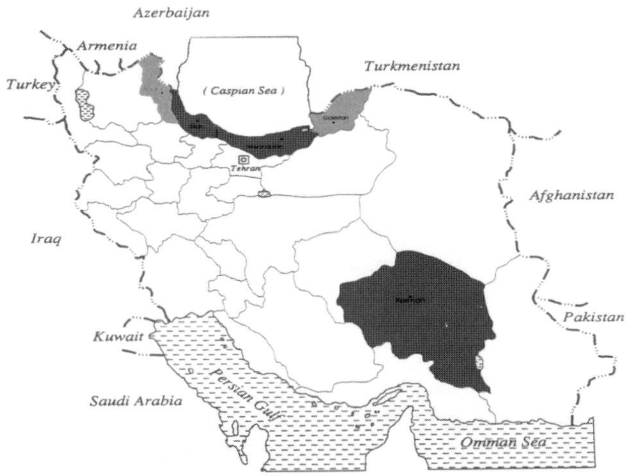

Figure 1. Ardabil, a high incidence area for gastric cancer in Iran.

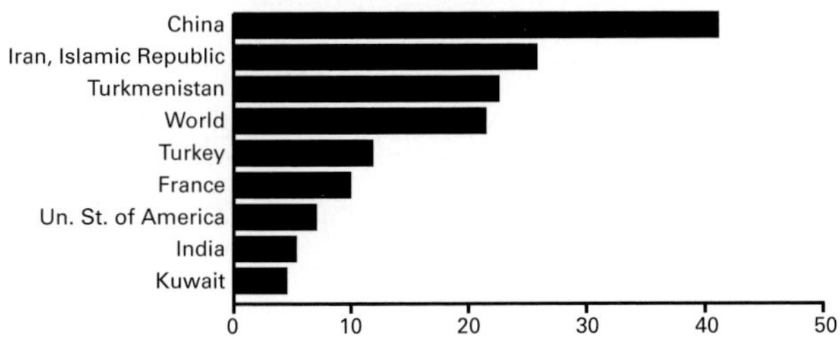

Figure 2. Comparison of Ardabil and other countries regarding the incidence of gastric cancer.

In a study 1,012 volunteer healthy Ardabil residents (40-65 years old) with no or minimal symptoms attributable to the upper GI tract, underwent upper GI endoscopy (UGIE) and protocol biopsies including biopsies from the gastric cardia (*Figure 3*). Thirty-five percent had esophagitis on endoscopy [14]. *Table I* shows the relation of *H. pylori* and inflammation at different parts of the stomach. As shown, the RR of carditis was 4.7 (95% CI: 2.6-8.5) in the presence of *H. pylori*. Therefore, in a high incidence area for cardia cancer, *H. pylori* has been shown to be independently related to carditis, a potential very early precursor in the pathway of carcinogenesis.

Table I. The relationship between *H. pylori* and carditis in Ardabil, Iran.

Biopsy site		*H. pylori*
Antrum	Bx 1	98.9 (22.6-432.6)
	Bx 2	16.1 (6.8-37.7)
	Bx 3	9.5 (5.0-18.1)
Corpus	Bx 4	5.6 (3.0-10.4)
	Bx 5	4.2 (2.3-7.4)
Cardia	Bx 6	4.7 (2.6-8.5)

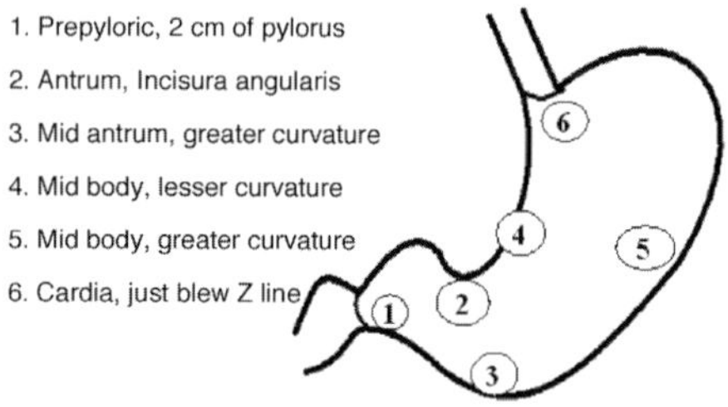

Figure 3. Sites of protocol biopsies in the Ardabil study.

In another ongoing study in Iran, the "Prospective Acid-Reflux Study of Iran, PARSI", a thousand patients with GERD have been enrolled (unpublished data). In addition to a detailed symptom registration, all have undergone UGIE with protocol biopsies including the cardia. *Table II* shows preliminary data from this ongoing study. As shown there 59.2% of those with carditis harbored *H. pylori* at the cardia as compared to only 1.9% of those without carditis ($p < 0.001$). When looking for *H. pylori* at any of the three gastric sites biopsied (i.e. antrum, corpus, and the cardia), 69.6% of those with carditis harbored *H. pylori versus* 12.4% of those without carditis ($p < 0.001$). When regression analysis was done on these data, *H. pylori* and age were the only independent risk factors for caditis. These data show that in a population of GERD patients, *H. pylori* is independently associated with carditis.

Table II. The relationship between *H. pylori* and carditis, the PARSI database (n: 522)

		Carditis		P-value
		Present	Absent	
H. pylori (%)	Cardia	59.2	1.9	< 0.001
	Body	53.6	4.6	< 0.001
	Antrum	58.2	11.2	< 0.001
	Any site	69.6	12.4	< 0.001
EE (%)		65.3	76.7	0.012
Mean age (yrs)		45.3	36.5	0.022

We conclude that *H. pylori* is an independent risk factor for development of inflammation at the cardia and that this process may differ in the west and the east.

References

1. Correa P, Haenszel W, Cuello C, et al. Gastric precancerous process in high risk population: cohort follow-up. Cancer Res 1990;50:4747.
2. Waterhouse J, Muir C, Correa P, et al. Cancer incidence in five continents. Vol III. IARC Scientific Publication no.15. International Agency for Research on Cancer, Lyon, 1976.
3. Kampschoer GH, Nakajima T, van de Velde CJ. Changing patterns in gastric adenocarcinoma. Br J Surg 1989;76(9):914-6.
4. El-Serag HB, Sonnenberg A. Opposing time trends of peptic ulcer and reflux disease. Gut 1998;43(3):327-33.
5. Malfertheiner P, Peitz U. The interplay between Helicobacter pylori, gastrooesophageal reflux disease, and intestinal metaplasia. Gut 2005;54;13-20.
6. Hansen S, Melby KK, Aase S, Jellum E, Vollset SE. Helicobacter pylori infection and risk of cardia cancer and non-cardia gastric cancer. A nested case-control study. Scand J Gastroenterol. 1999;34(4):353-60.
7. Helicobacter and Cancer Collaborative Group Gastric cancer and Helicobacter pylori: a combined analysis of 12 case control studies nested within prospective cohorts. Gut 2001;49;347-53.
8. Limburg P, Qiao Y, Mark S, et al. Helicobacter pylori seropositivity and subsite-specific gastric cancer risks in Linxian, China. J Natl Cancer Inst 2001;93(3):226-33.
9. Lagergren J, Bergstrom R, Lindgren A, Nyren O. Symptomatic gastroesophageal reflux as a risk factor for esophageal adenocarcinoma. N Engl J Med 1999;340(11):825-31.
10. Sadjadi AR, Malekzadeh R, Derakhshan MH, et al. Cancer Occurence in Ardabil: Results of a population-based cancer registry from Iran. Int J Cancer 2003;107:113-8.
11. Yazdanbod A, Arshi S, Derakhshan MH, Sadjadi AR, Malekzadeh R. Gastric cardia cancer; the most common type of upper gastrointestinal cancer in Adabil, Iran: an endoscopy clinic experience. Arch Irn Med 2001;4(2):76-9.
12. Yazdanbod A, Nasseri-Moghaddam S, Malekzadeh R. Upper gastro-intestinal cancer in Ardabil, North-west of Iran: A Review. Arch Irn Med 2004;7:173-7.
13. Jefferson G. The human stomach and the Canalis gastricus (Lewis). J Anat 1915;49:165-81.

Future antireflux therapy based on drugs targeting the lower esophageal sphincter

R. Penagini, A. Grigolon, C. Caparello (Milan)

Current treatment of gastroesophageal reflux disease (GERD) is based on inhibition of gastric acid secretion. Proton pump inhibitors (PPIs) are very effective in healing esophagitis and controlling symptoms [1,2].

Therapeutic success however does not occur in all patients. A minority remains unhealed and above all up to 30% have unsatisfactory symptom control. This occurs both in patients with esophagitis and in those with endoscopy negative reflux disease [2,3]. Which are the possible causes? On one side acid control is only partial with PPIs and there is room for faster and more profound inhibition of acid secretion, drugs being developed along this line [4], on the other development of prolonged intraluminal impedance recording has shown that symptoms may also occur during weakly acidic reflux episodes [5]. A recent paper has shown that about 40% of patients with GERD refractory to PPIs *bd* have a temporal relationship between their symptoms and weakly acidic reflux episodes [6].

Antireflux surgery achieves reflux control through its action on the mechanisms of reflux [7] and the possibility of shifting pharmacological treatment from acid control to reflux control is rather appealing. Which are the possible pharmacological targets for reflux control? To answer this question we need to understand the main mechanism of reflux. Prolonged lower esophageal sphincter (LES) recording with the use of a sleeve sensor have shown that the two main mechanisms are transient LES relaxation and low or absent LES pressure [8]. Whereas in patients with endoscopy negative reflux disease transient LES relaxation is predominant, a low LES tone becomes more important in patients with esophagitis and especially in those with severe mucosal lesions.

At the moment there is little evidence that an increase in LES pressure will decrease reflux [9] and above all there is no drug which, administered *per os*, consistently increases LES pressure in patients with GERD. On the contrary, stimulating data are available on inhibition of transient LES relaxation.

Transient LES relaxation is the spontaneous relaxation of the LES which allows us to belch (*Figure 1*). It is a vagavagal reflex triggered mainly by gastric distension although several other factors influence its frequency [10]. Patients with GERD have a similar rate of transient LES relaxation compared to healthy subjects [11] whereas the percentage of events associated with acid reflux is increased [10]. There are several validated targets for inhibition of transient LES relaxation (*Table I*): nitric oxide synthase, CCK1 receptor, muscarinic receptors, μ opioid receptor, cannabinoid 1 receptor, several metabotropic glutamate (mGlu) receptors and the γ-minobutyric acid $(GABA)_B$ receptor. Nitric oxide, CCK1 receptor, muscarinic receptors and some of the mGlu receptors stimulate transient LES relaxation and antagonists have been tested in order to inhibit transient LES relaxation whereas the μ opioid, cannabinoid 1, other mGlu and the $GABA_B$ receptor inhibit transient LES relaxation and agonists have been tested. For six of these targets there is evidence of effect in humans. As all these receptors are widespread along the neural pathways it is difficult to ascertain whether their effect on transient LES relaxation occurs at the level of the central nervous system or at the periphery. Furthermore it is obvious that such drugs

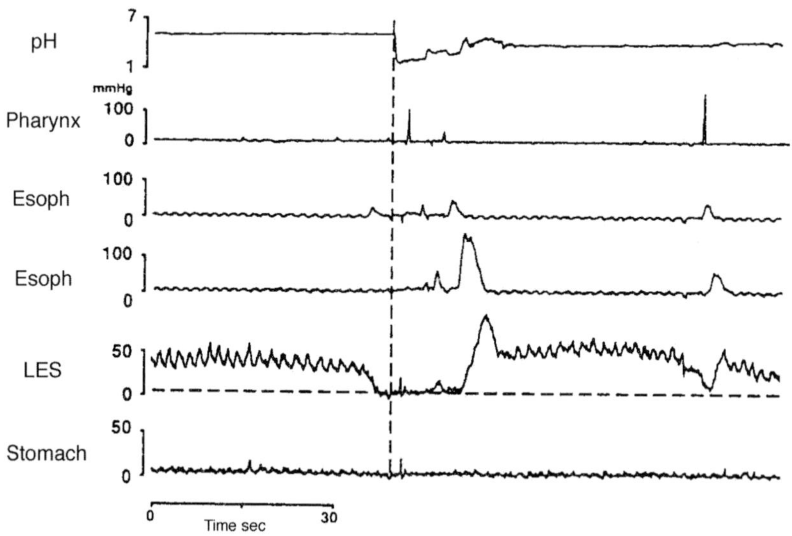

Figure 1. Episode of reflux during a transient LES relaxation. (Adapted from [23]).

Table I. Validated targets for inhibition of transient LES relaxation. (Adapted from [22]).

Target	Drugs used to verify target	Species	Proposed site of action	Effects on basal LESP
Nitric oxyde synthase	L-NAME, L-NMMA	Dog, human	Central	Increase
CCK1 receptor	Devazepide, loxiglumide	Dog, human	Peripheral	None
Muscarinic receptor(s)	Atropine	Human	Central	Decrease
μ opioid receptor	Morphine	Human	Central	None
CB1 receptor	WIN55, 212-2, Δ-9-tetrahydrocannabin	Dog, ferret, human	Central and/or peripheral	Decrease (humans)
mGluR5 receptor	MPEP, MTEP	Dog, ferret	Central and/or peripheral	Increase (ferrets) None (dogs)
mGluR group III receptors	L-AP4, (S)-3,4-DCPG	Ferret	Central and/or peripheral	None
$GABA_B$ receptor	Baclofen, CGP44532, SKF97541	Dog, ferret, cat, human	Central and/or peripheral	Increase (humans) None (dogs, ferrets)

may have side effects. $GABA_B$ and mGlu receptors are rather attractive because several recent data have shown that receptors located at the level of vagal afferents affect transient LES relaxation [12,13], thus suggesting that drugs which do not cross the blood brain barrier should be effective.

Knowledge of the role of the $GABA_B$ receptor is more advanced because we already have a drug approved for humans which is presently used in spasticity, i.e. baclofen. Several papers have shown that baclofen decreases the rate of transient LES relaxations and of reflux episodes in patients with GERD [14-18]. Furthermore placebo controlled studies have confirmed that both acute and chronic administration markedly decrease symptoms [17,19]. The central nervous system effects of baclofen however prevent its use in GERD except perhaps in patients partially refractory to PPIs with proven ongoing reflux and unwilling to undergo antireflux surgery, where baclofen can be tried by slowly increasing the dose. Studies are underway to assess the effectiveness/side effects balance in this group of patients.

Two further comments are worth to be done: the first one is that drugs which inhibit the rate of transient LES relaxations through the muscarinic, cannabinoid 1, μ opioid, $GABA_B$ and some of the mGlu receptors also decrease the rate of spontaneous swallowing and tend to increase acid clearance time, thus opposing the effect on esophageal acid exposure obtained by inhibition of transient LES relaxations. Effects on swallowing need therefore to be taken into account in the development of antireflux drugs.

The second one is that the effect on LES pressure is variable among different drugs which inhibit the rate of transient LES relaxations (*Table I*); theoretically a drug which also increases LES pressure should be more effective on reflux control.

The clinical settings where antireflux therapy could be useful are patients with extraesophageal symptoms where there is evidence of a possible role of weakly acidic reflux [20,21], pediatric patients where the main problem is volume regurgitation and, above all, those patients who are not completely satisfied with PPIs where antireflux therapy and PPIs could be administrated together. However, much work remains to be done in order to understand if antireflux therapy can really be useful in clinical practice. Firstly safe drugs with acceptable side effects and sufficiently powerful inhibition of transient LES relaxations need to be developed (it can be estimated from current data that at least 50% decrease in rate of transient LES relaxation should be obtained). Secondly eligible patient populations on which these drugs are tested need to be defined. Finally, appropriate large controlled clinical studies need to be designed in order to evaluate the degree of symptomatic improvement which can be obtained by reflux control.

References

1. Chiba N, De Gara CJ, Wilkinson JM, Hunt RH. Speed of healing and symptom relief in grade II to IV gastroesophageal reflux disease: a meta-analysis. Gastroenterology 1997;112:1798-810.
2. Richter JE, Kahrilas PJ, Johanson J, et al. Efficacy and safety of esomeprazole compared with omeprazole in GERD patients with erosive esophagitis: a randomized controlled trial. Am J Gastroenterol 2001;96:656-64.
3. Katz PO, Castell DO, Levine D. Esomeprazole resolves chronic heartburn in patients without erosive oesophagitis. Aliment Pharmacol Ther 2003;18:875-82.
4. Andersson K, Carlsson E. Potassium-competitive acid blockade: a new therapeutic strategy in acid-related diseases. Pharmacol Ther 2005;108(3):294-307.
5. Vela MF, Camacho-Lobato L, Srinivasan R, Tutuian R, Katz PO, Castell DO. Simultaneous intraesophageal impedance and pH measurement of acid and nonacid gastroesophageal reflux: effect of omeprazole. Gastroenterology 2001;120:1599-606.
6. Mainie I, Tutuian R, Shay S, et al. Acid and non-acid reflux in patients with persistent symptoms despite acid suppressive therapy: a multicentre study using combined ambulatory impedance-pH monitoring. Gut 2006;55:1398-402.
7. Ireland AC, Holloway RH, Toouli J, Dent J. Mechanisms underlying the antireflux action of fundoplication. Gut 1993;34:303-8.
8. Dent J, Holloway RH, Toouli J, Dodds WJ. Mechanisms of lower oesophageal sphincter incompetence in patients with symptomatic gastrooesophageal reflux. Gut 1988;29(8):1020-8.
9. Pehl C, Pfeiffer A, Wendl B, Stellwag B, Kaess H. Effect of erythromycin on postprandial gastroesophageal reflux in reflux esophagitis. Dis Esophagus 1997;10:34-7.
10. Mittal RK, Holloway RH, Penagini R, Blackshaw LA, Dent J. Transient lower esophageal sphincter relaxation. Gastroenterology 1995;109:601-10.
11. Sifrim D, Holloway RH. Transient lower esophageal sphincter relaxations: how many or how harmful? Am J Gastroenterol 2001;96(9):2529-32.
12. Page AJ, Blackshaw LA. GABA(B) receptors inhibit mechanosensitivity of primary afferent endings. J Neurosci 1999;19(19):8597-602.
13. Page AJ, Young RL, Martin CM, et al. Metabotropic glutamate receptors inhibit mechanosensitivity in vagal sensory neurons. Gastroenterology 2005;128(2):402-10.
14. Cange L, Johnsson E, Rydholm H, et al. Baclofen-mediated gastro-oesophageal acid reflux control in patients with established reflux disease. Aliment Pharmacol Ther 2002;16:869-73.
15. Koek GH, Sifrim D, Lerut T, Janssens J, Tack J. Effect of the GABA(B) agonist baclofen in patients with symptoms and duodeno-gastro-oesophageal reflux refractory to proton pump inhibitors. Gut 2003;52(10):1397-402.
16. van Herwaarden MA, Samsom M, Rydholm H, Smout AJ. The effect of baclofen on gastro-oesophageal reflux, lower oesophageal sphincter function and reflux symptoms in patients with reflux disease. Aliment Pharmacol Ther 2002;16(9):1655-62.
17. Vela MF, Tutuian R, Katz PO, Castell DO. Baclofen decreases acid and non-acid post-prandial gastro-oesophageal reflux measured by combined multichannel intraluminal impedance and pH. Aliment Pharmacol Ther 2003;17(2):243-51.
18. Zhang Q, Lehmann A, Rigda R, Dent J, Holloway RH. Control of transient lower oesophageal sphincter relaxations and reflux by the GABA(B) agonist baclofen in patients with gastro-oesophageal reflux disease. Gut 2002;50(1):19-24.
19. Ciccaglione AF, Marzio L. Effect of acute and chronic administration of the GABA B agonist baclofen on 24 hour pH metry and symptoms in control subjects and in patients with gastro-oesophageal reflux disease. Gut 2003;52(4):464-70.

20. Kawamura O, Aslam M, Rittmann T, Hofmann C, Shaker R. Physical and pH properties of gastroesophagopharyngeal refluxate: a 24-hour simultaneous ambulatory impedance and pH monitoring study. Am J Gastroenterol 2004;99(6):1000-10.
21. Sifrim D, Dupont L, Blondeau K, Zhang X, Tack J, Janssens J. Weakly acidic reflux in patients with chronic unexplained cough during 24 hour pressure, pH, and impedance monitoring. Gut 2005;54:449-54.
22. Lehmann A. Inhibitors of transient lower esophageal sphincter relaxations ("Reflux Inhibitors") in the future treatment of GERD. 2006;1:109-17.
23. Penagini R, Schoeman MN, Dent J, Tippett MD, Holloway RH. Motor events underlying gastro-oesophageal reflux in ambulant patients with reflux oesophagitis. Neurogastroenterol Motil 1996;8:131-41.

Does multiple rapid swallowing test improve the assessment of lower esophageal sphincter function?

R. Penagini, I. Bravi, P Cantù (Milan)

Achalasia is a primary motility disorder of the esophagus due to failing deglutitive inhibition [1] and characterized by incomplete swallow-induced lower esophageal sphincter (LES) relaxations and simultaneous or absent pressure waves in the esophageal body.

Denervation may be present to a variable degree as suggested by reports of apparent complete swallow induced LES relaxation and of transient LES relaxations in some patients [2,3]. One possible novel way of studying function of the inhibitory neural pathways in achalasia is to perform multiple rapid swallowing (MRS). MRS is a protracted inhibitory stimulus known to inhibit motility in the esophageal body of healthy subjects but not of patients with simultaneous esophageal contractions [4,5]. Furthermore, MRS has been found to induce complete LES relaxation in a pharmacological human model of incomplete LES relaxation [6]. Should MRS be able to inhibit or to delay onset of motor activity in the esophageal body of achalasia patients, it could also be a useful way to clarify if occurrence of simultaneous pressure waves in the esophageal body interferes with the evaluation of LES relaxations in response to single swallows: whereas after single swallows in healthy subjects the pressure wave usually reaches the LES when completion of relaxation has occurred [7,8], in achalasia patients the early arrival of a simultaneous wave may prematurely close the LES thus preventing its relaxation to reach completion.

Therefore we evaluated the motor response of achalasia patients to MRS with the hypothesis that MRS is more sensitive and/or accurate than single swallows in differentiating patients with residual activity of inhibitory neural pathways. We performed esophageal manometry in 20 consecutive untreated achalasia patients, 10 men, aged 23-81 years, median 54 years, using a multilumen polyvinyl assembly incorporating a sleeve sensor for the LES [9]. All patients took 6-8 single swallows with water (5 ml) at 30 seconds intervals and 2-3 MRS (5 swallaws, one every two seconds) while 10 ml of water was injected steadily into their mouth through a syringe [6]. The order of the single swallows and MRS series was randomized. Nadir LES pressure and duration of LES relaxation were measured.

According to a previous definition [8], nadir LES pressure was defined as the minimum pressure reached during relaxation, and complete relaxation was judged to have occurred when LES pressure fell to 1 mmHg of nadir pressure. Duration of LES relaxation was measured in the 16 achalasia patients who showed motor activity in the esophageal body after single swallows (see below) and defined as the time from pressure fall below the lowest point of the reference LES pressure (i.e. the LES pressure of the 5-10 seconds before

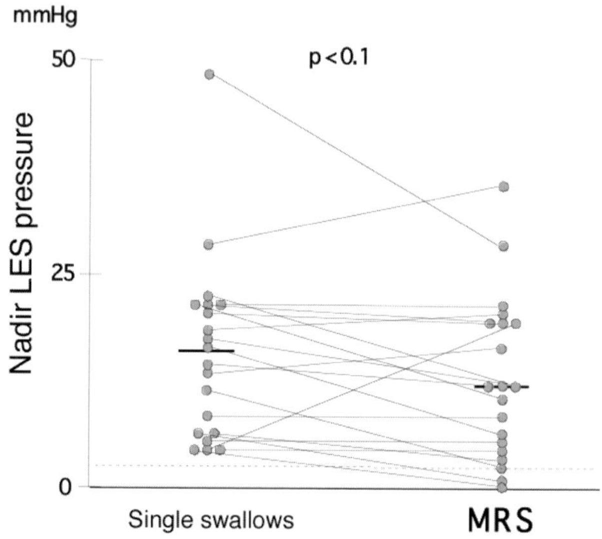

Figure 1. Nadir LES pressure after single swallows and MRS in the 20 achalasia patients. Horizontal bars represent medians and the dashed line the 90th percentile in a control population [11].

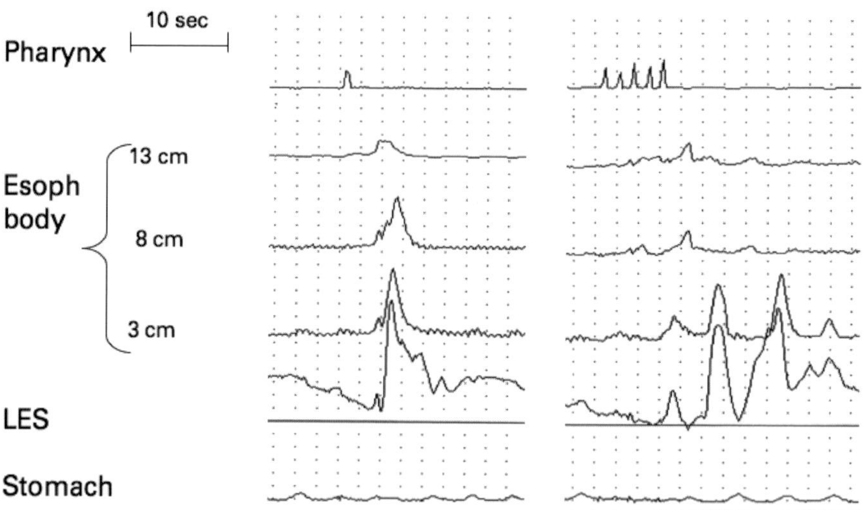

Figure 2. Tracings showing a single swallows and a MRS in one of the achalasia patients. The horizontal line in the LES channel represents the intragastric pressure. Vertical distance between two dots corresponds to 20 mmHg in the pharyngeal and esophageal body channels, whereas it corresponds to 10 mmHg in the LES and gastric channels. Note complete LES relaxation after MRS.

the swallow signal), to the time when pressure rose again above it [10]. On a few occasions contractions were recorded by the sleeve during relaxation; these were not considered to terminate the relaxation if LES pressure after the contraction remained lower that the reference LES pressure. Data were presented as median (IQ range) of the mean values in the 20 patients. Statistical significance was assessed by non parametric analysis.

Our results showed that overall nadir LES pressure tended to be lower during MRS compared to single swallows ($p < 0.1$, *Figure 1*). Looking at the individual patients in *Figure 1*, nadir LES pressure was lower in 12 and in 3 of them it reached < 3 mmHg (90th percentile of control values) [11]. These 3 patients tended to have a lower basal LES pressure, a smaller esophageal diameter and a shorter duration of symptoms compared to the remaining achalasia patients (median of 15 *versus* 25 mmHg, 2.5 *versus* 4.1 cm and 6 *versus* 12 months). The tracing of one of these three patients is shown in *Figure 2*.

With regards to the esophageal body, 4 patients had no motor activity both during single swallows and MRS. Of the remaining 16, 8 showed no motor activity in the esophageal body, i.e. deglutitive inhibition, during at least some of the MRS (4 of them during all MRS) whereas the remaining 8 patients always showed pressure waves (*Figure 3*). During MRS compared to single swallows nadir LES pressure tended to be lower and duration of LES relaxation was longer similarly in achalasia patients who showed deglutitive inhibition, 11 mmHg (4-19) *versus* 13 mmHg (6-17) p = NS and 6.5 sec. (3-8) *versus* 4.5 sec. (1.5-5) $p < 0.05$, and in those who did not 12 mmHg (5-13) *versus* 15 mmHg (7-19) p = NS and 6.5 sec. (6-7) *versus* 3.5 sec. (2-6) $p < 0.05$, suggesting that simultaneous pressure waves in the esophageal body did not interfere with evaluation of LES relaxation.

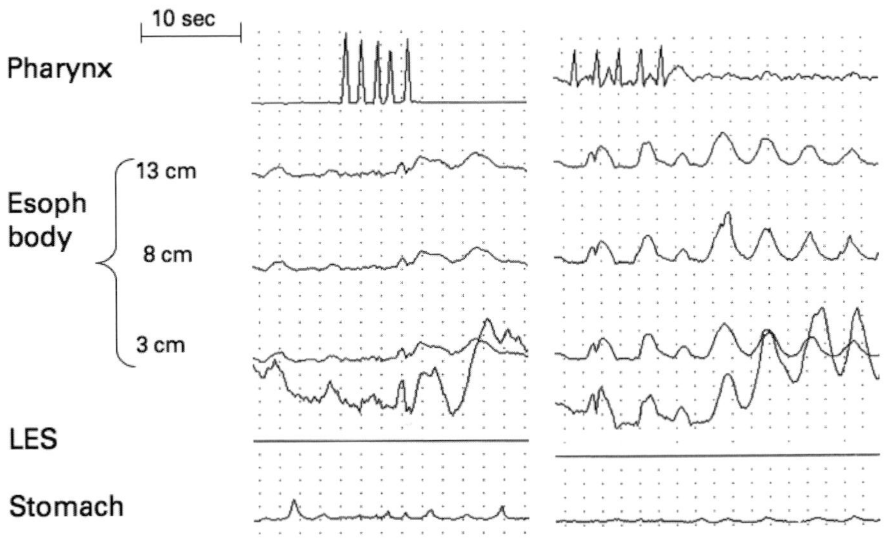

Figure 3. Tracings in two of the achalasia patients. The horizontal line in the LES channel represents the intragastric pressure. Vertical distance between two dots corresponds to 20 mmHg in the pharyngeal and esophageal body channels, whereas it corresponds to 10 mmHg in the LES and gastric channels. Note inhibition of motor activity in the esophageal body (patient on the left) and no inhibition (patient on the right).

In conclusion, our observations using MRS add further evidence to the hypothesis that idiopathic achalasia comprises several pathophysiologically different entities which manifest clinically with the same syndrome. Long term studies in larger series of achalasia patients after treatment will be able to tell us if inclusion of MRS in the diagnostic work-up has clinical usefulness in separating patients with different prognosis and/or with different therapeutic needs.

References

1. Sifrim D, Jannssens J, Vantrappen G. A wave of inhibition precedes primary peristaltic contractions in the human esophagus. Gastroenterology 1992;103:876-82.
2. van Herwaarden MA, Samsom M, Smout AJPM. Prolonged manometric recording of oesophagus and lower oesophageal sphincter in achalasia patients. Gut 2001;49:813-21.
3. Katz PO, Richter JE, Cowan R, Castell DO. Apparent complete lower esophageal sphincter relaxation in achalasia. Gastroenterology 1986;90:978-983.
4. Ask P, Tibbling L. Effect of time interval between swallows on esophageal peristalsis. Am J Physiol 1980;238:G485-90.
5. Vanek AW, Diamant NE. Responses of the human esophagus to paired swallows. Gastroenterology 1987;92:643-50.
6. Penagini R, Bianchi PA. Effect of morphine on gastroesophageal reflux and transient lower esophageal sphincter relaxation. Gastroenterology 1997;113:409-14.
7. Hollis JB, Castell DO. Effect of dry swallows and wet swallows of different volumes on esophageal peristalsis. J Appl Physiol 1975;38(6):1161-4.
8. Holloway RH, Penagini R, Ireland AC. Criteria for objective definition of transient lower esophageal sphincter relaxation. Am J Physiol 1995;268:G128-33.
9. Penagini R, Cantù P, Mangano M, Colombo P, Bianchi PA. Long-term effects of pneumatic dilatation on symptoms and lower oesophageal sphincter pressure in achalasia. Scand J Gastroenterol 2002;37:380-4.
10. Castell J, Boag Dalton C, Castell DO. On-line computer analysis of human lower esophageal sphincter relaxation. Am J Physiol 1988;255:G794-9.
11. Savojardo D, Mangano M, Cantù P, Penagini R. Multiple rapid swallowing in idiopathic achalasia: evidence for patients heterogeneity. Neurogastroenterol Motil 2007;19:263-9.

What are the drawbacks of the transnasal or transoral Bravo™ pH monitoring system?

J.E. Pandolfino (Chicago)

Catheter based ambulatory pH monitoring has significant methodological limitations. The nasally passed pH catheter is uncomfortable, cumbersome and conspicuous leading most patients to significantly restrict their daily activities or not complete the study [1]. In some instances patients may remain at home and consume a very limited diet while the catheter is in place. The resultant studies in these patients could potentially be "false negatives" if the limitations in activity and/or diet reduce their esophageal acid exposure to within the normal range. Other issues with catheter based pH monitoring are focused on accuracy and reproducibility. Position of the sensing electrode can be erroneous and either proximal or distal migration may alter the diagnosis in some patients. In addition, esophageal acid

Table I. Special considerations warranting preference for a wireless system or a catheter based system.

Special consideration	Bravo™	Catheter-based
Cost		++
Barrett's metaplasia		+
Bleeding diathesis		+
Known history of gastrointestinal stricture		+++
Zenker's diverticulum		+++
Previous nasal trauma	+++	
History of sinusitis	++	
Sensitive pharynx/active gag	+++	
Prior failed catheter study	+++	
Need for repeated studies	+++	
Need to assess non-acid reflux		+++*
+ weak preference, ++ moderate preference, +++ strong preference, *only with combined pH/impedance		

exposure may fluctuate from day to day [2] and 24-hour monitoring may not be an adequate period to document symptoms for correlation with reflux events.

Wireless pH monitoring was developed to circumvent many of the methodological limitations of catheter based pH monitoring. This pH system involves the attachment of a radiotelemetry pH sensing capsule to the mucosal wall of the esophagus 6 cm above the squamocolumnar junction (SCJ). The advantages of this system are improved comfort and patient acceptance. In addition, the pH indicator electrode position is fixed with respect to the esophageal mucosa and studies can be performed for longer time periods optimizing symptom-reflux correlation.

Placement of the Bravo™ pH capsule is a fast and relatively comfortable alternative to conventional transnasal catheter pH monitoring. It requires the same pre-procedure preparation as conventional catheter placement and only adds approximately 5 minutes to a standard endoscopy. The capsule is typically placed during endoscopy or shortly after endoscopy as long as measurement of the distance from the incisors to the SCJ has been made within a reasonable time period.

Disadvantages of the Bravo™ pH system

Esophageal discomfort

Improved tolerability is the main draw for the wireless pH monitoring system and has been assessed previously [2]. Only 4-14% of subjects, comprising healthy controls and gastroesophageal reflux disease (GERD) patients, reported throat discomfort with Bravo™ compared to 73-95% when catheter pH system was used. In opposition, esophageal discomfort was more common with the pH capsule at 33-34%, *versus* 17-18% reported for the catheter, but mostly in healthy controls rather than GERD patients. A small portion of patients (< 5-9%) developed severe odynophagia and chest pain warranting endoscopic removal of the capsule in less than 2% of cases [2,3]. Sporadic lesions at the attachment point can be seen on endoscopy in patients reporting chest discomfort after capsule dislodgment [4]. To what extent these symptoms affect diagnosis is unclear.

Additional procedures may be required for patients reporting severe chest pain, odynophagia or inability to tolerate food ingestion following capsule attachment [2,4]. Chest X-ray should rule out esophageal perforation as the cause of these symptoms, and if the capsule is still in place with no perforation, the symptoms may be controlled with a stomatitis cocktail containing viscous lidocaine or a carafate slurry. Repeat endoscopy is recommended as a last resort after failed conservative management and persistent symptoms after 48 hours. The majority of capsules detach within 5 days, hence, early endoscopy with the associated risk of perforation and capsule removal may be more harmful.

Accuracy

A major limitation of all single sensor pH monitoring devices is the inability to distinguish a "true" reflux event from artifact or swallowing. A recent study using combined MII-pH compared the accuracy of pH monitoring alone in detecting acid reflux to MII-pH [5]. Although pH monitoring alone was sensitive (100%) in detecting acid reflux, it lacked specificity (58% for abnormal percentage time of pH less than 4 and positive symptom index) offered by MII-pH. Eighty-one percent of acid reflux events were associated with swallows measurable by MII. This is an important observation as often patients sip acidic beverages (e.g. coffee, orange juice, cranberry juice, cola, soda) during the monitoring period without strict reporting of each sip. Hence, it is not surprising that over diagnosis of abnormal acid reflux occurred in up to 22% of patients in this study.

Inability to measure weakly-acidic/weakly-alkaline reflux

Although the clinical significance of weakly acidic or weakly alkaline reflux in generating symptoms is controversial, there is evidence to suggest that some patients do exhibit a correlation between symptoms and non-acid reflux events [6]. Thus, a main limitation of all pH monitoring systems is that they lack the ability to measure non-acid reflux. This was highlighted in a study that used combined MII-pH to compare the accuracy of pH monitoring alone in detecting acid and weakly acidic reflux to MII-pH [5]. pH alone had a sensitivity of 28% in detecting weakly acidic reflux with 83% of these events not coinciding with reflux detectable by MII. Thus, the Bravo™ system could not be used to assess the relationship between non-acid reflux and symptoms.

Summary

The Bravo™ pH monitoring system provides an answer to the limitations of catheter based systems, such as patients comfort, inconspicuousness and prolonged pH monitoring. Alas, this promising technique is not without shortcomings. Although chest pain and esophageal discomfort are drawbacks, the rate is low and most patients can be managed with reassurance and pain medication. Unfortunately, the major limitation of using esophageal acid exposure as a surrogate marker for gastroesophageal reflux remains can not be circumvented by the Bravo™ capsule as it stands. Whether this deficiency will dampen the enthusiasm for a catheter free system will depend on future studies documenting the importance of weakly acidic and weakly alkaline reflux.

References

1. Fass R, Hell R, Sampliner RE, et al. Effect of ambulatory 24-hour esophageal pH monitoring on reflux-provoking activities. Dig Dis Sci 1999;44:2263-9.
2. Pandolfino JE, Richter JE, Ours T, Guardino JM, Chapman J, Kahrilas PJ. Ambulatory esophageal pH monitoring using a wireless system. Am J Gastroenterol 2003;98:740-9.
3. Prakash C, Jonnalagadda S, Azar R, Clouse RE. Endoscopic removal of the wireless pH monitoring capsule in patients with severe discomfort. Gastrointest Endosc 2006;64:828-32.
4. Pandolfino JE. Bravo capsule pH monitoring. Am J Gastroenterol 2005;100:8-10.
5. Hila A, Agrawal A, Castell DO. Combined multichannel intraluminal impedance and pH esophageal testing compared to pH alone for diagnosing both acid and weakly acidic gastroesophageal reflux. Clin Gastroenterol Hepatol 2007;5:172-7.
6. Mainie I, Tutuian R, Shay S, et al. Acid and non-acid reflux in patients with persistent symptoms despite acid suppressive therapy: a multicentre study using combined ambulatory impedance-pH monitoring. Gut 2006;55:1398-402.

Do physiological interactions between the esophagus and stomach lay the foundation for overlap in disease?

F. Fornari, D. Sifrim (Leuven)

Although the esophagus looks like a mere tube for transportation of liquid and food to the stomach, esophageal malfunction and consequent disease have been a prevalent cause of quality of life impairment and economic burden. The prototype of this condition is gastroesophageal reflux disease (GERD), which has been extensively studied. Apart from morphological and functional abnormalities directly related with the esophagus, physiological interactions between the esophagus and other segments of the gastrointestinal (GI) tract including stomach, duodenum and colon seem to play a role in the genesis of gastroesophageal reflux (GER) and consequent esophageal reaction. Also important, bi-directional influences have been identified between the esophagus and the central nervous system, which in turn participates in the modulation of these complex esophagus-GI tract interactions.

Interactions between stomach and esophagus in patients with GERD rely mainly on the pattern of gastric acid secretion and gastric emptying, as well as the presence of *Helicobacter pylori* infection. Studies about gastric acid output in GERD patients are controversial. Initial evidence showed that a subgroup of GERD patients with heartburn refractory to H_2-blockers were hypersecretors of basal gastric acid, requiring increased acid-suppressive therapy [1]. However, a posterior study conducted in a large series of patients did not find differences either in fasting, basal or maximal gastric acid or pepsin secretion between patients with and without reflux esophagitis [2]. Another study evaluated possible differences in basal gastric acid secretion with regard to severity of GERD. Compared to normal subjects, mean acid secretion was significantly higher either in non erosive reflux disease (NERD), erosive reflux disease (ERD) or Barrett's esophagus patients. The latter group showed even more mean acid secretion when compared to NERD patients [3]. Recently, post-prandial integrated gastric acidity has been shown to be increased in patients with GERD when compared to normal individuals [4]. Taking these evidences into account, it seems that increased gastric acid secretion plays a role in the pathophysiology of GERD.

Additional finding linking the stomach with the esophagus is the recently described gastric acid pocket. Such phenomenon was originally recognized in healthy volunteers as a segment of post-prandial highly acidic unbuffered gastric juice present under the gastroesophageal junction [5]. Gastric acid pocket has been described to be larger in patients with severe GERD compared to healthy subjects, potentially contributing to the increased rate of acid reflux in the post-prandial period [6]. A critical analysis of this issue concluded that clarification of acidity levels at the gastric cardia has provided a plausible explanation for patterns of post-prandial reflux that appear superficially at odds with previous gastric pH measurements. The high levels of acidity at the gastric cardia appear likely to have a significant impact on acid exposure in the very distal esophagus and potentially on complications such as esophagitis and intestinal metaplasia and neoplasia. However, the relevance of the acid pocket, a phenomenon characterized by transient changes distal to the cardia to reflux disease remains unclear [7].

The pattern of gastric emptying after a meal has been implicated in GERD pathophysiology. Controversial evidences have risen from several studies showing delayed gastric emptying or no abnormality. In the light of more robust studies, it seems that delayed proximal gastric emptying plays a role at least in a subgroup of GERD patients, by increasing the number of reflux events and therefore total acid exposure [8,9]. Further evidence favouring a link between gastric emptying and GERD is provided by a study comparing proximal extent of GER in fasting, post-prandial and ambulant periods. Reflux episodes were more likely to reach the proximal esophagus during the early post-prandial period, particularly in ambulatory conditions [10]. This observation suggests that gastric fullness (meal volume related) and straining may correlate with the volume of the refluxate. Recently, it has been found that patients with GERD swallow air more frequently and belch more frequently than healthy subjects. However, air swallowing has not been considered as cause of increased reflux [11].

H. pylori infection of the gastric mucosa has been advocated as a protector condition for GERD [12]. Moreover, a recent analysis focused on more robust studies found no evidence that *H. pylori* eradication causes GERD or worsens GERD symptoms [13-16].

Interactions between duodenum and esophagus have been shown by infusing lipids or saline in the duodenal lumen and monitoring the effect on transient lower esophageal sphincter relaxations (TLESRs) and occurrence of acid reflux. Duodenal instillation with fat aggravates reflux in patients with GERD, by increasing the proportion of TLESRs accompanied by reflux [17]. Following this observation, a study showed that the infusion of fat into de duodenum can increase the rate of TLESRs in the post-prandial period. This phenomenon could be blocked by administering loxiglumide (CCK-A antagonist), suggesting that CCK mediates fat-induced TLESRs *via* a duodenal-esophageal reflex [18]. A more recent study found that duodenal infusion with lipids intensifies the perception of heartburn in patients with GERD [19]. Based on the aphorism that "the most common trigger for GERD symptoms is a meal" [20], it is clear that interactions involving the axis duodenum-esophagus-brain play a role in the pathophysiology of GERD.

The most distant interaction between the esophagus and GI organs was recently recognized in studies about colonic fermentation of carbohydrates and lower esophageal sphuncer (LES) function. Piche *et al.* assessed the effect of colonic infusion of lactose and short-chain fatty acids (SCFAs) on LES function in healthy volunteers. Both lactose and SCFA infusions increased the number of TLESRs as well as the proportion of TLESRs associated with acid reflux [21]. In a more recent study, colonic fermentation of indigestible carbohydrates reproduced these effects on LES function and worsened GERD symptoms. The integrated plasma response of glucagon-like peptide 1 (GLP-1) was significantly higher after carbohydrate administration, suggesting that excess release of GLP-1 might account for these effects [22].

The last and equally important interaction involving the esophagus is with the central nervous system. It is well known that visceral sensitivity can be modulated by central neural pathways and the esophagus does not escape the rule. First studies identified a link between neuropsychological behaviour and esophageal symptoms, particularly heartburn and chest pain. Disruptions in the central nervous function such as depression and anxiety have been described to provoke esophageal hypersensitivity, either for reaction to gastroesophageal reflux or esophageal motor activity. In many patients with negative findings following extensive investigation for esophageal diseases, central nervous system malfunction is the only abnormality that can be identified. More recent studies have reinforced the interaction between central nervous system and esophagus, assessing objective abnormalities either in humans or in animal models. In the light of reports showing an association between stress and increase in both gastric and colonic permeability, experimental studies done in our laboratory have found increased esophageal epithelium permeability induced uniquely by stress [23]. Increased epithelial permeability is believed to favour symptoms perception by facilitating the access of irritant components of the refluxate to neuronal endings [24]. In addition, since the neuronal endings are stimulated, the transmission and perception of the noxious stimulus seems to be facilitated by stress. These phenomenons can partially explain the occurrence of symptoms in GERD patients without macroscopic reflux-associated mucosa damage. Noteworthy, NERD patients account nowadays for the majority of GERD patients and therapeutic options are still a challenge.

Taking these considerations into account, physiological interactions between the esophagus and other GI segments lay the foundation for overlap in disease pathophysiology, particularly in GERD.

References

1. Collen MJ, Lewis JH, Benjamin SB. Gastric acid hypersecretion in refractory gastroesophageal reflux disease. Gastroenterology 1990;98:654-61.
2. Hirschowitz BI. A critical analysis, with appropriate controls, of gastric acid and pepsin secretion in clinical esophagitis. Gastroenterology 1991;101:1149-58.
3. Collen MJ, Johnson DA, Sheridan MJ. Basal acid output and gastric acid hypersecretion in gastroesophageal reflux disease. Correlation with ranitidine therapy. Dig Dis Sci 1994;39:410-7.
4. Gardner JD, Sloan S, Miner PB, Robinson M. Meal-stimulated gastric acid secretion and integrated gastric acidity in gastro-oesophageal reflux disease. Aliment Pharmacol Ther 2003;17:945-53.
5. Fletcher J, Wirz A, Young J, Vallance R, McColl KE. Unbuffered highly acidic gastric juice exists at the gastroesophageal junction after a meal. Gastroenterology 2001;121:775-83.

6. Clarke AT, Wirz AA, Manning JJ, Ballantyne SA, Alcorn DJ, McColl KE. Severe reflux disease is associated with an enlarged unbuffered proximal gastric acid pocket. Gut 2008;57:292-7.
7. Holloway RH, Sifrim DA. The acid pocket and its relevance to reflux disease. Gut 2008;57:285-6.
8. Buckles DC, Sarosiek I, McMillin C, McCallum RW. Delayed gastric emptying in gastroesophageal reflux disease: reassessment with new methods and symptomatic correlations. Am J Med Sci 2004;327:1-4.
9. Stacher G, Lenglinger J, Bergmann H, et al. Gastric emptying: a contributory factor in gastro-oesophageal reflux activity? Gut 2000;47:661-6.
10. Emerenziani S, Zhang X, Blondeau K, et al. Gastric fullness, physical activity, and proximal extent of gastroesophageal reflux. Am J Gastroenterol 2005;100:1251-6.
11. Bredenoord AJ, Weusten BL, Timmer R, Smout AJ. Air swallowing, belching, and reflux in patients with gastroesophageal reflux disease. Am J Gastroenterol 2006;101:1721-6.
12. Raghunath A, Hungin AP, Wooff D, Childs S. Prevalence of Helicobacter pylori in patients with gastro-oesophageal reflux disease: systematic review. Br Med J 2003;326:737.
13. Moayyedi P, Bardhan C, Young L, Dixon MF, Brown L, Axon AT. Helicobacter pylori eradication does not exacerbate reflux symptoms in gastroesophageal reflux disease. Gastroenterology 2001;121:1120-6.
14. Ott EA, Mazzoleni LE, Edelweiss MI, et al. Helicobacter pylori eradication does not cause reflux oesophagitis in functional dyspeptic patients: a randomized, investigator-blinded, placebo-controlled trial. Aliment Pharmacol Ther 2005;21:1231-9.
15. Schwizer W, Thumshirn M, Dent J, et al. Helicobacter pylori and symptomatic relapse of gastro-oesophageal reflux disease: a randomised controlled trial. Lancet 2001;357:1738-42.
16. Wu JC, Chan FK, Wong SK, Lee YT, Leung WK, Sung JJ. Effect of Helicobacter pylori eradication on oesophageal acid exposure in patients with reflux oesophagitis. Aliment Pharmacol Ther 2002;16:545-52.
17. Holloway RH, Lyrenas E, Ireland A, Dent J. Effect of intraduodenal fat on lower oesophageal sphincter function and gastro-oesophageal reflux. Gut 1997;40:449-53.
18. Zerbib F, Bruley des Varannes S, Scarpignato C, et al. Endogenous cholecystokinin in postprandial lower esophageal sphincter function and fundic tone in humans. Am J Physiol 1998;275:G1266-73.
19. Meyer JH, Lembo A, Elashoff JD, Fass R, Mayer EA. Duodenal fat intensifies the perception of heartburn. Gut 2001;49:624-8.
20. Fass R, Tougas G. Functional heartburn: the stimulus, the pain, and the brain. Gut 2002;51:885-92.
21. Piche T, Zerbib F, Bruley desVarannes SB, et al. Modulation by colonic fermentation of LES function in humans. Am J Physiol Gastrointest Liver Physiol 2000;278:G578-84.
22. Piche T, Bruley des Varannes S, Sacher-Huvelin S, Holst JJ, Cuber JC, Galmiche JP. Colonic fermentation influences lower esophageal sphincter function in gastroesophageal reflux disease. Gastroenterology 2003;124:894-902.
23. Farre R, De VR, Geboes K, et al. Critical role of stress in increased oesophageal mucosa permeability and dilated intercellular spaces. Gut 2007;56:1191-7.
24. Barlow WJ, Orlando RC. The pathogenesis of heartburn in nonerosive reflux disease: a unifying hypothesis. Gastroenterology 2005;128:771-8.

Controversies in Barrett's esophagus and Barrett's cancer

Pathologic findings in rat models of reflux-induced esophageal injury

E. Montgomery (Baltimore)

Details on the history, surgical techniques, and species of rat models are covered in other sections, and in this one, we will focus simply on the histology of selected reflux-induced rat models [1-7]. The findings in various rat models differ based on both surgical technique and animal subspecies [2-4,7-10], but there are certain common themes, namely that duodenal reflux appears to be a requirement to induce cancers in the absence of an exogenous carcinogen and that, in addition to Barrett-like lesions, squamous hyperproliferative lesions and squamous carcinomas are produced as well as adenocarcinomas. In addition, in contrast to human carcinomas, the lesions produced by these models have not been shown to metastasize so cannot be compared precisely to human carcinogenesis, but they have been prevented by COX-2 inhibitors [2,6]. These models allow us to explore esophageal carcinogenesis using modern techniques [1,11,12].

A striking lesion that we have observed is a squamous hyperproliferative one displaying extensive hyperkeratosis and parakeratosis in the presence of bile reflux [3] (*Figure 1*). This squamous hyperproliferative lesion is present in the background of other duodenal reflux models [2] that also produce a glandular lesion. The latter model produces zones that display striking resemblance to human Barrett's esophagus (*Figures 2 and 3*) and rare zones with features resembling dysplasia can be identified (*Figure 4*). In this background, some rats display tumors (*Figure 5*) having microscopic features similar to an esophageal adenocarcinoma (*Figures 6, 7 and 8*) but squamous carcinomas are also found (*Figure 9*).

In summary, these rat lesions share with human tumors squamous injury, intestinal metaplasia, and development of adenocarcinoma-like lesions but differ from human carcinogenesis by displaying squamous hyperproliferation, associated squamous carcinomas, and tumors that have not been shown to metastasize.

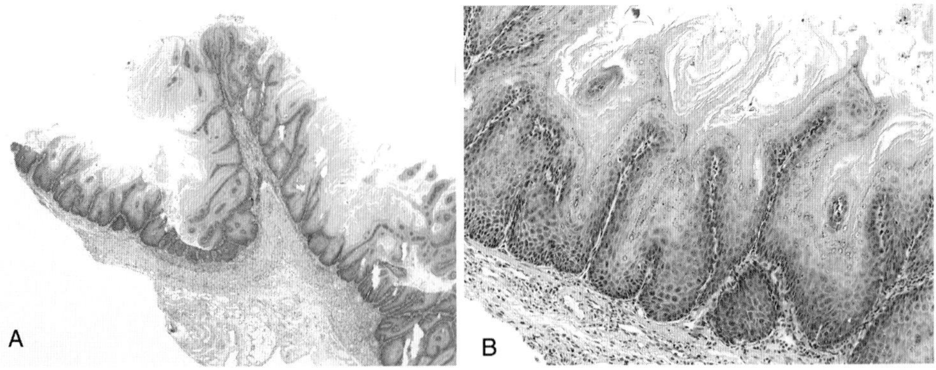

Figure 1. Squamous hyper-proliferative lesion induced by duodenal reflux displaying a papillary architecture (**A**) and prominent elongation of vascular papillae together with hyperkeratosis and parakeratosis (**B**). This epithelium was markedly acanthotic (thickened) compared to control animals. (See page XXI for colour figure).

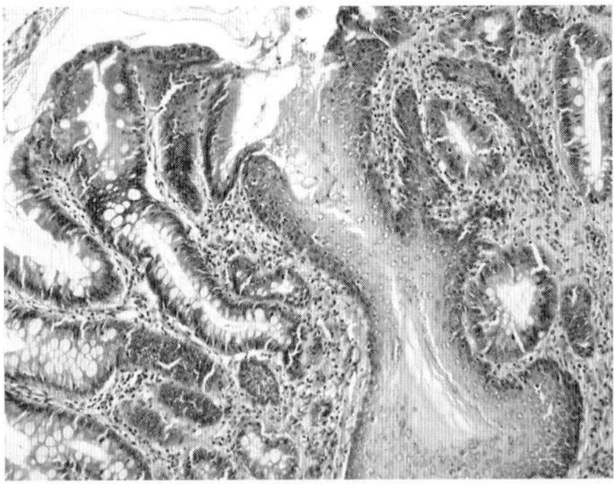

Figure 2. Lesion resembling Barrett's esophagus in duodenal reflux induced rat model. Patches of squamous mucosa are found on the right portion of this field and goblet cells are seen in the gland at the left. (See page XXI for colour figure).

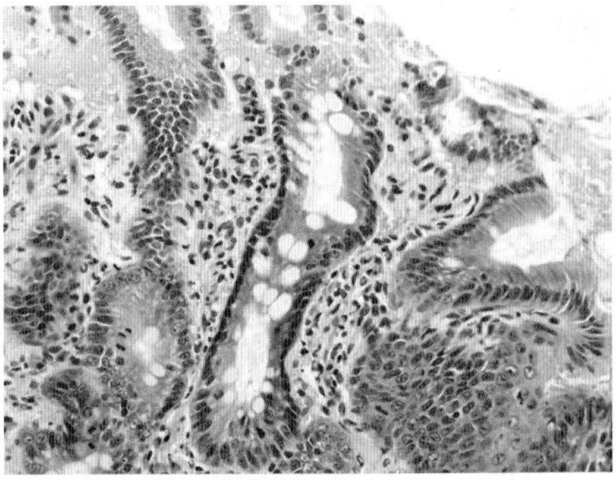

Figure 3. Higher-power view of the metaplastic focus depicted in *Figure 2*. Note the goblet cells in the gland in the center of the field. (See page XXI for colour figure).

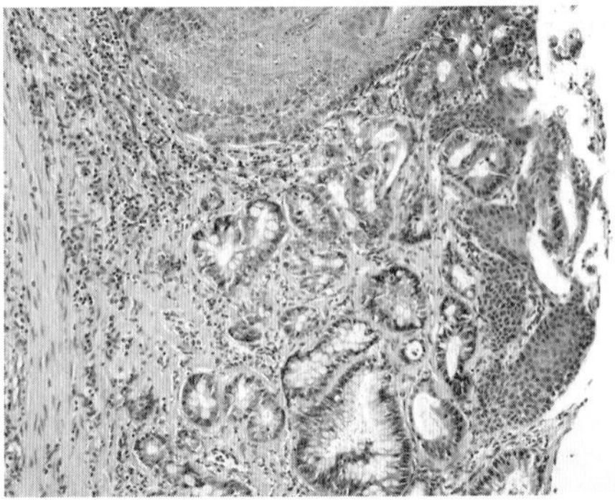

Figure 4. This lesion was found in a zone adjacent to a tumor and shows scattered glands having hyperchromatic nuclei, features similar to those found in dysplasia in Barrett's esophagus. (See page XXI for colour figure).

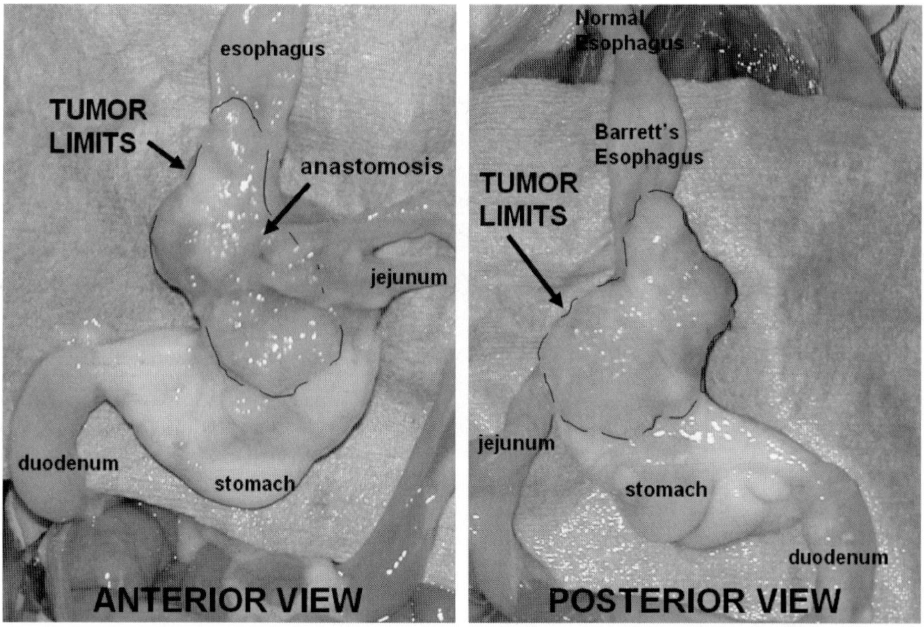

Figure 5. Gross dissections from animal models. (Courtesy of Dr, John Harmon). (See page XXII for colour figure).

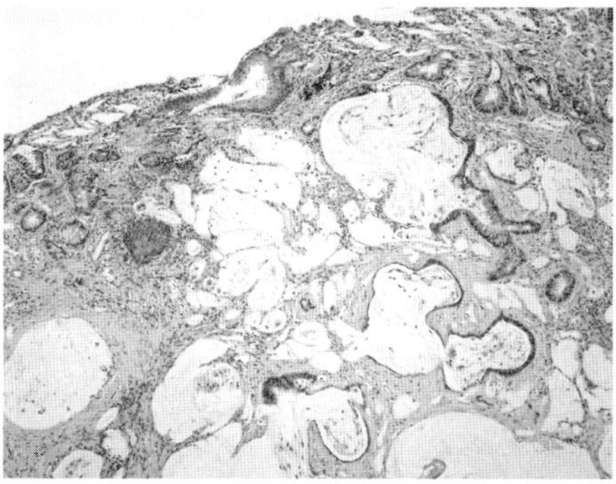

Figure 6. An adenocarcinoma-like lesion displaying an infiltrative growth pattern. (See page XXI for colour figure).

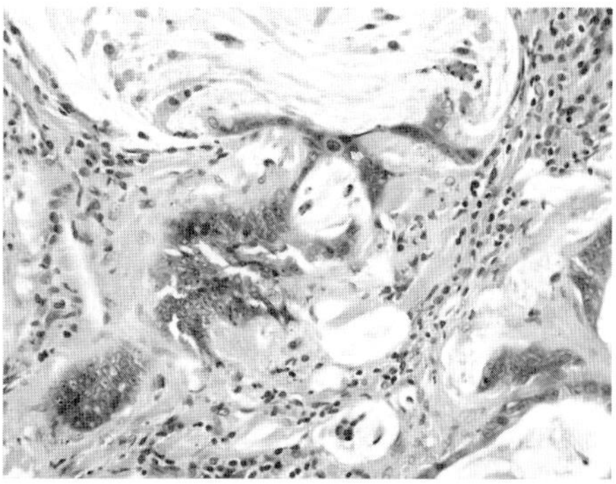

Figure 7. This adenocarcinoma-like lesion displays a dissecting growth pattern into surrounding connective tissue and an apparent tissue response. The proliferating nuclei appear enlarged and irregular. (See page XXII for colour figure).

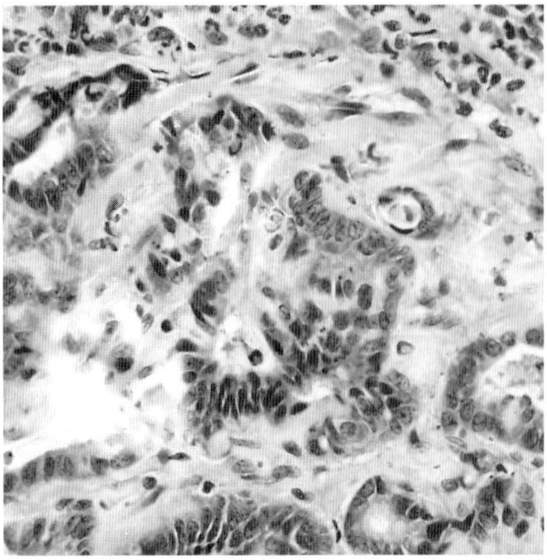

Figure 8. Another adenocarcinoma-like lesion displaying irregular nuclear contours and an apparent tissue response. (See page XXII for colour figure).

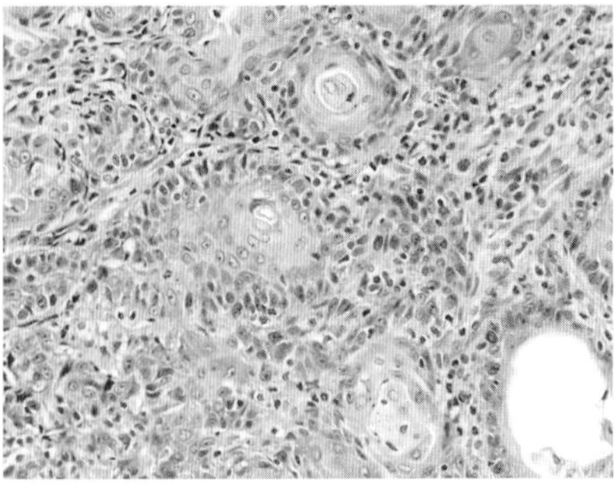

Figure 9. This tumor displays squamous differentiation, including keratinization and squamous "pearls". Some examples have adenosquamous features as well. (See page XXIII for colour figure).

References

1. Bonde P, Gao D, Chen L, et al. Duodenal reflux leads to down regulation of DNA mismatch repair pathway in an animal model of esophageal cancer. Ann Thorac Surg 2007;83(2):433-40.
2. Buttar NS, Wang KK, Leontovich O, et al. Chemoprevention of esophageal adenocarcinoma by COX-2 inhibitors in an animal model of Barrett's esophagus. Gastroenterology 2002;122(4):1101-12.
3. Byrnes CK, Bahadursingh A, Akhter N, et al. Duodenal reflux produces hyperproliferative epithelial esophagitis—a possible precursor to esophageal adenocarcinoma in the rat. J Gastrointest Surg 2003;7(2):172-80.
4. Miwa K, Hasegawa H, Fujimura T, et al. Duodenal reflux through the pylorus induces gastric adenocarcinoma in the rat. Carcinogenesis 1992;13(12):2313-6.
5. Miwa K, Hattori T, Miyazaki I. Duodenogastric reflux and foregut carcinogenesis. Cancer 1995;75:1426-32.
6. Miwa K, Oyama K, Fujimura T. A COX-2 inhibitor suppresses esophageal inflammation-metaplasia-adenocarcinoma sequence in rats. Nippon Rinsho 2005;63(8):1387-93.
7. Miwa K, Sahara H, Segawa M, et al. Reflux of duodenal or gastro-duodenal contents induces esophageal carcinoma in rats. Int J Cancer 1996;67(2):269-74.
8. Sato T, Miwa K, Sahara H, Segawa M, Hattori T. The sequential model of Barrett's esophagus and adenocarcinoma induced by duodeno-sophageal reflux without exogenous carcinogens. Anticancer Res 2002;22(1A):39-44.
9. Kumagai H, Mukaisho K, Sugihara H, et al. Cell kinetic study on histogenesis of Barrett's esophagus using rat reflux model. Scand J Gastroenterol 2003;38(7):687-92.
10. Pera M, Brito MJ, Poulsom R, et al. Duodenal-content reflux esophagitis induces the development of glandular metaplasia and adenosquamous carcinoma in rats. Carcinogenesis 2000;21(8):1587-91.
11. Sui G, Bonde P, Dhara S, et al. Epidermal growth factor receptor and hedgehog signaling pathways are active in esophageal cancer cells from rat reflux model. J Surg Res 2006;134(1):1-9.
12. Bonde P, Gao D, Chen L, et al. Selective decrease in the DNA base excision repair pathway in squamous cell cancer of the esophagus. J Thorac Cardiovasc Surg 2007;133(1):74-81.

Procarcinogenic signaling in Barrett's esophagus: do animals copy us? An overview of *in vivo* models

C. DeMars, N. Buttar (Rochester)

Animal models, by definition, are an approximation of reality. Several models of esophageal adenocarcinoma and Barrett's esophagus have been developed in last three decades. Correlations based upon pathophysiology, histology, immunohistochemistry, molecular and biochemical pathways are promising but also provide insights into the limitations as well as a need for improvement.

Models

The most widely used animal models of Barrett's esophagus include a rodent model, a murine model, and a canine model.

The first described animal model was a canine model in 1971. Dogs had surgically-induced esophageal reflux by creating a hiatal hernia and disrupting the lower esophageal sphincter, while acid hypersecretion was accomplished by giving animals histamine or pentagastrin. More recently, similar studies demonstrated a canine model where animals either had acid reflux *via* cardiectomy or bile reflux *via* total gastrectomy and esophagojejunostomy. The disadvantage of the canine model is that it takes years for Barrett's esophagus to develop.

The alternative animal models are the rat model and the mouse model. These models use surgical interventions with or without carcinogens and genetic manipulations. Typical surgical interventions to induce reflux include 1) gastrectomy plus esophagojejunostomy, 2) stomach and vagus preserving esophagojejunostomy or esophagoduodenostomy and 3) esophagogastroduodenostomy. Long-term bile acid supplementation is also proposed as a model. The rat and mouse models have the advantage of showing the development of Barrett's esophagus within the first 3-4 months of surgically-induced reflux and a high rate of esophageal adenocarcinoma.

Comparative studies and challenges

Unlike most other cancers, esophageal adenocarcinoma is unique in that it has features of columnar or glandular epithelium in an organ that is normally lined by squamous epithelium. Therefore, the models require a switch of squamous epithelium to columnar epithelium followed by signals which initiate cancer in this epithelium. Therefore, the challenge is two-fold, first to recognize the development of columnar metaplasia and next to undertake comparative studies for the adenocarcinoma.

Anatomy and pathophysiology

The forestomach in mice and rats, in contrast to humans, is lined by squamous epithelium, therefore the squamocolumnar junction is not at the end of the distal esophagus but rather in the mid-stomach body. Animals also lack submucosal glands in the esophagus, which is proposed to be one of the mechanisms that help in the development of columnar metaplasia. Most of the models have near neutral pH reflux, where injury is mainly induced by pancreatico-biliary contents. Acidification of drinking water to pH 4 along with surgical intervention to induce reflux can potentially recapitulate what is a more common subtype of reflux in patients with Barrett's esophagus and adenocarcinoma. One may argue that these differences are irrelevant because in the canine model either acid or bile salt reflux is sufficient to induce both Barrett's metaplasia and esophageal adenocarcinoma.

Histology

Barrett's metaplasia in animals appears as small foci and almost never has long-segments as seen in patients. However, the foci are periodic-acid Schiff (PAS) positive. The columnar mucosa in animals has goblet cells and is typically incomplete in nature. Similar to patients with Barrett's esophagus, multilayer epithelium and cells of ulcer associated lineage are also noted. Cellular features of dysplasia are present but flat dysplasia is less common. However, there is intense injury and inflammation which sometimes make it difficult to label mucosa as dysplastic. Adenocarcinoma is usually well-differentiated and exophytic. It does invade surrounding liver and is tumorigenic in nude mice. Tumors occasionally have adenosquamous phenotype particularly in animals that receive carcinogens in addition to surgical reflux. Surprisingly, the cell lines derived from the well differentiated adenocarcinomas in rats, when injected in nude mice, give rise to tumors with squamous cell cancer phenotype.

Immunohistochemistry, molecular and cell biochemical pathways

Several key pathways that have potential to promote carcinogenesis in Barrett's mucosa of patients are found to be up-regulated in the animal models of Barrett's esophagus. Immunohistochemistry, Western blotting, ELISA and EMSA suggest that surgically induced reflux activates PI3K, AKT, NFκB, cytosolic phospholipase A2, COX-2 and prostaglandin E2. When examined for mucin, CK7, CK20, Das1, villin, PS2/TFF1, c-myc, p-IKK (S181) and p-S6K1 (T389) and p53, Barrett's foci in animals also show marked similarities to patients with Barrett's esophagus. The challenge remains that several antibodies need to be developed due to the variability in the protein sequences between patients and animals.

Comparative oncogenomics

Preliminary studies show that there are similarities when the expression patterns of evolutionarily conserved genes are compared during progression from normal squamous epithelium to Barrett's mucosa and from Barrett's mucosa to adenocarcinoma in rats and humans.

Future directions

Several groups are working to develop novel models to understand the development of metaplasia and esophageal adenocarcinoma. Endodermal differentiation during early embryonic age in mice provides a model system to understand the development of Barrett's metaplasia. Xenograft models of cell lines and cancer are being investigated to recapitulate the complex multicellular and cell-extracellular matrix interactions that are involved in the initiation and progression of cancer. Nude rat and mice models are being developed to provide an alternative means to determine the causes of and treatments for esophageal malignancy. Adenoviral and retroviral infections and transgenic models are also being explored.

Summary

Animal models represent a resource of immense potential to unfold the development of Barrett's metaplasia and esophageal adenocarcinoma. The sophistication of modelling esophageal carcinogenesis in animals is slowly improving. This will allow investigators to observe and manipulate the complex process of carcinogenesis in a manner which is not possible to perform in patients.

Bibliography

- Bonde P, Sui G, Dhara S, et al. Cytogenetic characterization and gene expression profiling in the rat reflux-induced esophageal tumor model. J Thorac Cardiovasc Surg 2007;133:763-9.
- Buttar NS, Wang KK, Leontovich O, et al. Chemoprevention of esophageal adenocarcinoma by COX-2 inhibitors in an animal model of Barrett's esophagus. Gastroenterology 2002;122:1101-12.
- Fein M, Peters JH, Baril N, et al. Loss of function of Trp53, but not Apc, leads to the development of esophageal adenocarcinoma in mice with jejunoesophageal reflux. J Surg Res 1999;83:48-55.
- Milano F, Van Baal JWPM, Buttar NS, et al. Bone morphogenetic protein 4 expressed in esophagitis induces a columnar phenotype in esophageal squamous cells. Gastroenterology 2007;132:2412-21.
- Su Y, Chen X, Klein M, et al. Phenotype of columnar-lined esophagus in rats with esophagogastroduodenal anastomosis: similarity to human Barrett's esophagus. Lab Invest 2004;84:753-65.
- Yen CJ, et al. Cancer Res 2008 (in press).

Lessons from animal models: prevention of esophageal adenocarcinogenesis

K. Miwa (Uozu)

Esophageal adenocarcinoma arises in the Barrett's mucosa and is induced by reflux esophagitis. The metaplasia-adenocarcinoma sequence is possibly associated with duodenogastric reflux. In animal experiments, rats, which had undergone duodeno- or gastroduodenoesophageal reflux (DER or GDER) surgery, had columnar-lined epithelium and subsequent adenocarcinoma in the lower esophagus 50 weeks after surgery. This carcinogenesis did not arise due to the administration of carcinogens and was not observed in rats with gastroesophageal reflux (GER). The sequence looks remarkably like that of human esophageal adenocarcinogenesis. We investigated whether this rat carcinogenesis can be inhibited by some possible factors.

Animals and surgical procedure

Eight-week-old male Fisher 344 rats were used and given standard solid chow (CRF-1; Japan Charles River) and tap water. The animals were given no carcinogen.

Duodenoesophageal reflux

A rat surgical model for esophageal metaplasia-adenocarcinoma sequence induced by DER, which was established by our group in 1996 [1], was employed. Briefly, through an upper middle incision, total gastrectomy was performed. The duodenal stump was closed and then the esophageal stump was anastomosed to the jejunum approximately 4 cm distal to the Treitz's ligament in the end-to-side fashion. Finally, the oral jejunal cut end was anastomosed end-to-side with the jejunal loop approximately 4 cm distal to the esophago-jejunostoma. This surgery permitted only duodenal contents to flow back into the esophagus.

Duodenal switch

The animals with DER were relaparatomized and underwent a procedure which changed the reconstruction (the Schlatter type) into Roux-en-Y type to prevent DER.

Gastroduodenoesophageal reflux

The abdominal esophagus was transected under the diaphragm, and the distal cut end was closed with sutures. The esophageal stump was then anastomosed end-to-side to a loop of jejunum 4 cm distal to the Treitz's ligament in an ante-colic manner. This procedure allowed gastroduodenal contents to flow back into the esophagus.

Gastroesophageal reflux

The duodenum was cut off near the pylorus, and the distal duodenal stump was closed. The jejunum was transected approximately 4 cm distal to the Treitz's ligament, and the distal, cut end was closed with sutures. The proximal duodenal stump was anastomosed end-to-side with the distal jejunum near the sutures. Careful to preserve both vagus nerves, the abdominal esophagus was transected below the diaphragm, and the distal cut end was closed with sutures. The esophageal stump was anastomosed end-to-side to the distal jejunum approximately 4 cm distal to the gastro-jejunostoma. Finally, the proximal jejunal cut end was anastomosed end-to-side with the jejunal loop approximately 4 cm distal to the esophago-jejunostoma. This surgery permitted only gastric contents to flow back into the esophagus.

Approach to prevent esophageal adenocarcinogenesis

Biliary diversion

It is controversial whether antireflux surgery for Barrett esophagus and subsequent adenocarcinogenesis is effective or not. Though some authors indicated complete regression of Barrett's esophagus and a reduced risk of dysplasia and carcinoma, most papers demonstrated that antireflux surgery can not make the Barrett's esophagus regress. We aimed to examine whether biliary diversion surgery in rats with DER affects the development of columnar-lined epithelium and adenocarcinoma [2].

The animals with DER were divided into 5 groups: the DER20, DER30 and DER50 groups (the duodenoesophageal group; n = 80) were defined as subgroups of animals that were killed at 20, 30 and 50 weeks after surgery, respectively. The BD20 and BD30 groups (the biliary diversion procedure group; n = 80) were relaparatomized at 20 and 30 weeks after DER procedure, respectively, and received the duodenal switch procedure. The animals of the duodenal switch procedure groups were killed 50 weeks after the DER procedure. The incidence of columnar-lined epithelium was 100%, 92% and 94% in the animals in the DER 50, BD30 and DER30, respectively. These percentages were significantly higher than in animals in the DER20 (54%) and BD20 (62%) ($p < 0.01$). The incidence of columnar-lined epithelium in the BD30 and DER30 groups and in the BD20 and DER20 groups was similar. This implies that columnar-lined epithelium is irreversible, even if the causative factor is eliminated. On the other hand, the incidence of adenocarcinoma was significantly lower in the BD30 group (19%) and the BD20 group (3%) than in the DER50 group (60%). This means that reflux-preventing procedures can inhibit carcinogenesis. Conclusively, biliary diversion surgery prevented esophageal carcinogenesis but it did not make the columnar-lined epithelium regress.

Cyclooxygenase-2 inhibitors

Human esophagitis, Barrett's esophagus and adenocarcinoma contain up-regulated cyclooxygenase-2 (COX-2). COX-2 plays an important role in some aspects of tumorigenesis, such as the increase of cell proliferation, the reduction of apoptosis, and the promotion of angiogenesis. Furthermore, recent reports suggest the antitumor effect of selective inhibitors of COX-2 in esophageal carcinogenesis. This study is aimed to determine the association of COX-2 expression and DER, and the effect of a specific COX-

2 inhibitor in genesis of columnar-lined epithelium and esophageal adenocarcinoma in rats [3].

The DER rats were randomly divided into two groups: the control group (n = 60) rats were given commercial rat chow (CRF-1); the celecoxib group (n = 30) rats were given experimental rat chow premixed with celecoxib (500 ppm, 100 mg/Kg body weight/day). Celecoxib was obtained from SEARLE Company. An additional ten rats were monitored without any intervention and given commercial rat chow to obtain normal esophageal tissue. Randomly selected rats were killed by diethyl-ether inhalation at the 10th, 20th, 30th, and 40*th* week after surgery. Ten animals in the control group and five animals in the celecoxib group were killed every ten weeks until the 30th week after surgery. All remaining animals were sacrificed at the 40th week.

The distal portion of the esophagi in all the rats in the celecoxib group was smooth and without thickening though it was thickened and irregular in the control group. COX-2 expression of the mucosa after DER procedures markedly increased at 10 and 20 weeks and sequentially decreased at 30 and 40 weeks. However, there was no difference in the COX-2 expression between the celecoxib group and the control group. COX-2 immunoreactivity was observed in the stroma of epithelium with esophagitis, columnar-lined epithelium and adenocarcinoma. COX-2 mRNA expression was greater in the esophagi of rats with DER as compared to the results in the normal esophagi of those rats without surgical intervention ($p < 0.005$). The COX-2 stained cells were likely to be fibroblasts, infiltrating cells, and some Barrett's epithelial cells. The prostaglandin E2 level of the mucosa increased at 10 weeks and sequentially decreased at 20, 30 and 40 weeks after surgery. Compared with the control group, prostaglandin E2 induction at each week was significantly suppressed in the celecoxib group.

In the control group, columnar-lined epithelium and adenocarcinoma were observed first at 20 weeks and 30 weeks, respectively. Both incidences sequentially increased and at the 40th week reached 85% and 45%, respectively. On the other hand, in the celecoxib group, the esophagitis was mild and the incidence of columnar-lined epithelium was significantly lower for each group as compared with the control group, and adenocarcinoma was not observed throughout the experiment ($p < 0.05$).

In summary, there was a correlation between COX-2 expression and DER in rats. Esophagitis was related with the PGE2. Celecoxib is effective in preventing columnar-lined epithelium and adenocarcinoma by suppressing reflux esophagitis. Inhibition of COX-2 may be beneficial for patients with reflux-related metaplasia-adenocarcinoma sequence.

Nitrite scavenger

Thiazolidine-4-carboxylic acid, thioproline (TPRO), is a sulfur amino acid, a condensation product of cysteine and formaldehyde. In 1984 Tahira *et al.* described that thioproline acts as a nitrite scavenger and suppresses *in vivo* formation of carcinogenic N-nitroso compounds in the body [4]. Ingested thioproline, TPRO, effectively traps nitrites in the alimentary tract, and its nitrosated product, N-nitroso-thioproline (N-TPRO), is excreted from the body in the urine. Thus urinary N-TPRO is a sensitive probe for endogenous nitrosation. In 1998, Nakai, at that time a member of our department at Kanazawa University, observed that ingestion of thioproline increased the excretion of N-TPRO in the urine and decreased the incidence of gastric carcinoma in rats surgically induced by duodenogastric procedure [5]. These results showed that the development of gastric carcinomas in rats induced by DER is associated with endogenous nitrosation. With these items in mind our most recent model for the inhibition of carcinogenesis involved the use of thioproline [6]. A series of 200 male Fisher 344 rats received surgery to induce GDER. The control group rats were fed a standard diet. Others were fed a special diet containing 0.5% thioproline. The rats were sacrificed every 10 weeks from 25 weeks to 45 weeks after surgery. The macroscopic appearance indicated that the incidences of lesions in both groups increased in the later weeks, but the changes were similar for both groups over the duration of the experiment. Histological changes in the GDER rats included erosion, regenerative thickening and basal cell hyperplasia, all of which were present in all rats throughout the duration of the experiment. Columnar-lined epithelium was observed in both groups from 25 weeks to 45 weeks after surgery. At any given time during the experiment, the incidence of columnar-lined esophagus was almost the same for both groups. The incidence of adenocarcinoma in the lower esophagus for the TPRO and control groups was 0% and 0% at 25 weeks, 0% and 11% at 35 weeks, and 5% and 44% at 45 weeks, respectively. The occurrence of adenocarcinoma in the TPRO group was significantly lower than that in the control group at 45 weeks after surgery. In summary, the incidence of adenocarcinoma resulting from GDER was suppressed by oral administration of 0.5% thioproline during the progression from columnar-lined epithelium to adenocarcinoma. This fact indicates N-nitroso compounds, which are produced by endogenous nitrosation, play an important role in the formation of adenocarcinoma in a rat GDER model.

Conclusion

Valuable lessons learned from animal experiments suggest to us that reflux-induced esophageal carcinogenesis in rats is closely associated with endogenous nitrosation. The carcinogenesis can be inhibited by biliary diversion surgery, administration of COX-2 inhibitor or thioproline. We suggest thioproline administration, antireflux surgery and COX-2 inhibitor administration as possible approaches to prevent columnar-lined epithelium and adenocarcinoma.

References

1. Miwa K, Sahara M, Segawa M, et al. Reflux of duodenal or gastroduodenal contents induces esophageal carcinoma in rats. Int J Cancer 1996;67:269-74.
2. Nishijima K, Miwa K, Miyashita T, et al. Impact of the Biliary diversion procedure on carcinogenesis in Barrett's esophagus surgically induced by duodenoesophageal reflux in rats. Ann Surg 2004;240:57-67.
3. Oyama K, Fujimura T, Ninomiya I, et al. A COX-2 inhibitor prevents the esophageal inflammation-metaplasia-adenocarcinoma sequence in rats. Carcinogenesis 2005;26:565-70.
4. Tahira T, Tsuda M, Wakabayashi K, et al. Kinetics of nitrosation of thioproline, the precursor of a major nitroso compound in human urine, and its role as a nitrite scavenger. Gann 1984;75:889-94.
5. Nakai M, Inhibitory effect of thioproline on gastric carcinogenesis in rats with surgically induced duodenogastric reflux. J Juzen Med Soc 1996;105:648-57.
6. Sasaki S, Miwa K, Fujimura T, et al, Ingestion of Thioproline suppresses rat esophageal adenocarcinogenesis caused by duodenogastroesophageal reflux. Oncol Rep 2007;18(6):1443-9.

Synergistic interaction of low pH and bile acids

K. Dvorak, H.S. Garewal (Tucson)

Barrett's esophagus is a premalignant condition associated with the development of esophageal adenocarcinoma [4,5,10]. Patients with this cancer have a poor prognosis with a median survival of less than one year [3]. The precise mechanisms underlying the development of Barrett's esophagus and esophageal adenocarcinoma remain undefined.

Clinical studies have demonstrated that Barrett's esophagus patients have a higher acid exposure profile than patients with erosive esophagitis alone, regardless of the patients' position during the test [13,18]. Various factors, such as high prevalence of hiatal hernia [2], esophageal body motility abnormalities [11] and abnormally reduced lower esophageal sphincter basal pressure [16] may contribute to increased acid exposure and to an increase in esophageal mucosal contact time with refluxate. Although much of the focus has been on pH conditions (acid exposure), recently there has been increasing recognition of the potential role of other components of refluxate, especially bile acids, in the etiopathology of this condition. Nehra *et al.* showed that bile acids reflux into the esophagus concurrently with gastric acids [15]. Furthermore, they demonstrated that all Barrett's esophagus patients refluxed bile acids into the esophagus and that significantly higher levels of bile acids are present in the esophagi of patients with Barrett's esophagus than in controls [15]. Many studies have linked bile acids to colon carcinogenesis. Therefore bile acids may also play a crucial role in esophageal carcinogenesis.

Bile acids can be conjugated either with glycine or taurine. The solubility and cell damaging properties of different bile acids depend on their pKa and the ambient pH. At a pH corresponding to their pKa, 50% of a bile acid will be in the unionized form and 50% in the ionized form. Only the unionized bile acid can enter the cell through the cell membrane and influence intracellular pathways. At a significantly lower pH than its pKa, the bile acid irreversibly precipitates; at significantly higher pH than the pKa the bile acid is largely ionized and thus unable to penetrate the cell membrane. These basic chemical properties result in a profound effect of pH on the ability of a bile acid to influence cellular pathways.

We recently reported that patients with Barrett's esophagus have a longer duration of very low pH (pH $\leq$ 2] in the distal part of the esophagus, compared with erosive esophagitis patients [6]. Increased exposure to these very low pHs in Barrett's esophagus patients may have a direct injurious effect on the esophageal mucosa, which may also potentiate increased solubility, and thus the ability of certain bile acids with low pKa, such as taurodeoxycholic acid, to damage cells. Taurine conjugated bile acids are soluble and active at this very low pH, which is in fact the normal pH of the stomach (~2) since their pKa is approximately 2. In direct support of this, our data suggest that even a very brief exposure to the combination of 0.5 mM taurodeoxycholic acid (TDCA) and pH 2 is strongly associated with the induction of oxidative stress in the Seg-1 esophageal cell line (*Figure 1*). We used a dye that becomes fluorescent after oxidation, Hydroethidium, in conjunction with flow cytometry and fluorescence microscopy to study these effects. Reactive oxygen species (ROS) are generated after only a 60 second treatment with pH 2 in Seg-1 esophageal cells and the induction of ROS was significantly greater when the cells are

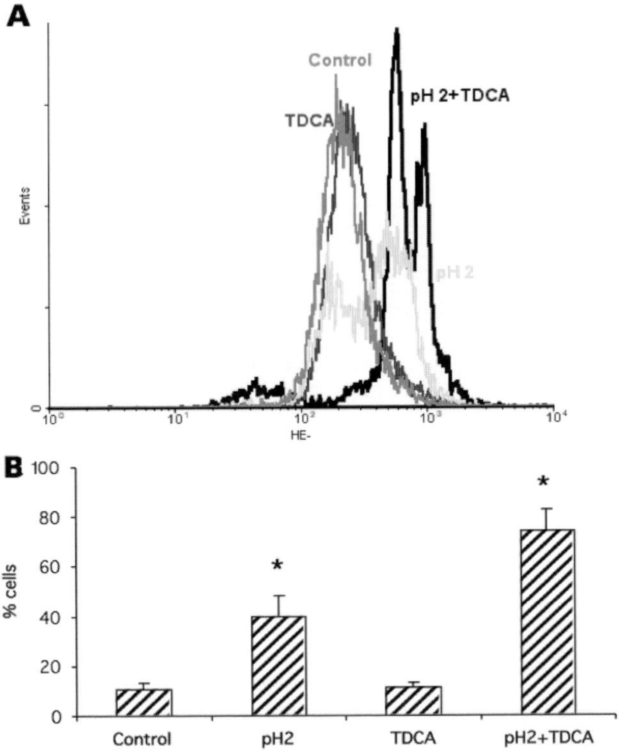

Figure 1. Levels of reactive oxygen species (by HE staining) in Seg-1 esophageal adenocarcinoma cells after exposure to low pH and/or TDCA. **A.** Histogram of untreated Seg-1 cells (control), cells treated with 0.5 mM TDCA at pH 7.4, cells treated with pH 2 and cells treated a combination of 0.5 mM TDCA and pH2 for 60 seconds, washed twice and stained with dihydroethidium (HE) as a measure of oxidative stress. **B.** Percentage of cells staining with HE in Seg-1 cells untreated (control) or treated with pH 2, 0.5mM TDCA or with a combination of 0.5 mM TDCA and pH 2. Asterisk indicates statistically significant difference compared to control.

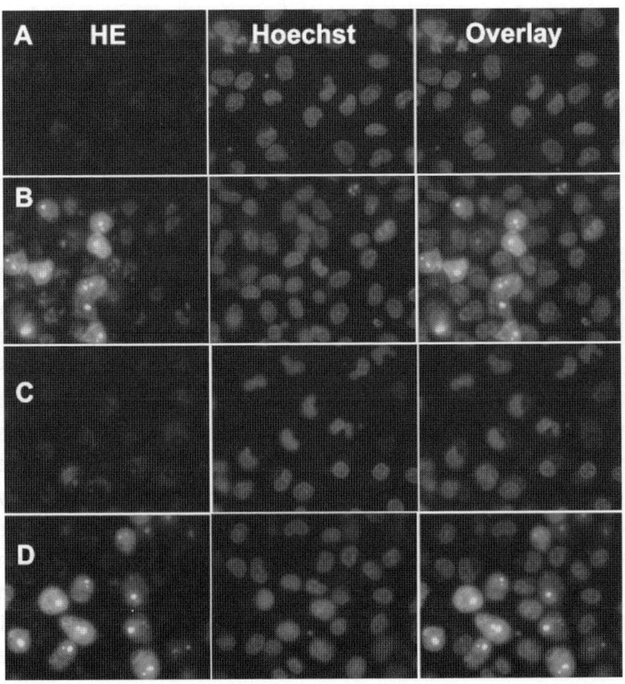

Figure 2. Oxidative stress in Seg-1 cells. Seg-1 cells were untreated (**A**) or exposed for 1 minute to pH 2 (**B**), 0.5 mM TDCA in neutral medium at pH 7.4 (**C**) or 0.5 mM TDCA in medium acidified to pH 2 (**D**), washed and stained with HE for 25 minutes and then with Hoechst 33342 for 5 minutes. The red signal represents oxidative damage (HE) while the blue signal represents nuclei (Hoechst 33342). (See page XXIII for colour figure).

treated with acidified medium containing 0.5 mM TDCA acid for 60 seconds (*Figures 1 and 2*). However, no increase in the level of ROS was observed if the cells were treated with TDCA alone at pH 7.4 (*Figures 1 and 2*). Pretreatment for 1 hour with antioxidants, such as 10 mM epigallocatechin galleate (EGCG) or N-acetylcysteine (NAC), inhibited the generation of ROS (*Figure 3*).

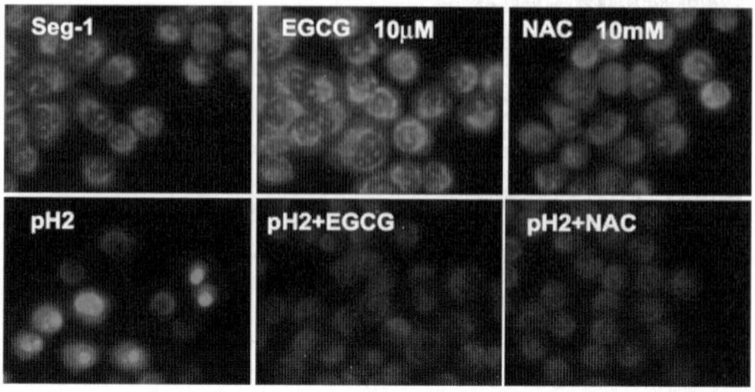

Figure 3. Oxidative stress induced in Seg-1 by pH 2 is inhibited by the pretreatment for 60 minutes with anti-oxidants such as EGCG or N-acetyl-cysteine (NAC). Red signal represents HE, a marker of oxidative stress. (See page XXIII for colour figure).

In contrast, at a higher pH (i. e. pH 4) glycine conjugated bile acids are soluble, unionized and thus active since their pKa is about 4. Glycine conjugated bile acids are the most prevalent bile acids in human bile and thus an increase of stomach pH, e.g. by proton pump inhibitor treatment to pH 4 may prevent normal precipitation of glycine-conjugated bile acids that would occur at pH 2. Theoretically this could lead to intracellular access and damage by these bile acids. In order to mimic the *in vivo* situation, we also used "bile acid cocktail" that reflects the composition of bile acids present in refluxate and showed that it induces oxidative DNA and mitochondrial damage *in vitro* in different esophageal cell lines, and *ex vivo* in esophageal biopsies [7]. The "bile acid cocktail" consisted of glycocholic acid, glycodeoxycholic acid, glychenodeoxycholic acid, taurocholic acid and deoxycholic acid. Oxidative stress was observed only when we used a combination of 0.1 mM bile acid cocktail and medium acidified to pH 4 with no effect being detected if the "bile acid cocktail" or acidified medium was used alone [7].

Gastric acid and bile acids have been shown to alter signaling pathways, such as the MAPK and NF-κB pathways [1,12,14,17]. These pathways are associated with increased proliferation and decreased apoptosis of esophageal cells. Indeed, we have shown that Barrett's esophagus cells are resistant to apoptosis [8]. Our group was also the first to show that IL-6/STAT3 signaling is elevated in Barrett's esophagus. IL-6 secretion is increased in Barrett's esophagus compared to squamous epithelium or duodenum. Both IL-6 and the IL-6 receptor are expressed in Barrett's esophagus epithelial cells [9]. This pro-survival cytokine activates the anti-apoptotic STAT3 pathway which results in increased expression of anti-apoptotic proteins such as survivin, Mcl-1 and Bcl-xL [8,9]. Our more recent experiments suggest that low pH and "bile acid cocktail" increase IL-6 protein secretion in Seg-1 esophageal cells. We also found that treatment with low pH and "bile acid cocktail" induces increased STAT3 translocation to the nucleus and increased expression of anti-apoptotic proteins (*Figure 4*). Importantly, increased nuclear staining of activated STAT3 was also detected in dysplastic Barrett's esophagus biopsies and in cancer tissues.

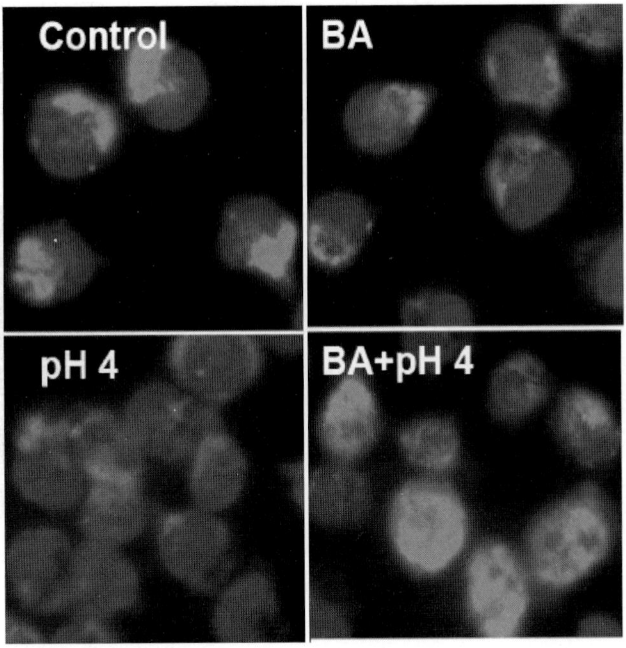

Figure 4. STAT3 translocation to the nucleus after 10 minutes treatment with 0.1 mM bile acid cocktail (BA) in acidified medium to pH4. The red signal represents STAT3, and the blue signal represents nucleus (DAPI staining). (See page XXIV for colour figure).

In summary, bile acids in combination with low pH induce oxidative stress and activate signaling pathways associated with resistance to apoptosis in esophageal cells. Chronic episodic exposure of the esophagus to bile acids and low pH as occurs in reflux episodes, may cause abnormal cell signaling leading to apoptosis resistance, increased proliferation and thus increased risk of developing esophageal adenocarcinoma. Bile acids appear to play a key role in this process.

References

1. Abdel-Latif MM, O'Riordan J, Windle HJ, et al. NF-kappaB activation in esophageal adenocarcinoma: relationship to Barrett's metaplasia, survival, and response to neoadjuvant chemoradiotherapy. Ann Surg 2004;239:491-500.
2. Cameron AJ. Barrett's esophagus: prevalence and size of hiatal hernia. Am J Gastroenterol 1999;94:2054-9.
3. DeMeester TR. Management of adenocarcinoma arising in Barrett's esophagus. Semin Thorac Cardiovasc Surg 1997;9:290-301.
4. Devesa SS, Blot WJ, Fraumeni JF Jr. Changing patterns in the incidence of esophageal and gastric carcinoma in the United States. Cancer 1998;83:2049-53.
5. Drewitz DJ, Sampliner RE, Garewal HS. The incidence of adenocarcinoma in Barrett's esophagus: a prospective study of 170 patients followed 4.8 years. Am J Gastroenterol 1997;92:212-5.
6. Dvorak K, Fass R, Dekel R, et al. Esophageal acid exposure at pH < or = 2 is more common in Barrett's esophagus patients and is associated with oxidative stress. Dis Esophagus 2006;19:366-72.
7. Dvorak K, Payne CM, Chavarria M, et al. Bile acids in combination with low pH induce oxidative stress and oxidative DNA damage: relevance to the pathogenesis of Barrett's Oesophagus. Gut 2007;56:763-71.
8. Dvorakova K, Payne CM, Ramsey L, et al. Apoptosis resistance in Barrett's esophagus: ex vivo bioassay of live stressed tissues. Am J Gastroenterol 2005;100:424-31.
9. Dvorakova K, Payne CM, Ramsey L, et al. Increased expression and secretion of interleukin-6 in patients with Barrett's esophagus. Clin Cancer Res 2004;10:2020-8.
10. Falk GW. Barrett's esophagus. Gastroenterology 2002;122:1569-91.
11. Kahrilas PJ, Dodds WJ, Hogan WJ. Effect of peristaltic dysfunction on esophageal volume clearance. Gastroenterology 1988;94: 73-80.

12. Kaur BS, Triadafilopoulos G. Acid- and bile-induced PGE(2) release and hyperproliferation in Barrett's esophagus are COX-2 and PKC-epsilon dependent. Am J Physiol Gastrointest Liver Physiol 2002;283:G327-34.
13. Martinez SD, Malagon IB, Garewal HS, Cui H, Fass R. Non-erosive reflux disease (NERD)—acid reflux and symptom patterns. Aliment Pharmacol Ther 2003;17:537-45.
14. Morgan C, Alazawi W, Sirieix P, Freeman T, Coleman N, Fitzgerald R. In vitro acid exposure has a differential effect on apoptotic and proliferative pathways in a Barrett's adenocarcinoma cell line. Am J Gastroenterol 2004;99:218-24.
15. Nehra D, Howell P, Williams CP, Pye JK, Beynon J. Toxic bile acids in gastro-oesophageal reflux disease: influence of gastric acidity. Gut 1999;44:598-602.
16. Parkman HP, Fisher RS. Contributing role of motility abnormalities in the pathogenesis of gastroesophageal reflux disease. Dig Dis 1997;15:40-52.
17. Souza RF, Shewmake K, Terada LS, Spechler SJ. Acid exposure activates the mitogen-activated protein kinase pathways in Barrett's esophagus. Gastroenterology 2002;122:299-307.
18. Vaezi MF, Richter JE. Role of acid and duodenogastroesophageal reflux in gastroesophageal reflux disease. Gastroenterology 1996;111:1192-9.

Induction of Barrett's metaplasia by acid and bile acid

N.J. Clemons, R. Fitzgerald (Cambridge)

Barrett's esophagus represents the first stage in the neoplastic sequence leading to esophageal adenocarcinoma. Once thought to be a congenital condition [1], Barrett's esophagus is now known to be an acquired condition that develops as a consequence of chronic reflux symptoms or gastroesophageal reflux disease (GERD). However, the aetiopathogenesis of Barrett's esophagus is currently unclear. Although reflux certainly plays an important role, it is likely that other environmental and genetic factors are also involved. An understanding of the development of Barrett's esophagus is likely to lead to a greater understanding of the pathogenesis of adenocarcinoma, and hence to the development of preventative and therapeutic strategies

Cell of origin

The conversion of squamous to columnar epithelium in the esophagus is a poorly understood process, particularly in comparison to epithelial metaplasias at other sites such as the cervix [2]. In particular, the cell of origin for Barrett's metaplasia is yet to be defined, although there are currently a number of theories:

- proximal migration of gastric or junctional columnar epithelium to replace the damaged epithelium (creeping substitution theory);
- stem cells in the basal layer of the inflamed mucosa or neck region of esophageal gland ducts undergoing altered programming;
- bone-marrow derived stem cells migrating to the esophagus;
- transdifferentiation of squamous epithelial cells;
- mesenchymal to epithelial transition (MET) of underlying stromal cells.

Of these theories, those implicating a multipotential stem cell are favoured since cell types not normally found in the esophagus, such as goblet and parietal cells, may be present in the metaplastic epithelium. The location of the squamous epithelium stem cell is likely to be in the basal layer between the papillae [3], or possibly in the neck region of submucosal gland ducts [4]. However, it is unclear whether Barrett's epithelium arises from the squamous stem cells. Successful induction of intestinal metaplasia in a canine model in which a ring of squamous epithelium had been removed to provide a barrier between the gastric cardia and the experimentally induced intestinal metaplasia, suggested that the cell of origin is intrinsic to the esophagus in contrast to the "creeping substitution" theory [5]. This hypothesis is supported by the presence of cytokeratin 13 in Barrett's epithelium, which is characteristic of squamous epithelia but is not present in the columnar epithelium of the cardia [6]. Thus, it is possible that the same stem cell may be responsible for the production of squamous epithelium under normal conditions and the columnar epithelium of Barrett's esophagus following chronic reflux. However, some recent preliminary evidence from rodent models show that both squamous epithelium [7,8] and Barrett's epithelium [9] regenerated following irradiation injury or surgically induced reflux respectively, are at least partly derived from progenitor cells derived from the bone marrow. This theory is supported by evidence from mouse models showing that bone marrow derived cells (BMDCs) may be responsible for a number of epithelial malignancies, particularly gastric cancer (reviewed in [10]). In the case of Barrett's esophagus, BMDCs also significantly contributed to the stroma of the new epithelium [9], however this work was only published in abstract form and there is yet to be any follow-up data from this group. Interestingly bone marrow derived myofibroblasts and fibroblasts have also been shown to contribute to the generation of a number of tissues including lung, stomach, skin and kidney and that this process is promoted by injury [7]. Once metaplasia is initiated in the esophagus, it is thought that columnar cells colonise the mucosa rapidly within 3 years, with only 5-10% of metaplasias increasing in surface area after that [11]. Others have reported that Barrett's esophagus develops in a matter of weeks [12].

The role of reflux in Barrett's metaplasia

It is well established that Barrett's esophagus develops as a consequence of chronic reflux and indeed, regardless of which theory for the cell of origin is correct, development of Barrett's esophagus depends upon reflux induced damage to initiate the metaplastic process. It has been proposed that stem cells are induced to undergo an altered programme of differentiation by extrinsic factors providing appropriate signals following chronic damage to the esophageal epithelium [13]. In support of this view, the prevalence of Barrett's esophagus is 1.2% in people without GERD, compared to 2.3% in those with GERD [14]. It seems unlikely that the squamous stem cells are directly exposed to the luminal environment, instead it would seem more likely that reflux induces alterations in cell signalling surrounding the stem cells, which could alter programming [3,15]. It has been suggested that when reflux exposure is repetitive and chronic, denuded areas of the esophagus may be replaced with metaplastic columnar epithelium as a protective mechanism. This new epithelium may be more acid resistant and pluripotent, thus it continues to regenerate in the presence of a toxic luminal environment. This is supported by evidence from a rat reflux model, in which damage to the esophagus was more readily repaired with columnar epithelium than with squamous epithelium, particularly under low pH conditions, suggesting that columnar cells are inherently more resistant to acid [16].

The refluxate is highly heterogeneous and its components can include saliva, food, acid, mucous and pepsin. In many patients with Barrett's esophagus, duodenal components including bile salts, trypsin, lipase and cholesterol are also present [17]. Of these components, most attention has been given to acid and bile in the development of Barrett's esophagus. A number of studies have used animal models to examine the potential of reflux to cause damage to the esophagus and lead to esophagitis and metaplasia reminiscent of Barrett's esophagus in humans. In a dog model, columnar regeneration occurred following exposure to acid or acid and bile in combination but not after exposure to bile alone [5]. In contrast, experiments in rodent models have demonstrated that gastroduodenoesophageal reflux (GDER) with its mix of acid, bile, pepsin and other components is more important than acid reflux alone in the pathogenesis of a Barrett's esophagus-like condition very similar to human Barrett's esophagus [18,19]. Similarly, in humans, while exposure to acid alone is sufficient to cause esophagitis, GDER appears to be required for the pathogenesis of Barrett's esophagus [20].

Acid and bile mediated events relevant to metaplasia

Growth control

Although the exact mechanisms by which reflux components promote the development of the metaplastic epithelium are presently unclear, there are a number of ways in which acid and bile may trigger metaplasia. For example, acid and bile in the extracellular environment promotes breakdown of the extracellular matrix [21]. In addition, cytoplasmic acid and bile affect growth control and differentiation status. In *in vitro* and *ex vivo* models, acid stimulates either proliferation or differentiation depending on the duration of acid exposure [22-24]. Current evidence shows that acid-induced proliferation *in vitro* occurs *via* sodium/hydrogen exchanger and MAPK mediated signalling pathways [24-26]. Low pH can also inhibit apoptosis *in vitro via* activation of the MAPK pathways [25] and down-regulation of the caspase cascade [27]. Similarly, bile acids have been shown to stimulate proliferation in Barrett's esophagus, although this effect was inhibited at low pH [28]. In contrast, at low pH, bile acids are soluble and non-polar and can accumulate in the cells where they can cause mitochondrial and DNA damage [29], demonstrating that the activity of bile acids is highly dependent on pH .

DNA damage

Acid and bile may also contribute to metaplasia *via* DNA damage mediated genetic alterations. The level of DNA strand breaks, but not oxidative damage, was found to be significantly higher in Barrett's mucosa compared to squamous mucosa from the same patient [30]. A number of recent studies have demonstrated that both acid and bile can induce DNA strand breaks [31] and oxidative damage in esophageal cell lines and tissue [32,33]. Both acid and bile induce the intracellular production of reactive oxygen species (ROS) and the anti-oxidant vitamin C can inhibit this damage, suggesting that ROS mediate acid and bile induced DNA damage [32,33]. High levels of nitric oxide (NO) are also generated in the lumen of the esophagus during bouts of reflux due to the reduction of salivary nitrite by acid and vitamin C in the refluxate [34]. Given the mutagenic potential of NO and its derivatives, it is tempting to speculate that luminal concentration of NO may also contribute to the generation of genetic abnormalities in the esophageal mucosa. However, whilst a Barrett's epithelium may contain a number of genetic abnormalities it is unknown whether these are causative or whether they occur after metaplasia has developed and thus may contribute to the progression of benign Barrett's esophagus to dysplastic tissue and beyond.

Effect of acid and bile on targets relevant to metaplasia

There are a number of studies demonstrating the effect of acid and bile on target genes that may be relevant to Barrett's metaplasia (*Table I*). Bile acid has also been shown to cause histone modification [35], activate NF-κB at neutral pH [36] and induce c-myc at acidic pH [37]. These data demonstrate the potential of bile to stimulate genes and signalling pathways that could play a role in metaplasia.

Table I. Effects of acid and bile on specific targets relevant to metaplasia.

Target	Acid	Bile
cdx1/2	*Via* NF-κB ?methylation	*Via* NF-κB and altered methylation
Integrins	*Via* MAPK	*Via* MAPK
Cytokines: TGFβ, IL-1β	Activated/↑expression ?methylation	Activated/↑expression ?methylation
Retinoic acid	?	Lithocholic acid binds promoter

Cdx1/2

Recent work has implicated the caudal-related homeobox genes *cdx1* and *cdx2* as possible drivers of metaplasia in Barrett's esophagus. The protein products of these genes are developmental transcription factors involved in specialisation of the gut during embryogenesis [38]. In adults, expression of Cdx1/2 protein is restricted to intestinal-type epithelium and is thus not normally expressed in the stomach or the esophagus. However, re-expression of Cdx1/2 in Barrett's epithelium has been reported by a number of groups [39-44]. Abnormal expression of Cdx2 mRNA has also been found in the squamous epithelium adjacent to Barrett's esophagus segments, leading to the suggestion that its expression may precede the morphological changes seen in Barrett's esophagus [39,42]. The argument for a causal role for Cdx1/2 in the development of Barrett's esophagus is strengthened by transgenic mouse studies in which targeted expression of Cdx2 in the stomach induced intestinal metaplasia and gastric carcinoma [45,46]. In addition, there is a link between expression of *cdx1/2* and reflux. Certain bile acids and chronic exposure to low pH lead to expression of *cdx2* in rat and mouse primary esophageal keratinocytes respectively [47,48]. Bile acid-induced *cdx2* expression appears to be through activation of NF-κB [47]. Ectopic expression of Cdx2 in rat esophageal keratinocytes also leads to the expression of the intestinal-type mucin, MUC2 [47]. Increased expression of *cdx1* in colorectal cancer cell lines and the squamous esophageal cell line KYSE30 following treatment with the inflammatory cytokines TNF-α and IL-1β has also been reported [44].

Furthermore, NF-κB mediates both cytokine and bile-induced *cdx1* expression in the colorectal cancer cell line C32 [44]. Interestingly, the expression of IL-1β is increased at the squamocolumnar junction in Barrett's esophagus and in esophagitis and its expression is increased by pulsatile exposure of Barrett's esophagus to acid and bile or by co-culturing squamous and columnar cell lines [49,50]. Recently, acid and bile were shown to result in *cdx2* promoter demethylation with subsequent increased gene expression in cell line models, demonstrating a further mechanistic link between reflux and *cdx* gene expression [51]. The importance of gene methylation is supported by the finding that tissue-specific expression of *cdx1* in the intestinal tract appears to be attributable to the methylation status of the promoter [44].

TGFβ

Alteration of the transforming growth factor β (TGFβ) signalling pathway by acid and bile may also play a role in the pathogenesis of Barrett's esophagus. Recent data shows that expression of SMAD2, 3 and 4, downstream components of the TGFβ signalling pathway, are downregulated in Barrett's esophagus compared to the normal squamous mucosa [52]. Downregulation of SMAD4 was found to occur *via* a number of different mechanisms including methylation and deletion. These alterations in Barrett's carcinogenesis lead to impaired TGFβ mediated growth suppression [52]. In addition, TGFβ is a well known inducer of epithelial to mesenchymal transition [53] and inhibition of this pathway can reverse this process *via* mesenchymal to epithelial transition (MET) [54]. It was also

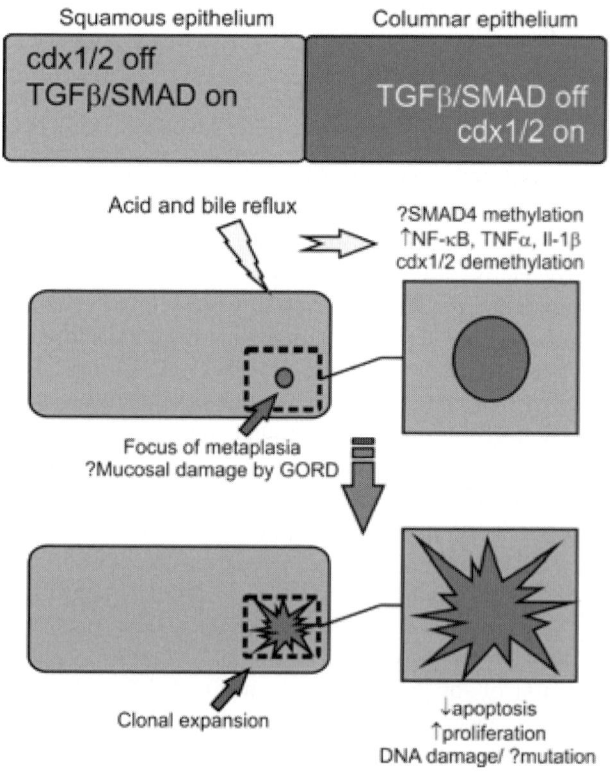

Figure 1. Proposed actions of acid and bile reflux in the pathogenesis of Barrett's esophagus.

demonstrated recently that activation of the TGFβ signalling pathway in Barrett's adenocarcinoma cells induces morphologic and molecular expression changes that are indicative of EMT, with promotion of *in vitro* invasion indices [55]. Interestingly, bile acids have been shown to stimulate intestinal epithelial cell migration and wound repair *via* NF-κB-mediated expression of TGFβ [56,57]. Given the potential of acid and bile to regulate signalling pathways through methylation and other genetic alterations and the impaired expression of SMADs in Barrett's esophagus, it is possible that MET *via* impaired TGFβ signalling may play a role in the pathogenesis of Barrett's esophagus.

In summary, while the pathogenesis of Barrett's esophagus is presently unclear, it is likely to be multifactorial and it is evident that factors other than reflux are also involved. We propose that the combination of these factors acting on the cell of origin produces a microenvironment that drives the generation and development of clones of cells that give rise to the metaplastic tissue (*Figure 1*).

References

1. Peters PM. The congenital short oesophagus. Thorax 1958;13:1-11.
2. Smedts F, Ramaekers FC, Vooijs PG. The dynamics of keratin expression in malignant transformation of cervical epithelium: a review. Obstet Gynecol 1993;82:465.
3. Seery JP, Watt FM. Asymmetric stem-cell divisions define the architecture of human oesophageal epithelium. Curr Biol 2000;10:1447-50.
4. Coad RA, Woodman AC, Warner PJ, Barr H, Wright NA, Shepherd NA. On the histogenesis of Barrett's oesophagus and its associated squamous islands: a three-dimensional study of their morphological relationship with native oesophageal gland ducts. J Pathol 2005;206:388-94.
5. Gillen P, Keeling P, Byrne PJ, West AB, Hennessy TP. Experimental columnar metaplasia in the canine oesophagus. Br J Surg 1988;75:113-5.
6. Salo JA, Kivilaakso EO, Kiviluoto TA, Virtanen IO. Cytokeratin profile suggests metaplastic epithelial transformation in Barrett's oesophagus. Ann Med 1996;28:305-9.
7. Direkze NC, Forbes SJ, Brittan M, et al. Multiple organ engraftment by bone-marrow-derived myofibroblasts and fibroblasts in bone-marrow-transplanted mice. Stem Cells 2003;21:514-20.
8. Epperly MW, Guo H, Shen H, et al. Bone marrow origin of cells with capacity for homing and differentiation to esophageal squamous epithelium. Radiat Res 2004;162:233-40.
9. Sarosi,GA, Brown G, Jaiswal K, et al. Reflux-damaged esophageal epithelium is replaced by cells derived from the bone marrow in a rat model of Barrett's esophagus. Gastroenterology 2004;126:A-35.
10. Li HC, Stoicov C, Rogers AB, Houghton J. Stem cells and cancer: evidence for bone marrow stem cells in epithelial cancers. World J Gastroenterol 2006;12:363-71.
11. Barrett MT, Sanchez CA, Prevo LJ, et al. Evolution of neoplastic cell lineages in Barrett oesophagus. Nat Genet 1999;22:106-9.
12. Cameron AJ, Lomboy CT. Barrett's esophagus: age, prevalence, and extent of columnar epithelium. Gastroenterology 1992;103:1241-5.
13. Jankowski JA, Wright NA, Meltzer SJ, et al. Molecular evolution of the metaplasia-dysplasia-adenocarcinoma sequence in the esophagus. Am J Pathol 1999;154:965-73.
14. Ronkainen J, Aro P, Storskrubb T, et al. Prevalence of Barrett's esophagus in the general population: an endoscopic study. Gastroenterology 2005;129:1825-31.
15. Seery JP. Stem cells of the oesophageal epithelium. J Cell Sci 2002;115: 1783-9.
16. Seto Y, Kobori O. Role of reflux oesophagitis and acid in the development of columnar epithelium in the rat oesophagus. Br J Surg 1993;80:467-70.
17. Wild CP, Hardie LJ. Reflux, Barrett's oesophagus and adenocarcinoma: burning questions. Nat Rev Cancer 2003;3:676-84.
18. Melo LL, Kruel CD, Kliemann LM, et al. Influence of surgically induced gastric and gastroduodenal content reflux on esophageal carcinogenesis—experimental model in Wistar female rats. Dis Esophagus 1999;12:106-15.
19. Xu X, LoCicero J 3rd, Macri E, Loda M, Ellis FH Jr. Barrett's esophagus and associated adenocarcinoma in a mouse surgical model. J Surg Res 2000;88:120-4.

20. Kauer WK, Peters JH, DeMeester TR, Ireland AP, Bremner CG, Hagen JA. Mixed reflux of gastric and duodenal juices is more harmful to the esophagus than gastric juice alone. The need for surgical therapy re-emphasized. Ann Surg 1995;222:525-33.
21. Mareel M, Leroy A. Clinical, cellular, and molecular aspects of cancer invasion. Physiol Rev 2003;83:337-76.
22. Fitzgerald RC, Omary MB, Triadafilopoulos G. Dynamic effects of acid on Barrett's esophagus. An ex vivo proliferation and differentiation model. J Clin Invest 1996;98:2120-8.
23. Fitzgerald RC, Omary MB, Triadafilopoulos G. Acid modulation of HT29 cell growth and differentiation. An in vitro model for Barrett's esophagus. J Cell Sci 1997;110:663-71.
24. Fitzgerald RC, Omary MB, Triadafilopoulos G. Altered sodium-hydrogen exchange activity is a mechanism for acid-induced hyperproliferation in Barrett's esophagus. Am J Physiol 1998;275:G47-55.
25. Souza RF, Shewmake K, Terada LS, Spechler SJ. Acid exposure activates the mitogen-activated protein kinase pathways in Barrett's esophagus. Gastroenterology 2002;122:299-307.
26. Souza RF, Shewmake, K, Pearson S, et al. Acid increases proliferation via ERK and p38 MAPK-mediated increases in cyclooxygenase-2 in Barrett's adenocarcinoma cells. Am J Physiol Gastrointest Liver Physiol 2004; 287:G743-8.
27. Morgan C, Alazawi W, Sirieix,P, Freeman T, Coleman N, Fitzgerald R. In vitro acid exposure has a differential effect on apoptotic and proliferative pathways in a Barrett's adenocarcinoma cell line. Am J Gastroenterol 2004;99:218-24.
28. Kaur BS, Ouatu-Lascar R, Omary MB, Triadafilopoulos G. Bile salts induce or blunt cell proliferation in Barrett's esophagus in an acid-dependent fashion. Am J Physiol Gastrointest Liver Physiol 2000;278:G1000-9.
29. Demeester SR, Peters JH, Demeester TR. Barrett's esophagus. Curr Probl Surg 2001;38:558-640.
30. Olliver JR, Hardie LJ, Dexter S, Chalmers D, Wild CP. DNA damage levels are raised in Barrett's oesophageal mucosa relative to the squamous epithelium of the oesophagus. Biomarkers 2003;8:509-21.
31. Jolly AJ, Wild CP, Hardie LJ. Acid and bile salts induce DNA damage in human oesophageal cell lines. Mutagenesis 2004;19:319-24.
32. Dvorak K, Payne CM, Chavarria M, et al. Bile acids in combination with low pH induce oxidative stress and oxidative DNA damage: relevance to the pathogenesis of Barrett's oesophagus. Gut 2007;56:763-71.
33. Jenkins GJ, D'Souza FR, Suzen HS, et al. Deoxycholic acid (DCA) at neutral and acid pH, is genotoxic to oesophageal cells through the induction of ROS: the potential role of antioxidants in Barrett's oesophagus. Carcinogenesis 2007;28:136-42.
34. Suzuki H, Iijima K, Scobie G, Fyfe V, McColl KE. Nitrate and nitrosative chemistry within Barrett's oesophagus during acid reflux. Gut 2005;54:1527-35.
35. Mano N, Kasuga K, Kobayashi N, Goto J. A nonenzymatic modification of the amino-terminal domain of histone H3 by bile acid acyl adenylate. J Biol Chem 2004;279:55034-41.
36. Jenkins GJ, Harries K, Doak SH, et al. The bile acid deoxycholic acid (DCA) at neutral pH activates NF-kappaB and induces IL-8 expression in oesophageal cells in vitro. Carcinogenesis 2004;25:317-23.
37. Tselepis C, Morris CD, Wakelin D, et al. Upregulation of the oncogene c-myc in Barrett's adenocarcinoma: induction of c-myc by acidified bile acid in vitro. Gut 2003;52:174-80.
38. Silberg DG, Swain GP, Suh ER, Traber PG. Cdx1 and cdx2 expression during intestinal development. Gastroenterology 2000;119:961-71.
39. Eda A, Osawa H, Satoh K, et al. Aberrant expression of CDX2 in Barrett's epithelium and inflammatory esophageal mucosa. J Gastroenterol 2003;38:14-22.
40. Groisman GM, Amar M, Meir A. Expression of the intestinal marker Cdx2 in the columnar-lined esophagus with and without intestinal (Barrett's) metaplasia. Mod Pathol 2004;17:1282-8.
41. Lord RV, Brabender J, Wickramasinghe K, et al. Increased CDX2 and decreased PITX1 homeobox gene expression in Barrett's esophagus and Barrett's-associated adenocarcinoma. Surgery 2005;138:924-31.
42. Moons LM, Bax DA, Kuipers,EJ, et al. The homeodomain protein CDX2 is an early marker of Barrett's oesophagus. J Clin Pathol 2004;57:1063-8.
43. Phillips RW, Frierson HF Jr, Moskaluk CA. Cdx2 as a marker of epithelial intestinal differentiation in the esophagus. Am J Surg Pathol 2003;27:1442-7.
44. Wong NA, Wilding J, Bartlett S, et al. CDX1 is an important molecular mediator of Barrett's metaplasia. Proc Natl Acad Sci USA 2005;102:7565-70.
45. Mutoh H, Sakurai S, Satoh K, et al. Development of gastric carcinoma from intestinal metaplasia in Cdx2-transgenic mice. Cancer Res 2004;64:7740-7.
46. Silberg DG, Sullivan J, Kang E, et al. Cdx2 ectopic expression induces gastric intestinal metaplasia in transgenic mice. Gastroenterology 2002;122:689-96.
47. Kazumori H, Ishihara S, Rumi MA, Kadowaki Y, Kinoshita Y. Bile acids directly augment caudal related homeobox gene Cdx2 expression in oesophageal keratinocytes in Barrett's epithelium. Gut 2006; 55:16-25.
48. Marchetti M, Caliot E, Pringault E. Chronic acid exposure leads to activation of the cdx2 intestinal homeobox gene in a long-term culture of mouse esophageal keratinocytes. J Cell Sci 2003;116:1429-36.
49. Fitzgerald RC, Abdalla S, Onwuegbusi BA, et al. Inflammatory gradient in Barrett's oesophagus: implications for disease complications. Gut 2002;51:316-22.
50. Fitzgerald RC, Onwuegbusi BA, Bajaj-Elliott M, Saeed IT, Burnham WR, Farthing MJ. Diversity in the oesophageal phenotypic response to gastro-oesophageal reflux: immunological determinants. Gut 2002;50:451-9.

51. Liu T, Zhang X, So CK, et al. Regulation of Cdx2 expression by promoter methylation, and effects of Cdx2 transfection on morphology and gene expression of human esophageal epithelial cells. Carcinogenesis 2007;28:488-96.
52. Onwuegbusi BA, Aitchison A, Chin SF, et al. Impaired transforming growth factor beta signalling in Barrett's carcinogenesis due to frequent SMAD4 inactivation. Gut 2006;55:764-74.
53. Thiery JP. Epithelial-mesenchymal transitions in development and pathologies. Curr Opin Cell Biol 2003;15:740-6.
54. Zeisberg M, Hanai J, Sugimoto H, et al. BMP-7 counteracts TGF-beta1-induced epithelial-to-mesenchymal transition and reverses chronic renal injury. Nat Med 2003;9:964-8.
55. Rees JR, Onwuegbusi BA, Save VE, Alderson D, Fitzgerald RC. In vivo and in vitro evidence for transforming growth factor-{beta}1-mediated epithelial to mesenchymal transition in esophageal adenocarcinoma. Cancer Res 2006;66:9583-90.
56. Strauch ED, Wang JY, Bass BL. Bile salt stimulates intestinal epithelial cell migration through TGF[beta] after wounding. J Surg Res 2001;97:49-53.
57. Strauch ED, Yamaguchi J, Bass BL, Wang JY. Bile salts regulate intestinal epithelial cell migration by nuclear factor-B-induced expression of transforming growth factor-? J Am Coll Surg 2003;197:974-84.

Immunohistochemistry in the study of columnar metaplasia

R.H. Riddell (Toronto)

To begin addressing the role of immunohistochemistry in Barrett's esophagus, it is first necessary to consider how many different types of epithelium can be found in the columnar-lined esophagus. They include:

- cardio-oxyntic mucosa;
- cardiac mucosa;
- intestinal metaplasia;
    • complete,
    • incomplete;
- pancreatic metaplasia.

It is self-evident that different types of mucosa will have the typical immunohistochemical staining patterns that are seen in the normal anatomical location of these types of mucosa in those that are metaplastic.

In **oxyntic mucosa** containing parietal cells, the later will have usual staining reactions for parietal cells (proton pump antigens, intrinsic factor, nitric oxide synthase), chief cells (pepsinogen-1), and possibly endocrine cells if they are present.

In **cardiac mucosa**, the usual mucin stains – whether histochemical, lectins, or MUC stains such as MUC5AC and 6 stains will be present.

In **pancreatic metaplasia**, when it is present, only the exocrine component is present, so that immunoreactivity for pancreatic exocrine stains will be present. These include tryptase, lipase, chymotrypsin, etc.

The **intestinal metaplasia** of Barrett's mucosa , the goblet stains will stain with any of the stains that usually stain intestinal goblet cells including appropriate lectins, CD10, villin, cdx-2, MUC6, etc. [1,2] (*Figure 1*). One problem for which there remains no good resolution is the ability to distinguish between intestinal metaplasia occurring in native cardiac mucosa from that occurring in Barrett's esophagus. About a decade ago the possibility that differential cytokeratin staining using CK7 and CK20 could do this was raised, but numerous studies have demonstrated that while overall this does seem to hold, that it does not have the positive predictive value to be used as a diagnostic tool [3] (*Figure 2*).

The pathway to carcinoma in Barrett's esophagus is almost certainly sequential with numerous processes that can result in the production of abnormal proteins or their loss through other mechanisms such as promoter methylation, mutations, loss of heterozygosity (LOH). The role of immunohistochemistry in this is in the detection of abnormal proteins or loss of normal proteins or of chromosomal abnormalities. However, the holy grail of immunohistochemistry in Barrett's esophagus is to find a marker for patients who are predestined to develop carcinoma. It matters little whether this is found at the stage of non-dysplastic Barrett's esophagus, or dysplastic Barrett's esophagus as long as it is both sensitive and specific, with a high enough positive predictive value to be of clinical value. Such a marker needs to be a marker that is has one of the following properties:

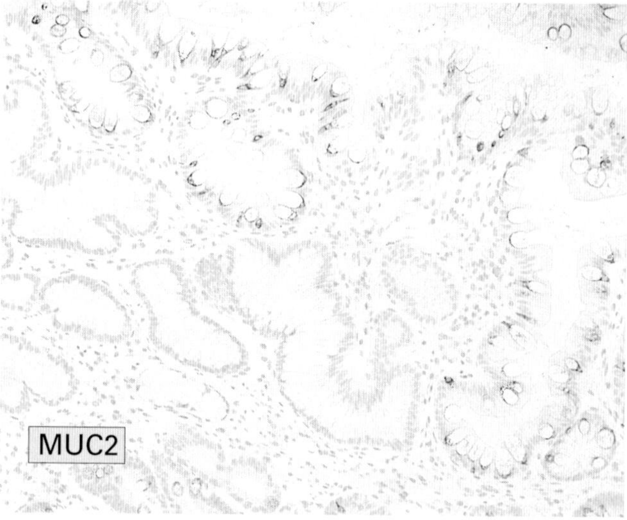

Figure 1. MUC6 which stains goblet cell mucin. (See page XXIV for colour figure).

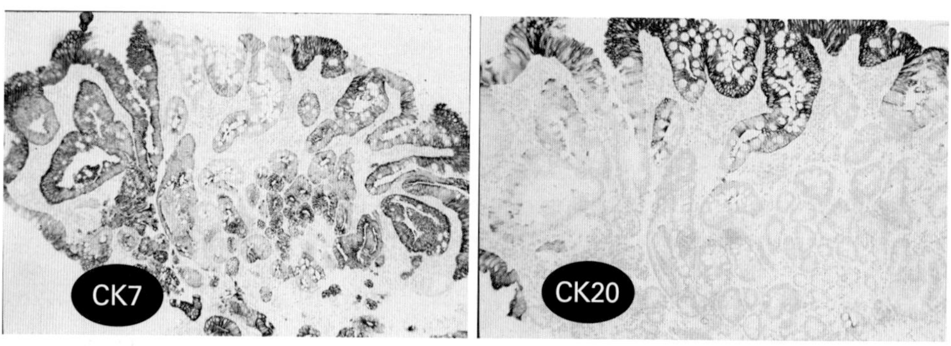

Figure 2. CK7 and CK20 in the "classical" cytokeratin pattern associated with Barrett's esophagus. CK7 stains both the surface and deep epithelium CK20 is limited to the superficial; part of the mucosa. (See page XXV for colour figure).

- identifies patients with non-dysplastic mucosa who are at increased risk of developing dysplasia, and presumably therefore at increased risk of developing carcinoma;
- identifies patients with dysplasia who form a subset of patients that are at increased risk of developing carcinoma over those with dysplasia that are at less risk, other than identification of high grade dysplasia (HGD) (or worse);
- is reproducible between centers.

Those that can be identified immunohistochemically include fall into two large categories:

- **FISH** (fluorescence *in situ* hybridization) that detect chromosomal gains, losses and translocations. This is therefore indicative of genomic instability. While studies on this are still in their infancy, there is the potential for this technique to detect some changes far earlier than those that can be appreciated by immunohistochemistry on tissue sections. However, it remains to be seen whether such abnormalities are dynamic and can come and go, and which are sustained and lead to populations of cells that can persist and are subject to further mutations [4-9]. Quantitative FISH (**QFISH**) can also be used, for example, to detect the decreasing telomere length that is usually associated with developing neoplasia [6];
- **tissue immunohistochemistry** that detects loss of, or abnormal, proteins – these are detected by immunohistochemistry on tissue sections.

• p53

It has long been recognized that dysplasia and carcinoma in Barrett's esophagus are invariably accompanied by mutations in the p53 gene that results in the production of abnormal proteins that have a longer 1/2 life and therefore accumulate in the cell where they can be detected by immunohistochemistry. Further, there is a disconnect between molecular abnormalities and the immunohistochemistry detection of p53, raising the possibility of other mechanisms being involved iincluding overproduction of wild-type p53. In patients with HGD p53 is common, but its frequency diminished in low grade dysplasia (LGD) and biopsies indefinite for dysplasia (IFD). In IFD there is a fairly typical pattern of immunoreactivity in which there is excess staining in the basal part of the mucosa with loss as the mucosa matures, although sometimes this extends quite close to the surface (*Figure 3*). However, the intriguing feature is that, primarily in patients with dysplasia on carcinoma elsewhere in the esophagus, the non-dysplastic mucosa may also be quite strongly immunoreactive. However this seems to be infrequent in biopsies [9-13].

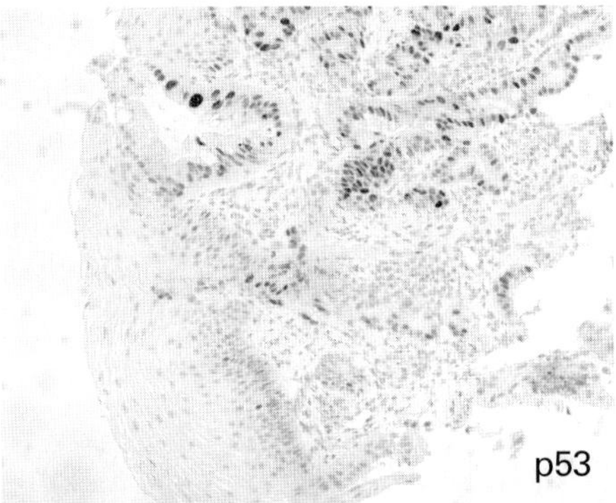

Figure 3. p53 immunostaining in a biopsy indefinite for dysplasia showing irregular immunoreactivity in the glandular mucosa extending close to the surface (left) adjacent to the squamous mucosa (left side). (See page XXV for colour figure).

• Cell cycle and proliferation markers
- Ki67 (proliferation marker): the mib-1 antibody that stains the Ki67 is useful in showing an extended proliferation zone, which is invariably present in neoplasia (*Figure 4*). However it is also present in reactive lesions so is of limited value [13,14];
- p16: loss of p16 appears to occur quite early in Barrett's neoplasia. The mechanism appears to be promoter methylation [13,15-20];
- p21: this does not seem to be a major player in the dysplasia-carcinoma pathway [10,21];
- p27: this is increased in dysplastic Barrett's esophagus but has not been seriously used for diagnostic purposes.

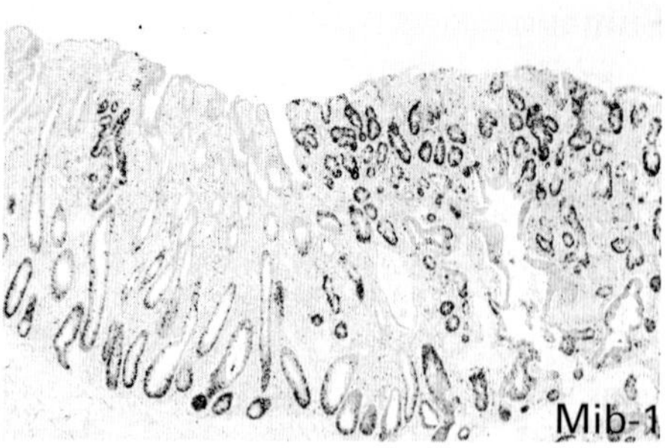

Figure 4. Mib-1 which stains the Ki-67 antigen associated with cell proliferation. On the left pits are stained primarily in the lower replicative zone except for one focus. However, on the right there is an area of dysplasia in which almost all of the cells are reactive virtually to the surface. Interestingly this virtually mirrored the p53 pattern of immunoreactivity. (See page XXV for colour figure).

• Markers of wnt pathway activation – β-catenin
Unfortunately this seems to activated late in the course of the dysplasia pathway so is unlikely to be of value as an early marker.
• Alpha-methylacyl-CoA racemase (AMACR) – usually simplified to "racemase" tends to be found in a variety of tumors, and is used immunohistochemically especially in the diagnosis of prostatic adenocarcinoma. However it is also emerging as a potential marker of dysplasia (*Figure 5*), but its positive predictive accuracy etc is unclear. It does seem to stain some lesions considered IFD, but it is also unclear whether these patients are at increased risk of developing carcinoma when compared with IFD without AMACR immunoreactivity [22-24]. Unfortunately most of the time when it is intense the histological diagnosis of dysplasia is not in question, but it may be of value, especially if combined with p53, in questionable dysplasia.

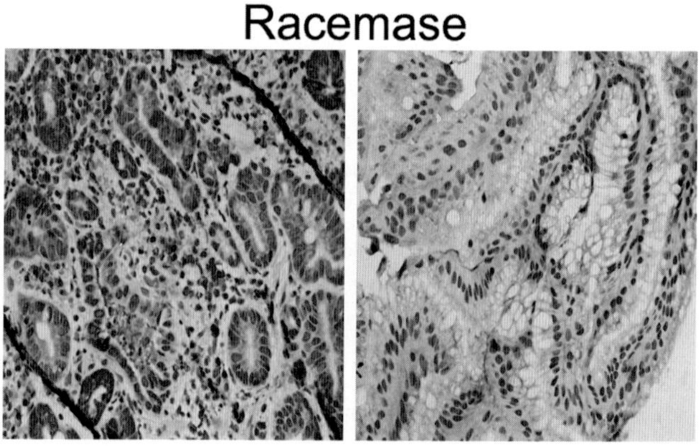

Figure 5. Racemase activity. Left shows strong staining in Barrett's esophagus with HGD and intramucosal carcinoma.) Right: non-dysplastic mucosa with minimal racemase immunoreactivity. (See page XXV for colour figure).

Summary

Immunohistochemistry plays a significant role in the diagnosis of Barrett's esophagus, but particularly in elucidating mechanisms by which dysplasia and carcinoma develop. This can be by using conventional immunohistochemistry on tissue sections, in which use of p53 in particular tends to be used to hold the hand of the pathologist in confirming their suspicion of dysplasia, especially HGD. However, increasingly, the use of immunohistochemistry for FISH and QFISH to detect chromosomal gains, losses, translocations, and aneuploidy, all of which tend to occur early in the course of the pathway to neoplasia, is being explored. Whether these will ever pan out to predict patients at particularly increased risk of dysplasia and carcinoma, and whether general or specific changes will prove of greatest value, remains to be elucidated.

References

1. Kerkhof M, Bax DA, Moons LM, et al. Does CDX2 expression predict Barrett's metaplasia in oesophageal columnar epithelium without goblet cells? Aliment Pharmacol Ther 2006;24(11-12):1613-21.
2. Pera M, Pera M, de Bolos C, et al. Duodenal-content reflux into the esophagus leads to expression of Cdx2 and Muc2 in areas of squamous epithelium in rats. J Gastrointest Surg 2007;11(7):869-74.
3. Nurgalieva Z, Lowrey A, El Serag HB. The use of cytokeratin stain to distinguish Barrett's esophagus from contiguous tissues: a systematic review. Dig Dis Sci 2007;52(5):1345-54.
4. Doak SH, Jenkins GJ, Parry EM, et al. Chromosome 4 hyperploidy represents an early genetic aberration in premalignant Barrett's oesophagus. Gut 2003;52(5):623-8.
5. Fahmy M, Skacel M, Gramlich TL, et al. Chromosomal gains and genomic loss of p53 and p16 genes in Barrett's esophagus detected by fluorescence in situ hybridization of cytology specimens. Mod Pathol 2004;17(5):588-96.
6. O'Sullivan JN, Finley JC, Risques RA, et al. Telomere length assessment in tissue sections by quantitative FISH: image analysis algorithms. Cytometry A 2004;58(2):120-31.
7. Peters FP, Krishnadath KK, Rygiel AM, et al. Stepwise radical endoscopic resection of the complete Barrett's esophagus with early neoplasia successfully eradicates pre-existing genetic abnormalities. Am J Gastroenterol 2007;102(9):1853-61.
8. Wongsurawat VJ, Finley JC, Galipeau PC, et al. Genetic mechanisms of TP53 loss of heterozygosity in Barrett's esophagus: implications for biomarker validation. Cancer Epidemiol Biomarkers Prev 2006;15(3):509-16.
9. Yang Y, Fruehauf J, Xiang S, Li CJ. Genomic instability in precancerous lesions before inactivation of tumor suppressors p53 and APC in patients. Cell Cycle 2006;5(13):1443-7.
10. Chatelain D, Flejou JF. High-grade dysplasia and superficial adenocarcinoma in Barrett's esophagus: histological mapping and expression of p53, p21 and Bcl-2 oncoproteins. Virchows Arch 2003;442(1):18-24.
11. Doak SH, Jenkins GJ, Parry EM, et al. Characterisation of p53 status at the gene, chromosomal and protein levels in oesophageal adenocarcinoma. Br J Cancer 2003;89(9):1729-35.
12. Fujii T, Nakagawa S, Hanzawa M, et al. Immunohistological study of cell cycle-related factors, oncogene expression, and cell proliferation in adenocarcinoma developed in Barrett's esophagus. Oncol Rep 2003;10(2):427-31.
13. Trudgill NJ, Suvarna SK, Royds JA, Riley SA. Cell cycle regulation in patients with intestinal metaplasia at the gastro-oesophageal junction. Mol Pathol 2003;56(6):313-7.
14. Griffiths EA, Pritchard SA, McGrath SM, et al. Increasing expression of hypoxia-inducible proteins in the Barrett's metaplasia-dysplasia-adenocarcinoma sequence. Br J Cancer 2007;96(9):1377-83.
15. Bian YS, Osterheld MC, Fontolliet C, Bosman FT, Benhattar J. p16 inactivation by methylation of the CDKN2A promoter occurs early during neoplastic progression in Barrett's esophagus. Gastroenterology 2002;122(4):1113-21.
16. Hardie LJ, Darnton SJ, Wallis YL, et al. p16 expression in Barrett's esophagus and esophageal adenocarcinoma: association with genetic and epigenetic alterations. Cancer Lett 2005;217(2):221-30.
17. Schulmann K, Sterian A, Berki A, et al. Inactivation of p16, RUNX3, and HPP1 occurs early in Barrett's-associated neoplastic progression and predicts progression risk. Oncogene 2005;24(25):4138-48.
18. Vieth M, Schneider-Stock R, Rohrich K, et al. INK4a-ARF alterations in Barrett's epithelium, intraepithelial neoplasia and Barrett's adenocarcinoma. Virchows Arch 2004;445(2):135-41.
19. Ellis FH Jr, Loda M. p27 and Barrett's esophagus: a review. Dis Esophagus 2004;17(2):113-7.
20. Umansky M, Yasui W, Hallak A, et al. Proton pump inhibitors reduce cell cycle abnormalities in Barrett's esophagus. Oncogene 2001;20(55):7987-91.
21. Villwock MM, Meurer L, Cavazzola LT, Gurski RR, Edelweiss MI, Schirmer CC. Prevalence of p21 immunohistochemical expression in esophageal adenocarcinoma. Arq Gastroenterol 2006;43(3):212-8.

22. Dorer R, Odze RD. AMACR immunostaining is useful in detecting dysplastic epithelium in Barrett's esophagus, ulcerative colitis, and Crohn's disease. Am J Surg Pathol 2006;30(7):871-7.
23. Lisovsky M, Falkowski O, Bhuiya T. Expression of alpha-methylacyl-coenzyme A racemase in dysplastic Barrett's epithelium. Hum Pathol 2006;37(12):1601-6.
24. Strater J, Wiesmuller C, Perner S, Kuefer R, Moller P. Alpha-methylacyl-CoA racemase (AMACR) immunohistochemistry in Barrett's and colorectal mucosa: only significant overexpression favours a diagnosis of intraepithelial neoplasia. Histopathology 2008.

Microarray technology in columnar metaplasia and carcinogenesis; excitement *versus* reality

E. Montgomery (Baltimore)

For years, before Lagergren *et al.* proved on epidemiologic grounds that reflux is a risk factor for esophageal adenocarcinoma [1], most practicing gastroenterologists, surgeons, and pathologists who dealt with esophageal diseases have believed that esophageal adenocarcinomas proceed through a series of histologically defined precursor lesions. These include Barrett's esophagus, Barrett's esophagus with columnar epithelial dysplasia, and finally esophageal adenocarcinoma [2,3] as progressive genetic alterations were acquired.

Years later, after many hours of research, as cutting edge techniques exploiting gene array technology have come into their own, the shocking conclusion, in papers that often have more than twenty authors and involve expensive work, is that Barrett's metaplasia is an early intermediate stage in esophageal adenocarcinogenesis [4]! Obviously, it is far less expensive to review a glass slide, as imperfect as that analysis can be.

As cutting edge technology has come our way, may laboratories have used new gene array technology to compare the genetic signature of normal esophageal mucosa to that of carcinomas and precursors. Each laboratory arrives at a different set of molecular targets depending on which tumors and cell lines are tested [5-11]. As of this writing, not a single one of these trumps "antiquated" histology as a tool for day-to-day management of patients. The bloom has faded on hopes concerning the speed with which the use of array technology will change the way we practice medicine but ultimately the study of cancer as a genetic disease should lead to improved treatments.

Typically, array technology yields a long list of potential targets. These must be then validated at the protein level, usually by immunohistochemistry [9,12]. This technique is most easily accomplished using paraffin block arrays, in which many small samples are placed in one tissue block to only one slide need be stained to test a large number of lesions for the given protein.

As an example, in our hands differential gene expression analysis revealed an upregulation of 560 genes and a downregulation of 148 genes comparing esophageal adenocarcinoma to normal esophageal mucosa scrapings [7]. Validation of these findings was performed using tissue microarrays composed of the spectrum of lesions associated with esophageal adenocarcinoma progression, including Barrett esophagus of the distinctive type and dysplastic epithelia. Squamous mucosa was also represented on the tissue arrays. We used normal squamous mucosa rather than glandular mucosa (such as gastric cardiac type mucosa) for the control normal esophageal tissue in gene array component of the study, but we still found differential expression on validated molecules in the various adenocarcinoma precursors. Two of the proteins – Igfbp3 and Cdc5 – whose transcripts were upregulated in esophageal adenocarcinomas were validated using this progression model. These markers demonstrated minimal baseline expression in normal gastric and esophageal mucosa. Igfbp3 demonstrated a stepwise increase in tissue expression, with a large increase between low-grade dysplasia (14%) and high-grade dysplasia (HGD) (50%), and again between HGD (50%) and adenocarcinoma (95%) and metastases (95%), suggesting distinct regulatory mechanisms of this molecule with cancer progression. Similarly, Cdc5 demonstrated a stepwise increase in expression, although a large increase was primarily identified between adenocarcinoma (34%) and lymph node metastases (52%), suggesting a possible role for Cdc5 in metastatic spread. Neither of these molecules has been previously studied in esophageal adenocarcinoma.

Of the molecules validated, Cdc2/Cdk1 (the human homolog of p34 in yeast) demonstrated the greatest utility both as a clinicopathologic marker and as a potential chemotherapeutic target. Dysregulation of cell cycle mediators has been proposed to play a pivotal role in the development and progression of many human cancers [13]. Cdc2/Cdk1 is a member of the cyclin-dependent kinases (CDK) family, which regulates phase transitions and checkpoints within the cell cycle. Cdc2/Cdk1 is a highly conserved molecule that undergoes cell cycle-dependent tyrosine phosphorylation, which controls subcellular localization. Cdc2/Cdk1 binds to cyclin B, forming an active complex that leads to the phosphorylation of cell cycle regulatory elements, as well as other substrates. The recent of CDC2/CDK1 inhibitors has offered new inroads in the examination and possible treatment of cancers overexpressing this molecule. In our hands, in fact, esophageal adenocarcinoma cells lines were inhibited by the specific inhibitor. However, there is no practical method to administer this inhibitor to the esophagus.

Epigenetics offers some new hope in the search for prognosticators [8,14-19] and study of promoter methylation yields some predictive value in assigning patients to higher and lower risk. Unfortunately, it, like image analysis [20], does not presently offer sufficient advantages over conventional histology to be used clinically.

One problem with gene array technology is that the genes studies must be known and of course, only genes represented on any given array can be studied. This may not matter in some cases but it is critical in others. For example, we now know that uterine cervical cancer is driven by a virus in the vast majority of cases, but generally viral genes are not included on gene arrays. To circumvent these shortcomings, the wave of the future will revolve around serial analysis of gene expression (SAGE) [21].

Essentially, three principles underlie the SAGE methodology:

- a short sequence tag (10-14 bp) contains sufficient information to uniquely identify a transcript provided that that the tag is obtained from a unique position within each transcript;
- sequence tags can be linked together to from long serial molecules that can be cloned and sequenced;
- quantitation of the number of times a particular tag is observed provides the expression level of the corresponding transcript.

The SAGE technique offers the opportunity to overcome limitations of current array technology. However, once esophageal carcinomas have been fully evaluated by SAGE, there will remain the long tedious task of validating any interesting molecules. Watch this space but expect to wait many years to change your practice!

References

1. Lagergren J, Bergstrom R, Lindgren A, Nyren O. Symptomatic gastroesophageal reflux as a risk factor for esophageal adenocarcinoma. N Engl J Med 1999;340(11):825-31.
2. Montgomery E, Bronner MP, Goldblum JR, et al. Reproducibility of the diagnosis of dysplasia in Barrett esophagus: a reaffirmation. Hum Pathol 2001;32(4):368-78.
3. Reid BJ, Haggitt RC, Rubin CE, et al. Observer variation in the diagnosis of dysplasia in Barrett's esophagus. Hum Pathol 1988;19(2):166-78.
4. Wang S, Zhan M, Yin J, et al. Transcriptional profiling suggests that Barrett's metaplasia is an early intermediate stage in esophageal adenocarcinogenesis. Oncogene 2006;25(23):3346-56.
5. Brabender J, Marjoram P, Salonga D, et al. A multigene expression panel for the molecular diagnosis of Barrett's esophagus and Barrett's adenocarcinoma of the esophagus. Oncogene 2004;23(27):4780-8.
6. McManus DT, Olaru A, Meltzer SJ. Biomarkers of esophageal adenocarcinoma and Barrett's esophagus. Cancer Res 2004;64(5):1561-9.
7. Hansel DE, Wilentz RE, Yeo CJ, Schulick RD, Montgomery E, Maitra A. Expression of neuropilin-1 in high-grade dysplasia, invasive cancer, and metastases of the human gastrointestinal tract. Am J Surg Pathol 2004;28(3):347-56.
8. Powell EL, Leoni LM, Canto MI, et al. Concordant loss of MTAP and p16/CDKN2A expression in gastroesophageal carcinogenesis: evidence of homozygous deletion in esophageal noninvasive precursor lesions and therapeutic implications. Am J Surg Pathol 2005;29(11):1497-504.
9. Hansel DE, Dhara S, Huang RC, et al. CDC2/CDK1 expression in esophageal adenocarcinoma and precursor lesions serves as a diagnostic and cancer progression marker and potential novel drug target. Am J Surg Pathol 2005;29(3):390-9.
10. Maley CC, Galipeau PC, Finley JC, et al. Genetic clonal diversity predicts progression to esophageal adenocarcinoma. Nat Genet 2006;38(4):468-73.
11. Sui G, Zhou S, Wang J, et al. Mitochondrial DNA mutations in preneoplastic lesions of the gastrointestinal tract: a biomarker for the early detection of cancer. Mol Cancer 2006;5:73.
12. Montgomery E, Mamelak AJ, Gibson M, et al. Overexpression of claudin proteins in esophageal adenocarcinoma and its precursor lesions. Appl Immunohistochem Mol Morphol 2006;14(1):24-30.
13. Swanton C. Cell-cycle targeted therapies. Lancet Oncol 2004;5(1):27-36.
14. Barrett MT, Sanchez CA, Prevo LJ, et al. Evolution of neoplastic cell lineages in Barrett oesophagus. Nat Genet 1999;22(1):106-9.
15. Eads CA, Lord RV, Kurumboor SK, et al. Fields of aberrant CpG island hypermethylation in Barrett's esophagus and associated adenocarcinoma. Cancer Res 2000;60(18):5021-6.
16. Krishnadath KK, Wang KK, Taniguchi K, et al. Persistent genetic abnormalities in Barrett's esophagus after photodynamic therapy. Gastroenterology 2000;119(3):624-30.
17. Hamilton JP, Sato F, Jin Z, et al. Reprimo methylation is a potential biomarker of Barrett's-Associated esophageal neoplastic progression. Clin Cancer Res 2006;12(22):6637-42.
18. Schulmann K, Sterian A, Berki A, et al. Inactivation of p16, RUNX3, and HPP1 occurs early in Barrett's-associated neoplastic progression and predicts progression risk. Oncogene 2005;24(25):4138-48.
19. Kawakami K, Brabender J, Lord RV, et al. Hypermethylated APC DNA in plasma and prognosis of patients with esophageal adenocarcinoma. J Natl Cancer Inst 2000;92(22):1805-11.
20. Sabo E, Beck AH, Montgomery EA, et al. Computerized morphometry as an aid in determining the grade of dysplasia and progression to adenocarcinoma in Barrett's esophagus. Lab Invest 2006;86(12):1261-71.
21. Velculescu VE, Zhang L, Vogelstein B, Kinzler KW. Serial analysis of gene expression. Science 1995;270(5235):484-7.

What are the minimal criteria for the diagnosis of low-grade dysplasia in Barrett's mucosa?

E. Montgomery (Baltimore)

Conventional histopathologic evaluation of biopsies

Using histopathologic criteria suggested in 1988 [1], we derived an algorithm for assessment of biopsies in Barrett's esophagus [2].Our algorithm was based on 4 mucosal features in Barrett's esophagus:

1: SURFACE MATURATION compared to the underlying glands;
2: ARCHITECTURE of the glands;
3: CYTOLOGIC FEATURES;
4: INFLAMMATION and erosions/ulcers.

Applying the algorithm, we classified "indefinite for dysplasia" and "low grade dysplasia" (LGD) as follows.

Barrett's esophagus, indefinite for dysplasia

Using the algorithm, we included cases which had deeper cytologic changes suggestive of dysplasia but which showed surface maturation in the indefinite category [2] whereas other observers have used the indefinite category as a "wastecan" [1]. Cases in the indefinite category (*Figures 1, 2 and 3*) could have normal architecture or some degree of glandular crowding. On cytologic evaluation, lesions could have hyperchromasia, nuclear membrane irregularities, and increased mitoses in the deeper aspects and these matured to the surface. Loss of nuclear polarity was not a feature. In the presence of inflammation, more striking architectural abnormalities were to be included in the indefinite category. Some cases display peculiar morphology and it is unclear whether they are neoplastic or reparative.

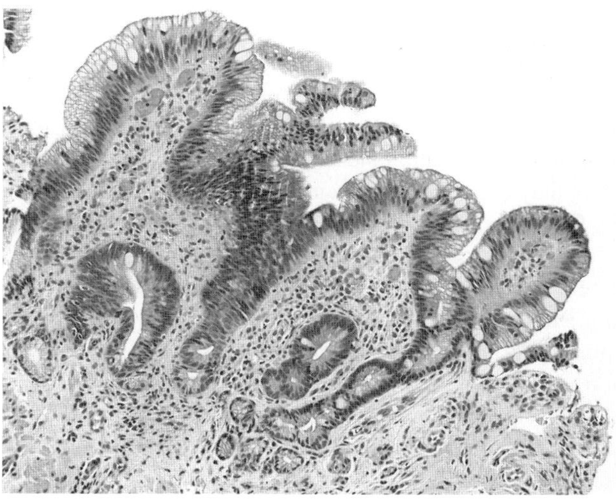

Figure 1. Indefinite for dysplasia. This focus has many intraepithelial neutrophils and merges with surrounding columnar epithelium that clearly lacks dysplasia. (See page XXVI for colour figure).

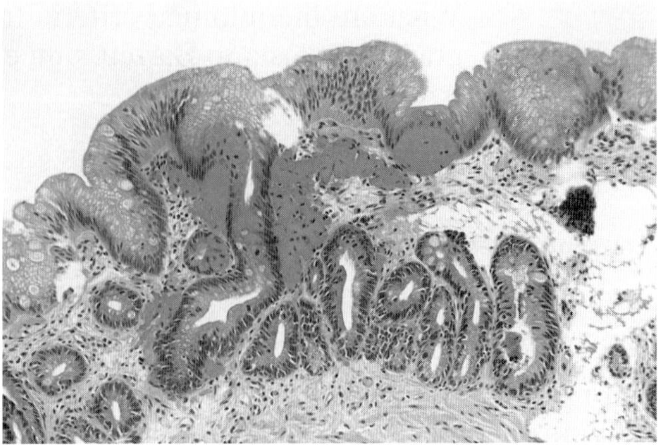

Figure 2. Indefinite for dysplasia. This focus lacks an abrupt transition with surrounding areas. (See page XXVI for colour figure).

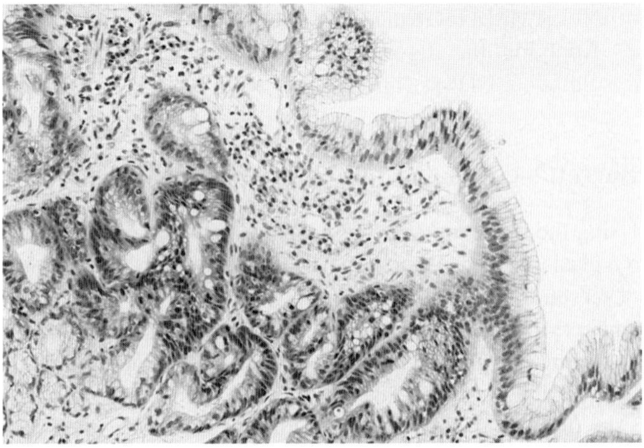

Figure 3. Indefinite for dysplasia. This lesion has too much surface maturation to be regarded as dysplastic. (See page XXVI for colour figure).

Barrett's esophagus, low-grade dysplasia

In Barrett's esophagus with LGD, the surface appears similar to the underlying glands at low magnification or displays only slight maturation. The architecture may be mildly to markedly distorted with glandular crowding although lamina propria should be identifiable between glands. The cytologic features are important and the changes should extend at least focally to the surface (*Figures 4 and 5*). These include nuclear hyperchromasia with some chromatin clumping. The nuclei show nuclear membrane irregularities but not pronounced nuclear enlargement, although there may be focal marked enlargement if the other features support an interpretation of LGD. Of course Lomo *et al.* have described cases of columnar epithelial dysplasia that display surface maturation, but such cases are in the minority [3]. Nucleoli are not typically prominent in LGD. Loss of nuclear polarity is not a feature of LGD, though nuclear stratification similar to that seen in colonic adenomas is within the spectrum of LGD and may be present at the surface. Inflammation is typically minimal; cases with abundant inflammation and the other features of LG are usually best classified in the IND category. If tangential embedding precludes evaluation of the surface, LGD can be diagnosed if there are dysplastic features in the deep aspects in the absence of inflammation provided that the features of high-grade dysplasia are lacking.

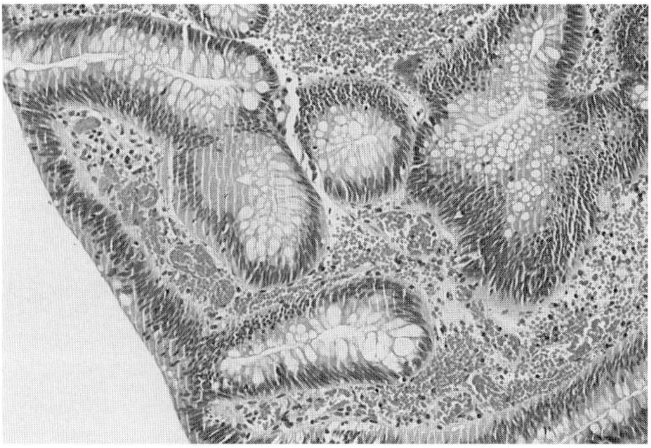

Figure 4. Occasional cases of low-grade dysplasia are indistinguishable from colon adenomas. (See page XXVII for colour figure).

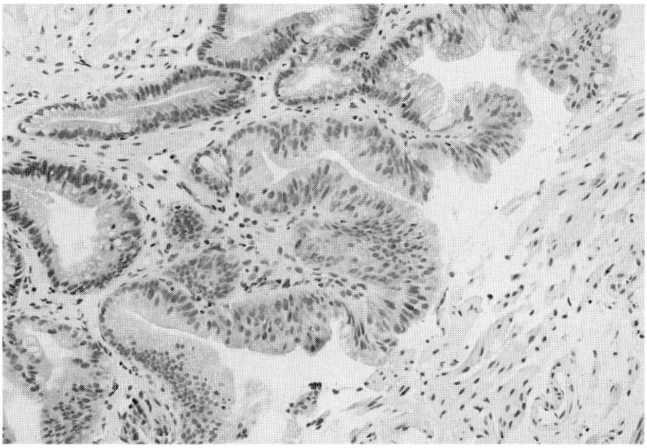

Figure 5. Another example of low-grade dysplasia. Changes extend to the epithelial surface and are homogeneous. (See page XXVII for colour figure).

To define the "line" between "indefinite" and "low-grade" is somewhat arbitrary, however, and it is certainly well-known that there is observer variation in separating these lesions at the low end of the spectrum [2,4]. This is partly the result of the task assigned to pathologists of separating lesions into 6 categories (negative, indefinite, low-grade, high-grade, intramucosal carcinoma, submucosal invasive carcinoma) and partly since the categories are in a spectrum and sometimes difficult to categorize. When simpler distinctions are asked (such as the difference between hyperplastic polyps and adenomas), excellent observer agreement is generally afforded [5] whereas, when there are more categories, agreement diminishes, such as in pancreatic intra-epithelial neoplasia [6].

However, at our institution, we see many examples of dysplastic Barrett's esophagus and separate indefinite lesions from LGD by requiring an abrupt transition to a "clone" of hyperchromatic cells that appear distinct from the adjacent Barrett's mucosa (*Figures 6, 7, 8 and 9*). Unfortunately, there are no good data that indicate that such findings place the patient in a higher risk category than those with "indefinite" features alone.

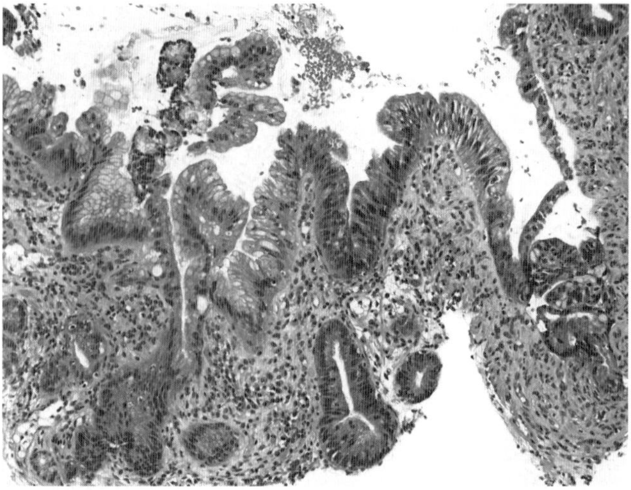

Figure 6. "Early" low-grade dysplasia. Note the abrupt transition between the dysplastic focus and the adjoining epithelium. (See page XXVII for colour figure).

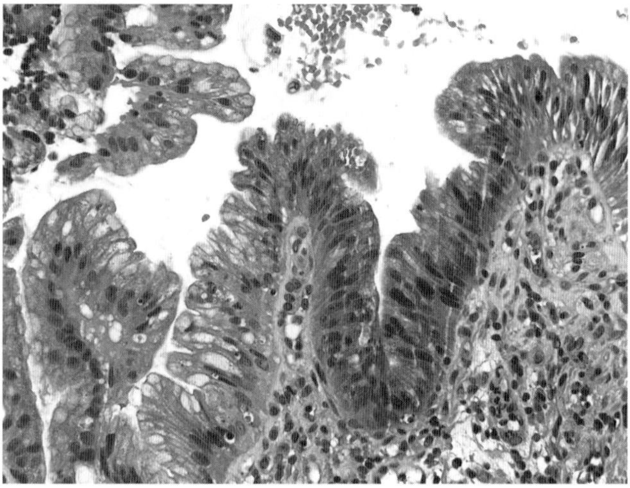

Figure 7. Higher magnification of the focus in *Figure 6*. (See page XXVIII for colour figure).

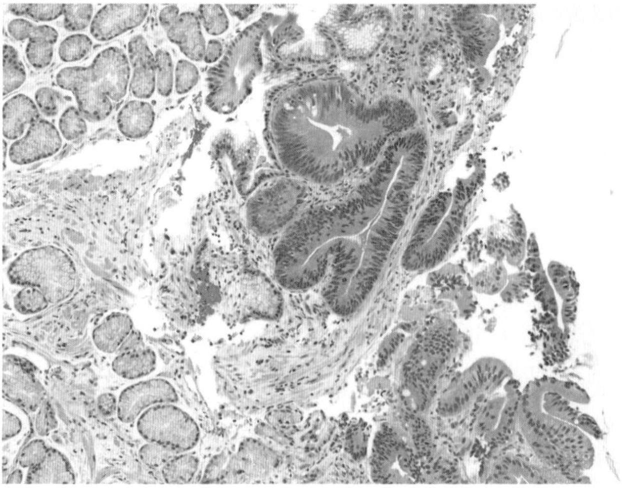

Figure 8. Another example of low-grade dysplasia in which the dysplastic focus is sharply distinct from surrounding tissue, appearing "clonal". (See page XXVIII for colour figure).

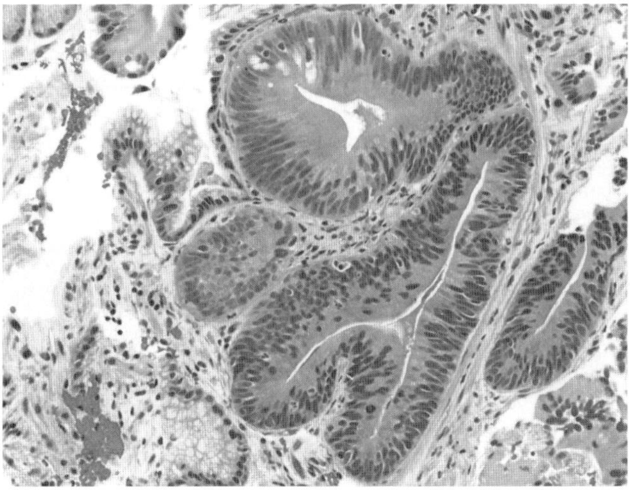

Figure 9. Higher magnification of Figure 8. (See page XXVIII for colour figure).

References

1. Reid BJ, Haggitt RC, Rubin CE, et al. Observer variation in the diagnosis of dysplasia in Barrett's esophagus. Hum Pathol 1988;19(2):166-78.
2. Montgomery E, Bronner MP, Goldblum JR, et al. Reproducibility of the diagnosis of dysplasia in Barrett esophagus: a reaffirmation. Hum Pathol 2001;32(4):368-78.
3. Lomo LC, Blount PL, Sanchez CA, et al. Crypt dysplasia with surface maturation: a clinical, pathologic, and molecular study of a Barrett's esophagus cohort. Am J Surg Pathol 2006;30(4):423-35.
4. Montgomery E. Is there a way for pathologists to decrease interobserver variability in the diagnosis of dysplasia? Arch Pathol Lab Med 2005;129(2):174-6.
5. Cross SS, Betmouni S, Burton JL, et al. What levels of agreement can be expected between histopathologists assigning cases to discrete nominal categories? A study of the diagnosis of hyperplastic and adenomatous colorectal polyps. Mod Pathol 2000;13(9):941-4.
6. Hruban RH, Adsay NV, Albores-Saavedra J, et al. Pancreatic intraepithelial neoplasia: a new nomenclature and classification system for pancreatic duct lesions. Am J Surg Pathol 2001;25(5):579-86.

What are the minimal criteria for the diagnosis of high-grade dysplasia in Barrett's mucosa?

H.D. Appelman (Ann Arbor)

Dysplasia in Barrett's mucosa is recognized morphologically by combinations of cytologic changes that deal with the appearance of individual cells especially their nuclei, and architectural changes that deal with the relationship of cells to each other and the variety of structures that they form. *Table I* has a limited list of twelve such cytologic and architectural features. If each of these twelve features is graded on a scale of 0 to 3 and all ten are added

Table I. An abbreviated list of ten cytologic and architectural features that occur in dysplastic epithelium.

- Cytologic abnormalities
  - Nuclear variations from normal
    - Enlargement with increased nuclear to cytoplasmic ratio
    - Hyperchromatism (darkly staining nuclei)\
    - Pleomorphism (variation in size and shape of nuclei)\
    - Mitoses
      - Too many mitoses (more mitoses than in non-dysplastic epithelium)
      - Mitoses in the superficial mucosa where they do not normally occur
      - Abnormal mitoses (the shapes of the mitotic figures are peculiar)
  - Cytologic: loss of maturation, mainly decrease or total loss of mucin content

- Architectural
  - Cellular (the ways that cells relate to each other in tissues
    - Crowding (the cells are closer together)
    - Stratification (the cells and their nuclei are not at the base of the cells but are higher up)
  - Pattern of growth of cells (what kinds of structures do they form)
    - Tubules that are crowded, generally superficially beneath the surface
    - Formation of villi (long slender projections) on the surface
    - Complexity of the tubules (they are not simple round or elongated structures, but they have peripheral buds or branches or there are bridges of epithelium that cross and subdivide them, the cribriform pattern)

for every epithelium in Barrett's mucosa that is found on a biopsy, the totals will range from 0 to 36. At the lowest end of the total score, that is a score of zero, the Barrett's epithelium, which is metaplastic to begin with and therefore abnormal, has not a single dysplastic feature, and it is formally designated as negative for dysplasia. In contrast at the highest end, where every single feature has the highest score and where the total score for the epithelium is 36, the epithelium is the highest of high-grade dysplasias (HGD). Somewhere in between are those epithelia that are considered to be indefinite for dysplasia and those thought to have low-grade dysplasia (LGD). As the total score for those epithelia that are considered to be negative for dysplasia increases, there must come a point or a score beyond which the epithelium qualifies as indefinite for dysplasia. Similarly there must be a total score that indicates the epithelium is no longer indefinite but is now LGD, and there must be a score which indicates that the epithelium has crossed from LGD to HGD. What we must remember is that the changes mentioned above do not occur at the same rate or with the same weight in every dysplasia. Ideal LGD might have nuclei confined to the basal half of the cells with little pleomorphism and satisfactory cytoplasmic maturation, and the architecture might be that of slight villous exaggeration on the surface or increased numbers of superficial tubules which continue to have lamina propria separating them. But perhaps some LGDs have a higher pleomorphism score but a lower stratification score. Ideal HGD is likely to have full thickness nuclear stratification, hyperchromatism and pleomorphism with atypical mitoses and no cytoplasmic maturation, and the architecture is likely to have an exaggerated villous surface and/or very crowded superficial tubules separated by little lamina propria. But some HGDs may have a lower architectural score with higher stratification hyperchromatism scores. What we want to know is what we need to add, in terms of scores of any of the dysplastic features, to typical LGD to make it just barely more than LGD, that is, the lowest end of HGD. We can assume that such changes include, beginning on the low-grade side, gradually increasing nuclear size, hyperchromatism, pleomorphism, stratification, and diminished cytoplasmic maturation, all while the architecture is becoming gradually more complex. Clearly, defining that specific set of morphologic characteristics which identify the crossing from highest end of low-grade to lowest end of HGD is a subjective microscopic interpretation that is likely to vary dramatically from one pathologist to another, even the most experienced pathologists.

Are there any published criteria for minimal HGD? In a paper by Snell *et al.* on the long-term nonsurgical management of Barrett's esophagus with HGD, mention was made that "the interpretation of the microscopic findings was based on previously established definitions", and the reference was to a paper published in 1983 by Riddell *et al.* that dealt with colitis, not with Barrett's mucosa [1,2]. Furthermore, that paper does not give solid diagnostic criteria. In a paper by Skacel *et al.* covering the diagnosis of LGD in Barrett's esophagus, mention was made that "each biopsy was classified ... using previously published criteria modified...", also citing the Riddell *et al.* paper with the same limitations [3]. Montgomery *et al.*, in a publication on the reproducibility of the diagnosis of dysplasia in Barrett's esophagus mentioned that "the participants were familiar with the criteria proposed in 1988 and used these as a general basis for their interpretations" [4]. This reference was to a paper by Reid *et al.* on observer variation in the diagnosis of dysplasia in Barrett's esophagus [5] This was a study of multiple cases by gastrointestinal pathologists from four centers in the United States and Canada. The diagnostic features were separated into two types, architectural and nuclear (cytologic), and these features were recognized as being those of dysplasia in general, not specifically any grade. Architectural features included the following:

- budded, branched, crowded or irregularly-shaped glands;
- papillary extensions in the gland lumina;
- villiform configuration of the mucosa.

Nuclear changes included:

- marked variation in size and shape;
- nuclear and/or nucleolar enlargement;
- increased nuclear/cytoplasmic ratio;
- hyperchromatism;
- increased numbers of abnormal mitoses (which presumably assumed that there were normal numbers of abnormal mitoses).

Furthermore, in this study, the following statement was made: "the diagnosis of low-grade dysplasia or high-grade dysplasia is based on the severity of both architectural and cytologic criteria... although either architectural or cytologic abnormalities may predominate, high-grade dysplasia is diagnosed if either one is sufficiently prominent." Unfortunately, there is no definition of how prominent is "sufficiently" prominent in separating the highest side of LGD from the lowest side of HGD. Therefore, this widely quoted paper does not tell us how to make these distinctions.

In a publication by Buttar *et al.,* on the extent of HGD in Barrett's esophagus, HGD was also defined by criteria originally established by Reid *et al.* with the same limitations mentioned above [6]. Back to the paper by Montgomery *et al.* on reproducibility of dysplasia diagnoses, HGD was described as having no surface maturation [4]. The architecture may show crowding or be markedly distorted with glandular crowding and little lamina propria. However, there is no definition for the words "may", "markedly", and "little". Furthermore, also in that paper it was mentioned that "nuclei may have either delicately-clumped dark heterochromatin and inconspicuous nucleoli or prominent irregular nuclei with irregularly-clumped chromatin and irregular nuclei. Markedly enlarged hyperchromatic nuclei are a feature of high-grade dysplasia and these may extend to the surface. Loss of nuclear polarity is seen. Mitoses are readily identified." This sounds like a solid definition, but it includes numerous words that are not defined such as "may", "delicately", "inconspicuous", "irregular", "markedly", "readily identified". There is no mention of how we tell markedly from less than markedly and regularly from irregularly. Not only do these recent publications fail to tell us where LGD ends and HGD begins, but none of the established textbooks in gastrointestinal pathology are also of any help. The illustrations in those textbooks of dysplasia tend to be typical LGDs or typical HGDs which clearly don't look anything alike.

In summary, how do we tell the difference between LGDs and HGDs? There are no specific rules just suggestions. From a practical standpoint, we look at epithelium and try to determine if it looks bad enough to be HGD, or we show it to other experienced pathologists to see if they think it looks bad enough to be HGD. What we really need is a HGD stain or some clear-cut marker, either protein or genetic, that will tell us where LGD ends and HGD begins. At the moment, the answer to the question posed by the title at the beginning of this presentation is that the minimal criteria for the diagnosis of HGD exist in the eyeballs of the pathologists and in their ocular-cerebral reflexes. These changes are not defined anywhere, and as far as I can tell, there are no reproducible studies of diagnoses in this intermediate dysplasia area.

References

1. Snell TG, Sontag SJ, Chejfec G, et al. Long-term nonsurgical management of Barrett's esophagus with high-grade dysplasia. Gastroenterology 2001;120:1607-19.
2. Riddell RH, Goldman H, Ransohoff DF, et al. Dysplasia in inflammatory bowel disease: Standardized classification with provisional clinical applications. Hum Pathol 1983;14:931-68.
3. Skacel M, Petras RE, Gramlich TL, et al. The diagnosis of low-grade dysplasia in Barrett's esophagus and its implications for disease progression. Am J Gastroenterol 2000;95:3383-7.
4. Montgomery E, Bronner MP, Goldblum JR. Reproducibility of the diagnosis of dysplasia in Barrett's esophagus: a reaffirmation. Hum Pathol 2001;32:368-78.
5. Reid BJ, Haggitt RC, Rubin CE, et al. Observer variation in the diagnosis of dysplasia in Barrett's esophagus. Hum Pathol 1988;19:166-78.
6. Buttar NS, Wang KK, Sebo TJ, et al. Extent of high-grade dysplasia in Barrett's esophagus correlates with risk of adenocarcinoma. Gastroenterology 2001;120:1630-9.

What is the reproducibility of diagnosis of Barrett's metaplasia/dysphagia in images submitted to a panel of pathologists?

G. Chejfec, S. Sontag, T. Schnell (Chicago)

Case 1: dormant high grade dysplasia

Question: can you have Barrett esophagus with persistent high grade dysplasia for 12 years without developing cancer?

A 63-year-old white male with typical symptoms of gastroesophageal reflux (GERD) for 35 years was first seen in 1992 with perfectly flat Barrett mucosa, extending from 18-40 cm (*Figure 1*). There was no dysplasia; these findings were confirmed in 1994 (*Figure 2*). A subsequent endoscopy and biopsy in 1996 revealed high grade dysplasia (HGD) for the first time (*Figure 3*). He was placed on a strict observation program, comprising endoscopy and biopsy every 3 months for 1 year ("the hunt"). The HGD remained unchanged for one year. He then entered a surveillance protocol until the present time. The esophageal mucosa has remained flat, and periodic examinations have not shown any progression to adenocarcinoma (*Figures 4, 5, 6 and 7*). Clinically, he is doing very well and continues on medical management consisting of proton pump inhibitors (PPIs).

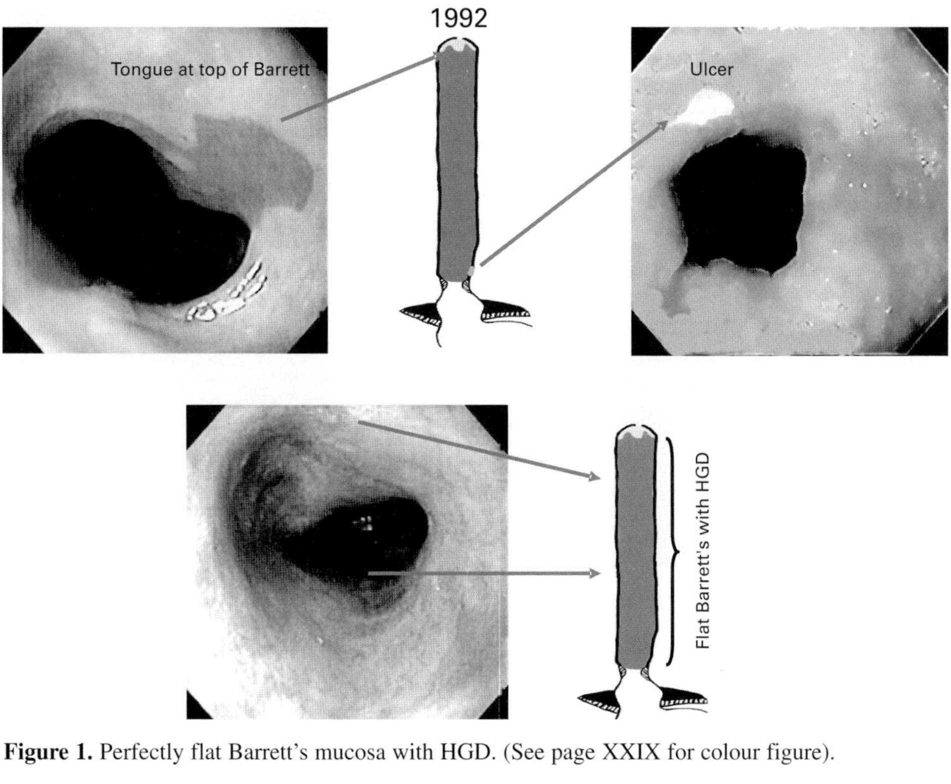

Figure 1. Perfectly flat Barrett's mucosa with HGD. (See page XXIX for colour figure).

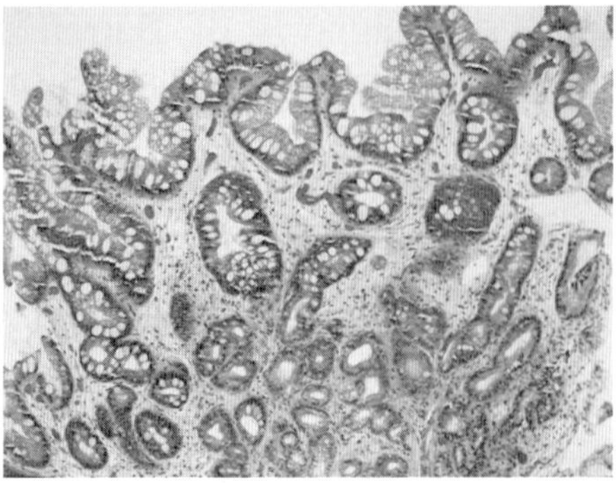

Figure 2. February 1994. (See page XXIX for colour figure).

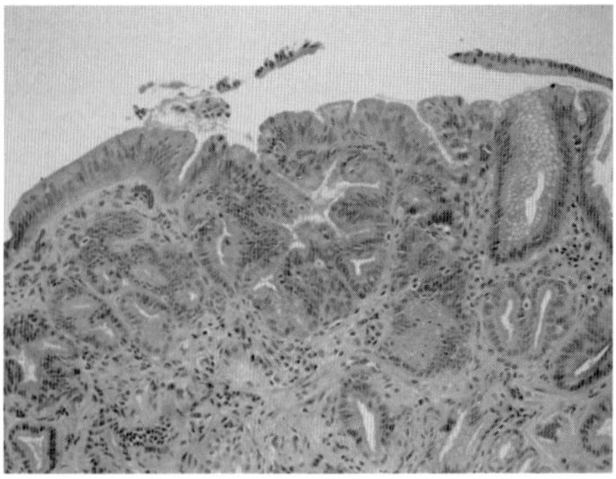

Figure 3. January 1996. (See page XXIX for colour figure).

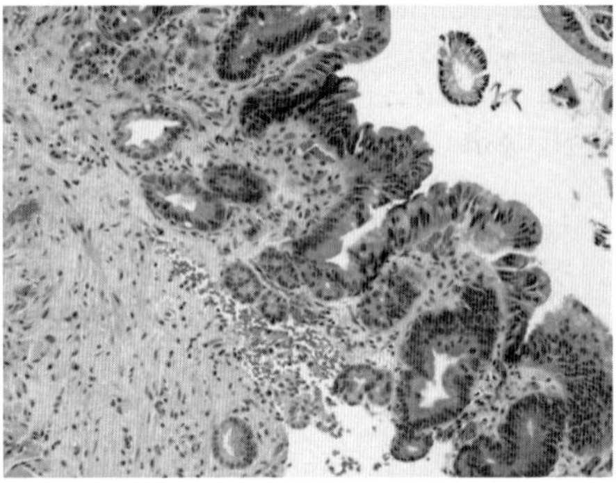

Figure 4. April 1999. (See page XXIX for colour figure).

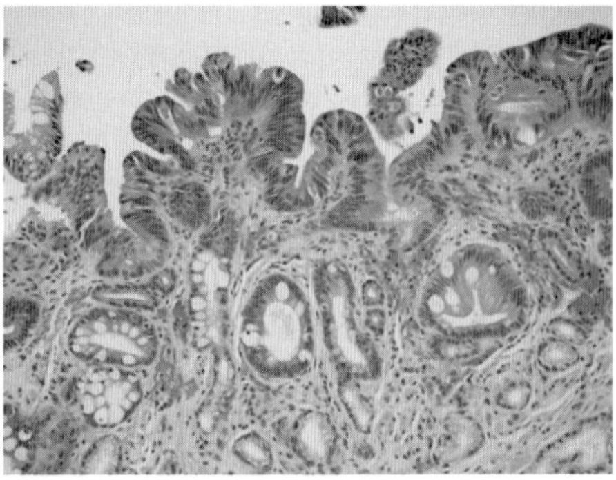

Figure 5. October 2002. (See page XXIX for colour figure).

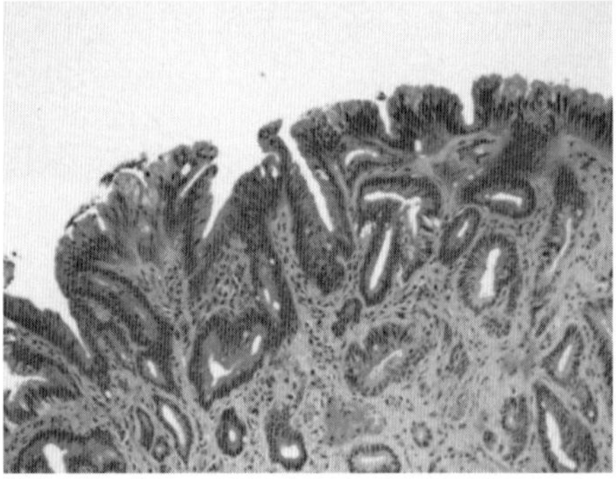

Figure 6. June 2005. (See page XXX for colour figure).

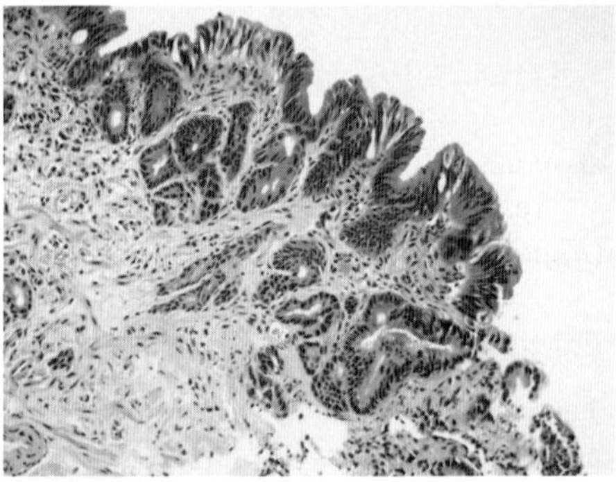

Figure 7. April 2006. (See page XXX for colour figure).

Discussion

Although the duration of follow up in this case is unique, HGD in Barret esophagus has been observed to persist for protracted periods of time. We [1] and others [2] have identified such patients enrolled in a surveillance program.

In our program patients with HGD are enrolled only after 4 endoscopic procedures in a period of 1 year have failed to detect adenocarcinoma. Using this protocol for more than 20 years we diagnosed HGD in 7.2% of 1,099 patients with Barrett esophagus.

In this group of 79 patients with HGD, 34 had HGD on first endoscopy and 45 developed HGD during surveillance for lesser grades of dysplasia. Four of 34 with HGD on first endoscopy were found with adenocarcinoma during "the hunt" period. Adding the 30 patients who remained during "the hunt" to the 45 patients who developed HGD during routine surveillance, a total of 75 patients remained. In 12 of these 75 patients (16%), adenocarcinoma developed in a 7.3 year surveillance period. Eleven of the 12 patients were cured with surgical or ablation therapy, and the remaining 63 continue on surveillance.

The reasons for the persistence of HGD remain an enigma. Several studies have proposed the use of biomarkers to identify patients at risk of progressing to cancer. Flow cytometry has yielded the most consistent results. Thus, aneuploidy or 4N present in HGD were found in over half of the patients developing cancers during a 5 year surveillance period [2]. Similar flow cytometry findings were observed by other investigators [3-5]. Whether our patients with HGD had such cytometric abnormalities remains unknown. Assuming, however, that all of our patients who developed cancer actually had aneuploidy or 4N present in the HGD, would the absence of aneuploidy be sufficient to allow us to conclude that the "fixed" status of HGD will remain fixed?

As of now this question remains unanswered.

Case 2: vanishing high grade dysplasia

Question: can high grade dysplasia completely regress?

A 66-year-old white male with a 15 year history of dyspepsia and heartburn. Endoscopy demonstrated a perfectly flat Barrett's mucosa (*Figure 8*). Biopsy revealed HGD (*Figure 9*). Repeat biopsy 2 weeks later yielded Barrett mucosa without dysplasia (*Figure 10*). A third biopsy, 2 weeks later, again showed HGD (*Figure 11*). Three months later there was no evidence of HGD (*Figure 12*).

Yearly examinations for the next 6 years showed only Barrett mucosa without dysplasia (*Figures 13 and 14*). The patient continues to do clinically well until the present.

Discussion

There are two explanations for the vanishing HGD. First, epithelial dysplasias are focal in nature. The most logical explanation for the disappearance of HGD in this patient would be that the biopsy sites were the only exhibiting HGD and all such tissue was actually removed with the endoscopic biopsies.

Second, spontaneous regression of dysplasia has been described in the uterine cervix. In a cohort of 17,000 women with pap smears showing a spectrum of dysplasias from mild to severe, the majority of mild and moderate dysplasias regressed. The risk of progression from moderate to severe dysplasia was found to be 16% within 2 years and 25% within

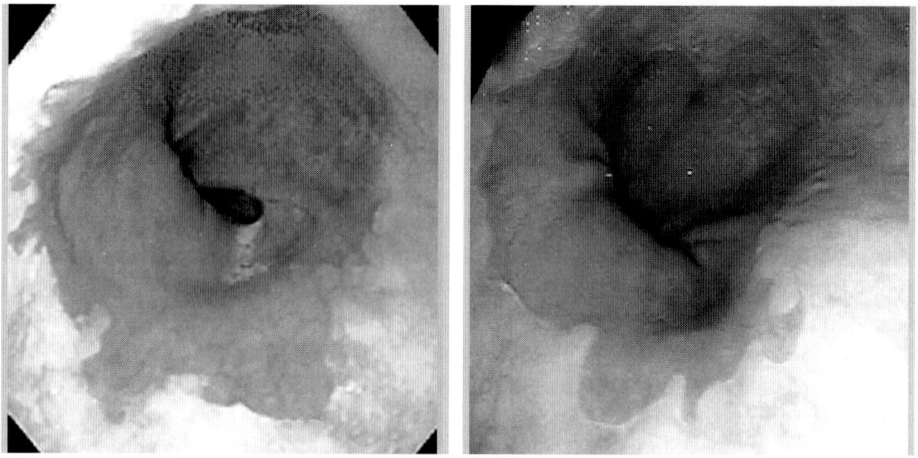

Figure 8. Perfectly flat Barrett's mucosa. (See page XXX for colour figure).

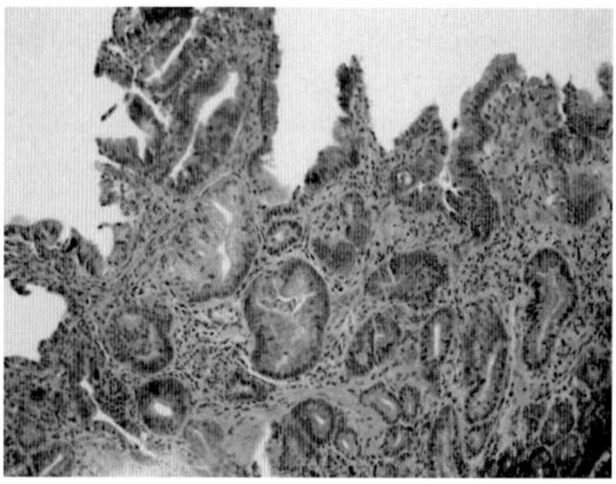

Figure 9. September 5, 2000. (See page XXX for colour figure).

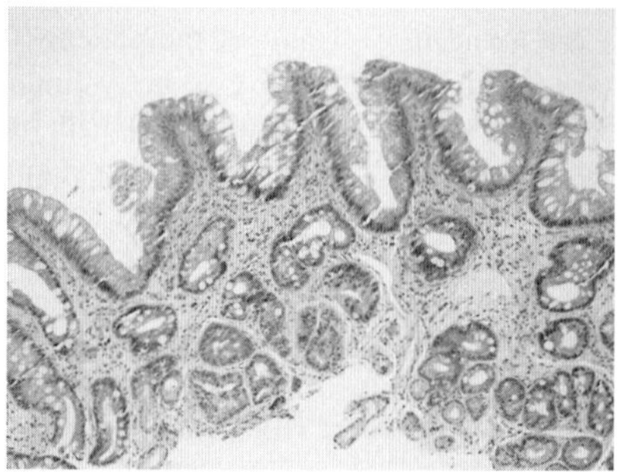

Figure 10. October 3, 2000. (See page XXX for colour figure).

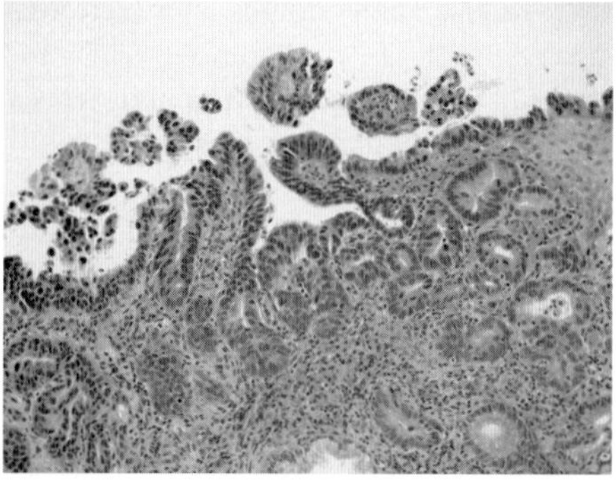

Figure 11. October 16, 2000. (See page XXXI for colour figure).

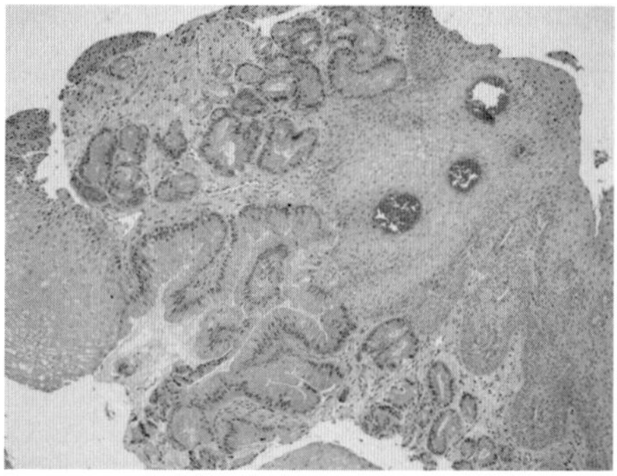

Figure 12. December 10, 2000. (See page XXXI for colour figure).

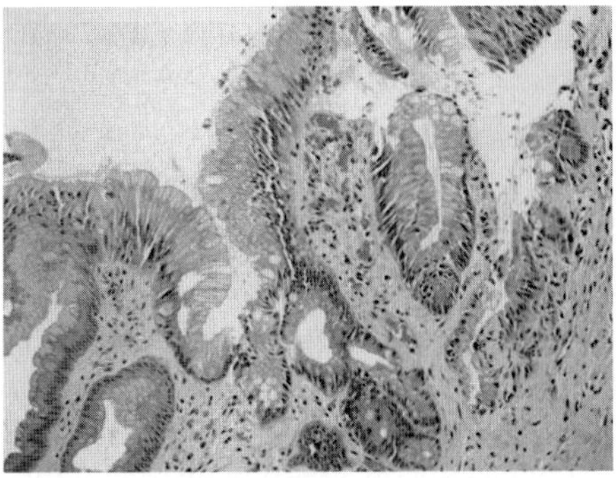

Figure 13. 2002. (See page XXXI for colour figure).

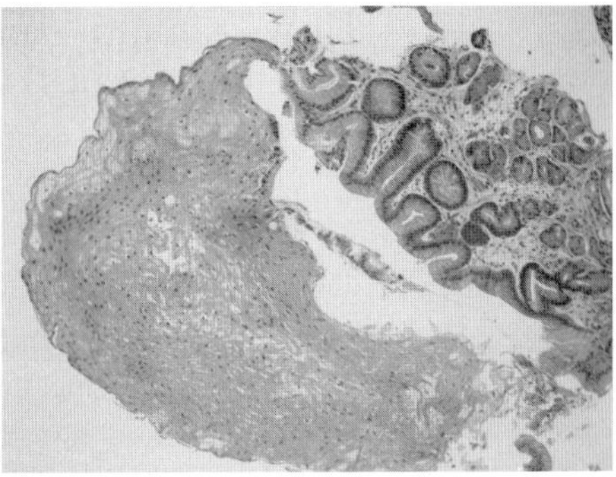

Figure 14. 2006. (See page XXXI for colour figure).

5 years of diagnosis. Most untreated mild dysplasias regressed to normal within 2 years [6]. The natural history of severe (high grade) dysplasia in these reports could not be determined since patients with severe dysplasia were treated surgically.

In our experience, HGD either bounced from HGD to low grade dysplasia (LGD) and back again, reverted to LGD and remained, or developed into adenocarcinoma. For certain, most of the HGD patients discovered by our group did not require surgery and many are living out their old age in retirement or nursing homes.

Finally, only one of our HGD patients has died from Barrett's cancer and this one had a diagnosis for 10 years of HGD, only to return with brain metastasis.

References

1. Schnell T, Sontag SJ, Chejfec G, et al. Long term non-surgical management of Barrett's esophagus with high grade dysplasia.Gastroenterology 2001;120:1607-19.
2. Reid BJ, Levine S, Longton G, et al. Predictors of progression to cancer in Barrett's esophagus: Baseline histology and flow cytometry identify low and high risk patient subsets. Am J Gastroenterol 2000;95:1669-76.
3. Fennerty MB, Sampliner RE, Way D, et al. Discordance between flow cytometric abnormalities and dysplasia in Barrett's esophagus. Gastroenterology 1989;97:815-20.
4. Gareval HS, Sampliner RE, Fennerty MB. Flow cytometry in Barrett's esophagus. Dig Dis Sci 1991;36:548-51.
5. Teodoric L, Gohde W, Persiani M, et al. DNA / protein flow cytometry as a predictive marker of malignancy in dysplasia-free Barrett's esophagus. Cytometry 1998;34:257-63.
6. Holowaty P, Miller AB, Rohan T. Natural history of dysplasia of the uterine cervix. J Natl Cancer Inst 1999;91:252-8.
7. Savage GF, McConnell KJ, Kulasingam SL. Risk of cervical cancer associated with extending the interval between cervical – cancer screenings. N Engl J Med 2003;349:1501-9.

How should acid suppression be done in the management of Barrett's esophagus?

C. Scarpignato, S. Contini (Parma)

Gastric juice that refluxes into the esophagus can injure esophageal squamous epithelium. When the injury heals through a metaplastic process in which an abnormal columnar epithelium replaces the injured squamous one, the resulting condition is called Barrett's esophagus [1]. Barrett's esophagus is therefore a complication of gastroesophageal reflux disease (GERD) that however develops in a minority of patients.

The abnormal columnar epithelium is an incomplete form of intestinal metaplasia, containing several columnar cell types with gastric, small intestinal, or colonic features. Although this so-called specialized intestinal metaplasia may be more resistant to gastroesophageal reflux (GER) than the native squamous mucosa, the metaplastic cells are predisposed to malignancy. Indeed, GERD and Barrett's esophagus are the most important risk factors for esophageal adenocarcinoma, a tumor whose frequency has increased dramatically during the last two decades in Western countries [2].

The pathogenesis of Barrett's metaplasia is not yet precisely understood; in particular, the key factors favoring its development are not known. Barrett's metaplasia is an acquired condition, clearly associated with severe GER. Compared with patients with erosive and non erosive GERD without Barrett's esophagus, patients with columnar-lined esophagus typically have greater esophageal acid exposure based on 24-hour pH monitoring [3-6]. However, there is some overlap and some studies found no difference in intraesophageal acid exposure time between Barrett's patients and patients with high-grade esophagitis [7]. Part of the increase in acid exposure in Barrett's patients may be related to the almost uniform presence of a hiatal hernia, which is typically longer and associated with larger defects in the hiatus than controls or patients with esophagitis alone [8]. In addition, patients with Barrett's esophagus have a lower basal esophageal sphincter pressure (LESP) compared with GERD patients without columnar metaplasia [4].

It has long been known that acid GER is accompanied by the reflux of duodenal contents, and there is increasing evidence from animal and human studies that duodenogastroesophageal reflux (DGER), consisting mainly of bile and pancreatic juice, might play a significant role in the development of Barrett's metaplasia and Barrett's carcinoma [9-11]. Several studies using ambulatory 24-hour bilirubin monitoring (i.e. bilimetry [12]) have provided important insights into the role of DGER in causing esophageal mucosal injury in humans. These studies showed a significant but graded increase in both acid and DGER from normal controls to esophagitis and Barrett's esophagus patients, with the highest values in patients with Barrett's esophagus. Furthermore, it appears that DGER occurs most commonly in association with acid reflux. A pivotal study of Vaezi and Richter [13] in patients with and without complications of Barrett's esophagus found increased reflux of bile and acid into the lower esophagus of both groups compared to healthy controls. More importantly, reflux of acid paralleled DGER, and both were significantly higher in patients with complicated Barrett's esophagus than in the uncomplicated group. Other investigators [*for review see* 10] have subsequently confirmed the results of these studies.

Barrett's disease and the underlying GERD are intensively treated with the aim of reducing mortality from cancer arising from columnar metaplasia. Several management strategies have been proposed:

- antireflux therapy [14] or antireflux surgery [15] to reduce or even abolish GER and DGER;
- endoscopic ablation of Barrett»s epithelium [16,17];
- the use of non-steroidal anti-inflammatory drugs (NSAIDs) to inhibit cyclo-oxygenase (COX) isoenzymes and their effect on cellular proliferation [18,19];
- regular endoscopic (and histologic) surveillance [20,21].

Although each strategy has a plausible rationale and some indirect evidence to support it, none has proved to reduce deaths from cancer in Barrett's esophagus. Furthermore, each entails expense, inconvenience, and variable risk [22]. Among the preventive strategies for cancer, only regular endoscopic surveillance has been recommended for routine clinical use by several medical societies, including the American Gastroenterological Association [23], the British Society of Gastroenterology [24] and the American College of Gastroenterology [25].

Is gastric acid secretion increased in patients with Barrett's esophagus?

The presence of basal acid hypersecretion in a small group of patients with Barrett's esophagus was first reported by Mulholland *et al.* [26]. Although in this patient population meal-stimulated secretion was comparable to that of healthy controls, gastrin (G-17-I)-induced acid hypersecretion was significantly higher when compared with controls. However, parietal cell sensitivity to gastrin, expressed as the concentration causing half-maximal acid secretion, was not significantly different (i.e. 56.8 ± 5.5 fmol/ml *versus* 63.6 ± 6.9 fmol/ml, respectively) [26]. In this study no data were provided on how many patients were true hypersecretors (i.e. with basal acid output, BAO, higher than 10 mEq/h) and how many had concomitant esophagitis and/or duodenal ulcer.

In a subsequent larger study, Collen *et al.* [27] reported that patients with Barrett's esophagus display – as a group – a significantly higher BAO than healthy controls. Many patients however had their value in the normal range. Only 15 out of 42 patients with Barrett's esophagus (i.e. 36%) had BAO higher than 10 mEq/h. There was a significant correlation between BAO and the daily ranitidine dose, required for esophageal mucosal healing and complete symptom control. Although in a previous study of the same group of investigators [28] no difference between patients with Barrett's esophagus and those with reflux esophagitis (without columnar metaplasia), in either BAO mean values and proportion of subjects with BAO higher than 10 mEq/h, was found, Stein *et al.* [29] reported that basal and pentagastrin-stimulated acid secretion were in Barrett's patients significantly higher than those found in symptomatic patients with erosive esophagitis. Different selection criteria of the patient populations may explain the different findings of the two investigations. In studying acid secretion, there are indeed many confounding influences, such as gender (male secrete more than females) and the presence or esophagitis, duodenal ulcer or Zollinger-Ellison syndrome (ZES) [30].

In a landmark study which adopted appropriate controls (i.e. patients with esophagitis, but not columnar-lined esophagus, who were matched for age, sex and presence or absence of duodenal ulcer or ZES), Hirschowitz [31] did unquestionably show that there is no significant difference in both basal and stimulated secretion between patients with esophagitis and those who have, in addition, Barrett's esophagus.

The presence of complications (e.g. stricture, ulceration, dysplasia or cancer) does not seem to influence either acid secretion and the proportion of Barrett patients with hypersecretion [32]. The available results from gastric secretory studies, including the proportion of patients with basal acid hypersecretion, are summarized in *Table I* [33].

Table I. Basal and stimulated acid secretion in patients with Barrett's esophagus (from [33]).

Year	Authors	BAO	MAO/PAO	Patients with acid hypersecretion
1989	Mulholland *et al.* [26]	Increased	Normal	NA
1992	Collen & Johnson [27]	Increased	NA	15/42 (36%)
1995	Stein *et al.* [29]	Increased	Increased	11/23 (48%)
1996	Hirschowitz [31]	Normal	Normal	7/30 (24%)
BAO = basal acid output; MAO/PAO = maximal acid output/peak acid output; NA = not available				

The role of pepsin has not been explored extensively in Barrett's esophagus. Activation of pepsin requires a pH of less than 3 [34]; thus, separating the role of pepsin from acid alone is difficult. One early study [35] reported an increased gastric juice concentration of pepsin, but it is flowed by methodological drawbacks. An indeed, Hirschowitz [31] could not find any difference in pepsin output between patients with Barrett's esophagus and appropriate controls.

The gastric pH profile in this patient population was first studied in 1985 by Stein *et al.* [29] who found that – compared to patients with esophagitis – those with columnar metaplasia displayed a marked shift of the recorded pH values towards a more acidic range.

The development of better computer programs to quantitate and analyze 24-hour pH recordings has allowed Savarino *et al.* [36] to study thoroughly the intragastric acidity pattern of patients with Barrett's esophagus. They found no difference in the 24-hour and daytime patterns of gastric pH between patients and healthy subjects, a finding recently confirmed by Fein *et al.* [37]. However, during the night, acidity was significantly lower in Barrett's patients.

It must be emphasized that almost all the above secretory studies have been performed before the "*Helicobacter* revolution" [33]. And the more recent pH-metric investigations did not specifically look at the *Helicobacter* status, which does markedly influence the acid secretory capacity of the stomach [38,39] as well as the effect of antisecretory drugs, mainly proton pump inbitors (PPIs) [40,41]. Furthermore, although still debated, *H. pylori* infection may protect against the development of esophagitis by decreasing the potency of the gastric refluxate in patients with corpus-predominant gastritis [42,43]. It is therefore evident that further studies taking into account the *Helicobacter* status are needed to definitely establish whether patients with Barrett's esophagus have a gastric secretory pattern different from that seen in patients with GERD or healthy controls.

Why should acid suppression be used in patients with Barrett's esophagus?

Although not a constant finding, gastric acid hypersecretion is relatively common in patients with Barrett's esophagus, irrespective of the presence of esophagitis. This finding, however, could be simply attributed to the frequent but coincidental presence of duodenal ulcer [30,31]. Indeed, studies, which adopted appropriate controls, failed to show any difference in gastric secretory states.

Available data are consistent with the idea that a defective gastroesophageal barrier is the predominant factor for the development of complications in both GERD and Barrett's esophagus [44]. Indeed, in a population of 75 GERD patients (including 13 patients with columnar-lined esophagus), gastric hypersecretion was a less frequent finding than a mechanically defective lower esophageal sphincter (LES) [45]. In the presence of normal gastric secretion, complications occurred in 18% of those with a normal sphincter and 77% of those with a defective sphincter while, in the presence of hypersecretion, the complication rate was 40% and 82%, respectively [45]. In addition, although abnormal esophageal exposure to acid (which correlates to abnormal sphincter pressure [46]) was detected in almost all (i.e. 93%) Barrett patients, gastric hypersecretion was present only in 44% of them [32]. All these findings suggest that the development of reflux complications (including Barrett's esophagus) is mainly dependent on the presence of a defective barrier rather than of acid hypersecretion. Finally, the low prevalence of columnar metaplasia in patients with ZES [47], whose acid secretion is more than 8 folds that of healthy subjects, emphasizes once again the limited role of gastric hypersecretion alone in the pathogenesis of Barrett's esophagus. Nonetheless, inhibition of acid secretion still remains a cornerstone of the therapy due to its ability to reduce the aggressive power of the refluxate [23-25,48,49].

Aims of the pharmacological treatment of Barrett's esophagus

The primary goals of antireflux therapy, irrespective of the presence of Barrett's esophagus, are elimination of the symptoms and signs of reflux esophagitis, and prevention of GERD complications, such as peptic esophageal stricture and adenocarcinoma. Antireflux lifestyle modifications have traditionally been recommended for patients with GERD, including elevation of the head of the bed, avoidance of recumbency for several hours after meals, reduction in fat intake, and cessation of smoking, but little published data support the efficacy of these modifications [50]. And indeed the Genval Workshop Report [51] on reflux disease stated that there is currently a significant overestimation of the likelihood that patients will derive adequate relief through alterations in lifestyle factors.

Modern medical therapy for GERD focuses on the suppression of gastric acid secretion through histamine H_2-receptor antagonist (H_2RA) or PPI therapy [52-55], whereas surgical therapy is directed at correcting the underlying diathesis by creating a barrier to GER through fundoplication [56,57]. Medical and surgical therapies have been shown to be effective for healing the symptoms and signs of reflux esophagitis, and for limiting the peptic complications of GERD, although antireflux surgery is not devoid of morbidity [58] and, although very rarely, of mortality [56].

Both medical [59] and surgical [15,60] therapy may induce some regression of the Barrett metaplasia, but neither approach has been proved to decrease the risk of esophageal adenocarcinoma, even if the incidence of developing dysplasia or cancer following fundoplication appears to be less than that observed with antisecretory treatment [61].

Antisecretory drugs for Barrett's esophagus: how much are they effective?

H_2RAs and PPIs represent the two classes of antisecretory drugs today available. Although both have been used in GERD, PPIs are clearly the winner. Indeed, a large meta-analysis [62] clearly showed a distinct advantage – either in terms of healing and symptom relief – of PPIs over H_2RAs, a finding confirmed in a more recent Cochrane Review [63].

The reasons for the PPI superiority over H_2RAs rely on the different pharmacological properties of these compounds [64,65]. H_2RAs have a short duration of action, produce incomplete inhibition of post-prandial acid secretion and tolerance to standard doses usually develop within 2 weeks. In contrast, PPIs control both basal and food-stimulated acid secretion and produce more complete and longer lasting acid suppression than H_2-blockers [64,65]. Such acid inhibition virtually abolishes the damaging peptic activity of gastric juice. In addition, tolerance to PPIs has not been observed, an advantage presumably attributable to the fact that they act at the final site of acid production, thereby blocking the effects of any compensatory mechanisms promoting acid secretion [64,65].

Conventional-dose antisecretory therapy reduces, but fails to abolish, gastric acid secretion in most patients with Barrett's esophagus. Furthermore, the effect of this therapy of GERD symptoms in these patients does not accurately reflect the degree of acid suppression. Indeed, symptom control is not so difficult in patients with columnar metaplasia since they seem to display low esophageal sensitivity to endogenous acid [66], which confer them an impaired ability to recognize acid reflux. Barrett's patients have actually less sensitivity than GERD patients for similar acid exposure. In these patients normal esophageal motility is associated with the poorest sensitivity and the presence of increased acid exposure is required in order to achieve sensitivity levels comparable with GERD patients [67].

Esophageal pH monitoring studies frequently reveal pathologic acid reflux in patients with Barrett's esophagus rendered asymptomatic by PPIs administered in conventional dosages [68]. Persistent acid reflux on PPI therapy is common in these patients [69,70]. Approximately 80% of patients with Barrett's esophagus treated with a PPI twice daily experience nocturnal acid breakthrough (NAB), which is often associated with episodes of acid reflux [71]. In addition, 50% of patients asymptomatic under PPI therapy still display abnormal esophageal exposure to acid (*Figure 1*) [72]. It is worth mentioning that PPI efficacy in suppressing esophageal acidification may decrease over time, as suggested by a recent investigation showing a significant rise in acid exposure after 2-years of continuous drug treatment [73].

The more effective and predictable acid control achieved with esomeprazole compared with other PPIs [74,75] translates into a better therapeutic efficacy in GERD. Three meta-analyses have indeed shown not only that esomeprazole achieves the highest healing rates of reflux esophagitis in the short-term [76,77] but also that esomeprazole 20 mg is the only step-down dose PPI able to show a significantly higher proportion of patients in remission of reflux compared with lansoprazole 15 mg [78]. However, although this PPI proved to be more effective than lansoprazole in reducing esophageal acid exposure in patients with Barrett's esophagus [79], up to 62% of patients had abnormal esophageal pH profiles

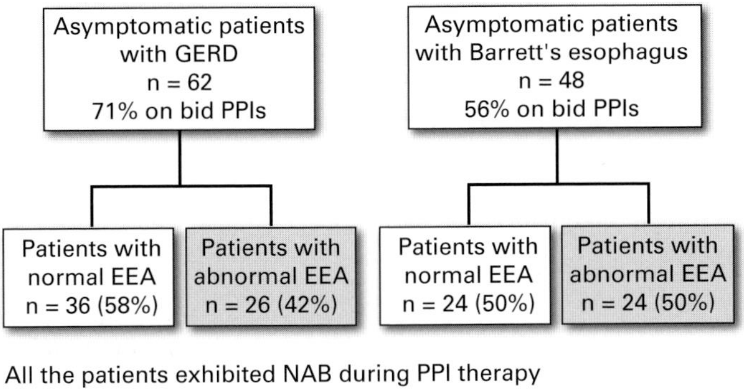

Figure 1. Failure of current PPI regimens to normalize esophageal exposure to acid (EEA) in patients with GERD or Barrett's esophagus despite symptom control (from [72]).

despite being asymptomatic [80]. Even with a very high dose regimen (namely 120 mg daily), 16-23% of patients continued to have an abnormal esophageal acidification [81]. Adding an H_2RA at bedtime to a twice daily PPI regimen can improve nocturnal acid control [82], but such a benefit is not long-lasting because of the development of tolerance [83].

Predicting the normalization of esophageal acid exposure after acid suppression in patients with Barrett's esophagus is extremely difficult. Factors such as age, length of the columnar-lined epithelium or hiatal hernia size cannot be used to predict the persistence of abnormal esophageal acid exposure after PPIs (*Table II*) [84]. Tailoring acid control individually with the help of pH-monitoring is therefore needed. It is feasible and effective and may also result on decreased length and development of squamous islands in patients with Barrett's epithelium [85].

Table II. Clinical, endoscopic and ambulatory 24-hour pH characteristics of the Barrett's patients, whose esophageal exposure to acid was normalized by PPI treatment or remained still abnormal during therapy (from [75]).

	Normal pH study (n = 34)	Abnormal pH study (n = 12)	p value
Age (years)	64 (44-84)	58 (42-75)	0.075
Sex male female	33 1	11 1	0.458*
Hiatal hernia size (cm)	3 (0-6)	3 (2-5)	0.513
Barrett's esophagus length (cm)	3 (2-6)	3 (2-6)	0.765
Helicobacter pylori infection	3	0	
Total time pH < 4 (%)	0.2 (0-3.6)	9.3 (4.5-29.9)	
Supine time pH < 4 (%)	0 (0-12.9)	11.3 (0-47.2)	
Upright time pH < 4 (%)	0.2 (0-4.2)	10.1 (1.2-47.9)	

Values within parentheses denote range. Abnormal 24-hour pH study was defined as intra-esophageal pH < 4 for longer than 4.2% of the total monitoring period. Except for gender, all numbers are medians. There was no statistically significant differences between the two groups for age, hiatal hernia size, Barrett's esophagus length and *H. pylori* infection. All continuous variables were compared using the Wilcoxon rank sum test.
* Variables that were compared with the Fisher's exact test.

Although the best way of decreasing DGER is a surgical procedure that corrects the defective antireflux barrier, acid suppression therapy with omeprazole 20 mg orally twice daily increases gastric pH, decreases gastric volume, and diminishes DGER to a similar degree of antireflux surgery [86-89], an effect shared also by pantoprazole [90] (*Table III*) and probably by the other PPIs [91]. The most likely mechanism by which PPIs reduce DGER is by decreasing the volume of gastric secretions, with less fluid available in the stomach to mix with the relatively small volumes of duodenal contents that would be transported up into the esophagus, especially in presence of low LESP [*for review see* 91].

Table III. Inhibitory effect of PPIs on DGER (measured by bilirubin monitoring) in adults (modified from [91]).

Authors	Year	PPI	Dose	DGER
Champion *et al.* [86]	1994	Omeprazole	20 mg bid	⇓
Marshall *et al.* [87]	1998	Omeprazole	20 mg bid	⇓
Stein *et al.* [88]	1998	Omeprazole	20 mg bid	⇓
Menges *et al.* [89]	2001	Omeprazole or pantoprazole	40 mg od or 40 mg bid	⇓
Netzer *et al.* [90]	2001	Pantoprazole	40 mg od	⇓
⇓ = decrease				

Although reduction of esophageal acidification always paralleled inhibition of biliary reflux [91], normalization of esophageal exposure to acid does not guarantee control of DGER in patients with Barrett's esophagus (*Figure 2*) [92,93], despite being asymptomatic after therapy [92].

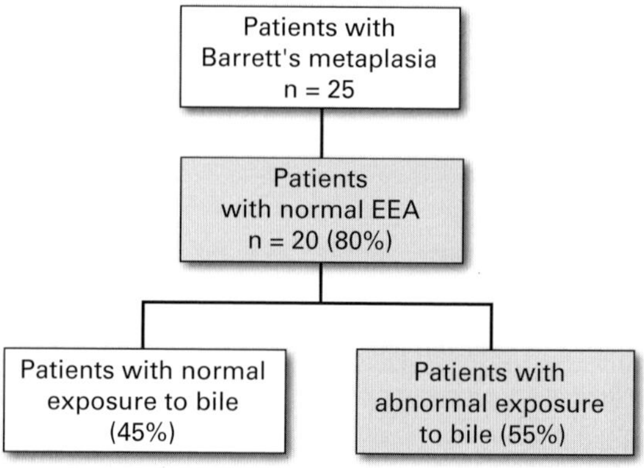

Figure 2. Presence of DGER in patients with Barrett's esophagus during PPI therapy despite control of symptoms and esophageal exposure to acid (EEA) (from [93]).

Healing of coexistent esophagitis is an important goal of treatment in patients with Barrett's esophagus. Elimination of erosive esophagitis or erythema of the esophagus permits better delineation of the metaplastic epithelium and facilitates the recognition of dysplasia. In these patients PPIs do heal mucosal lesions although less quickly than in patients with erosive esophagitis [94]. Indeed, results of the ProGERD study [95] have shown that healing rates at four and eight weeks are considerably lower for patients with Barrett's esophagus than for those without, whatever the diagnostic methodology (endoscopy combined with histology or endoscopy alone) of columnar metaplasia adopted (*Figure 3*). As expected, Barrett's patients with Los Angeles (LA) grade A/B esophagitis had higher healing rates at both four and eight weeks (64.5% and 78.6%, respectively) than those with grade C/D esophagitis (45.0% and 63.0%, respectively) [95].

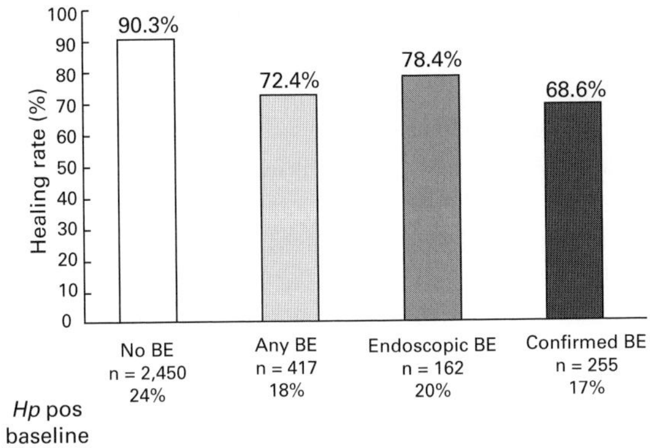

Figure 3. Endoscopic healing rates (%) at eight weeks for erosive reflux disease patients according to method of diagnosis of Barrett's esophagus: no Barretts' esophagus, any Barretts' esophagus (endoscopic + confirmed), endoscopic Barretts' esophagus, confirmed Barretts' esophagus (from [95]).
$p = 0.03$ for endoscopic Barretts' esophagus *versus* confirmed Barretts' esophagus;
$p < 0.0001$ for no Barretts' esophagus *versus* any Barretts' esophagus, endoscopic Barretts' esophagus, or confirmed Barretts' esophagus.

In Barrett's patients, ulcers are located either within the metaplastic columnar mucosa, typically in the lower part of the esophagus, or higher up in the distal portion of the squamous esophagus near the squamometaplastic junction [96]. Regardless of their location, these ulcers cause reflux symptoms in 70% of cases, may contribute to anemia and gastrointestinal bleeding in 50% [96] and may actually result in a life-threatening esophagobronchial fistula [97]. PPIs heal these ulcers in 80-90% of cases, but recurrences are common [96].

Besides healing of esophagitis and ulcers, PPIs proved to be superior to H_2RAs also in the prevention of recurrence [98] and of peptic stricture formation [99,100], which may occur in up to 70% of the patients with Barrett's ulcer at the squamometaplastic junction.

In summary, PPIs represent the cornerstone of the therapy of patients with Barrett's esophagus since they control symptoms, heal esophagitis and ulcers, and prevent recurrence and strictures [94]. Although some regression of the metaplastic epithelium can occur during long-term (more than 2 years) treatment with PPIs [59], to this aim they are best viewed as adjuvant therapy after endoscopic ablation of the columnar epithelium [101]. Use of ongoing PPI therapy appears beneficial in the prevention of dysplasia [102,103] and adenocarcinoma [102,104] in patients with Barrett's esophagus. Nevertheless, the impact of PPI therapy on the natural history and evolution of Barrett's esophagus towards dysplasia and adenocarcinoma is still unclear and further long-term studies with complete suppression of intraesophageal acid and bile reflux will be necessary [18,94].

Adequate acid suppression in Barrett's esophagus: an unmet clinical need

Both available literature and clinical practice clearly show that "standard" PPI therapy is unable to normalize esophageal exposure to acid in the vast majority of patients with Barrett's esophagus. Profound and individually tailored acid suppression is needed not only to control GER [85] but also to achieve a chemopreventive effect [18,19,49].

Although effective and safe, currently available PPIs are still far from the ideal antisecretory compound. Currently available PPIs have notable limitations [105]. These drugs exhibit substantial inter-patient variability in pharmacokinetics and some may have clinically significant interactions with other drugs. The time of dosing and ingestion of meals may also influence the pharmacokinetics of these agents as well as their ability to suppress gastric acid secretion. First-generation PPIs (i.e. omeprazole, pantoprazole and lansoprazole) have a relatively slow onset of pharmacological action and may require several doses to achieve maximum acid suppression and symptom relief, possibly limiting their usefulness in on-demand GERD therapy. All the available compounds may also fail to provide 24-hour suppression of gastric acid, and nocturnal acid breakthrough (NAB, defined as a drop of intragastric pH under 4 for more than 1 hour) can occur even with twice-daily dosing [105]. Furthermore, there is increasing evidence of both inappropriate prescribing and inappropriate use of these drugs. Only seldom, indeed, primary care physicians give their patients advice on when and how to take their medication [65]. Despite the dramatic success of pharmacological acid suppression, a number of challenges remain in the management of acid-related disorders [106] and full acid control in Barrett's esophagus represents clearly a major unmet clinical need. Taking all the above considerations into account, it is clear that there is room for improvement. In this connection, new formulations and/or novel PPIs could be able to overcome the limitations of the currently available compounds.

New formulations

Extended-release formulations of PPIs will become an increasingly important strategy used by Pharmaceutical Companies, as they will be useful for the potential treatment of NAB because of their controlled and sustained release [65]. This is a strategy that is being adopted by AGI Therapeutics, who is developing in cooperation with Axcan Pharma **AGI-010**, a delayed and controlled-release (ChroNAB technology) formulation of omeprazole. This is also a strategy that has been used by TAP Pharmaceuticals for its modified release version of dex-lansoprazole (**TAK-390MR**) [65]. The preliminary results of a pharmacokinetic and pharmacodynamic evaluation have just been presented at the past Digestive Disease Week [107]. The study showed that TAK-390MR has an extended drug exposure compared to the parent compound (i.e. lansoprazole). 24-hour intragastric pH recording also showed across all doses levels (60, 90 and 120 mg) a prolonged acid inhibition. Eisai too is developing an extended-release version of Pariet/Aciphex (rabeprazole) for the treatment of upper GI disorders, which is however still in Phase I [108].

Currently available PPIs are orally administered as gastroprotected preparations. The different enteric coatings (granules encapsulated in a gelatine shell, tablets or multiple unit pellet system – MUPS), which are necessary to protect the acid-labile PPI from acid degradation within the stomach, have the potential disadvantage of delaying PPI absorption and, as a consequence, the available PPI formulations are considered delayed-release (DR) preparations. The recently FDA-approved **immediate-release (IR) omeprazole** formulation displays a different pharmacokinetics and pharmacodynamics compared with the standard, DR preparation [109]. This formulation (available as sachets, capsules or chewable tablets) consists of pure, non-enteric-coated omeprazole powder (40 mg or 20 mg per unit dose) along with 1,680 mg of sodium bicarbonate (containing 460 mg of sodium). The antisecretory effect of IR omeprazole is quicker than that observed with classical DR formulation while the duration of the acid lowering activity is similar [109]. The early increase in intragastric pH is likely due to the neutralizing capacity of sodium bicarbonate, which also accelerates and enhances absorption of omeprazole whose increased bioavailability translates into a more profound acid suppression.

Vecta Ltd (an Israeli Company) is currently investigating **Vecam** (VB101) for the potential treatment of GERD. Vecam is a combination of a PPI with a chemical "acid pump activator" to allow a meal-independent antisecretory effect. In order to identify compounds that induce acid secretion in humans, Vecta screened several small molecules that were known to have acid-promoting properties. VB101 was chosen because oral administration of the compound in humans displays the same acid stimulating activity of pentagastrin (http://www.vecta.co.il/products_vecam.html).

Novel proton pump inhibitors

Several new PPIs have been synthesized since the discovery of omeprazole. The majority of them is still in preclinical development or have been abandoned [65]. **Ilaprazole** (compound marked IY-81149) is a benzimidazole compound synthesized at Il-Yang (South Korea) and presently developed by TAP Pharmaceuticals. Its antisecretory activity proved to be 2-3 times higher and its half-life 2-3 times longer than that of omeprazole. Although the drug is already on the market in South Korea, a phase II clinical trials is ongoing in United States (http://www.clinicaltrials.gov).

Allergan is developing a pro-drug (**AGN 201904**), which is actually the acid stable sodium salt of a sulfonamide of omeprazole. This compound was designed to have delayed absorption in order to prolong the plasma residence time and thus increase the number of proton pumps within the gastric secretory canaliculus that might be inhibited. In an ambulatory 24-hour intragastric pH recording in healthy, *Helicobacter pylori*-negative male subjects [110], AGN 201904 was shown to provide faster and more profound acid suppression than esomeprazole on day 1 and day 5. Nocturnal acid suppression was also greater by > 2 pH units after 5 days, and the median pH never dropped below 5.0 with AGN. This medication may therefore be useful for patients with nocturnal symptoms or perhaps even for patients who need rapid and robust acid suppression, such as those with PU-related bleeding.

Tenatoprazole (compound also marked TU-199) has been developed by Mitsubishi Pharma in Japan and is now under active development by NEGMA-Gild (France) & SIDEM (Luxenbourg). Conversely from all the other PPIs, this compound is not a benzimidazole derivative, consisting of one imidazopyridine ring connected to a pyridine ring by a sulfinylmethyl chain. It represents therefore a new chemical entity. The inhibitory activity of this novel compound on gastric H^+,K^+-ATPase has been thoroughly characterized by George Sachs' Team [111]. Like the other PPIs, tenatoprazole is a prodrug (pKa = 4.04), which is converted to the active sulfenamide or sulfenic acid by acid in the secretory canaliculus of the stimulated parietal cell of the stomach. This active species binds to luminally accessible cysteines of the gastric H^+,K^+-ATPase resulting in disulfide formation and acid secretion inhibition. The binding sites of tenatoprazole were at Cys813 and Cys822 as shown by tryptic and thermolysin digestion of the ATPase labelled by tenatoprazole. Both of these sites are located in the proton transport pathway, though cysteine 822 is found deeper in the TM5/6 membrane domain than cysteine 813 [111].

Pharmacokinetics studies revealed that tenatoprazole displays a long half-life (8.7 ± 2.6 hours for repeated administration of 40 mg) and pharmacodynamic investigations on the same subjects have shown an increase of intragastric pH with tenatoprazole (40 mg daily for seven days) significantly higher ($p < 0.05$) than that observed with the same regimen of esomeprazole, the median pH being respectively [112]. A further investigation [113] did confirm and extended previous data showing the prolonged duration of acid suppression with tenatoprazole.

Like the other PPIs, tenatoprazole is a racemic mixture of two stereoisomers, which derive from the chiral nature of the sulphur atom of the sulfinyl group. Therefore, in order to exploit the features of stereoselective catabolism, the S-isomer was selected for further development. A careful pharmacokinetic and structural study [111] showed that the oral bioavailability of S-tenatoprazole sodium salt hydrate is almost twice that of S-tenatoprazole free form. The difference in bioavailability can be explained by the better solubility of the sodium salt due to its peculiar crystal structure. The crystal form of S-tenatoprazole sodium salt hydrate is indeed quite different from that of S-tenatoprazole free form. In the crystal of S-tenatoprazole, sodium salt hydrate there is a loose packing structure of molecules, which results in rapid water access and hence greater solubility. The pharmacokinetics of S-tenatoprazole sodium was then studied in healthy volunteers and proved to be linear with a dose-related increase in both C_{max} and AUC (Ficheux *et al.*, unpublished observations). The results of a dose-ranging (30, 60 and 90 mg daily) pharmacodynamic study have recently been presented [114] and show that all the doses of S-tenatoprazole Na resulted in a higher median pH on day 5 compared to esomeprazole (40 mg daily). The drug provided significant greater and more prolonged and dose-dependent acid suppression than the comparator (namely esomeprazole) either during the day and the night. A still unpublished study from Professor Galmiche's Team (Nantes, France) compared this compound (60 mg once daily) with esomeprazole (40 mg twice daily). The duration of acid suppression achieved with S-tenatoprazole Na once daily was similar to that observed after esomeprazole 40 mg twice daily, but the first drug did show a carry-over effect, the intragastric pH control being significantly higher 3 days after stopping treatment (*Figure 4*).

All these data clearly show that – compared to the existing PPIs – tenatoprazole has a longer half-life and a longer duration of the antisecretory action, in agreement with the current knowledge according to which the antisecretory effect is proportional to the AUC [115]. Although these properties should theoretically translate into a better therapeutic efficacy, no randomized clinical trials in acid-related diseases are available as yet. However, the available studies point out both pharmacokinetic and pharmacodynamic advantages of tenatoprazole over esomeprazole. Since this last compound provides – amongst the members of the class – the most effective control of intragastric pH whatever the parameter considered [75], it is conceivable that tenatoprazole could similarly be better than the other existing PPIs. S-tenatoprazole sodium then appears a promising PPI for the treatment of acid-related diseases (including GERD and its complications), where it has the

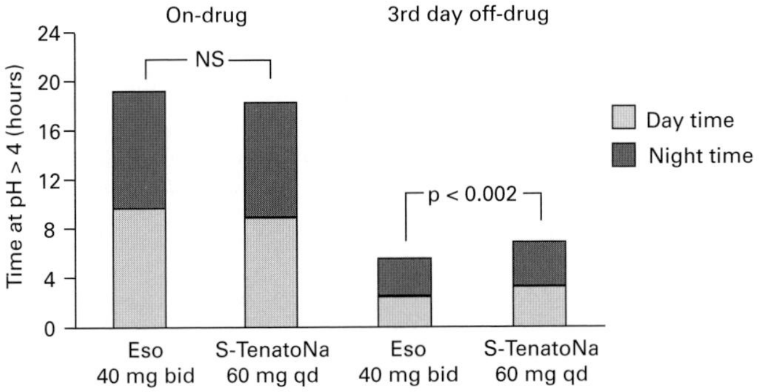

Figure 4. Intragastric 24-hour pH-recording in healthy volunteers given esomeprazole (40 mg bid) or S-tenatoprazole Na (60 mg qd) (from Galmiche *et al.*, unpublished results).

potential to address unmet clinical needs [116]. In patients with Barrett's esophagus this compound should be capable to fully control both day-time and night-time acid secretion and virtually abolish esophageal exposure to acid, thus allowing not only healing of esophageal lesions but also exerting a true chemopreventive effect.

References

1. Spechler SJ, Goyal RK. The columnar lined esophagus, intestinal metaplasia, and Norman Barrett. Gastroenterology 1996;110:614-21.
2. Shaheen N, Ransohoff DF. Gastroesophageal reflux, Barrett esophagus, and esophageal cancer: scientific review. JAMA 2002;287:1972-81.
3. Neumann CS, Cooper BT. 24 hour ambulatory oesophageal pH monitoring in uncomplicated Barrett's oesophagus. Gut 1994;35:1352-5.
4. Singh P, Taylor RH, Colin-Jones DG. Esophageal motor dysfunction and acid exposure in reflux esophagitis are more severe if Barrett's metaplasia is present. Am J Gastroenterol 1994;89:349-56.
5. Oberg S, DeMeester TR, Peters JH, et al. The extent of Barrett's esophagus depends on the status of the lower esophageal sphincter and the degree of esophageal acid exposure. J Thorac Cardiovasc Surg 1999;117:572-80.
6. Vaezi MF, Richter JE. Role of acid and duodenogastroesophageal reflux in gastroesophageal reflux disease. Gastroenterology 1996;111:1192-9.
7. Coenraad M, Masclee AA, Straathof JW, Ganesh S, Griffioen G, Lamers CB. Is Barrett's esophagus characterized by more pronounced acid reflux than severe esophagitis? Am J Gastroenterol 1998;93:1068-72.
8. Cameron AJ. Barrett's esophagus: prevalence and size of hiatal hernia. Am J Gastroenterol 1999;94:2054-9.
9. Vaezi MF, Richter JE. Double reflux: double trouble. Gut 1999;44:590-2.
10. Richter JE. Importance of bile reflux in Barrett's esophagus Dig Dis 2001;18:208-16.
11. Gutschow CA, Schroder W, Holscher AH. Barrett's esophagus: what is the poison - alkaline, biliary or acidic reflux? Dis Esophagus 2002;15:5-9.
12. Bechi P, Cianchi F. Technical aspects and clinical indications of 24-hour intragastric bile monitoring. Hepatogastroenterology 1999;46:54-9.
13. Vaezi MF, Richter JE. Synergism of acid and duodenogastroesophageal reflux in complicated Barrett's esophagus. Surgery 1995;117:699-704.
14. Fitzgerald RC, Lascar R, Triadafilopoulos G. Review article: Barrett's oesophagus, dysplasia and pharmacologic acid suppression. Aliment Pharmacol Ther 2001;15:269-76.
15. DeMeester TR. Surgical therapy for Barrett's esophagus: prevention, protection and excision. Dis Esophagus 2002;15:109-16.
16. Walker SJ, Selvasekar CR, Birbeck N. Mucosal ablation in Barrett's esophagus. Dis Esophagus 2002;15:22-9.
17. Urosevic P, Kiroff GK. Ablation of Barrett's epithelium: the promise and the problems. Dis Esophagus 2002;15:30-8.
18. Fennerty MB, Triadafilopoulos G. Barrett's-related esophageal adenocarcinoma: is chemoprevention a potential option? Am J Gastroenterol 2001;96:2302-5.
19. Fennerty MB. Barrett's-related esophageal cancer: has the final hurdle been cleared, now paving the way for human chemoprevention trials? Gastroenterology 2002;122:1172-5.
20. Sontag SJ. Preventing death of Barrett's cancer: does frequent surveillance endoscopy do it? Am J Med 2001;111:137S-41S.

21. Craanen ME, Blok P, Meijer GA, Meuwissen SG. Surveillance in Barrett's oesophagus: a critical reappraisal. Scand J Gastroenterol 2002;37:4-8.
22. Spechler SJ. Managing Barrett's esophagus. Decisions have to be based on indecisive data. Br Med J 2003;326:892-4.
23. Sharma P, McQuaid K, Dent J, et al.; AGA Chicago Workshop. A critical review of the diagnosis and management of Barrett's esophagus: the AGA Chicago Workshop. Gastroenterology 2004;127:310-30.
24. British Society of Gastronterology. Guidelines for the diagnosis and management of Barrett's columnar-lined oesophagus. A report of the Working Party of the British Society of Gastroenterology, August 2005 [http://www.bsg.org.uk]
25. Wang KK, Sampliner RE. Updated guidelines 2008 for the diagnosis, surveillance and therapy of Barrett's esophagus. Am J Gastroenterol 2008;103:788-97.
26. Mulholland MW, Reid BJ, Levine DS, Rubin CE. Elevated gastric acid secretion in patients with Barrett's metaplastic epithelium. Dig Dis Sci 1989;34:1329-34.
27. Collen MJ, Johnson DA. Correlation between basal acid output and daily ranitidine dose required for therapy in Barrett's esophagus. Dig Dis Sci 1992;37:570-6.
28. Collen MJ, Johnson DA, Sheridan MJ. Basal acid output and gastric acid hypersecretion in gastroesophageal reflux disease. Correlation with ranitidine therapy. Dig Dis Sci 1994;39:410-7.
29. Stein HJ, Hoeft S, DeMeester TR. Functional foregut abnormalities in Barrett's esophagus. J Thorac Cardiovasc Surg 1993;105:107-11.
30. Hirschowitz BI. A critical analysis with appropriate controls of gastric acid and pepsin secretion in clinical esophagitis. Gastroenterology 1991;101:1149-58.
31. Hirschowitz BI. Gastric acid and pepsin secretion in patients with Barrett's esophagus and appropriate controls. Dig Dis Sci 1996;7:1384-91.
32. DeMeester TR, Attwood SE, Smyrk TC, Therkildsen DH, Hinder RA. Surgical therapy in Barrett's esophagus. Ann Surg 1990;212:528-40.
33. Scarpignato C, Pelosini I, Contini S. How abnormal is gastric function in patients with Barrett's esophagus? In: Giuli R, Siewert JR, Couturier D, Scarpignato C, eds, Barrett's esophagus. 250 questions, 250 answers, Volume 1. Paris: John Libbey Eurotext, 2003:26-34.
34. Berstad A. Effect of storage on peptic activity of human gastric juice. Scand J Gastroenterol 1970;5:525-7.
35. Gotley DC, Morgan AP, Ball D, Owen RW, Cooper MJ. Composition of gastro-oesophageal refluxate. Gut 1991;32:1093-9.
36. Savarino V, Mela GS, Zentilin P, et al. Time pattern of gastric acidity in Barrett's esophagus. Dig Dis Sci 1996;41:1379-83.
37. Fein M, Fuchs KH, Freys SM. Is gastric secretion different in Barrett patients and in patients with reflux esophagitis? In: Giuli R, Siewert JR, Couturier D, Scarpignato C, eds. Barrett's esophagus. 250 questions, 250 answers. Paris: John Libbey Eurotext, 2003:179-82.
38. Calam J. Helicobacter pylori modulation of gastric acid. Yale J Biol Med 1999;72:195-202.
39. McColl KE, el-Omar E, Gillen D. Helicobacter pylori gastritis and gastric physiology. Gastroenterol Clin North Am 2000;29:687-703.
40. Smout AJ. Is the sensitivity to gastric acid inhibition Helicobacter pylori status-dependent? Scand J Gastroenterol 1998;33:32-5.
41. Scarpignato C, Pelosini I. Antisecretory drugs for eradication of Helicobacter pylori: Antibacterial activity and synergism with antimicrobial agents. Progr Basic Clin Pharmacol 1999;11:135-78.
42. Dent J. Review article: Is Helicobacter pylori relevant in the management of reflux disease? Aliment Pharmacol Ther 2001;15:16-21.
43. Sharma P, Vakil N. Review article: Helicobacter pylori and reflux disease. Aliment Pharmacol Ther2003;17:297-305.
44. Buttar NS, Falk GW. Pathogenesis of gastroesophageal reflux and Barrett esophagus. Mayo Clin Proc 2001;76:226-34.
45. Barlow AP, DeMeester TR, Ball CS, Eypasch EP. The significance of the gastric secretory state in gastroesophageal reflux disease. Arch Surg 1989;124:937-40.
46. Boesby S. Relationship between gastro-oesophageal acid reflux, basal gastro-oesophageal sphincter pressure, and gastric acid secretion. Scand J Gastroenterol 1977;12:547-51.
47. Strader DB, Benjamin SB, Orbuch M, et al. Esophageal function and occurrence of Barrett's esophagus in Zollinger-Ellison syndrome. Digestion 1995;56:347-56.
48. Scarpignato C. Acid-lowering drugs in the treatment of gastroesophageal reflux disease: an overview. Front Gastrointest Res 1992;20:129-52.
49. Raj A, Jankowski J. Acid suppression and chemoprevention in Barrett's oesophagus. Dig Dis 2004;22:171-80.
50. Meining A, Classen M. The role of diet and lifestyle measures in the pathogenesis and treatment of gastroesophageal reflux disease. Am J Gastroenterol 2000;95:2692-7.
51. Dent J, Brun J, Fendrick AM, et al. An evidence-based appraisal of reflux disease management: Genval Workshop Report. Gut 1999;44:1-16.
52. Peterson WL. Improving management of GERD. Evidence-based therapeutic strategies. Bethesda: AGA Press, 2002:1-28.
53. Katelaris P, Holloway R, Talley N, Gotley D, Williams S, Dent J; Digestive Health Foundation of the Gastroenterological Society of Australia. Gastro-oesophageal reflux disease in adults: Guidelines for clinicians. J Gastroenterol Hepatol 2002;17:825-33.
54. Armstrong D, Marshall JK, Chiba N, et al; Canadian Association of Gastroenterology GERD Consensus Group. Canadian Consensus Conference on the management of gastroesophageal reflux disease in adults - update 2004. Can J Gastroenterol 2005;19:15-35.

55. DeVault KR, Castell DO. American College of Gastroenterology. Updated guidelines for the diagnosis and treatment of gastroesophageal reflux disease. Am J Gastroenterol 2005;100:190-200.
56. Watson DI, Jamieson GG. Antireflux surgery in the laparoscopic era. Br J Surg 1998;85:1173-84.
57. Triadafilopoulos G. Endotherapy and surgery for GERD. J Clin Gastroenterol 2007;41:S87-96.
58. Bruley des Varannes S, Gharib H. Reflux gastro-oesophagien: contreparties fonctionnelles de la chirurgie anti-reflux. Gastroenterol Clin Biol 2000;24:B17-23.
59. Sampliner RE. Reduction of acid exposure and regression of Barrett's esophagus. Dig Dis 2000-2001;18:203-7.
60. Gurski RR, Peters JH, Hagen JA, et al. Barrett's esophagus can and does regress after antireflux surgery: a study of prevalence and predictive features. J Am Coll Surg 2003;196:706-12.
61. Klaus A, Hinder RA. Medical therapy versus antireflux surgery in Barrett's esophagus: what is the best therapeutic approach? Dig Dis 2000;18:224-31.
62. Chiba, N, De Gara, CJ, Wilkinson, JM, Hunt, RH. Speed of healing and symptom relief in grade II to IV gastroesophageal reflux disease: a meta-analysis. Gastroenterology 1997;112:1798-810.
63. van Pinxteren B, Numans ME, Bonis PA, Lau J. Short-term treatment with proton pump inhibitors, H2-receptor antagonists and prokinetics for gastro-oesophageal reflux disease-like symptoms and endoscopy negative reflux disease (Cochrane Review). Cochrane Database Syst Rev 2001;CD002095.
64. Huang JQ, Hunt RH. Pharmacological and pharmacodynamic essentials of H2-receptor antagonists and proton pump inhibitors for the practising physician. Best Pract Res Clin Gastroenterol 2001;15:355-70.
65. Scarpignato C, Pelosini I, Di Mario F. Acid suppression therapy: where do we go from here? Dig Dis 2006;24:11-46.
66. Johnson DA, Winters C, Spurling TJ, Chobanian SJ, Cattau EL Jr. Esophageal acid sensitivity in Barrett's esophagus. J Clin Gastroenterol 1987;9:23-7.
67. Byrne PJ, Mulligan ED, O'Riordan J, Keeling PW, Reynolds JV. Impaired visceral sensitivity to acid reflux in patients with Barrett's esophagus. The role of esophageal motility. Dis Esophagus 2003;16:199-203.
68. Ouatu-Lascar R, Triadafilopoulos G. Complete elimination of reflux symptoms does not guarantee normalization of intraesophaeal acid reflux in patients with Barrett's esophagus. Am J Gastroenterol 1998;93:711-6.
69. Basu KK, Bale R, West KP, de Caestecker JS. Persistent acid reflux and symptoms in patients with Barrett's oesophagus on proton-pump inhibitor therapy. Eur J Gastroenterol Hepatol 2002;14:1187-92.
70. Gerson LB, Shetler K, Triadafilopoulos G. Control of intra-oesophageal and intra-gastric pH with proton pump inhibitors in patients with Barrett's oesophagus. Dig Liver Dis 2005;37:651-8.
71. Katz PO, Anderson C, Khoury R, Castell DO. Gastro-oesophageal reflux associated with nocturnal gastric acid breakthrough on proton pump inhibitors. Aliment Pharmacol Ther 1998;12:1231-4.
72. Gerson LB, Boparai V, Ullah N, Triadafilopoulos G. Oesophageal and gastric pH profiles in patients with gastro-oesophageal reflux disease and Barrett's oesophagus treated with proton pump inhibitors. Aliment Pharmacol Ther 2004;20:637-43.
73. Frazzoni M, Manno M, De Micheli E, Savarino V. Efficacy in intra-oesophageal acid suppression may decrease after 2-year continuous treatment with proton pump inhibitors. Dig Liver Dis 2007;39:415-21.
74. Tonini M, Vigneri S, Savarino V, Scarpignato C. Clinical pharmacology and safety profile of esomeprazole, the first enantiomerically pure proton pump inhibitor. Dig Liver Dis 2001;33:600-6.
75. Miner P Jr, Katz PO, Chen Y, Sostek M. Gastric acid control with esomeprazole, lansoprazole, omeprazole, pantoprazole, and rabeprazole: a five-way crossover study. Am J Gastroenterol 2003;98:2616-20
76. Edwards SJ, Lind T, Lundell L. Systematic review: proton pump inhibitors (PPIs) for the healing of reflux oesophagitis - a comparison of esomeprazole with other PPIs. Aliment Pharmacol Ther 2006;24:743-50.
77. Gralnek IM, Dulai GS, Fennerty MB, Spiegel BM. Esomeprazole versus other proton pump inhibitors in erosive esophagitis: a meta-analysis of randomized clinical trials. Clin Gastroenterol Hepatol 2006;4:1452-8.
78. Edwards SJ, Lind T, Lundell L. Systematic review of proton pump inhibitors for the maintenance of healed reflux oesophagitis. J Drug Ass 2002:5:165-78.
79. Frazzoni M, Manno M, De Micheli E, Savarino V. Intra-oesophageal acid suppression in complicated gastro-oesophageal reflux disease: esomeprazole versus lansoprazole. Dig Liver Dis 2006;38:85-90.
80. Yeh RW, Gerson LB, Triadafilopoulos G. Efficacy of esomeprazole in controlling reflux symptoms, intraesophageal, and intragastric pH in patients with Barrett's esophagus. Dis Esophagus 2003;16:193-8.
81. Spechler SJ, Sharma P, Traxler B, Levine D, Falk GW. Gastric and esophageal pH in patients with Barrett's esophagus treated with three esomeprazole dosages: a randomized, double-blind, crossover trial. Am J Gastroenterol 2006;101:1964-71.
82. Xue S, Katz PO, Banerjee P, Tutuian R, Castell DO. Bedtime H2 blockers improve nocturnal gastric acid control in GERD patients on proton pump inhibitors. Aliment Pharmacol Ther 2001;15:1351-6.
83. Fackler WK, Ours TM, Vaezi MF, Richter JE. Long-term effect of H2RA therapy on nocturnal gastric acid breakthrough. Gastroenterology 2002;122:625-32.
84. Wani S, Sampliner RE, Weston AP, et al. Lack of predictors of normalization of oesophageal acid exposure in Barrett's oesophagus. Aliment Pharmacol Ther 2005;22:627-33.
85. Srinivasan R, Katz PO, Ramakrishnan A, Katzka DA, Vela MF, Castell DO. Maximal acid reflux control for Barrett's oesophagus: feasible and effective. Aliment Pharmacol Ther 2001;15:519-24.
86. Champion G, Richter JE, Vaezi MF, Singh S, Alexander R. Duodenogastroesophageal reflux: relationship to pH and importance in Barrett's esophagus. Gastroenterology 1994;107:747-54.

87. Marshall RE, Anggiansah A, Manifold DK, Owen WA, Owen WJ. Effect of omeprazole 20 mg twice daily on duodenogastric and gastro-oesophageal bile reflux in Barrett's oesophagus. Gut 1998;43:603-6.
88. Stein HJ, Kauer WK, Feussner H, Siewert JR. Bile reflux in benign and malignant Barrett's esophagus: effect of medical acid suppression and Nissen fundoplication. J Gastrointest Surg 1998;2:333-41.
89. Menges M, Muller M, Zeitz M. Increased acid and bile reflux in Barrett's esophagus compared to reflux esophagitis, and effect of proton pump inhibitor therapy. Am J Gastroenterol 2001;96:331-7.
90. Netzer P, Gut A, Brundler R, Gaia C, Halter F, Inauen W. Influence of pantoprazole on oesophageal motility, and bile and acid reflux in patients with oesophagitis. Aliment Pharmacol Ther 2001;15:1375-84.
91. Scarpignato C, Pelosini I, Contini S. How can reduction of duoedenogastroesophageal reflux following medical acid suppression by proton pump inhibitors be explained? In: Giuli R, Scarpignato C., Collard JM, Richter JE, eds. The duodenogastroesophageal reflux. 125 questions, 125 answers. Paris: John Libbey Eurotext, 2006:262-71.
92. Sarela AI, Hick DG, Verbeke CS, Casey JF, Guillou PJ, Clark GW. Persistent acid and bile reflux in asymptomatic patients with Barrett esophagus receiving proton pump inhibitor therapy. Arch Surg 2004;139:547-51.
93. Todd JA, Basu KK, de Caestecker JS. Normalization of oesophageal pH does not guarantee control of duodenogastro-oesophageal reflux in Barrett's oesophagus. Aliment Pharmacol Ther 2005;21:969-75.
94. Triadafilopoulos G. Proton pump inhibitors for Barrett's oesophagus. Gut 2000;46:144-6.
95. Malfertheiner P, Lind T, Willich S, et al. Prognostic influence of Barrett's oesophagus and Helicobacter pylori infection on healing of erosive gastro-oesophageal reflux disease (GORD) and symptom resolution in non-erosive GORD: report from the ProGORD study. Gut 2005;54:746-51.
96. Ollyo JB, Monnier PH, Fontolliet CH, et al. L'ulcère de Savary : une nouvelle complication du reflux gastro-oesophagien. Schweiz Med Woschenschr 1988;118:823-7.
97. Nigro JJ, Bremner RM, Fuller CB, Theisen J, Ma Y, Starnes VA. Perforating Barrett's ulcer resulting in a life-threatening esophagobronchial fistula. Ann Thorac Surg 2002;73:302-4.
98. Vigneri S, Termini R, Leandro G, et al. A comparison of five maintenance therapies for reflux esophagitis. N Engl J Med 1995;333:1106-10.
99. Smith PM, Kerr GD, Cockel R, et al., & the RESTORE Investigator Group. A comparison of omeprazole and ranitidine in the prevention of recurrence of benign esophageal stricture. Gastroenterology 1994;107:1312-8.
100. Swarbrick ET, Gough AL, Foster CS, Christian J, Garrett AD, Langworthy CH. Prevention of recurrence of oesophageal stricture, a comparison of lansoprazole and high-dose ranitidine. Eur J Gastroenterol Hepatol 1996;8:431-8.
101. Overholt BF. Acid suppression and reepithelialization after ablation of Barrett's esophagus. Dig Dis 2000-2001;18:232-9.
102. Hillman LC, Chiragakis L, Shadbolt B, Kaye GL, Clarke AC. Proton-pump inhibitor therapy and the development of dysplasia in patients with Barrett's oesophagus. Med J Aust 2004;180:387-91.
103. El-Serag HB, Aguirre TV, Davis S, Kuebeler M, Bhattacharyya A, Sampliner RE. Proton pump inhibitors are associated with reduced incidence of dysplasia in Barrett's esophagus. Am J Gastroenterol 2004;99:1777-83.
104. Cooper BT, Chapman W, Neumann CS, Gearty JC. Continuous treatment of Barrett's oesophagus patients with proton pump inhibitors up to 13 years: observations on regression and cancer incidence. Aliment Pharmacol Ther 2006;23:727-33.
105. Tytgat GN. Shortcomings of the first-generation proton pump inhibitors. Eur J Gastroenterol Hepatol 2001;13: S29-33.
106. Hunt RH. Review article: the unmet needs in delayed-release proton-pump inhibitor therapy in 2005. Aliment Pharmacol Ther 2005;22:10-9.
107. Zhang W, Wu J-T, Atkinson S. Pharmacokinetic (PK), pharmacodynamic (PD), and safety of single and multiple 60 Mg, 90 Mg, and 120 Mg oral doses of modified release TAK-390 (TAK-390mr) and 30 mg oral doses of lansoprazole (Lan) in healthy subjects. Gastroenterology 2007;132:A-487.
108. Data Monitor. Pipeline Insight: Upper GI Disorders, 2007;1-226.
109. Howden CW. Review article: immediate-release proton-pump inhibitor therapy - potential advantages. Aliment Pharmacol Ther 2005;22:25-30.
110. Hunt RH, Armstrong D, Yaghoobi M, et al. Inhibition of acid secretion by a novel proton pump inhibitor. Gastroenterology 2007;132:A-486.
111. Shin JM, Homerin M, Domagala F, Ficheux H, Sachs G. Characterization of the inhibitory activity of tenatoprazole on the gastric H+,K+-ATPase in vitro and in vivo. Biochem Pharmacol 2006;71:837-49.
112. Galmiche JP, Bruley Des Varannes S, Ducrotte P, et al. Tenatoprazole, a novel proton pump inhibitor with a prolonged plasma half-life: effects on intragastric pH and comparison with esomeprazole in healthy volunteers. Aliment Pharmacol Ther 2004;19:655-62.
113. Hunt RH, Armstrong D, James C, et al. Effect on intragastric pH of a PPI with a prolonged plasma half-life: comparison between tenatoprazole and esomeprazole on the duration of acid suppression in healthy male volunteers. Am J Gastroenterol 2005;100:1949-56.
114. Hunt RH, Armstrong D, Yaghoobi M, James C, Chen Y. S-tenatoprazole-Na 30 mg, 60 mg and 90 mg versus esomeprazole (ESO) 40 mg in healthy male volunteers (HMVs). Gastroenterology 2007;132:A-488.
115. Junghard O, Hassan-Alin M, Hasselgren G. The effect of the area under the plasma concentration vs time curve and the maximum plasma concentration of esomeprazole on intragastric pH. Eur J Clin Pharmacol 2002;58:453-8.
116. Scarpignato C, Pelosini I. Review article: the opportunities and benefits of extended acid suppression. Aliment Pharmacol Ther 2006;23:23-34.

Does normalization of esophageal pH with proton pump inhibitors induce regression of metaplasia and reduce the risk of adenocarcinoma?

V. Mokkala, C.J. DeMars, N. Buttar (Rochester)

Acid suppression with proton pump inhibitors (PPI) is a common practice in patients with Barrett's esophagus. The proposed rationale behind this approach is that acid suppression has a potential to regress Barrett's esophagus or prevent the development of cancer. In the following discussion, we will briefly examine the existing literature that supports or refutes this rationale.

Endoscopic observations of neosquamous islands in patients with Barrett's metaplasia on PPIs led to several retrospective studies to examine the role of acid suppression in regression of Barrett's metaplasia. Cooper *et al.* followed a large cohort of patients ranging from 1 to 13 years [1]. The patients received omeprazole 20 to 40 mg or lansoprazole 30 to 60 mg. Baseline and follow-up endoscopies were compared in these patients to examine if there was regression of Barrett's esophagus. In 76 patients, who had 1-3 years of follow-up, the length of Barrett's metaplasia did not change significantly with the use of PPIs. Similarly, 7 patients who were followed for almost 13 years did not show any significant regression of Barrett's metaplasia. The caveat here is that these patients were not investigated as to whether they really had the acid reflux controlled by PPIs. A prospective, long-term follow-up of patients with Barrett's esophagus receiving high dose PPI to normalize esophageal pH also failed to show any regression of Barrett's metaplasia [2]. The weakness of the study is that there were only 13 participants; however, the strength is that the pH was monitored and the follow-up was quite long. Another retrospective analysis found that the Barrett's length at initial endoscopy in patients who were not on PPI was significantly higher than the patients who were on a PPI [3]. Although this study does not address whether the acid suppression decreases the length of Barrett's esophagus, it does suggest that those patients with reflux who receive long-term acid suppression using PPIs have a shorter length of Barrett's esophagus when Barrett's develops.

A randomized controlled trial was recently conducted where the percent change in the length of Barrett's mucosa was endoscopically examined at 0, 3, 9, 15, and 24 months to address the effect of acid suppression on the regression of Barrett's esophagus [4]. Twenty-six patients in profound acid suppression arm (omeprazole 40 mg bid) and 27 patients in mild acid suppression arm (ranitidine 150 mg bid) completed the study. Patients receiving omeprazole had a 6% decrease in the length of Barrett's esophagus, which was significantly more than in patients who received ranitidine. The interobserver and intraobserver variation in length determination ranged from 5 to 6%. Therefore, it remains unclear whether this truly represents a regression or a sampling error. A recent metaanalysis failed to show that the PPI results in the regression of Barrett's metaplasia. Therefore, we can conclude that there is a lack of evidence to support the rationale to use PPI as an approach to regress Barrett's metaplasia.

The other proposed rationale to use PPI in patients with Barrett's esophagus is that acid suppression may prevent the development of cancer. This is supported by epidemiological studies that suggest a strong association between chronic gastroesophageal reflux disease and adenocarcinoma of the esophagus [5-7]. In addition, preclinical studies provide mechanistic explanation into the role of acid and bile reflux in esophageal carcinogenesis. Contents of reflux lead to chronic injury, induce oxidative stress and up-regulate several pro survival signaling pathways [8]. Extracellular acid exposure causes intracellular acidification *via* Cl^-/HCO_3^- exchanger, which triggers the mitogen activated protein kinase (MAPK) signaling and proliferation in Barrett's epithelial cells [9,10]. Acid induced MAPK signaling can also up-regulate the pro-carcinogenic arachidonic acid pathway [10].

Patients on PPIs have decreased expression of proteins that promote the transit of cells through the cell cycle and have a higher expression of cell cycle inhibitors like p16, p21, and p27 [11]. The use of PPIs also results in a decreased proliferation and higher differentiation in the Barrett's epithelial cells [12]. Lao-Sirieix prospectively investigated the effect of acid suppression on the molecular predictors of esophageal cancer. Barrett's esophageal biopsies from patients were assessed for Mcm2 protein, 3 months prior to pH monitoring, and 4 and 12 months after pH monitoring In 32 patients that had successful acid inhibition based on pH monitoring, there was a significant drop in the Mcm2 protein. On the other hand, 19 patients who failed acid inhibition showed progressive increase in Mcm2 protein over 4 and 12 months of follow-up [13]. Based on these preclinical studies, it appears that acid suppression may have a role in the prevention of development of carcinogenesis.

Recently, retrospective studies have provided additional preliminary evidence that patients who use PPIs are at lower risk of progression to dysplasia or cancer [14,15]. El-Serag *et al.* showed in 236 patients that the cumulative incidence of dysplasia was significantly lower among patients who received PPI after Barrett's esophagus diagnosis than in those who received no therapy or H_2RA. Furthermore, among those on PPIs, a longer duration of use was associated with less frequent occurrence of dysplasia. In multivariate analysis, the use of PPI after Barrett's esophagus diagnosis was independently associated with reduced risk of dysplasia, hazards ratio: 0.25 (95% CI 0.13-0.47) [14]. In another study, Hillman *et al.* followed 350 patients and found that the patients who delayed using a PPI for 2 years or more after diagnosis with Barrett's esophagus had 5.6 times (95% CI, 2.0-15.7) the risk of developing low-grade dysplasia (LGD) at any given time as those who used a PPI in the first year. Similar results were found for the risk of developing high-grade dysplasia (HGD) or adenocarcinoma (hazard ratio, 20.9; 95% CI, 2.8-158) [15]. Unfortunately, the majority of the patients who progressed in these studies were diagnosed with LGD, a histologic diagnosis which is not as robust as HGD or cancer. These studies also had the inherent problem of being retrospective [14,15].

One of the possible reasons for the controversy regarding the chemopreventive potential of acid suppression is that complete symptom eradication with PPI use does not guarantee normalization of intraesophageal pH in Barrett's esophagus patients. This is supported by the finding that when patients on PPIs are monitored using 24-hour pH testing, there is decreased proliferation and improved differentiation in the group of patients that have adequate acid suppression [13,16].

Based on existing data, it appears that PPI use for acid suppression does not result in regression of Barrett's. There is some preclinical and epidemiological data to suggest that PPI therapy may reduce the risk of adenocarcinoma; however, this needs to be investigated, and there are currently patients undergoing trials to investigate this issue.

References

1. Cooper BT, et al. Continuous treatment with omeprazole 20 mg daily for up to 6 years in Barrett's oesophagus. Aliment Pharmacol Ther 1998;12(9):893-7.
2. Sharma P, Sampliner RE, Camargo EZ. Normalization of esophageal pH with high-dose proton pump inhibitor therapy does not result in regression of Barrett's esophagus. Am J Gastroenterol 1997;92(4):582-5.
3. El-Serag HB, et al. The length of newly diagnosed Barrett's oesophagus and prior use of acid suppressive therapy. Aliment Pharmacol Ther 2004;19(12):1255-60.
4. Peters FT, et al. Endoscopic regression of Barrett's oesophagus during omeprazole treatment; a randomised double blind study. Gut 1999;45(4):489-94.
5. Lagergren J, et al. Symptomatic gastroesophageal reflux as a risk factor for esophageal adenocarcinoma. N Engl J Med 1999;340(11):825-31.
6. Champion G, et al. Duodenogastroesophageal reflux: relationship to pH and importance in Barrett's esophagus. Gastroenterology 1994;107(3):747-54.
7. Stein HJ, et al. Bile reflux in benign and malignant Barrett's esophagus: effect of medical acid suppression and nissen fundoplication. J Gastrointestin Surg 1998;2(4):333-41.
8. Buttar NS, Wang KK. Mechanisms of diseases: carcinogenesis in Barrett's esophagus. Nat Clin Pract Gastroenterol Hepatol 2004;1:106-12.
9. Sarosi GA Jr, et al. Acid increases MAPK-mediated proliferation in Barrett's esophageal adenocarcinoma cells via intracellular acidification through a Cl-/HCO3- exchanger. Am J Physiol Gastrointest Liver Physiol 2005;289(6):G991-7.
10. Souza RF, et al. Acid exposure activates the mitogen-activated protein kinase pathways in Barrett's esophagus. Gastroenterology 2002;122(2):299-307.
11. Umansky M, et al. Proton pump inhibitors reduce cell cycle abnormalities in Barrett's esophagus. Oncogene 2001;20(55):7987-91.
12. Ouatu-Lascar R, Fitzgerald RC, Triadafilopoulos G. Differentiation and proliferation in Barrett's esophagus and the effects of acid suppression. Gastroenterology 1999;117(2):327-35.
13. Lao-Sirieix P, et al. Effect of acid suppression on molecular predictors for esophageal cancer. Cancer Epidemiol Biomarkers Prev 2006;15(2):288-93.
14. El-Serag HB, et al. Proton pump inhibitors are associated with reduced incidence of dysplasia in Barrett's esophagus. Am J Gastroenterol 2004;99(10):1877-83.
15. Hillman LC, et al. Proton-pump inhibitor therapy and the development of dysplasia in patients with Barrett's oesophagus. Med J Aust 2004;180(8):387-91.
16. Ouatu-Lascar R, Fitzgerald RC, Triadafilopoulos G. Differentiation and proliferation in Barrett's esophagus and the effects of acid suppression. Gastroenterology 1999;117(2):327-35.

What information on the potential for malignant progression in Barrett's metaplasia can be derived from biomarkers of DNA damage?

A.G. Casson (Saskatoon)

Supported in part by the Nova Scotia Health Research Foundation; the Capital Health Research Fund; and the National Cancer Institute of Canada with funds from the Canadian Cancer Society. AGC is supported by a Senior Clinical Research Scholarship from the Dalhousie University Faculty of Medicine.

Esophageal adenocarcinomas are thought to arise from Barrett's esophagus, an acquired condition in which the normal esophageal squamous epithelium is replaced by a specialized metaplastic columnar cell-lined epithelium [1,2]. Progression of Barrett's esophagus to invasive malignancy is reflected histologically by the metaplasia-dysplasia-adenocarcinoma sequence [3]. As gastroesophageal reflux disease (GERD) is a risk factor for Barrett's esophagus, there is a plausible link between GERD, Barrett's esophagus and esophageal adenocarcinoma [4]; it is hypothesized that GERD results in acute mucosal injury (esophagitis), promotes cellular proliferation, and induces specialized columnar metaplasia of the normal squamous epithelium lining the esophagus. Dysplasia is widely regarded as the precursor of invasive cancer, and high-grade dysplasia (HGD) in Barrett's epithelium is frequently associated with esophageal adenocarcinoma. The recent identification of molecular markers associated with Barrett metaplasia-dysplasia-adenocarcinoma progression will likely offer further insight into the molecular pathogenesis of this disease, and may well have potential clinical application to identify those individuals with Barrett's esophagus at increased risk for progression to invasive adenocarcinoma [3,5-7]. This short review will discuss, based on current evidence, selected molecular biomarkers associated with Barrett's esophagus that may have future clinical application to the management of this disease.

Barrett's esophagus

It is currently unclear whether the prevalence of Barrett's esophagus is increasing, or whether this diagnosis is being made more frequently because of widespread use endoscopy [8,9]. Preliminary data from the UK, adjusting for increasing numbers of endoscopic procedures, suggests a real increase in prevalence of Barrett's esophagus [10]. The American College of Gastroenterology currently defines Barrett's esophagus as "a change in the esophageal epithelium of any length that can be recognized at endoscopy and is confirmed to have intestinal metaplasia by biopsy" [11,12]. Goblet cells are the hallmark of intestinal metaplasia, and must be diagnosed histologically using hematoxylin and eosin staining of tissue sections [13,14]. As goblet cells contain acidic mucin, alcian blue staining may be used to complement the histologic diagnosis. Immunohistochemical studies using monoclonal antibodies to cytokeratin (CK) 7 and 20 are increasingly used to differentiate between esophageal and cardia intestinal metaplasia [15]: in esophageal intestinal metaplasia, CK 7 positivity is found in superficial and deep glands, whereas CK 20 positivity is limited to superficial glands only (Barrett CK 7/20 pattern). In cardia intestinal metaplasia, CK 7 immunoreactivity is absent (or weak or patchy), but CK 20 positivity is seen in both superficial and deep glands.

Dysplasia may be identified histologically on the basis of phenotypic nuclear alterations resulting from DNA abnormalities, and is classified as indefinite, low-grade, or high-grade. The histologic diagnosis of dysplasia is largely subjective and considerable intra- and inter-observer variation is reported. Furthermore, dysplastic change should be interpreted with caution when atypical epithelial cells (arising from a background of active inflammation) are present. Low-grade dysplasia (LGD) is generally distinguished from HGD based on nuclear localization in relation to the luminal surface of the cell. Although the natural history of dysplasia is not known, HGD is currently regarded as the most reliable predictor for progression to invasive cancer, and is frequently associated with esophageal adenocarcinoma [16,17].

Pathogenesis

The precise etiology and natural history of Barrett's esophagus is still unknown. It is generally accepted that Barrett's esophagus is an acquired condition resulting from GERD. Clinical and experimental studies of patients with Barrett's esophagus (with and without reflux-related symptoms) have demonstrated several physiological abnormalities including increased acid exposure, a defective lower esophageal sphincter (length, pressure and both), and impared motility and clearance from the esophageal body, compared with normal subjects [18]. Reflux of duodenal contents has been suggested as an important contributing factor in the pathogenesis of esophagitis and Barrett's esophagus, an obsevation supported by clinical [19] and experimental animal models of duodenoesophageal reflux [20]. It is hypothesized that GERD results in acute mucosal injury (esophagitis), promotes cellular proliferation, and induces specialized columnar metaplasia (Barrett's epithelium) of the normal squamous epithelium lining the esophagus, although the precise biological mechanism is still unknown. Barrett's esophagus has been shown to be hyperproliferative, reflected by an increased S-phase fraction on flow cytometry [21] and immunohistochemically using monoclonal antibodies to proliferating cell nuclear antigen (PCNA) [22,23] and Ki67, a cell nuclear proliferation-associated antigen [24]. Whereas PCNA immunostaining is normally seen in the basal layer of metaplastic Barrett's epithelia, in HGD, it is seen to extend to more superficial layers. Similar patterns of staining were seen for Ki-67, suggesting a functional instability of Barrett's mucosa.

Molecular biology

Several molecular alterations have been reported in Barrett's esophagus and are implicated in the molecular pathogenesis of esophageal adenocarcinoma [3,5-7]. Many such biomarkers have been proposed to have potential clinical application, in areas such as molecular diagnosis for early detection, to predict risk for disease progression in endoscopic surveillance programs, for staging and prognosis, to predict chemosensitivity, as intermediate biomarkers in chemoprevention studies, and as novel targets for anticancer therapies. However, relatively few will ultimately prove to be clinically useful, and the introduction of tumor markers into clinical practice has been poorly controlled [25].

To facilitate the translation of recent advances in basic science into clinical practice, the National Cancer Institute Early Detection Research Network (NCI-EDRN) proposed five phases to validate novel biomarkers used in screening and surveillance for the early detection of cancer [26]. As these were developed as a conceptual framework for coordinating biomarker research, not all biomarkers need to progress consecutively through each of the following five phases before recommendations are made as to potential clinical application. Briefly, the aim of phase 1, or preclinical exploratory studies, is to identify novel biomarkers in tumor tissues, using matched histologically normal tissues for comparison. Biomarkers identified by such phase 1 studies, considered to be potentially useful in clinical practice, are subject to phase 2 studies, primarily to validate assays and to estimate true- and false-positive rates. Secondary aims of phase 2 are to optimize assay conditions, to compare assay techniques, and to explore associations between a biomarker and selected clinicopathologic factors in patients with cancer (e.g. tumor histology, grade, etc.) and normal controls (e.g. gender, age, smoking history, etc.). Phase 3 are retrospective longitudinal repository studies, utilizing banked tissues to evaluate the capacity of a biomarker to detect preclinical disease, and to define criteria for a positive screening test in preparation for phase 4. The ability of a biomarker to predict disease is determined by prospective screening studies (phase 4), which should also consider potential benefits of early detection, the feasibility and costs of implementing a screening program. The final phase (cancer control studies; phase 5) addresses whether biomarker-based screening will reduce cancer mortality.

To date, no potential biomarker associated with Barrett esophagus has been evaluated in a phase 5 study. As several biomarkers have been identified in Barrett esophagus, and many implicated in disease progression, the reader is referred to recent reviews summarizing the results of selected phase 1 and 2 studies [3,5-7]. The following sections will therefore summarize the results of a limited number of phase 3 and 4 studies which have evaluated selected biomarkers identified as having potential clinical application in the management of Barrett esophagus.

Ploidy

Several phase 1-3 studies have now clearly demonstrated that abnormal cell nuclear DNA content (aneuploidy) in Barrett epithelia is associated with risk for progression to malignancy, and that the prevalence of aneuploidy appears to increase with the degree of dysplasia determined using tissue histology [21,27-30]. Using a well established endoscopic biopsy protocol to optimize tissue diagnosis, compelling evidence for utilizing flow cytometry to determine tissue ploidy was recently published from an ongoing phase 4 study, which has now prospectively evaluated over 300 patients over a fifteen year interval [32-34]. In summary, patients with Barrett's esophagus whose baseline biopsy demonstrated no, indefinite or LGD with a diploid cell population (without aneuploidy or increased 4N fraction) appeared to be at low risk for malignant progression [32]. For this group of patients, endoscopic surveillance at intervals up to 5-years was proposed. More frequent surveillance was recommended for patients whose baseline biopsies had aneuploidy, tetraploidy (4N) or HGD with 5-year cancer incidences of 43%, 56% and 59%, respectively. Patients who did not have aneuploidy or tetraploidy defined by flow cytometry, but who progressed to invasive esophageal adenocarcinoma, all had HGD at baseline biopsy [32]. It was subsequently reported that specific ploidy variables determined by flow cytometry (aneuploid DNA content > 2.7N; 4N fraction > 6%) were even more highly predictive of cancer progression [34].

p53

The p53 tumor suppressor gene, located on chromosome 17p13, encodes a 53 kd polypeptide (TP53) that regulates cell cycle progression, DNA repair, apoptosis, and neovascularization in normal and malignant cells *via* highly complex DNA and protein interactions [35]. TP53 mediates cell cycle arrest in part by inducing the expression of p21 (WAF-1) which sequesters a variety of cyclin-dependent kinases (CDK) facilitating G_1 as well as G_2/M arrest. Loss of p53 function by point mutation is a common mechanism of inactivation, and over 90% of p53 mutations have been found locate in the conserved DNA binding domain (exons 5 to 8). p53 appears to have a central role in human malignancy, and has been characterized extensively over the past decade [36].

p53 gene mutations were initially reported in primary esophageal adenocarcinomas and associated Barrett's epithelium in 1991 [37]. These findings were subsequently confirmed in several phase 1 and 2 studies, and the spectrum of p53 alterations in Barrett's esophagus has been described [38]. The finding of p53 mutations in non-dysplastic Barrett's epithelia suggests that p53 may be altered early in the metaplasia-dysplasia-carcinoma sequence, and may therefore be a useful biomarker in endoscopic surveillance programs. In a ten-year prospective study of surgically resected esophageal adenocarcinomas, p53 mutations were associated with poor tumor differentiation, and reduced disease-free and overall survival following surgical resection [39]. Of particular biologic interest was the observation that patterns of p53 mutations in esophageal adenocarcinomas were predominantly G:C to A:T transitions at CpG dinucleotides, suggesting that p53 mutations result from endogenous mechanisms, likely involving spontaneous deamination into thymine of the 5'methylated cytosine that frequently occurs at CpG dinucleotides. As this mechanism is enhanced by exposure to oxyradicals and nitroradicals, we hypothesised that local overproduction of nitric oxide, a consequence of chronic GERD, may enhance the rate of formation of spontaneous p53 mutations in Barrett's esophagus.

Although no phase 4 studies have evaluated p53 mutations or protein overexpression in Barrett's epithelia as predictors of malignant progression, loss of heterozygosity (LOH) of 17p (inclusive of p53) was evaluated in one phase 4 study in conjunction with flow cytometry [33]. The prevalence of 17p LOH ranged from 6% in non-dysplastic Barrett epithelia, to 57% in HGD, and was a significant independent predictor of progression to esophageal adenocarcinoma, with a relative risk of 16. In this study of 325 patients with Barrett esophagus, only six of 26 patients who progressed to malignancy did not have 17p LOH. 17p LOH was also associated with increased risk for aneuploidy, tetraploidy, and HGD, with relative risks of 7.5, 6.1, and 3.6, respectively.

Cyclin D1

Cyclin D1, encoded by the CCND1 gene located on chromosome 11q13, is a key regulator of cell cycle progression, particularly the transition from G_1 to S phase [40]. Several phase 1 and 2 studies have implicated cyclin D1 in esophageal malignancy, and overexpression of cyclin D1 protein has been reported in up to 64% of adenocarcinomas and associated Barrett epithelia [41]. In a recent phase 3 case-control study, immunohistochemical overexpression of cyclin D1 in patients with Barrett esophagus was associated with a six-fold increased risk for progression to esophageal adenocarcinoma.

It has recently been reported that a common polymorphism (G870A) in exon 4 of CCND1 creates an alternative splice site, encoding a truncated protein isoform with an altered C-terminal domain that has been implicated in neoplastic transformation [42]. In a prospective case-control (phase 4) study, we found that individuals with the CCND1 A/A genotype are at increased risk for GERD, Barrett esophagus, and esophageal adenocarcinoma, supporting the hypothesis that this polymorphism is an individual susceptibility factor in the molecular progression of esophageal adenocarcinoma [42].

p16INK4a

The INK4a gene, localized to chromosome 9p21, encodes a protein, p16, that belongs to a family of CDK inhibitors. p16 binds to and inhibits CDK4/6, resulting in reduced phosphorylation of Rb and inhibition of cell-cycle progression through G_1. An alternative transcript, p14ARF, functions to sequester MDM2, thereby stabilizing the p53 tumor suppressor gene. Alterations of p16 are reported frequently in various human malignancies, but mechanisms of p16 inactivation appear to vary between tumor type. While point mutations in Barrett esophagus and esophageal adenocarcinoma are relatively uncommon, 9p LOH, p16 mRNA overexpression and promoter hypermethylation appear to be frequent mechanisms of p16 inactivation [43,44]. While the subject of phase 1 and 2 studies only, p16 alterations are increasingly recognized as critical early molecular lesions associated with clonal proliferation within Barrett's epithelia [43].

Summary

Although several molecular alterations have been described in Barrett esophagus, and have been suggested as clinically useful biomarkers to predict progression to invasive esophageal adenocarcinoma, it is anticipated that relatively few will ultimately prove to be of value. To date, only a limited number of phase 3 and 4 studies (as defined by the NCI-EDRN) of biomarkers associated with Barrett esophagus have been completed. Biomarkers which currently appear to predict of progression of Barrett's esophagus to invasive esophageal adenocarcinoma (other than HGD) include aneuploidy (DNA content > 2.7N; 4N fraction > 6%; or both) [32,34], 17p LOH (further implicating the p53 tumor suppressor gene) [33] , and cyclin D1 protein overexpression [41] , and with further validation will most likely be incorporated into routine clinical practice. Additional biomarkers of interest include p16 [43,44] and the CCND1 G870A polymorphism [42]. However, as it is unlikely that a single biomarker will be utilized to predict risk, it is anticipated that models incorporating objective scores of sociodemographic and lifestyle risk factors (ie. age, gender, body mass index), severity of reflux symptoms, endoscopic and histologic findings, and an assessment of a panel of biomarkers, will be developed to further define subsets of patients with Barrett esophagus at increased risk for malignant progression, thereby permitting the development of more rational endoscopic surveillance and screening programs.

References

1. Enzinger PC, Mayer RJ. Esophageal cancer. N Engl J Med 2003;349:2241-52.
2. Specher SJ. Clinical practice. Barrett's esophagus. N Engl J Med 2002;346:836-42.
3. Jankowski JA, Wright NA, Meltzer SJ, et al. Molecular evolution of the metaplasia-dysplasia-adenocarcinoma sequence in the esophagus. Am J Pathol 1999;154:965-73.
4. Shaheen N, Ransohoff DF. Gastroesophageal reflux, Barrett's esophagus and esophageal cancer. JAMA 2002;287:1972-81.
5. Casson AG. Role of molecular biology in the follow-up of patients who have Barrett's esophagus. Chest Surg Clin N Am 2002;12:93-111.
6. Reid BJ, Blount PL, Rabinovitch PS. Biomarkers in Barrett's esophagus. Gastrointest Clin N Am 2003;13:369-97.
7. McManus DT, Olaru A, Meltzer SJ. Biomarkers of esophageal adenocarcinoma and Barrett's esophagus. Cancer Res 2004;64:1561-69.
8. Conio M, Cameron AJ, Romero Y, et al. Secular trends in the epidemiology and outcomes of Barrett's oesophagus in Olmsted County, Minnesota. Gut 2001;48:304-9.
9. Prach AT. Increasing incidence of Barrett's esophagus: education, enthusiasm, or epidemiology? Lancet 1997;350:933.
10. Caygill CPJ, Reed PI, Johnston BJ, et al. A single centre's 20 year experience of columnar-lined (Barrett's) oesophagus diagnosis. Eur J Gastroenterol Hepatol 1999;11:1355-8.
11. Sampliner RE. Practice guidelines on the diagnosis, surveillance, and therapy of Barrett's esophagus. Am J Gastroenterol 1998;93:1028-32.
12. Spechler SJ. Columnar-lined esophagus. Definitions. Chest Surg Clin N Am 2002;12:1-13.
13. Haggitt RC. Barrett's esophagus, dysplasia, and adenocarcinoma. Hum Pathol 1994;25:983-93.
14. Antonelli DA, Wang HH. Morphology of Barrett's esophagus and Barrett's-associated dysplasia and adenocarcinoma. Gastroenterol Clin N Am 1997;26:495-506.
15. Ormsby AH, Vaezi MF, Richter JE, et al. Cytokeratin immunoreactivity patterns in the diagnosis of short-segment Barrett's esophagus. Gastroenterology 2000;119:683-90.
16. McArdle JE, Lewin KJ, Randall G, et al. Distribution of dysplasias and early invasive carcinoma in Barrett's esophagus. Hum Pathol 1992;23:479-82.
17. Buttar NS, Wang KK, Sebo TJ, et al. Extent of high-grade dysplasia in Barrett's esophagus correlates with risk of adenocarcinoma. Gastroenterology 2001;120:1630-9.
18. DeMeester SR, DeMeester TR. Columnar mucosa and intestinal metaplasia of the esophagus. Fifty years of controversy. Ann Surg 2000;3:303-21.
19. Champion G, Richter JE, Vaezi MF, et al. Duodenogastroesophageal reflux: relationship to pH and importance in Barrett's esophagus. Gastroenterology 1994;107:747-54.
20. Goldstein SR, Yang G, Curtis SK, et al. Development of esophageal metaplasia and adenocarcinoma in a rat surgical model without the use of a carcinogen. Carcinogenesis 1997;18:2265-70.
21. Reid BJ, Blount PL, Rubin CE, et al. Flow-cytometric and histological progression to malignancy in Barrett's esophagus: prospective endoscopic surveillance of a cohort. Gastroenterology 1992;102:1212-9.
22. Gray MR, Hall PA, Nash J, et al. Epithelial proliferation in Barrett's esophagus by proliferating cell nuclear antigen immunolocalization. Gastroenterology 1992;103:1769-76.
23. Gillen P, McDermott M, Grehan D, et al. Proliferating cell nuclear antigen in the assessment of Barrett's mucosa. Br J Surg 1994;81:1766-8.
24. Hong MK, Laskin WB, Herman BE, et al. Expansion of the Ki-67 proliferative compartment correlates with degree of dysplasia in Barrett's esophagus. Cancer 1995;75:423-9.
25. Hayes DF, Bast RC, Desch CE, et al. Tumor marker utility grading system: a framework to evaluate clinical utility of tumor markers. J Natl Cancer Inst 1996;88:1456-66.
26. Pepe MS, Etziomi R, Feng Z et al. Phases of biomarker development for early detection of cancer. J Natl Cancer Inst 2001;93:1054-61.
27. Menke-Pluymers MB, Mulder AH, Hop WC et al. Dysplasia and aneuploidy as markers of malignant degeneration in Barrett's esophagus. The Rotterdam Oesophageal Tumor Study Group. Gut 1994;35:1348-51.
28. Galipeau PC, Cowan DS, Sanchez CA, et al. 17p (p53) allelic losses, 4N (G2/tetraploid) populations, and progression to aneuploidy in Barrett's esophagus. Proc Natl Acad Sci USA 1996;93:7081-4.
29. Montgomery EA, Hartmann DP, Carr NJ, et al. Barrett esophagus with dysplasia. Flow cytometric DNA analysis of routine, paraffin-embedded mucosal biopsies. Am J Clin Pathol 1996;106:298-304.
30. Tedori L, Gohde W, Persiani M, et al. DNA/protein flow cytometry as a predictive marker of malignancy in dysplasia-free Barrett's esophagus: thirteen-year follow-up study of a cohort of patients. Cytometry 1998;34:257-63.
31. Reid BJ, Blount PL, Feng Z, et al. Optimizing endoscopic biopsy detection of early cancers in Barrett's high-grade dysplasia. Am J Gastroenterol 2000;95:3089-96.
32. Reid BJ, Levine DS, Longton G, et al. Predictors of progression to cancer in Barrett's esophagus: baseline histology and flow cytometry identify low- and high-risk patient subsets. Am J Gastroenterol 2000;95:1669-76.

33. Reid BJ, Prevo LJ, Galipeay PC, et al. Predictors of progression in Barrett's esophagus II: Baseline 17p (p53) loss of heterozygosity identifies a patient subset at increased risk for neoplastic progression. Am J Gastroenterol 2001;96:2839-48.
34. Rabinovitch PS, Longton G, Blount PL, et al. Predictors of progression in Barrett's esophagus III: Baseline flow cytometric variables. Am J Gastroenterol 2001;96:3071-83.
35. Sengupta S, Harris CC: p53: traffic cop at the crossroads of DNA repair and recombination. Nature Rev 2005;6:44-55.
36. Wallace-Brodeur RR, Lowe SW. Clinical implications of p53 mutations. Cell Mol Life Sci 1999;54:64-75.
37. Casson AG, Mukhopadhyay T, Cleary KR, et al. p53 gene mutations in Barrett's epithelium and esophageal cancer. Cancer Res 1991;51:4495-9.
38. Schneider PM, Casson AG, Levin B, et al. Mutations of p53 in Barrett's esophagus and Barrett's cancer: a prospective study of 98 cases. J Thorac Cardiovasc Surg 1996;111:323-33.
39. Casson AG, Evans SC, Gillis A, et al. Clinical implications of p53 tumor suppressor gene mutation and protein expression in esophageal adenocarcinoma: results of a 10-year prospective study. J Thorac Cardiovasc Surg 2003;125:1121-31.
40. Murray AW. Recycling the cell cycle: cyclins revisited. Cell 2004;116:221-34.
41. Bani-Hani K, Martin IG, Hardie LJ, et al. Prospective study of cyclin D1 overexpression in Barrett's esophagus: Association with increased risk of adenocarcinoma. J Natl Cancer Inst 2000;92:1316-21.
42. Casson AG, Zheng Z, Evans SC, et al. Cyclin D1 polymorphism G870A and risk for esophageal adenocarcinoma. Cancer 2005;104:730-9.
43. Maley CC, Galipeau PC, Li X, et al. Selectively advantageous mutations and hitchhikers in neoplasma: p16 lesions are selected in Barrett's esophagus. Cancer Res 2004;64:3414-27.
44. Hardie LJ, Darnton SJ, Wallis YL et al. p16 expression in Barrett esophagus and esophageal adenocarcinoma: association with genetic and epigenetic alterations. Cancer Lett 2005;217:221-30.

Are genetic alterations observed in non-dysplastic Barrett's epithelium?

H. Garewal, K. Dvorak (Tucson)

The answer to the above question is an unequivocal "YES". As illustrated further below, although a specific alteration may be observed with increasing frequency with greater degrees of dysplasia, a number of cases of non-dysplastic epithelium displaying the change is virtually always present in reported data. It is tempting to think that these findings might be a result of the well known inter-observer and intra-observer discrepancies in pathologic readings of dysplasia, i.e. the non-dysplastic epithelium displaying a genetic alteration is not really "non-dysplastic". However, this is unlikely to be the whole story and the reports generally indicate involvement of an "expert pathologist". One clinical goal of this exercise is to develop so called "biomarkers", which may augment the ability to predict the course of a patient beyond what was achievable histologically. Thus far, however, this remains to be demonstrated for any single genetic change or grouping of changes. Nevertheless, their presence in non-dysplastic epithelium, together with the inverse, i.e. absence in dysplasia, holds the promise that such a biomarker role may some day add to histology alone in assessing cancer risk.

A fundamental question is what constitutes a change? In other words, what tissue is to be used as a control for comparison purposes? For changes such as mutations, deletions, other structural alterations, etc., a reasonable comparison would be with the normal genotype from the same patient, perhaps determined using white blood cells or control, normal gastrointestinal (GI)-tissue biopsies. Nonetheless, it is apparent that intestinal metaplasia is a somewhat unique type of tissue not normally present and, therefore, must have a different pattern of expression of genetic material to create its configuration, compared with any other "control" normally present epithelium. Thus it would be different from that required for generating squamous esophageal epithelium, sometimes used as a control, or even columnar upper GI epithelium from other sites, such as stomach or small intestine. With the availability of increasingly powerful tools for genetic analysis, such as microarray comparisons, there are increasing numbers of reports of such studies comparing Barrett's epithelium with some form of a control. In this setting, it is the rule to find a relatively large number of genes that are expressed differently and expected to do so. In this discussion, however, we will limit ourselves to specific alterations reported in studies prior to such broad microarray type of comparisons. These are more than sufficient to support the statement that genetic alterations are found in non-dysplastic Barrett's epithelium.

There are basically three main approaches that have been used in studying the genetics of Barrett's epithelium over the past decades (*Table I*). Using classical cytogenetic techniques our group was the first to report on chromosomal changes in Barrett's epithelium, including non-dysplastic ones [1]. Loss of chromosome Y was frequently observed, much more so than would be expected by aging alone. Furthermore, this was limited to the Barrett's tissue as it was absent from control buccal smears. In addition, somatic chromosomal changes were also described, both numerical as well as structural. Interestingly, this was one of the first reports of cytogenetic changes in pre-cancerous lesions. The finding of extra copies of chromosome 7 was especially

Table I. Approaches used to study genetic alterations in Barrett's esophagus.

Classical cytogenetics (plus FISH and/or comparative genomic hybridization)
DNA Content (fuelgen, flow cytometry)
Specific genetic alterations, e.g. p53

Interesting as the gene for epidermal growth factor receptor (EGFR) resides on this chromosome. At this time the significance of EGFR in carcinogenesis was just being appreciated and its finding in a pre-malignant lesion attracted particular attention. Subsequently, this has become one of the most significant chromosomal changes studied in pre-cancerous lesions from numerous epithelia. Other investigators have since studied the cytogenetics of Barrett's epithelium in larger groups of patients [2]. The loss of chromosome Y has been uniformly confirmed. Although it increases with grades of dysplasia, the phenomenon is observed in non-dysplastic Barrett's epithelium also. The availability of chromosomal probes allowed subsequent investigators to target specific chromosomes or chromosomal abnormalities in larger numbers of patients without the need for tissue culture and the inherent risk of introducing abnormalities artificially. Nonetheless, the findings were sustained.

DNA content abnormalities have been the target of investigations with flow cytometric techniques being the most commonly used approach. Other methods have used specific DNA staining, such as with the Fuelgen stain, and quantitation of its intensity. Aneuploidy is the prototype abnormality using such methods. Other criteria for abnormality, using more quantitatively based rather than qualitative changes, have also been proposed, especially by one group of investigators [3]. This included an increased percentage of S phase and G_2M phase cells. In the initial report, this investigative group reported virtually a 100% relationship between dysplasia and one or the other of the flow cytometric changes [3]. However, our group was unable to reproduce this at such a level of correlation [4]. This was especially true for the quantitative S phase percentage. Even on a theoretical basis, quantitation of a phase is always open to question, since the biopsy being studied will contain variable numbers of epithelial cells, presumably the cells of interest, *versus* other cells in the biopsy, such as stromal or inflammatory cells. For example, one could easily distort quantitation by having a large cluster of inflammatory cells, such as lymphocytes. This could easily influence the percentage of S-phase cells that the flow cytometer detects as it would count all nuclei present. As controls in our initial study, we did a large number of biopsies from presumably normal tissues, such as stomach and small bowel, and found significant numbers that had elevated S phases, or even increased G_2M phases, well above the proposed threshold. Thus, many investigators, including our group, have restricted themselves to studying aneuploidy only. Even with this as the sole criterion, it is clear that aneuploid clones can be observed in histologically non-dysplastic Barrett's epithelium. Summarizing data from a number of reports, approximately 5%-20% of non-dysplastic epithelium, 30%-50% of dysplastic (both high grade and low grade) and greater than 70% of cancers display aneuploidy.

There is considerable interest in determining whether a single aneuploid biopsy means anything clinically significant. Although the number of reported cases is just a handful, it does appear that multiple aneuploid clones or repeated demonstrations of aneuploid in serial endoscopies may be a more ominous sign of progression towards cancer than if a single biopsy, amongst several, is aneuploid. Nevertheless, the fact remains that aneuploidy can be observed in histologically non-dysplastic biopsies.

Finally, there have been a number of reports regarding specific genetic alterations, often selected because of their role and significance in cancer at other sites. It is not possible to include every one of these in this brief discussion. In *Table II* there is a very abbreviated listing of some of the changes reported. In each case, non-dysplastic Barrett's epithelium also displays the particular abnormality, albeit in a much smaller percentage of cases than in high-grade dysplasia (HGD) for example. One of the first and most frequently reported on change relates to p53, studied either by immunohistochemistry, molecular techniques or 17p allelic loss (loss of heterozygosity, LOH). There have been well over 25 reports on p53 related changes in Barrett's epithelium, the majority correlating the change with various grades of dysplasia. Overall again, the frequency of the abnormality increases with the degree of dysplasia, but it is not absent in non-dysplastic Barrett's epithelium. As an average, about 5%-10% of non-dysplastic

Table II. Examples of genetic changes observed in Barrett's esophagus.

Loss of Y, other numerical/structural changes
Aneuploidy
Growth factor related genes (EGFR, TGF)
↑ Proliferation related genes
↑ Cox-2
p53 (17 p LOH), p63, p73
p16 (9p21), promoter methylation
FHIT (fragile histidine triad gene)

biopsies display the abnormality, as opposed to 30%-40% in low-grade dysplasia, and 70%-75% in HGD or cancer. In addition to the pathology reading, the method used for p53 analysis is of obvious importance in arriving at a number in a particular study. But even acknowledging this, a number of non-dysplastic Barrett's epithelial biopsies show the abnormality.

In summary, genetic changes, much like other potential "biomarkers", are observed in Barrett's epithelium. As expected, the studies have focused on changes of potential interests in the carcinogenesis process. Some of these are listed in *Table II*, which is by no means exhaustive. Dysplasia is defined on a histologic basis using criteria developed over the years. It is by no means a "perfect", reproducible description. Genetic alterations have been studied mainly with two objectives in mind. Which are to try and understand the mechanisms involved in the evolution of this condition and to develop a clinically applicable biomarker that will help identify patients at greater risk to target with focused surveillance. For the latter purpose, it is actually encouraging that alterations can be observed in histologically "benign" looking, non-dysplastic Barrett's epithelium. This raises the possibility of predicting clinical behavior more so than by histology alone. However, multicenter, blinded efforts will need to be launched to definitively such a role for any alteration. Perhaps the most developed situation is with flow cytometry where the need for initial correlative, technique development studies has been fulfilled. To move this field further along and prove that there is an added clinical value of flow cytometry over histology and dysplasia assessment alone will require such a collaborative effort.

References

1. Garewal HS, Sampliner RE, Liu Y, Trent JM. Chromosomal rearrangements in Barrett's esophagus: a premalignant lesion of esophageal adenocarcinoma. Cancer Genet Cytogenet 1989;42:281-96.
2. Krishnadath KK, Tilanus HW, van Blankenstein M, et al. Accumulation of genetic abnormalities during neoplastic progression in Barrett's esophagus. Cancer Res 1995;55:1971-6.
3. Reid BJ, Haggitt RC, Rubin CE, Rabinovitch PS. Barrett's esophagus: correlation between flow cytometry and histology in detection of patients at risk for adenocarcinoma. Gastroenterology 1987;93:1-11.
4. Fennerty MB, Sampliner RE, Way D, Riddell R, Steinbronn K, Garewal HS. Discordance between blow cytometric abnormalities and dysplasia in Barrett's esophagus. Gastroenterology 1989;97:815-20.

Are there specific biomarkers of genetic damage that correlate with different grades of dysplasia?

P. Lao-Sirieix, R. Fitzgerald (Cambridge)

Although great efforts are currently being made to improve the outcomes for patients with esophageal adenocarcinoma, through optimisation of current treatment modalities and development of novel approaches, the prognosis of these individuals remains dismal [1].

The rates of success for treatments of cancer patients could be greatly increased by early detection of tumours [2]. In view of the development in genomics and proteomics and the improvement of immunological techniques, new molecular targets have become available. These new biomarkers are defined as a characteristic that is measured or evaluated as an indicator of a pathological process or as a response to a therapeutic intervention [3].

In the context of cancer research, both predictive and prognostic markers may be identified. Predictive markers are used to predict the differential efficiency of a particular therapy that is based on marker status. Prognostic markers are testable and indicative of a relevant biological aspect of cancer [4]. Such markers allow for segregation between patients who progress towards a defined stage of a disease and those who do not. The stage of interest could be the development of cancer or the apparition of metastases. In the case of Barrett's esophagus, most studies related to biomarkers have been carried out with the aim of identifying prognostic markers for early detection and/or stratification of the risk of progression.

In an effort to coordinate research between groups interested in early detection of cancers, the National Cancer Institute, has created the Early Detection Research Network (EDRN) [5]. In 2001 the EDRN published guidelines suggesting that an approach similar to drug discovery should be used for the development and validation of the usefulness of biomarkers. The different phases of biomarker development are summarized as follows (for a complete explanation of the 5 phases, refer to Sullivan-Pepe *et al.,* [6]):

- phase 1: pre-clinical and exploratory studies. Expression of a marker at different stages of the disease;
- phase 2: clinical assay development for clinical disease. Development of a sampling method: determination of sensitivity, specificity, positive and negative predictive values;
- phase 3: retrospective longitudinal repository studies to determine the degree of prediction of disease progression;
- phase 4: large prospective studies to test the biomarker;
- phase 5: large, long term study to estimate the reduction in cancer mortality afforded by the biomarker.

In the case of Barrett's esophagus carcinogenesis, phase 1 and 2 studies represent the bulk of the publications with more than 60 potential targets identified (refer to [7-9] for more details). In the majority of these studies, the expression of a marker is analysed in the Barrett's esophagus-dysplasia-adenocarcinoma sequence without normal controls from the squamous epithelium and other columnar tissue like the gastric antrum and the duodenum. Conclusions about the clinical relevance of a given marker with increased or decreased expression with progression from Barrett's esophagus to adenocarcinoma need to be interpreted with caution. A number of these abnormalities may not be causally related to the disease pathogenesis and are hence termed "hitchhiker" lesions [10,11]. Ideally a biomarker should have biological relevance in disease progression. Phase 3 and 4 studies are required to more accurately determine the clinical utility of a given biomarker. To date, very few biomarkers have been evaluated in phase 3 and 4 in the context of screening and/or surveillance programmes for Barrett's esophagus.

The prognostic biomarker with the most supportive evidence in the context of Barrett's esophagus is dysplasia. The presence of low grade dysplasia (LGD) is sufficient to increase the frequency of surveillance biopsies and a diagnosis of high grade dysplasia (HGD) may result in a therapeutic intervention including an esophagectomy [12]. Nevertheless, a diagnosis of dysplasia is highly subjective with substantial inter- and intra-observer variation [13,14]. Furthermore, the data substantiating the increased risk of cancer progression in dysplastic tissue is not very strong. The reported risk of progression to adenocarcinoma in a LGD and HGD background has been shown to be between 2-3% and 9-59% respectively [15-19] and spontaneous regression from LGD to non-dysplastic Barrett's esophagus is not a rare occurrence [20]. It remains unconvincing to date if dysplasia would be validated as prognostic biomarker if an investigator were to follow the strict EDRN guidelines.

The only molecular markers to reach phase 4 is the panel identified by the group led by Brian Reid in Seattle. Over the past 20 years, this group has led the field for early detection of cancer in Barrett's esophagus. They have set up a stratification method by two-parameter flow cytometry (DNA content and Ki-67 expression to tag the proliferative cells) followed by detection of epigenetic and genetic abnormalities on chromosome 17p (locus for p53) and chromosome 9p (locus for p16). The two-parameter flow cytometry approach allows the analysis of proliferation, cell cycle phase and aneuploidy while keeping the DNA intact for subsequent mutational, methylation and loss of heterozygosity (LOH) analysis [21]. Although aneuploidy, tetraploidy and 17p LOH were proven to be individual markers of risk of progression, it has been suggested that a combination of markers might increase the capacity to stratify patients at risk further and hence this might prove to be a usable surveillance tool [22]. In a cohort of 267 patients with Barrett's esophagus followed up for 1,180 patient years, the length of the clone carrying p53 LOH or ploidy abnormalities was predictive. The associated risk was 1.27^x (95% interval 1.07-1.50) and 1.31^x (95% interval 1.07-1.60) for p53 LOH and ploidy abnormalities respectively where x is the length of the clone bearing the abnormality [23]. The aim of research on biomarkers in a premalignant disease such as Barrett's esophagus is to identify a marker or combination of markers that accurately predict which patients will progress to adenocarcinoma. In these terms, the combination of markers identified by the Reid group has proven successful since their panel of markers offers a sensitivity and specificity for the risk of cancer development of 95% [22]. Before this panel of markers enters mainstream clinical practice it needs to be validated by other laboratories, ideally in a non-tertiary referral centre. Furthermore, the technology required to carry out the Reid protocol is not available in many hospitals, as well as being time consuming and expensive. Unless alternative technology becomes available, it is unlikely that those markers will be used in routine surveillance or screening programmes in the near future.

No other phase 4 markers have been identified yet, although a number of phase 3 studies using immunohistochemistry of cell cycle linked biomarkers exist. The expression levels of cyclin D1 have been shown to increase with progression to cancer and were proposed to be of predictive value in determining patients at risk for progression to neoplasia in a retrospective, longitudinal case-control study. The risk of cancer progression in patients positive for cyclin D1nwas 6.85 times (95% CI: 1.57-29.91) that of patients negative for cyclin D1 [24]. A later study in a nested-case control population (population of 1.7 million) failed to show any association between cyclin D1 and the risk of progression to adenocarcinoma. The presence of diffuse or intense p53 staining in this large patient cohort was associated with a higher risk of developing adenocarcinoma (odds ratio of 11.7; 95% CI 1.93-71.4) although this staining pattern was only found in 32% of the progressors. In this same cohort, increased expression of both p53 and Cox-2 was associated with OR of 27.3 (95% CI 2.89, 257.0) although only 15% of the progressors expressed both [25]. This study underlines a very important point. Although some markers may be associated with increased OR, their expression is only detectable in a small proportion of the progressors. In order to successfully stratify Barrett's esophagus patients, a marker should be expressed in every progressor prior to the development of a malignancy. Our laboratory has carried out a systematic phase 1/2 study of cell cycle markers, including proliferation markers, Minichromosome maintenance protein 2 (Mcm2) and Ki-67 as well as cell cycle phases specific markers cyclin D1 (G1 phase), cyclin A (S and G2 phases), cyclin B1 (G2 phase) and phosphorylated histone H3 (M phase) [26,27]. Both Mcm2 and cyclin A showed promise and were integrated into a phase 3 study. Ectopic expression at the luminal surface of mcm2 and cyclin A in non-dysplastic Barrett's esophagus was associated with an increased risk of progression to adenocarcinoma with an odds ratio of 136 (95% CI:7.2-2465, $p < 0.0001$) and 7.6 (95% CI:1.6-37.0, $p < 0.012$) respectively. Eighty-nine percent and 93.8% of the progressors had ectopic expression of Mcm2 and cylin A respectively at the luminal surface [27,28]. We have also demonstrated that both markers could be applied to endoscopic cytological brushings to stratify patients according to their risk of progression. This methodology is cheap and simple, negating the risks of multiple biopsy protocols. The large confidence interval associated with Mcm2 as a prognostic marker makes it relatively unreliable unlike cyclin A whose confidence interval is tight enough [28] to give hope that the associated risk of progression would hold true in a larger cohort of patients.

In addition to the Reid panel of biomarkers and the cell cycle/proliferation linked markers, two studies investigated the value of epigenetic markers. Promoter methylation of 10 putative markers was first examined in a phase 1 study and then promising methylated targets were tested in phase 3 case-control study with 8 patients who progressed to HGD or adenocarcinoma and 45 controls. HPP1, RUNX3 and p16 methylation were all associated with an increased risk of progression with odds ratios of 1.77 (95% CI:1.06-2.81), 1.80 (95% CI:1.08-2.81) and 1.74 (95% CI:1.33-2.20) respectively [29]; however, methylation of p16 promoter was not found to be prognostic of progression by the Reid group [23] .The second smaller study of just 12 progressors and 16 controls suggested that methylation of APC, TMIP3 and TERT were risk factors of cancer progression [30]. Epigenetic alterations provide another approach to biomarkers, which include analyses of global epigenetic changes.

All phase 3/4 markers were assessed with cancer, or at least HGD, as an endpoint. Although biomarker research in Barrett's has more than more than 20 years of history, only one panel of markers has made it to phase 4. The relative low incidence of adenocarcinoma does not make biomarker research as simple as one might hope and it appears increasingly necessary to pool resources in order to discover biomarker(s) that would allow for accurate risk stratification of Barrett's esophagus patients. Research is still needed in order to understand the driving forces behind Barrett's carcinogenesis and to develop clinically applicable algorithms so that molecular biomarkers can enter mainstream diagnostic use.

References

1. Enzinger PC, Mayer RJ. Esophageal cancer. N Engl J Med 2003;349:2241-52.
2. Fountoulakis A, Zafirellis KD, Dolan K, et al. Effect of surveillance of Barrett's oesophagus on the clinical outcome of oesophageal cancer. Br J Surg 2004;91:997-1003.
3. McManus DT, Olaru A, Meltzer SJ. Biomarkers of esophageal adenocarcinoma and Barrett's esophagus. Cancer Res 2004;64:1561-9.

4. Park JW, Kerbel RS, Kelloff GJ, et al. Rationale for biomarkers and surrogate end points in mechanism-driven oncology drug development. Clin Cancer Res 2004;10:3885-96.
5. Srivastava S, Kramer BS. Early detection cancer research network. Lab Invest 2000;80:1147-8.
6. Sullivan Pepe M, Etzioni R, Feng Z, et al. Phases of biomarker development for early detection of cancer. J Natl Cancer Inst 2001;93:1054-61.
7. Reid BJ, Blount PL, Rabinovitch PS. Biomarkers in Barrett's esophagus. Gastrointest Endosc Clin N Am 2003;13:369-97.
8. Caygill CP, Watson A, Lao-Sirieix P, Fitzgerald RC. Barrett's oesophagus and adenocarcinoma. World J Surg Oncol 2004;2:12.
9. Koppert LB, Wijnhoven BP, van Dekken H, Tilanus HW, Dinjens WN. The molecular biology of esophageal adenocarcinoma. J Surg Oncol 2005;92:169-90.
10. Maley CC, Galipeau PC, Finley JC, , et al. Genetic clonal diversity predicts progression to esophageal adenocarcinoma. Nat Genet 2006;38:468-73.
11. Maley CC, Galipeau PC, Li X, et al. Selectively advantageous mutations and hitchhikers in neoplasms: p16 lesions are selected in Barrett's esophagus. Cancer Res 2004;64:3414-27.
12. Sampliner RE. Updated guidelines for the diagnosis, surveillance, and therapy of Barrett's esophagus. Am J Gastroenterol 2002;97:1888-95.
13. Reid BJ, Haggitt RC, Rubin CE, et al. Observer variation in the diagnosis of dysplasia in Barrett's esophagus. Hum Pathol 1988;19:166-78.
14. Montgomery E, Goldblum JR, Greenson JK, et al. Dysplasia as a predictive marker for invasive carcinoma in Barrett esophagus: a follow-up study based on 138 cases from a diagnostic variability study. Hum Pathol 2001;32:379-88.
15. Schnell TG, Sontag SJ, Chejfec G, et al. Long-term nonsurgical management of Barrett's esophagus with high-grade dysplasia. Gastroenterology 2001;120:1607-19.
16. Weston AP, Banerjee SK, Sharma P, et al. p53 protein overexpression in low grade dysplasia (LGD) in Barrett's esophagus: immunohistochemical marker predictive of progression. Am J Gastroenterol 2001;96:1355-62.
17. Buttar NS, Wang KK, Sebo TJ, et al. Extent of high-grade dysplasia in Barrett's esophagus correlates with risk of adenocarcinoma. Gastroenterology 2001;120:1630-9.
18. Reid BJ, Levine DS, Longton G, Blount PL, Rabinovitch PS. Predictors of progression to cancer in Barrett's esophagus: baseline histology and flow cytometry identify low- and high-risk patient subsets. Am J Gastroenterol 2000;95:1669-76.
19. Weston AP, Sharma P, Topalovski M, et al. Long-term follow-up of Barrett's high-grade dysplasia. Am J Gastroenterol 2000;95:1888-93.
20. van Sandick JW, van Lanschot JJ, Kuiken BW, et al. Impact of endoscopic biopsy surveillance of Barrett's oesophagus on pathological stage and clinical outcome of Barrett's carcinoma. Gut 1998;43:216-22.
21. Paulson TG, Galipeau PC, Reid BJ. Loss of heterozygosity analysis using whole genome amplification, cell sorting, and fluorescence-based PCR. Genome Res 1999;9:482-91.
22. Galipeau PC, Li X, Longton G, et al. A panel of molecular and cytmoteric markers in Barrett's Esophagus (BE) predicts progression to esophageal adenocarcinoma (AC). Gastroenterology 2004;126:A-822.
23. Maley CC, Galipeau PC, Li X, et al. The combination of genetic instability and clonal expansion predicts progression to esophageal adenocarcinoma. Cancer Res 2004;64:7629-33.
24. Bani-Hani K, Martin IG, Hardie LJ, et al. Prospective study of cyclin D1 overexpression in Barrett's esophagus: association with increased risk of adenocarcinoma. J Natl Cancer Inst 2000;92:1316-21.
25. Murray L, Sedo A, Scott M, et al. TP53 and progression from Barrett's metaplasia to oesophageal adenocarcinoma in a UK population cohort. Gut 52006;5:1390-7.
26. Lao-Sirieix P, Brais R, Lovat L, Coleman N, Fitzgerald RC. Cell cycle phase abnormalities do not account for disordered proliferation in Barrett's carcinogenesis. 2004;Neoplasia 6:751-60.
27. Sirieix P, O'Donovan M, Brown J, et al. Surface expression of mini-chromosome maintenance proteins provides a novel method for detecting patients at risk for developing adeocarcinoma in Barrett's oesophagus. Clin Cancer Res 2003;9:2560-6.
28. Lao-Sirieix P, Lovat L, Fitzgerald RC. Cyclin A immunocytology as a risk stratification tool for Barrett's oesophagus surveillance. Clin Cancer Res 2007;13:659-65.
29. Schulmann K, Sterian A, Berki A, et al. Inactivation of p16, RUNX3, and HPP1 occurs early in Barrett's-associated neoplastic progression and predicts progression risk. Oncogene 2005;24:4138-48.
30. Clement G, Braunschweig R, Pasquier N, Bosman FT, Benhattar J. Methylation of APC, TIMP3, and TERT: a new predictive marker to distinguish Barrett's oesophagus patients at risk for malignant transformation. J Pathol 2006;208:100-7.

What is the best way to measure the length of Barrett's metaplasia

R.K.H. Wong (Washington)

The best way to determine the length of the Barrett's epithelial segment is dependent on several factors. These factors include:

- shortening of the esophagus from contraction of the longitudinal muscle during swallowing or with secondary peristalsis;
- shortening of the esophagus in patients with large hiatal hernias from hyperinflation of the stomach during endoscopy (*Figure 1*);
- peristalsis of the distal esophagus which unfolds the distal Z line making it difficult to measure the length of the esophagus and identify a normal Z-line;
- difficulty in identifying the squamocolumnar junction;
- large separation of distance markers on the shaft of the endoscope;
- a bite block which is not inserted so that the teeth are flushed a against the outer barrier of the bite block;
- intra and inter observer variation.

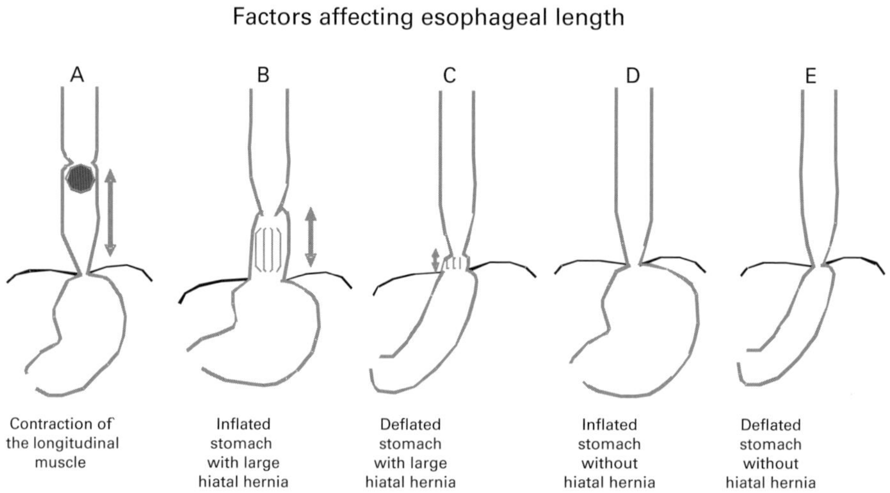

Figure 1. These are factors which affect the length of the esophagus and possibly the measured length of Barrett's epithelium. **A.** During contraction there is shortening of the esophagus. **B.** With a large hiatal hernia and an inflated stomach the esophagus will shorten. **C.** With a deflated stomach and a large hiatal hernia, the true esophageal length is noted. **D.E.** With no hiatal hernia, an inflated or deflated stomach does not affect esophageal length.

One study has shown that in a large population of severe gastroesophageal reflux disease (GERD) patients who underwent endoscopy, biopsy and manometry 6 weeks apart, there was a change of ≥ 4 cm in the length of the esophagus relating to both endoscopic and manometric findings. This resulted in an 18% apparent change in the diagnosis of Barrett's esophagus [1]. In another *in vitro* study, a model of the esophagus was fashioned with 10 fixed lengths of Barrett's like inserts measuring between 2-7.5 cm being placed in the distal esophagus. Only 16% of endoscopists were accurate in their measurement with 37% over estimating and 28% underestimating the actual Barrett's length with variability in the range of 7 cm and a mean error rate of 1 cm [2]. Another study developed a novel computer program to measure the area of Barrett's epithelium and compared it to actual endoscopic photographs of Barrett's esophagus [3]. The correlation between observer was very high when endoscopic photos were obtained at 1, and 2 cms ($r = 0.96$) and between the models and the actual esophagus ($r = 0.99$). Sharma *et al.* [4] showed that narrow band imaging (NBI) has allowed for better identification of intestinal metaplasia in the esophagus and likely a better location of the Barrett's epithelium. Finally, Amano *et al.* [5] noted that the use of a new classification of Barrett's (Prague C&M) allowed for a closer correlation between investigators when describing Barrett's epithelium.

In conclusion, the best way to measure the length of the Barrett's esophagus is to:
- be sure that the outer guard of the bite block is inserted tightly against the teeth;
- calibrating the distance markers on the endoscope to reflect 1 cm increments between 25-50 cm;
- decrease peristalsis in the esophagus;
- not to over inflate the stomach;
- possibly use stains such as Lugol's, methylene blue or newer endoscopic techniques such as narrow band imaging to better identify the squamocolumnar junction or the Barrett's epithelium;
- use of the new Prague C&M criteria for determining the location and length of Barrett's epithelium [5-11].

References

1. Kim SL, Waring JP, Spechler SJ, et al. Diagnostic inconsistencies in Barrett's esophagus. Gastroenterology 1994;107(4):945-9.
2. Guda NM, Partington S, Vakil N. Inter- and intra-observer variability in the measurement of length at endoscopy: Implications for the measurement of Barrett's esophagus. Gastrointest Endosc 2004;59(6):655-8.
3. Kim R, Baggott BB, Rose S, et al. Quantitative endoscopy: precise computerized measurement of metaplastic epithelial surface area in Barrett's esophagus. Gastroenterology 1995;108(2):360-6.
4. Sharma P, Bansal A, Mathur S, et al. Barrett's esophagus. The utility of novel narrow band imaging endoscopy system in patients with Barrett's esophagus. Gastrointest Endosc 2006;64(2):167-75.
5. Amano Y, Ishimura N, Furuta K, et al. Which landmark results in a more consistent diagnosis of Barrett's esophagus, the gastric folds or the palisade vessels? Gastrointest Endosc 2006;64(2):206-11.
6. Herlihy KJ, Orlando RC, Bryson JC, Bozymski EM, Carney CN, Powell DW. Barrett's esophagus: clinical, endoscopic, histologic, manometric, and electrical potential difference characteristics. Gastroenterology 1984;86:436-43.
7. Bombeck CT, Dillard DH, Nyhus LM. Muscular anatomy of gastroesophageal junction an role of phrenoesophageal ligament. Ann Surg 1966;164:643-52.
8. McClave SA, Boyce Jr HW, Gottfried MR. Early diagnosis of columnar-lined esophagus: a new endoscopic diagnostic criterion. Gastrointest Endosc 1987;33:413-41.
9. Chobanian SJ, Cattau Jr EL, Winters Jr C, et al. In vivo staining with toluidine blue as an adjunct to the endoscopic detection of Barrett's esophagus. Gastrointest Endosc 1987;33:99-101.

10. Katzka D, Plotkin A, Saul S, et al. A controlled study of toluidine blue staining in patients with Barrett's metaplasia of the esophagus. Gastroenterology 1986;90:1485.
11. Stevens PD, Lightdale CJ, Green PHR, et al. Combined magnification endoscopy with chromoendoscopy for the evaluation of Barrett's esophagus. Gastrointest Endosc 1994;40:747-9.

Detection of high-grade dysplasia in Barrett's esophagus using narrow band imaging

G.W. Falk (Cleveland)

Barrett's esophagus is a clear risk factor for the development of esophageal adenocarcinoma. Current practice guidelines recommend endoscopic surveillance of patients with Barrett's esophagus in an attempt to detect cancer at an early and potentially curable stage. Endoscopic surveillance relies on white light endoscopy and has numerous shortcomings as currently practiced. Dysplasia and early adenocarcinoma are endoscopically indistinguishable from intestinal metaplasia without dysplasia. The distribution of dysplasia and cancer is highly variable, and even the most thorough biopsy surveillance program has the potential for sampling error. There are considerable interobserver variability and quality control problems in the interpretation of dysplasia in both the community and academic settings. Current surveillance programs are expensive and time consuming. Furthermore, most patients do not have dysplasia and will never develop cancer.

High-grade dysplasia (HGD) in Barrett's esophagus is the best recognized risk factor for the development of adenocarcinoma [1-3]. The presence of HGD is a threshold for intervention in Barrett's esophagus patients be it surgical, endoscopic or simply intensified surveillance. Unfortunately, HGD is often invisible with white light endoscopy. However, when HGD is associated with mucosal abnormalities there is an even greater risk for the development of cancer [1].

In order to make surveillance techniques more effective, new approaches are necessary. A variety of endoscopic techniques are under development in an attempt to improve the efficiency and sampling in surveillance programs. All of these techniques are based on the principle that benign and malignant tissues have different optical qualities. In theory, this would permit optical sampling of larger areas of the columnar-lined esophagus and improve the efficiency of biopsies by targeting areas thought to harbor dysplasia or cancer. Narrow band imaging is one such technique which is now widely commercially available.

What is narrow band imaging?

Narrow band imaging is a new imaging technique based on the principle that the depth of light penetration into tissue is dependent on its wavelength. Short wavelength blue light has a shallow depth of penetration compared to long wavelength red light. The selective use of blue light, by applying filters to conventional white light, provides enhanced imaging of superficial mucosal and vascular patterns without the need for applying dyes such as indigo carmine or methylene blue [4]. By narrowing the wavelength of light to 415 nm, which corresponds to the peak absorption spectrum of hemoglobin, structures with high hemoglobin content such as superficial vessels appear darker than the surrounding mucosa. Current instrumentation permits the endoscopist to switch between conventional white light and narrow band imaging with a switch on the endoscope or processor.

Narrow band imaging has several potential advantages compared to standard white light endoscopy. First, it permits contrast enhancement without the need for administering staining agents. It is user friendly, simply requiring the touch of a button on the endoscope or light processor. Narrow band imaging can provide a wide area overview, but can also be used with magnification endoscopy for more detailed inspection of suspicious areas. Finally, this technique is now widely available commercially. However, limited information is available about the utility of narrow band imaging in Barrett's esophagus patients with HGD.

Narrow band imaging for the detection of high-grade dysplasia

To date, several studies have examined the utility of narrow band imaging for the detection of HGD in Barrett's esophagus. Kara *et al.* compared high resolution white light endoscopy + indigo carmine chromoendoscopy to high resolution white light endoscopy + narrow band imaging in 28 Barrett's esophagus patients referred for the management of endoscopically inconspicuous HGD or early adenocarcinoma [5]. In this randomized crossover study, a total of 14 cases of HGD or early adenocarcinoma were found in the study population. High resolution endoscopy + indigo carmine chromoendoscopy detected 13 of 14 (93%) of the cases compared to 12 of 14 (86%) with high resolution white light endoscopy + narrow band imaging. Furthermore, 9 additional lesions were detected with narrow band imaging compared to 4 additional lesions by indigo carmine chromoendoscopy. These findings provided proof of principle of "electronic chromoendoscopy" as a technique for the detection of intraepithelial neoplasia.

Kara *et al.* subsequently expanded their findings to a much larger group of Barrett's esophagus patients [6]. After first undergoing high resolution white light endoscopy, narrow band imaging was used in conjunction with magnification endoscopy in 63 Barrett's esophagus patients undergoing surveillance endoscopy with or without a prior diagnosis of dysplasia. Of note, random areas were examined with magnification endoscopy and biopsies were obtained. HGD and intraepithelial neoplasia were characterized by three abnormalities with narrow band imaging: irregular/disrupted mucosal patterns, irregular vascular patterns and abnormal blood vessels. All areas of HGD or intraepithelial neoplasia had at least one of these abnormalities.

Similarly, Sharma *et al.* examined the utility of narrow band imaging in 51 consecutive Barrett's esophagus patients without dysplasia or obvious mass lesions in a veterans administration setting [7]. Only seven patients had HGD. An irregular/distorted mucosal pattern or abnormal vascularity was encountered in all of the patients with HGD.

Finally, narrow band imaging has been used in conjunction with autofluorescence endoscopy by Kara *et al.* in 20 high risk patients with either a recent diagnosis of endoscopically inconspicuous HGD, or follow-up after endoscopic therapy of HGD [8].

Patients first underwent endoscopy with a prototype videoendoscope with high resolution white light endoscopy followed by switching to autofluorescence mode. During endoscopy with the autofluorescence mode, suspicious lesions appear blue/violet in color while nondysplastic epithelium has a green appearance. The location of all suspicious areas was documented, the instrument was then withdrawn and replaced by a narrow band videoendoscope with zoom capabilities of 115X magnification. This scope was also fitted with a cap to permit fixation of mucosal areas of interest prior to biopsies. The narrow band scope was utilized with moderate or high magnification in order to determine the mucosal and vascular appearance of the abnormal areas detected by the autofluorescence mode. The worst diagnosis found in the 20 patients studied was HGD in 14, low-grade dysplasia (LGD) in 1, indefinite for dysplasia in 1 and intestinal metaplasia without dysplasia in 4. A total of 47 suspicious areas were identified with autofluorescence of which 28 were confirmed to have HGD. All 28 of these confirmed abnormalities were also abnormal by narrow band imaging criteria. However, 14/19 false positive autofluorescence findings were normal on narrow band imaging thereby reducing the number of false positive lesions from 19 (40%) to 5 (10%) of the initial 47 autofluorescence lesions. This study used the concept of multimodal imaging, which takes advantage of wide area viewing for an initial overview of at risk mucosa obtained by autofluorescence followed by more in depth imaging of high-risk mucosa by narrow band imaging.

Summary

Narrow band imaging clearly enhances mucosal and vascular patterns without the need for chromoendoscopy. The data presented are very encouraging and exciting for the detection of HGD in Barrett's esophagus. Studies to date have been small and all have required the use of magnification endoscopy to evaluate the mucosal pattern, making the technique more amenable to small area imaging in contrast to a broad area imaging technique such as autofluorescence endoscopy. Some of the studies have concentrated on high risk patient groups which may not be generalizable to the routine Barrett's population. There is a need for a common terminology to describe narrow band imaging abnormalities and a critical need for adequate training in such a language. We already know that there is considerable interobserver variability with respect to detection of mucosal patterns with magnification endoscopy using white light [9]. It is anticipated that a combination of techniques that permit efficient sampling of a wide surface area of involved mucosa accompanied by deep tissue penetration and high cellular resolution will be the most useful strategy in the future for the surveillance of Barrett's esophagus.

References

1. Buttar NS, Wang KK, Sebo TJ, et al. Extent of high-grade dysplasia in Barrett's esophagus correlates with risk of adenocarcinoma. Gastroenterology 2001;120:1630-9.
2. Reid BJ, Levine DS, Longton G, Blount PL, Rabinovitch PS. Predictors of progression to cancer in Barrett's esophagus: baseline histology and flow cytometry identify low- and high-risk patient subsets. Am J Gastroenterol 2000;95:1669-76.
3. Schnell TG, Sontag SJ, Chejfec G, et al. Long-term nonsurgical management of Barrett's esophagus with high-grade dysplasia. Gastroenterology 2001;120:1607-19.
4. Wani S, Sharma P. Endoscopic surface imaging of Barrett's esophagus: an optimistic view. Gastroenterology 2007;133:11-3.

5. Kara MA, Peters FP, Rosmolen WD, et al. High-resolution endoscopy plus chromoendoscopy or narrow-band imaging in Barrett's esophagus: a prospective randomized crossover study. Endoscopy 2005;37:929-36.
6. Kara MA, Ennahachi M, Fockens P, ten Kate FJ, Bergman JJ. Detection and classification of the mucosal and vascular patterns (mucosal morphology) in Barrett's esophagus by using narrow band imaging. Gastrointest Endosc 2006;64:155-66.
7. Sharma P, Bansal A, Mathur S, et al. The utility of a novel narrow band imaging endoscopy system in patients with Barrett's esophagus. Gastrointest Endosc 2006;64:167-75.
8. Kara MA, Peters FP, Fockens P, ten Kate FJ, Bergman JJ. Endoscopic video-autofluorescence imaging followed by narrow band imaging for detecting early neoplasia in Barrett's esophagus. Gastrointest Endosc 2006;64:176-85.
9. Sharma P. Magnification endoscopy. Gastrointest Endosc 2005;61:435-43.

Epithelial types in columnar metaplasia in magnification and narrow band imaging

G. Triadafilopoulos (Stanford)

Current issues in Barrett's esophagus

Currently, there are several issues in the management of Barrett's esophagus. First, it is still a challenge to identify Barrett's intestinal metaplasia unless a careful endoscopy and multiple biopsies are performed in subjects with chronic gastroesophageal reflux disease (GERD). The recognition of the salmon-colored epithelium, typically in the distal esophagus, still requires histological confirmation of the presence of goblet cells using Alcian blue staining in representative biopsies taken from the entire surface of the Barrett's esophagus [1]. Further, the identification of Barrett's low- or high-grade dysplasia (LGD or HGD) depends not only on the acquisition of four-quadrant biopsies taken from each 1 cm of the Barrett's esophagus surface using large capacity forceps but also on an accurate pathologic interpretation. Hence it is the combination of endoscopic and histological assessment that Barrett's esophagus can be validated and appropriately managed. Once this is accomplished, the identification of those patients who may already harbor cancer within the Barrett's esophagus surface can be challenging unless a careful endoscopic evaluation, matched with the necessary biopsies, is performed. Predicting those patients who will progress to cancer still remains an elusive goal since no single biomarker other the histological presence of HGD, has been identified as carrying enough reliability and specificity in predicting such outcome.

Increasingly, the management of HGD is non surgical. Endoscopic mucosal resection (EMR) [2], photodynamic therapy (PDT) [3] and radiofrequency ablation using the HALO balloon-based system (BARRx Medical, Inc.) [4] have been associated with favorable rates of technical success, safety and durability of effect while they provide significantly less morbidity and mortality than esophagectomy. Although all these modalities deliver a quick and largely successful elimination of the metaplastic and dysplastic epithelia, they require concomitant proton pump inhibition (PPI) therapy that will provide the necessary pH milieu for effective re-epithelialization by squamous mucosa. Esophagectomy, with its ability to remove the entire metaplastic and dysplastic changes, remains the gold standard and should always be explored as an option, particularly in fit patients with HGD or intra-mucosal carcinoma.

Endoscopy in Barrett's esophagus

Standard endoscopy without biopsies can detect columnar-lined esophagus but cannot confirm specialized intestinal metaplasia or detect early neoplasia (dysplasia). Multiple, 4-quadrant, large-capacity biopsy specimens obtained at 1-cm intervals is the current standard in the diagnosis and surveillance of patients with Barrett's esophagus [5]. New techniques for the detection of Barrett's esophagus and early neoplasia are increasingly utilized and validated either singly or in combination. These techniques include magnification chromo-endoscopy, methylene blue or indigo carmine chromoscopy, acetic acid instillation, narrow band imaging (NBI), and high-resolution/magnification endoscopy [6-9]. However, because these techniques require time, expertise and special equipment, they have not yet been widely adopted by the general practicing gastroenterologists who conduct the majority of screening and surveillance endoscopy in patients with GERD and Barrett's esophagus.

High-resolution, magnification and chromo-endoscopy

An improved ability to discriminate between two points on the endoscopic field offers new horizons in the recognition and regular surveillance of Barrett's esophagus. High-resolution endoscopes discriminate lesions 10 to 71 μm apart (conventional 125 to 165 μm). Resolution reflects pixel density. Standard endoscopes have pixel densities of 100-200,000; magnification endoscopes reach pixel densities of 850,000. During magnification endoscopy, a movable lens -controlled by the operator- varies the degree of magnification from 1.5x to 115x. The combination strategy of magnification chromoendoscopy implies that magnified images are further enhanced by the topical application of stains or pigments. Equipment and experience with all these modalities are evolving and they may improve the diagnostic accuracy in Barrett's esophagus, dysplasia and early neoplasia [10,11]. In terms of technique, magnification and staining take additional 5-10 minutes, and methylene blue, indigo carmine, or acetic acid are the most commonly used agents. Ideally chromoscopy requires special catheter spraying of 5-10 ml (distal to proximal) and should be done with the head of the bed elevated in order to reduce the risk of aspiration [12,13].

Methylene blue chromoendoscopy is used to detect specialized columnar epithelium since the stain is preferentially taken up by the non-dysplastic columnar tissue. Seven studies have reported high sensitivity (91%-98%) and variable specificity (43%-97%) while another four studies reported unsatisfactory sensitivity (53%-72%) and specificity (32%-51%) [14]. When used to improve the diagnosis of dysplasia in Barrett's esophagus, two studies showed MB-directed biopsy to be better than random biopsy, but 3 others did not.

In a study of 80 patients with suspected Barrett's esophagus, indigo carmine magnification chromoendoscopy revealed the following mucosal patterns: 17%, circular pattern and 97%, ridged/villous pattern. In 6 patients with HGD, all (100%) revealed an irregular/distorted pattern [8]. In acetic acid magnification chromoendoscopy, the acetic acid opacifies the epithelial surface masking the sub-epithelial vascular network and making the surface appear white. Two to three minutes later, the esophagus remains white while the gastric epithelium and Barrett's mucosa become red [15]. When acetic acid magnification chromoendoscopy was used in 195 patients without obvious Barrett's esophagus, intestinal metaplasia of the gastric cardia was found in 44%. Further, 4 patterns (% IM yield) were recognized: round pits (0%), reticular (5%), villous (56%), and ridged (96%) [9]. In another study of acetic acid chromoendoscopy, 67 symptomatic patients revealed 39% yield of intestinal metaplasia in the esophagus or gastroesophageal junction with resulting sensitivity of 89%, specificity of 90%, positive predictive value of 85%, and negative predictive value of 93% [15]. These authors also proposed a classification of surface pattern of Barrett's epithelium and esophagogastric junctional mucosa by enhanced magnifying endoscopy with gyrus, villous and mixed gyrus and villous patterns reflecting histological intestinal metaplasia.

Issues with inter-observer reliability remain. When 51 patients with GERD underwent magnification chromoendoscopy using acetic acid or methylene blue and their videotapes were randomly reviewed by 4 endoscopists, intestinal metaplasia was detected in 61% and there was a high-level of inter-observer variability (Kappa < 0.4). The overall accuracy was only 50% and no differences observed before or after acetic acid or methylene blue. However, variable levels of inter-observer variability have been described [16,17].

In summary, magnification chromoendoscopy is still evolving but it improves the identification of mucosal abnormalities and may guide biopsies. The technique cannot yet replace histology as a final diagnostic tool and there is still a need for guidelines on when and what to stain and a better standardization of the observed patterns, while the involved costs and time are impediments to a wider use and applicability [18].

Narrow band imaging

NBI enhances the fine structure of the mucosal surface without the use of dyes. The technique is based upon a light source with sequential red-green-and-blue (RGB) illumination; blue light penetrates only superficially, whereas red light penetrates into deeper layers. NBI enables better visualization of the mucosa because blue light allows for optimal superficial imaging and it reveals the superficial vasculature because of absorption of the blue light by hemoglobin [19]. A key advantage of the technique is that it can be easily applied by an easy switch between standard and NBI-mode in the new generation of endoscopes. Various morphologic abnormalities in patients with Barrett's esophagus have been described by NBI: regular villous and gyrus-forming mucosal and vascular patterns, villi of various sizes and shapes, blood vessels between mucosal ridges, flat-type mucosa without pits or villi and regular, long-branching vessels [20] (*Figure 1*). In contrast, features suggestive of HGD and cancer are multiple spiral vessels of variable caliber, numerous small, isolated blood vessels, irregular or disrupted mucosal patterns, irregular vascular patterns, or remnants of villous or gyrus-forming mucosal patterns [21]. Overall, NBI requires no special dyes, is operator-friendly, evaluates both mucosa and vascular bed, can help target biopsies. However, the technology is still available only at few centers and there is still need for image recognition training and standardization.

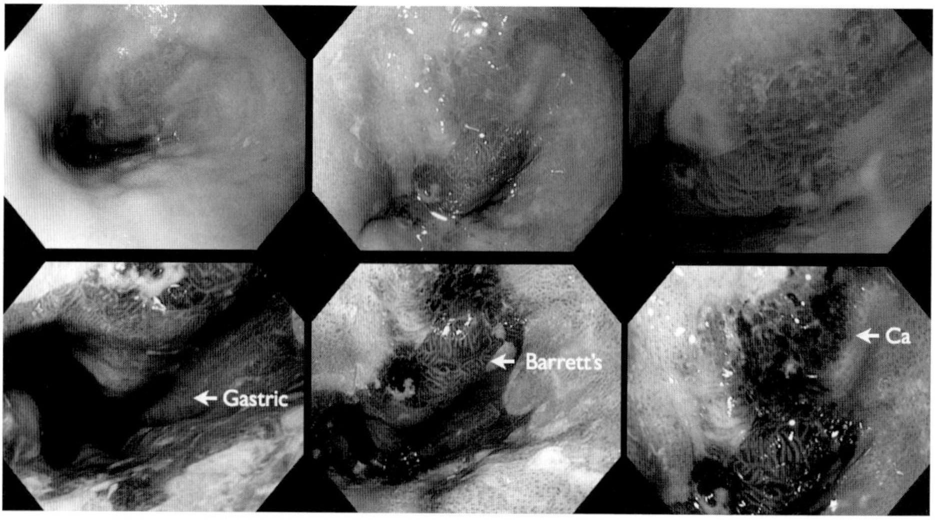

Figure 1. NBI in early esophageal adenocarcinoma (Courtesy: Roy Soetikno, MD, Stanford, CA). (See page XXXII for colour figure)

The future

Unquestionably, there is a need to study the incremental benefit of these novel advanced imaging techniques to the endoscopic diagnosis of Barrett's esophagus provided by high-resolution endoscopy alone. There is also a need for randomized validation studies after initial pilot and prospective cohort studies, followed by studies of the reliability and cost-effectiveness. There is also need for a consensus on terminology and techniques as well as on necessary training and credentialing. Nevertheless, all these techniques have already provided an extra dimension in our recognition of metaplasia and dysplasia in Barrett's esophagus and have brought forward a level of alertness that enhances patient care.

References

1. Johansson J, Håkansson HO, Mellblom L, et al. Diagnosing Barrett's oesophagus: factors related to agreement between endoscopy and histology. Eur J Gastroenterol Hepatol 2007;19(10):870-7.
2. Soehendra N, Seewald S, Groth S, et al. Use of modified multiband ligator facilitates circumferential EMR in Barrett's esophagus (with video). Gastrointest Endosc 2006;63(6):847-52.
3. Overholt BF, Wang KK, Burdick JS, et al. International Photodynamic Group for High-Grade Dysplasia in Barrett's Esophagus. Five-year efficacy and safety of photodynamic therapy with Photofrin in Barrett's high-grade dysplasia. Gastrointest Endosc 2007;66(3):460-8.
4. Roorda AK, Marcus SN, Triadafilopoulos G. Early experience with radiofrequency energy ablation therapy for Barrett's esophagus with and without dysplasia. Dis Esophagus 2007;20(6):516-22.
5. Sharma P, Sampliner RE. Barrett esophagus. Curr Opin Gastroenterol 2002;18(4):471-8.
6. Canto MI, Setrakian S, Willis J, et al. Methylene blue-directed biopsies improve detection of intestinal metaplasia and dysplasia in Barrett's esophagus. Gastrointest Endosc 2000;51(5):560-8.
7. Endo T, Awakawa T, Takahashi H, et al. Classification of Barrett's epithelium by magnifying endoscopy Gastrointest Endosc 2002;55(6):641-7.
8. Sharma P, Weston AP, Topalovski M, Cherian R, Bhattacharyya A, Sampliner RE. Magnification chromoendoscopy for the detection of intestinal metaplasia and dysplasia in Barrett's oesophagus. Gut 200;52(1):24-7.
9. Guelrud M, Herrera I, Essenfeld H, Castro J. Enhanced magnification endoscopy: a new technique to identify specialized intestinal metaplasia in Barrett's esophagus. Gastrointest Endosc 2001;53(6):559-65.
10. ASGE technology status evaluation report. GIE 2000; 52: 864–866.

11. Kiesslich R, Jung M. Magnification endoscopy: does it improve mucosal surface analysis for the diagnosis of gastrointestinal neoplasias? Endoscopy 2002;34(10):819-22.
12. Guelrud M, Herrera I. Acetic acid improves identification of remnant islands of Barrett's epithelium after endoscopic therapy. Gastrointest Endosc 1998;47(6):512-5.
13. Canto MI, Yoshida T, Gossner L. Chromoscopy of intestinal metaplasia in Barrett's esophagus Endoscopy 2002;34(4):330-6.
14. Canto MI, Kalloo A Chromoendoscopy for Barrett's esophagus in the twenty-first century: to stain or not to stain? Gastrointest Endosc 2006;64(2):200-5.
15. Guelrud M, Herrera I, Essenfeld H, Castro J, Antonioli DA. Intestinal metaplasia of the gastric cardia: A prospective study with enhanced magnification endoscopy. Am J Gastroenterol 2002;97(3):584-9.
16. Toyoda H, Rubio C, Befrits R, Hamamoto N, Adachi Y, Jaramillo E. Detection of intestinal metaplasia in distal esophagus and esophagogastric junction by enhanced-magnification endoscopy. Gastrointest Endosc 200;59(1):15-21.
17. Meining A, Rösch T, Kiesslich R, Muders M, Sax F, Heldwein W. Inter- and intra-observer variability of magnification chromoendoscopy for detecting specialized intestinal metaplasia at the gastroesophageal junction. Endoscopy 2004;36(2):160-4.
18. Mayinger B, Oezturk Y, Stolte M, et al. Evaluation of sensitivity and inter- and intra-observer variability in the detection of intestinal metaplasia and dysplasia in Barrett's esophagus with enhanced magnification endoscopy. Scand J Gastroenterol 200;41(3):349-56.
19. Kiesslich R, Jung M, DiSario JA, Galle PR, Neurath MF. Perspectives of chromo and magnifying endoscopy: how, how much, when, and whom should we stain? J Clin Gastroenterol 2004;38(1):7-13.
20. Gono K, Obi T, Yamaguchi M, et al. Appearance of enhanced tissue features in narrow-band endoscopic imaging. J Biomed Opt 2004;9(3):568-77.
21. Kara MA, Peters FP, Fockens P, ten Kate FJ, Endoscopic video-autofluorescence imaging followed by narrow band imaging for detecting early neoplasia in Barrett's esophagus.

How might gastroesophageal reflux disease promote carcinogenesis in Barrett's esophagus?

K. Dvorak, H. Garewal (Tucson)

Barrett's esophagus is a condition where normal squamous epithelium is replaced by metaplastic, specialized columnar epithelium. This lesion is associated with the development of esophageal adenocarcinoma, a cancer with a poor prognosis and a median survival of less than one year [5,6,11].

Barrett's esophagus arises as a consequence of chronic gastroesophageal reflux disease (GERD). In this paper we discuss some of our proposed hypotheses and mechanisms that might be involved. Overall, we hypothesize that Barrett's esophagus is formed in response to stress, injury and repair induced by the refluxate to which the normal squamous epithelium in the distal esophagus is exposed. For decades after the recognition of the link between GERD and Barrett's esophagus, it was assumed that the main, perhaps the only, injurious component of refluxate was acidity or low pH. However, in recent years, we and others have paid increasing attention to other components of refluxate. One such component is bile acids, whose DNA damaging and carcinogenic role we had recognized and studied mainly in colorectal cancer [3]. Of course, the nature and properties of bile acids are influenced by pH, among other factors. In this brief overview our focus will be on recent work on the combination of bile acids in producing the deleterious effects of refluxate together with the potential role of pH in modulating this.

There is substantial, emerging evidence that the combination of acid and bile acids, as present in the refluxate, is more injurious to the esophageal epithelium than either acid alone or bile acids alone [14,16,19,20,25]. The predominant bile acids in the refluxate of patients with GERD include mostly the conjugated bile acids: glycocholic acid, taurocholic acid, glycodeoxycholic acid and glycochenodeoxycholic acid [12-14]. Of considerable interest is the observation that unconjugated bile acids, such as deoxycholic acid, are present in the refluxate ofpatients taking proton pump inhibitors [24]. Bile acids conjugated with glycine are toxic at pH 4 since their pKa is ~ 4. At this pH, these bile acids are partly non-ionized and thus they may penetrate through the cell membrane and disrupt intracellular pathways. Relative to their pKa, at lower pH they precipitate, and at higher pH, they are ionized and thus unable to interact with the lipid bi-layer of the cell membrane. The total bile acid concentrations in the refluxate of Barrett's esophagus patients varies and median bile acid concentrations are in the range 0.2-1.4 mM [12,19]. However, concentrations of bile acids as high as 7.6 mM have been reported [12].

Acute exposure to bile acids may induce oxidative stress, mitochondrial damage, activation of pro-apoptotic pathways and consequently cell death, depending on the nature and concentration of the bile acids as well as the pH (*Figure 1*) [4,21,22,26]. However, chronic exposure under varying conditions of concentration of bile acids and pH may lead to sub-lethal damage, such as increased oxidative stress that activates the ERK, p38 MAPK and NF-κB pathways. These signaling pathways are associated with increased proliferation and decreased apoptosis of esophageal cells (*Figure 1*) [1,7,15,18]. Thus, we hypothesize that after prolonged sublethal episodic exposure, a relatively apoptosis-resistant metaplastic epithelium emerges by natural selection to replace the normal squamous epithelium, most likely as a protective mechanism against a hostile environment. But, as perhaps an "unwanted" consequence, the epithelial cells in this new tissue with decreased apoptotic ability accumulate DNA damage leading to mutation, thereby being more prone to cancer development (*Figure 1*). Intuitively, the balance between proliferation and apoptosis within a tissue would be very important in controlling its overall growth. In addition, the ability to undergo programmed cell death is important for the elimination of cells with damaged DNA [17]. A reduction in apoptotic ability results in the retention of cells with unrepaired

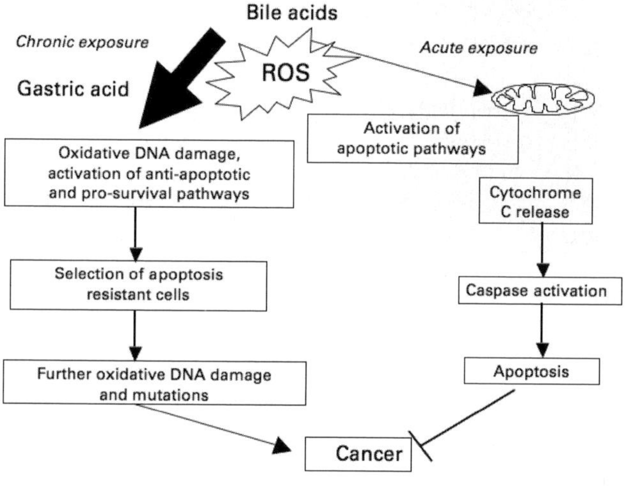

Figure 1. Chronic exposure to pulses of bile acids and gastric acid results in the oxidative damage, DNA mutations, activation of pro-survival and anti-apoptotic pathways and the selection of epithelial cells resistant to apoptosis, finally leading to cancer.

DNA damage and a consequent increase in genomic instability. Possibly, acquisition and retention of other properties associated with malignancy, such as tissue invasion and ability to metastasize and grow at other sites, occurs in emerging clones as a consequence of mutations and selection in response to further exposure to bile acids and gastric acid. Our data suggest that brief exposures to low pH and/or bile acids, that mimic esophageal reflux, induce oxidative stress in cells. Oxidative stress was detected by flow cytometry or fluorescent microscopy using nonfluorescent dyes, such as Hydroethidium or MitoSOX Red that are oxidized by ROS and form highly fluorescent dyes in different esophageal cell lines including immortalized Barrett's esophagus cells (CP-D, kindly provided by Dr. Rabinovitch), normal squamous epithelial cells (Het1A), (*Figure 2*), and Barrett's esophagus adenocarcinoma cells (Seg1, data not shown) [8]. Furthermore, immunohistochemical studies revealed that Barrett's esophagus tissue, stressed *ex vivo* for only 10 minutes with a combination of bile acids and acid show evidence of increased oxidative DNA damage (*Figure 3*) [8].

Oxidative stress is associated with activation of signal transduction pathways that can upregulate expression of anti-apoptotic, pro-survival and angiogenic proteins [2,27]. These include, for example, the NF-κB, JAK-STAT and MAPK pathways. Activation of these pathways and expression of anti-apoptotic proteins is increased in Barrett's esophagus [1,10,23]. Conversely, the levels of proapoptotic markers are low [9]. Thus, chronic oxidative stress induced by the components of refluxate, bile acids and gastric acid, may result in oxidative DNA damage, mutations, activation of prosurvival and anti-apoptotic pathways and the selection of epithelial cells resistant to apoptosis (*Figure 1*). Accumulating DNA damage and mutations in these apoptosis-resistant cells is a clearly dangerous situation.

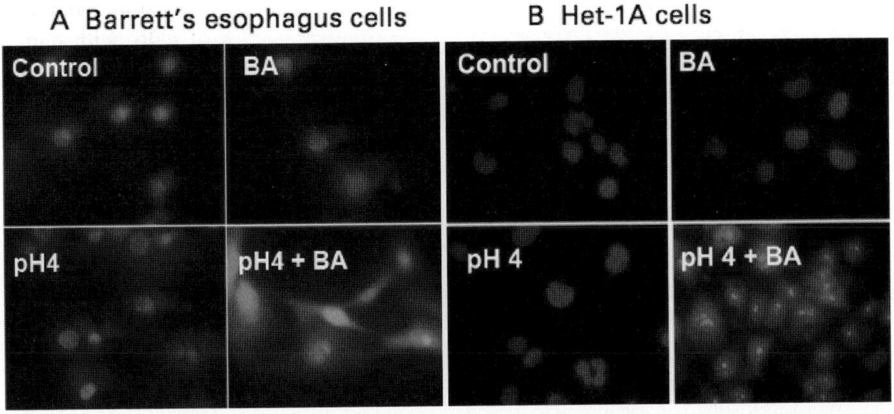

Figure 2. Detection of mitochondrial superoxide in Barrett's esophagus cells (CP-D cells) and HET-1A cells after treatment with pH 4 and/or bile acid cocktail by fluorescence microscopy. Cells were treated for 5 or 1.5 minutes, respectively, with control medium (pH 7.4), medium containing 0.1 mM bile acids cocktail (BA), medium acidified to pH 4 and medium acidified to pH 4 and containing bile acid cocktail. The cells were then washed and stained with 5 μM MitoSOX Red to measure mitochondrial superoxide (red signal). Cells were also stained with 10 μM Hoechst 3222 to visualize the nuclei (blue signal). Panel A shows Barrett's esophagus cells immortalized by hTERT transfection, panel B shows HET-1A cells. (See page XXXI for colour figure).

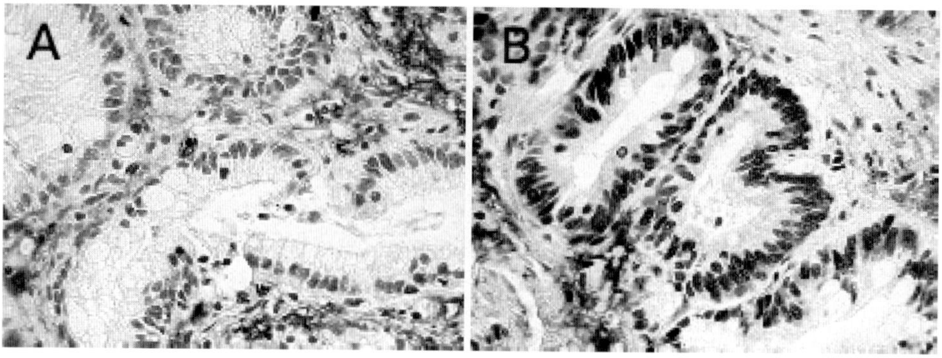

Figure 3. Immunohistochemical staining pattern of 8-OH-dG in Barrett's esophagus tissues. Barrett's esophagus biopsies were incubated in control medium **(A)** or medium acidified to pH 4 and supplemented with 0.5mM bile acid cocktail **(B)**. Note the intense nuclear staining of 8-OH-dG in epithelial cells after incubation with pH 4 and bile acid cocktail. (See page XXXII for colour figure).

In summary, GERD appears to be the cause of most cases of Barrett's esophagus and esophageal adenocarcinoma. We have focused on the hypothesis that increased oxidative stress, and oxidative DNA damage, contribute to this process resulting in mutations, genomic instability, abnormal cell signaling and apoptosis resistance. These alterations likely have a role in the progression to cancer.

References

1. Abdel-Latif MM, O'Riordan J, Windle HJ, et al. NF-kappaB activation in esophageal adenocarcinoma: relationship to Barrett's metaplasia, survival, and response to neoadjuvant chemoradiotherapy. Ann Surg 2004;239:491-500.
2. Angelo LS, Talpaz M, Kurzrock R. Autocrine interleukin-6 production in renal cell carcinoma: evidence for the involvement of p53. Cancer Res 2002;62:932-40.
3. Bernstein H, Bernstein C, Payne CM, Dvorakova K, Garewal H. Bile acids as carcinogens in human gastrointestinal cancers. Mutat Res2005;589:47-65.
4. Bernstein H, Payne CM, Bernstein C, Schneider J, Beard SE, Crowley CL. Activation of the promoters of genes associated with DNA damage, oxidative stress, ER stress and protein malfolding by the bile salt, deoxycholate. Toxicol Lett 1999;108:37-46.
5. DeMeester TR. Management of adenocarcinoma arising in Barrett's esophagus. Semin Thorac Cardiovasc Surg 1997;9:290-301.
6. Drewitz DJ, Sampliner RE, Garewal HS. The incidence of adenocarcinoma in Barrett's esophagus: a prospective study of 170 patients followed 4.8 years. Am J Gastroenterol 1997;92:212-5.
7. Duggan SP, Gallagher WM, Fox EJ, Abdel-Latif MM, Reynolds JV, Kelleher D. Low pH induces co-ordinate regulation of gene expression in oesophageal cells. Carcinogenesis 2006;27:319-27.
8. Dvorak K, Payne CM, Chavarria M, et al. Bile acids in combination with low pH induce oxidative stress and oxidative DNA damage: relevance to the pathogenesis of Barrett's Oesophagus. Gut 2007;56:763-71.
9. Dvorakova K, Payne CM, Ramsey L, et al. Apoptosis resistance in Barrett's esophagus: ex vivo bioassay of live stressed tissues. Am J Gastroenterol 2005;100:424-31.
10. Dvorakova K, Payne CM, Ramsey L, et al. Increased expression and secretion of interleukin-6 in patients with Barrett's esophagus. Clin Cancer Res 2004;10:2020-8.
11. Falk GW. Barrett's esophagus. Gastroenterology 2002;122:1569-91.
12. Iftikhar SY, Ledingham S, Steele RJ, et al. Bile reflux in columnar-lined Barrett's oesophagus. Ann R Coll Surg Engl 1993;75:411-6.
13. Kauer WK, Peters JH, DeMeester TR, et al. Composition and concentration of bile acid reflux into the esophagus of patients with gastroesophageal reflux disease. Surgery 1997;122:874-81.
14. Kauer WK, Peters JH, DeMeester TR, Ireland AP, Bremner CG, Hagen JA. Mixed reflux of gastric and duodenal juices is more harmful to the esophagus than gastric juice alone. The need for surgical therapy re-emphasized. Ann Surg 1995;222:-525-33.

15. Kaur BS, Triadafilopoulos G. Acid- and bile-induced PGE(2) release and hyperproliferation in Barrett's esophagus are COX-2 and PKC-epsilon dependent. Am J Physiol Gastrointest Liver Physiol 2002;283:G327-34.
16. Lang J, Blikslager A, Regina D, Eisemann J, Argenzio R. Synergistic effect of hydrochloric acid and bile acids on the pars esophageal mucosa of the porcine stomach. Am J Vet Res 1998;59:1170-6.
17. Lips J, Kaina B. DNA double-strand breaks trigger apoptosis in p53-deficient fibroblasts. Carcinogenesis 2001;22:579-85.
18. Morgan C, Alazawi W, Sirieix P, Freeman T, Coleman N, Fitzgerald R. In vitro acid exposure has a differential effect on apoptotic and proliferative pathways in a Barrett's adenocarcinoma cell line. Am J Gastroenterol 2004;99:218-24.
19. Nehra D, Howell P, Williams CP, Pye JK, Beynon J. Toxic bile acids in gastro-oesophageal reflux disease: influence of gastric acidity. Gut 199944:598-602.
20. Oh DS, Hagen JA, Fein M, et al. The impact of reflux composition on mucosal injury and esophageal function. J Gastrointest Surg 2006;10:787-97.
21. Qiao L, Studer E, Leach K, et al. Deoxycholic acid (DCA) causes ligand-independent activation of epidermal growth factor receptor (EGFR) and FAS receptor in primary hepatocytes: inhibition of EGFR/mitogen-activated protein kinase-signaling module enhances DCA-induced apoptosis. Mol Biol Cell 2001;12:2629-45.
22. Sokol RJ, Winklhofer-Roob BM, Devereaux MW, McKim JM Jr. Generation of hydroperoxides in isolated rat hepatocytes and hepatic mitochondria exposed to hydrophobic bile acids. Gastroenterology 1995;109:1249-56.
23. Souza RF, Shewmake K, Terada LS, Spechler SJ. Acid exposure activates the mitogen-activated protein kinase pathways in Barrett's esophagus. Gastroenterology 2002;122:299-307.
24. Theisen J, Nehra D, Citron D, et al. Suppression of gastric acid secretion in patients with gastroesophageal reflux disease results in gastric bacterial overgrowth and deconjugation of bile acids. J Gastrointest Surg 2000;4:50-4.
25. Vaezi MF, Richter JE. Role of acid and duodenogastroesophageal reflux in gastroesophageal reflux disease. Gastroenterology 1996;111:1192-9.
26. Washo-Stultz D, Crowley-Weber CL, Dvorakova K, et al. Role of mitochondrial complexes I and II, reactive oxygen species and arachidonic acid metabolism in deoxycholate-induced apoptosis. Cancer Lett 2002;177:129-44.
27. Yu H, Jove R. The STATs of cancer--new molecular targets come of age. Nat Rev Cancer 2004;4:97-105.

Is chemoprevention of Barrett's esophagus a feasible strategy?

S.J. Sontag (Chicago)

The management of Barrett's esophagus is controversial. Preventing the development of Barrett's esophagus is even more controversial, as the mechanism by which Barrett's develops as well as the time of development are complete enigmas. Therefore, emphasis is necessarily placed on preventing esophageal cancer once Barrett's esophagus is detected. Current surveillance recommendations for patients with documented Barrett's esophagus are predicated on the hope that Barrett's cancer either can be prevented or can be detected early enough so that therapy prevents death from the cancer. The frequency of surveillance endoscopies needed to accomplish this goal remains as unknown today as it did a generation ago. Frequency intervals vary from every 3 months for Barrett's with high-grade dysplasia (HGD) to every 3-5 years for Barrett's without dysplasia. Thus, the goal of treatment can be either detection of early esophageal cancer followed by some type of curative intervention, or prevention of cancer development altogether. With either goal, knowledge of the natural history of the disease is important, and some type of follow-up will be necessary for years to come.

It is generally accepted that the development of Barrett's cancer follows a dysplasia-carcinoma sequence: intestinal metaplasia without dysplasia progresses to intestinal metaplasia with low-grade dysplasia (LGD) to intestinal metaplasia with HGD to cancer [1]. The factors that encourage or discourage the leap to cancer remain unidentified, and the timeframe in which this progression occurs is unknown. A few facts, however, are generally accepted:

The vast majority of patients with uncomplicated Barrett's esophagus is rather healthy, and thus remains undiagnosed. The vast majority of patients with Barrett's cancer comes to endoscopy when it is too late.

Based on our 25-year Hines VA database, the prevalence and incidence of Barrett's esophagus and Barrett's cancer are as follows:

- prevalence:
  - 15% of all adults with gastroesophageal reflux (GER) symptoms have Barrett's esophagus,
  - 0.7% of all adults with GER symptoms will have Barrett's cancer at first endoscopy;
- incidence:
  - 2% of all Barrett's esophagus patients will develop Barrett's cancer during a mean of 10 years (0.3% per year),
  - 15% of all Barrett's HGD patients will develop Barrett's cancer during a mean of 10 years (2.2% per year).

Based on national statistics, the importance of esophageal cancer is as follows:

- esophageal cancer represents about 1% of all new cancers;
- esophageal cancer represents about 2% of all cancer deaths;
- esophageal cancer results in death in 97% of its victims.

Indeed, only 12,000 new cases of esophageal cancer are diagnosed each year: Half are squamous cell carcinomas and half are adenocarcinoma. Of the half that are adenocarcinoma, only half of these are actually Barrett's esophagus cancers. The remaining half are adenocarcinoma (probably of the gastroesophageal junction), but without goblet cells and thus, not considered to be Barrett's esophagus. Thus, of the 12,000 new esophageal cancers diagnosed each year, only one-quarter are due to Barrett's esophagus.

From these statistics, it appears that only a small minority of patients with Barrett's esophagus will ever go on to develop HGD and eventually cancer.

It seems, therefore, that if any major decrease in the mortality of Barrett's cancer is to be achieved, it will be brought about only by the large-scale identification of patients with Barrett's esophagus who do not yet have cancer. At the present time, such identification could occur only by massive screening of individuals at high risk for Barrett's and cancer. Such individuals are otherwise healthy, although heartburn symptoms may help in their identification. Indeed, a recent study from Sweden showed that the presence of heartburn, regurgitation or both at least one time per week increases the risk of esophageal cancer 8-fold [2]. If the symptoms are frequent, severe and of long duration, the cancer risk increases 44-fold. In order to substantially reduce the esophageal cancer death rate, this group would need to be targeted for early endoscopic examination. Anything short of a full-blown attack on this group with symptomatic gastroesophageal reflux (GER) will necessarily fail to achieve that goal. On the other hand, a full-blown attack on this group would require massive investment of time and energy by currently available endoscopists. On the negative side, only half the patients who present with advanced esophageal adenocarcinoma admit to ever having experienced GER symptoms.

Given the high prevalence of symptomatic GER in the general population, the low prevalence of Barrett's esophagus in the symptomatic GER population, the very low Barrett's esophagus diagnosis rate in the total Barrett's population, the minuscule incidence of cancer in the Barrett's population, and the dismal survival rate of patients with Barrett's cancer, it is unlikely that a major decrease in mortality from Barrett's cancer will occur in the near future. There is, however, a possibility that a completely different form of therapy may have an impact in the morbidity and mortality of esophageal cancer.

A different approach

If we must question the wisdom of spending a hunk of our resources on a disease in which 97% of its victims are "goners" from the time of first diagnosis, and less than 3% are potentially treatable or curable, then perhaps we might find some hope in the concept of chemoprevention. Although of still unproven efficacy, chemoprevention – in the form of food derivatives and synthetic pharmaceuticals – are now being studied for the prevention and regression of colon polyps and the prevention and regression of Barrett's esophageal dysplasia.

Free radicals, antioxidants and chemoprevention

The concept of chemoprevention of cancer rests on fairly well documented studies that demonstrate the production of "free radical" molecules during our every-day normal life processes. The free radical is an oxygen molecule with a missing electron, and in constant search to find an electron mate – from any source. Unfortunately, the peacefully paired electrons in our normal resting cells are fair game. In the process, the free radical kidnaps the peaceful electrons, destroying the friendly cell and injuring the DNA.

Free radicals, therefore, are biochemical terrorists that systematically and on a regular basis attack our normal cells, including our DNA, on an average of 10,000 hits per day. Such internal weapons of mass destruction – through a process known as oxidative stress - are thought to be responsible for up to three-quarters of all our diseases – especially those of the so-called degenerative diseases of aging, which includes the following:
- aging;
- cancer;
- cardiovascular disease;
- immune system decline;
- brain dysfunction;
- cataracts.

Sources of free radical production include the following:
- endogenous:
    - normal aerobic respiration (e.g. eating),
    - phagocyte activities against infections,
    - fatty acid degradation,
    - cytochrome p450 enzyme actions;
- exogenous:
    - cigarette smoke,
    - toxins.

There are several customs means by which free radicals can be reduced. Such means include the following:
- ingestion of anti-oxidant enzymes;
- ingestion of anti-oxidants;
- ingestion of vitamin C, vitamin E, carotenoids;
- ingestion of crucifers.

Increasing our antioxidant intake requires an increase in our daily intake of phytonutrients, which are found in fruits and vegetables. Among this class are the polyphenols, which are in large part responsible for the different colors seen in plants, fruits and vegetables, and the bioflavonoids. Some of the best sources of bioflavonoids include the following fruits:
- berries (strawberries, blueberries, blackberries, cranberries);
- grapes;
- pomegranates;
- citrus fruits;
- green tea leaves.

Increasing our consumption of certain fish has also been shown to have antioxidant effects, and the health industry has made available the two most important of the fish oils: EPA (eicosapentanoic acid) and DHA (docosahexanoic acid). These polyunsaturated fish oils have multiple benefits on human cells, one of which is the enhancement of free radical scavenging in tissues and organs.

In addition, NSAIDs and statins have been shown to offer protection against the effects of free radicals. The mechanisms by which these two agents reduce the harmful effects are as follows:
- decrease cellular proliferation;
- increase apoptosis;
- decrease tissue invasion;
- decrease angiogenesis.

It is evident that we cannot stop the natural production of free radicals. We need to eat, and thus we will always produce these cellular terrorists. Furthermore, because of our lifestyles, it is often difficult to get sufficient antioxidants form our current food supply. With this in mind, numerous health industries have sprung up to offer additional antioxidants from supplements in the form of powder or capsules. Such blends of natural foods may well prove beneficial in preventing the development of certain diseases, including cancer.

Barrett's cancer chemoprevention

The theoretical goal of cancer chemoprevention is to inhibit or reverse pre-invasive carcinogenesis before the development of clinical cancer. The goals of current clinical studies, funded by both private industry and government grants, are to demonstrate:
- regression of existing neoplasia;
- prevention of recurrent neoplasia;
- prevention of first-time neoplasia.

The genetic targets for chemoprevention are genetic damage and genetic defects. The results of these studies, as well as the verdict itself, will be available in the near future.

Meanwhile, if chemoprevention eventually proves to be a reliable discipline in the reversal of dysplasia or the prevention of the ultimate dysplasia — cancer — its eventual impact would depend completely on how the medical community and the public at large responds to the following question:

If physicians and their patients with Barrett's esophagus could be relatively certain that esophageal cancer would not develop – regardless of the current grade of dysplasia – would they be satisfied with and compliant with life-long ingestion of antioxidant supplements or other chemopreventive agents in lieu of repeated endoscopies, endoscopic therapies, and surgical resection. The answer is blowing in the wind.

References

1. Lagergren J, Bergstrom R, Lindgren A, et al. Symptomatic gastroesophageal reflux as a risk factor for esophageal adenocarcinoma. N Engl J Med 1999;340:825-31.
2. Jemal A, et al. American Cancer Society. Cancer statistics. CA Cancer J Clin 2007;57:43-66.

What is the outcome of radiofrequency ablation of Barrett's esophagus?

G. Triadafilopoulos (Stanford)

For the practicing endoscopist, the key issues in the management of Barrett's esophagus are: the identification of dysplasia either endoscopically or histologically (or both), the identification of patients who already harbor invasive cancer, the ability to predict those patients who will progress to cancer and the ability to treat high-grade dysplasia (HGD) non-surgically, either by endoscopic mucosal resection (EMR), or by any of the available ablation methods, such as photodynamic therapy (PDT), thereby avoiding esophagectomy with its associated morbidity and mortality (*Figure 1*).

- Identify Barrett 's dysplasia
  - Endoscopically
  - Histologically
- Identify those who already harbor cancer
- Predict those who will progress to cancer
- Treat high-grade dysplasia non-surgically
  - EMR
  - Ablation

  + twice daily proton pump inhibition therapy
- Esophagectomy

Figure 1. Key issues in the management of Barrett's esophagus.

The aims of any ablation method for Barrett's esophagus are twofold: first, to achieve a complete, endoscopic and histologic elimination of Barrett's esophagus without residual overt or "buried" metaplasia (ablation of metaplasia), and, second, to achieve a complete, endoscopic and histologic elimination of dysplasia and early cancer without surrounding residual "overt" or "buried" Barrett's metaplasia (ablation of dysplasia and early cancer) [1]. Obviously, the latter aim is more urgent and important than the former. Both aims are difficult to accomplish universally, and many methods, thermal and non-thermal, have been used in conjunction with either medical or surgical gastroesophageal reflux control with variable success rates and complications [2]. "Ideal" ablation objectives would involve a peroral endoscopic approach, the ability to remove dysplasia in addition to all existing intestinal metaplasia, a circumferential ablation, a quick and well-tolerated procedure that accomplishes a uniform and reproducible ablation depth (targeting ablation down to the level of muscularis mucosae without injury to submucosa or deeper structures), a very low risk of immediate (bleeding, perforation) or late (stricture formation) complications and a near 0% risk for adenocarcinoma development over the lifetime of the patient (*Figure 2*).

- Single-session intervention
- Operator-independent
- 100% effective in eliminating metaplasia and dysplasia
- No complications
- Lifetime guarantee of no recurrence
- 0% risk for adenocarcinoma

Figure 2. Ideal therapy for Barrett's esophagus

The radiofrequency ablation system Halo^{360} (BARRX, Inc. Sunnyvale, CA) has been recently introduced for the treatment of Barrett's esophagus with and without HGD/early cancer. Thus far, experience with this system has demonstrated feasibility and efficacy with a very low rate of complications. The technique uniformly treats large surface areas of Barrett's epithelium with maximum ablation depth to the muscularis mucosae, while it allows for secondary treatments to manage recurrent (new) or persistent Barrett's esophagus over the lifetime of the patient. Further, the technique is nearly operator-independent, in regards to dosing, depth of ablation, and targeting [1,3].

The BARRX ablation system is a balloon-based electrode that, since it received FDA clearance in 2001, has been successfully used in clinical trials as well as community practice in the US. The bipolar electrode delivers 350 W power at 465 kHz frequency and creates an "even" target of ablation. Multiple treatments are given as short radiofrequency energy bursts (~300 msec), while the distended balloon ensures a standardized energy density and controls the depth of ablation enabling a uniform mucosal ablation and eliminating the point-and-shoot approach of other ablation strategies previously used (*Figures 3 and 4*).

An early key study determined the optimal ablation parameters for human esophageal epithelium using the Halo^{360} balloon-based electrode [4]. Immediately prior to esophagectomy, subjects underwent esophagoscopy and ablation of two separate, 3-cm long, circumferential segments of non-tumor-bearing esophageal epithelium. Thirteen subjects were randomized to one of three energy density groups: 8, 10, or 12 J/cm^2. RF energy was applied one time (1x) proximally and two times (2x) distally. Following resection, sections from each ablation zone were evaluated using H&E and diaphorase. Histological endpoints were complete epithelial ablation, maximum ablation depth, and

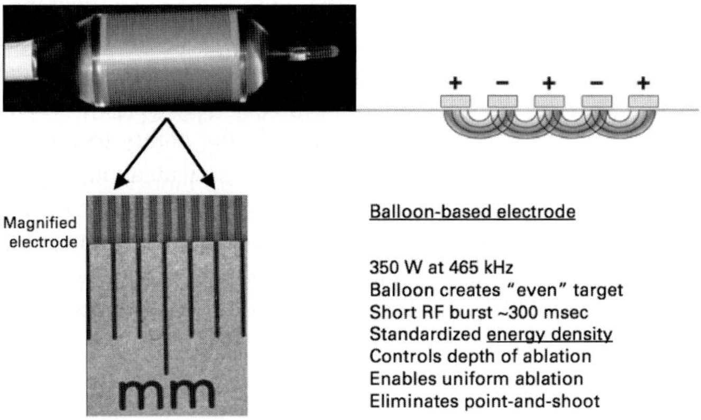

Figure 3. Balloon-based Halo^{360} electrode.

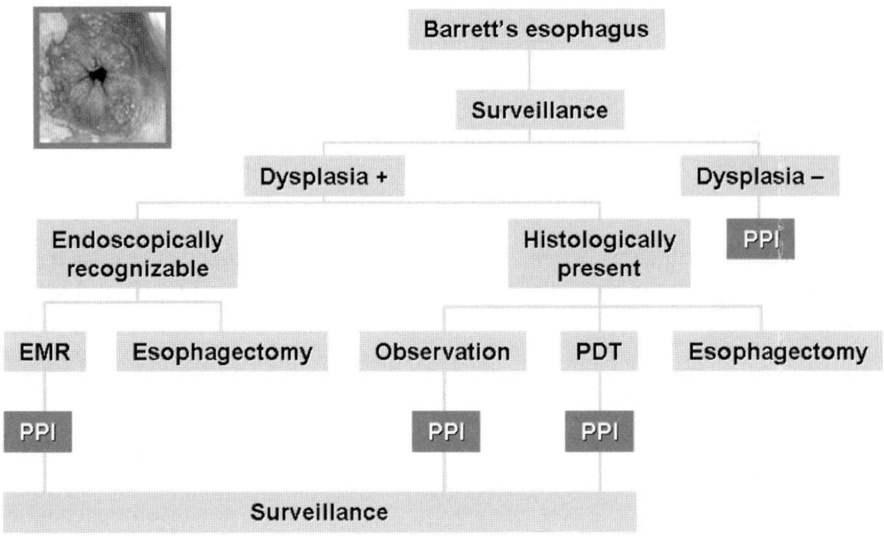

Figure 4. Algorithm for management of Barrett's esophagus.

residual ablation thickness. Outcomes were compared according to energy density group after one (1x) or two applications (2x). Complete epithelial ablation occurred in the following zones: 10 J/cm^2 (2x) and 12 J/cm^2 (1x and 2x) and the maximum depth of injury was the muscularis mucosae with a maximum thickness of residual ablation after tissue slough of 35 microns.

More recently, two ablation of intestinal metaplasia (AIM) multicenter clinical trials were reported from eight US sites. Both trials involved patients with non-dysplastic specialized intestinal metaplasia: AIM-I evaluated dose-response and safety of 6-12 J/cm^2; AIM-II evaluated safety and effectiveness of 10 J/cm^2 (two applications per session). To date, 28 of 32 patients (90%) in AIM-I have completed one-year follow-up and 67 of 70 patients (96%) in AIM-II have achieved 6 months follow-up. The primary histological endpoint for both AIM trials was the clearance of intestinal metaplasia. After treatment with the HALO^{360} system patients underwent follow-up endoscopy with biopsy sampling at 1, 3, 6 and 12 months. The biopsy protocol consisted of 4-quadrant tissue samples using maximum capacity endoscopic forceps, at a minimum of every 2 cm, from the Barrett's region. In addition, all non-squamous appearing islands are sampled. The AIM-I trial has generated 1,300 f/u biopsies from 32 patients while the AIM-II trial has generated 3,007 follow-up biopsies from 70 patients. Overall, 59-69% of all follow-up biopsy specimens demonstrated complete clearance of intestinal metaplasia and there were no biopsy specimens with signs of "buried glands" (defined as intestinal metaplasia overlain exclusively by reconstituted esophageal squamous epithelium) [5]. Current stricture rate including all patients (N = 600) treated in clinical studies and post-clinical studies is about 1 %.

In another US multicenter trial, the Halo^{360} system was used in 22 patients with HGD using 12 J/cm^2. The follow-up at 3-15 months has shown a mean regression of Barrett's esophagus of 96% and complete regression of metaplasia in 50% of cases. Complete regression of HGD occurred in 73% (50% to normal; 18% to metaplasia and 5% to low-grade dysplasia). Residual (unaffected) HGD was seen only in 5 patients, one of them with T1 cancer. There were no complications with the procedure.

As mentioned above, the ideal therapy for Barrett's esophagus should involve a single-session intervention, should be operator-independent, 100% effective in eliminating metaplasia and dysplasia, carry no complications and provide lifetime guarantee of no recurrence and 0% risk for cancer development (*Figure 2*). Although the Halo^{360} system appears very promising in many of these regards, further studies and long-term follow-up will be needed to validate its role in the management of Barrett's esophagus and where it fits amidst other available ablation or resection endoscopic techniques. Nevertheless, the proof of principle has been established that radiofrequency ablation can effectively eliminate metaplasia and dysplasia in the majority of patients and deserves our attention and early implementation in clinical practice. On the basis of this, we propose an algorithm for the overall management of Barrett's esophagus with and without dysplasia (*Figure 5*).

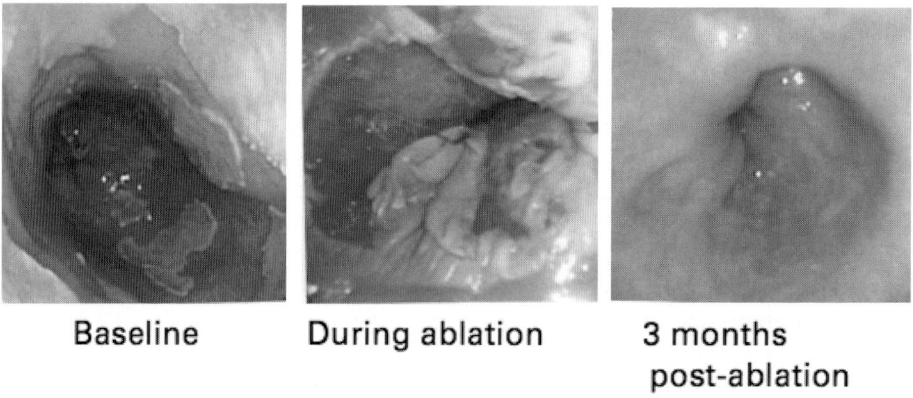

Figure 5. Long-segment Barrett's esophagus before, during and after radiofrequency ablation using Halo^{360} balloon system. (See page XXXII for colour figure).

References

1. Yeh RW, Triadafilopoulos G. Endoscopic therapy for Barrett's esophagus. Gastrointest Endosc Clin N Am 2005;15:377-97.
2. Sharma P, Wani S, Weston AP, et al. A randomized controlled trial of ablation of Barrett's esophagus with multipolar electrocoagulation versus argon plasma coagulation in combination with acid suppression: long term results. Gut. 2006;55:1233-9.
3. Panjehpour M, Overholt BF. Porfimer sodium photodynamic therapy for management of Barrett's esophagus with high-grade dysplasia. Lasers Surg Med. 2006;38:390-5.
4. Dunkin BJ, Martinez J, Bejarano PA, Smith CD, Chang K, Melvin WS. Thin-layer ablation of human esophageal epithelium using a bipolar radiofrequency balloon device (BARRX). Surg Endosc 2006;20:125-30.
5. Sharma VK, Wang KK, Overholt BF, et al. Circumferential endoscopic ablation of Barrett esophagus using a balloon-based system: 1-year follow-up of 100 patients. Gastrointest Endosc 2007;65:185-95.

Is it unequivocally necessary to combine laser ablation with antireflux surgery?

C.J. Lightdale (New York)

It has been well demonstrated since the early 1990's that endoscopic ablation of Barrett's mucosa combined with suppression of acid reflux can result in healing with squamous mucosa [1,2]. If Barrett's mucosa was the result of chronic injury by acid refluxate, ablating the Barrett's, a reversal injury, by laser or other means, seemed a logical therapy. The origin of the new squamous mucosa is presumed to be from pluripotential cells or stem cells perhaps in the submucosal glands or perhaps recruited from circulating stem cells originating in the bone marrow [3]. In theory, in the presence of acid, Barrett's mucosa is produced after injury; in the absence of acid, regeneration occurs with normal squamous mucosa.

Multiple methods useful for ablation of Barrett's mucosa have been developed in recent years. Lasers have been one method, and multiple lasers producing a thermal or heat ablation effect have been utilized. These include argon lasers, Nd:YAG lasers, and KTP-YAG lasers. Other methods resulting in thermal ablation that have been used to remove Barrett's mucosa include multipolar coagulation, argon plasma coagulation, and radiofrequency ablation. Freezing using liquid gas, most recently liquid nitrogen sprays, have also been employed. Photodynamic therapy, a photochemical ablation, using a systemic light sensitize drug activated by a low power laser, most recently diode lasers, have been extensively studied with impressive results in preventing esophageal cancer mortality in patients with Barrett's esophagus and high-grade dysplasia (HGD) [4,5].

From the beginning of ablation therapy for Barrett's esophagus, there have been questions regarding the level of acid suppression needed to achieve the best results of complete restoration of squamous mucosa and the avoidance of the development of new Barrett's mucosa. Medical acid suppression with proton pump inhibitor (PPI) medications have been used extensively. Some studies have measured esophageal pH to confirm acid suppression, while others have utilized high dose therapy, at least twice daily, and some even higher doses to ensure acid suppression [5].

Antireflux surgery has also been used with ablation to achieve and secure normal squamous epithelium following ablation therapy for Barrett's esophagus. The potential benefits of anitreflux surgery over PPIs include better acid reflux control and the elimination of gastroduodenal refluxate with other potential injurious agents, such as bile salts. The potential problems of antireflux surgery are the initial small risks of anesthesia and surgery (now usually laparoscopic), the possibility of decreased reflux control with time, and if surgery is performed before ablation, there is the possibility that complete ablation might be technically more difficult.

Ablation of Barrett's esophagus using a variety of thermal ablation methods combined with antireflux surgery has been reported to be successful in multiple small case series [6-11]. Salo reported in 1998 complete replacement of Barrett's mucosa with squamous epithelium in 9/11 patients treated with Nd:YAG laser ablation and antireflux surgery, and Bowers reported in 2003 similar success in 8/9 patients using KTP laser [6,8].

Multiple studies have shown that acid suppression with PPIs combined with ablation can be successful. The randomized trail of photodynamic therapy for Barrett's esophagus with HGD showed that twice daily doses of 20 mg omeprazole could be successful in achieving ablation of Barrett's esophagus with HGD [12]. Most recently, a complete ablation of Barrett's mucosa was achieved in 60/61 (98%) of patients treated with radiofrequency ablation combined with esomeprazole 40 mg twice daily at 2.5 years follow-up [13].

Is it unequivocally necessary to combine laser ablation with antireflux surgery? Unequivocally no! Ablation combined with antireflux surgery is feasible and safe, but PPI therapy has also been safe and successful combined with ablation in replacing Barrett's mucosa with normal squamous mucosa. Whether antireflux surgery is superior to PPI therapy in achieving complete elimination of Barrett's mucosa and preventing recurrence after ablation therapy remains an open question, however, and demands a randomized comparative trial.

References

1. Berenson MM, Johnson TD, Markowitz NR, et al. Restoration of squamous mucosa after ablation of Barrett's esophageal epithelium. Gastroenterology 1993;104:1855-8.
2. Sampliner RE, Hixson LJ, Fennerty MB, Garewal HS. Regression of Barrett's esophagus buy laser ablation in an anacid environment. Dig Dis Sci 1993;38:365-8.
3. Houghton J, Stoicov C, Nomura S, et al. Gastric cancer originating from bone marrow-derived cells. Science 2004;306:1455-7.
4. Sampliner RE. Ablative therapies for the columnar-lined esophagus. Gastroenterol Clin North Am 1997;26:685-94.
5. Spechler SJ. Thermal ablation of Barrett's esophagus: a heated debate. Am J Gastroenterol 2006;101:1770-2.
6. Salo JA, Salminen JT, Kiviluoto TA, et al. Treatment of Barrett's esophagus by endoscopic laser ablation and antireflux surgery. Ann Surg 1998;227:40-4.
7. Montes CG, Brandalise NA, Deliza R, et al. Antireflux surgery followed by bipolar Electrocoagulation in the treatment of Barrett's esophagus. Gastrointest Endosc 1999;50:173-7.
8. Bowers SP, Mattear SG, Waring PJ, et al. KTP laser ablation of Barrett's esophagus after anti-reflux surgery results in long-term loss of intestinal metaplasia. Surg Endosc 2003;17:49-54.
9. Morino M, Rebecchi F, Giaccone C, et al. Endoscopic ablation of Barrett's esophagus using argon plasma coagulation (APC) following surgical laparoscopic fundoplication. Surg Endosc 2003;17:539-42.
10. Pagani M, Granelli P, Chella B, et al. Barrett's esophagus: combined treatment using argon plasma coagulation and laparoscopic antireflux surgery. Dis Esoph 2003;16:279-83.

11. Pinotti AC, Cecconello T, Filho FM, et al. Endoscopic ablation of Barrett's esophagus using argon plasma coagulation: a prospective study after fundoplication. Dis Esoph 2004;17:243-6.
12. Overholt BF, Lightdale CJ, Wang KK, et al. Photodynamic therapy with porfimer sodium for ablation of high-grade dysplasia in Barrett's esophagus: international, partially blinded, randomized phase III trial. Gastrointest Endosc 2005;62:499-503.
13. Fleischer DE, Overholt BF, Sharma VK, et al. Long-term (2,5 year) follow-up of the AIM-II trial for ablation of Barrett's esophagus: results after primary circumferential ablation followed by secondary focal ablation. Gastrointest Endosc 2007;65:AB135.

High rate of lymph node metastasis in submucosal Barrett's cancer. Consequences for choice of therapy

A.H. Hölscher, E. Bollschweiler (Köln)

Lymphatic spread of mucosal and submucosal adenocarcinomas of the esophagus is strongly correlating with the deepness of wall infiltration. Therefore it is appropriate to differentiate early cancer in mucosal and submucosal carcinomas. Further mucosa as well as submucosa should be subdivided concerning three thirds of deepness of infiltration (*Figure 1*). The resulting six tissue layers m1, m2, m3, sm1, sm2, sm3 allow a more detailed evaluation of lymph node metastasis in early esophageal cancer. The frequency of patients with early adenocarcinoma of the esophagus according to the above mentioned classification is shown in *Table I*. According to the current surgical literature mucosal and submucosal cancers are distributed about half to half. This will change in the future in favour of submucosal adenocarcinoma in the surgical series as mucosal lesions are more and more treated endoscopically. Within the submucosal layer sm1 and sm3 cancers are nearly equally distributed whereas sm2 is quite rare.

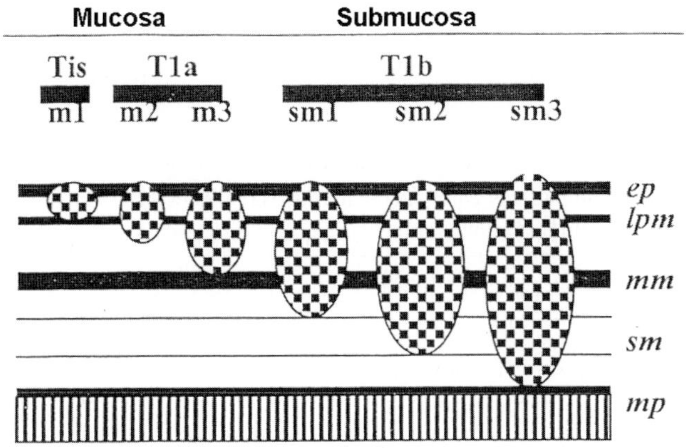

Figure 1. Early carcinoma: depth of tumor infiltration.

Table I. Frequency of patients with early adenocarcinoma of the esophagus.

	pT1 m/sm	sm1 n (%)	sm2 n (%)	sm3 n (%)
Liu 2005 [5]	53/37	12 (8%)		25 (36%)
Westerterp 2005 [6]	54/66	25 (0%)	23 (35%)	18 (67%)
Bollschweiler 2006 [1]	26/26	10 (20%)	6 (0%)	10 (70%)
Total	133/129	47 (18%)	29 (11%)	53 (20%)
%	51%/49%			

Concerning the question of lymph node metastasis in the different layers of early esophageal adenocarcinoma we analysed our own material of 54 patients [1]. Forty-six of these cases had transthoracic esophagectomy and 6 transhiatal esophagectomy. The average number of resected lymph nodes was 29 with a range of 13 to 45. The R0 resection rate was 100%. Twenty-six patients had mucosal cancer (pT1a) and another 26 had submucosal carcinoma (pT1b). None of the patients with mucosal cancer had lymph node metastasis. The rate of lymph node metastasis in patients with submucosal cancer however was 35% (n = 9) [1]. The frequency of lymph node metastasis in sm1 (n = 10) was 20%, in sm2 (n = 6) 0% and in sm3 (n = 10) 70%. The distribution of the lymph node metastasis of the 26 submucosal cancer was 36.4% abdominal lymph nodes, 4.6% infrabifurcal lymph nodes, 9.1% lymph nodes at the bifurcation and 4.6% above the bifurcation. No patient had lymph nodes along the recurrent laryngeal nerve chain.

The comparison of the data to the literature shows in the analysis of 246 patients with mucosal adenocarcinoma of the esophagus only 2% lymph node metastasis (*Table II*). The analysis of 3 reports on detailed differentiation of the 3 submucosal layers in 129 patients results in 7% lymph node metastasis for patients with sm1, 29% for sm2 and 53% for sm3 (*Table III*).

Table II. Lymph node-metastasis in patients with pT1a (mucosa) adenocarcinoma of the esophagus.

Author	Mucosa	Lymph node metastasis
Van Sandick 2000 [7]	12	0 (0%)
Hagen 2001 [8]	16	0 (0%)
Rice 2001 [9]	53	2 (4%)
Stein 2003 [10]	27	0 (0%)
Liu 2005 [5]	53	2 (4%)
Westerterp 2005 [6]	54	1 (2%)
Bollschweiler 2006 [1]	26	0 (0%)
Oh 2006 [11]	23	1 (4%)
Total	246	6 (2%)

Table III. Lymph node metastases (LNM) in patients with pT1b (submucosa) adenocarcinoma of the esophagus, submucosa divided in 3 thirds: sm1, sm2 and sm3.

Authors	Mucosa (% LNM)	sm1 (% LNM)	sm2 (% LNM)	sm3 (% LNM)
Liu 2005 [5]	53 (4%)	12 (8%)	–	25 (36%)
Westerterp 2005 [6]	54 (2%)	25 (0%)	23 (35%)	18 (67%)
Bollschweiler 2006 [1]	22 (0%)	10 (20%)	5 (0%)	10 (70%)
Total	131 (2%)	47 (7%)	28 (29%)	53 (53%)

The rate of lymph node metastasis in patients with submucosal esophageal cancer is depending on the radicality of surgical resection and especially the extent of lymphadenectomy. Four series with 2-field or 3-field lymphadenectomy in the frame of transthoracic en bloc-esophagectomy give a frequency of lymph node metastasis in pT1b adenocarcinoma of 31% to 50% (*Table IV*). On the contrary three series with limited lymphadenectomy by transhiatal esophagectomy or just distal esophageal resection (Merendino operation) show 0 to 30% lymph node metastasis (*Table V*). In conclusion only series with at least 2-field lymphadenectomy and transthoracic esophagectomy are appropriate to show the real status of lymph node metastasis in submucosal esophageal cancer.

Table IV. Lymph node metastases (LNM) in patients with pT1b adenocarcinoma of the esophagus.

	Therapy	Nb of patients	Frequency of LNM
Altorki 2000 [12]	TTE + 3-field LAD	4	50%
Lerut 2004 [13]	TTE + 3-field LAD	23	35%
Hagen 2001 [8]	TTE + 2-field LAD	16	31%
Bollschweiler 2006 [1]	TTE + 2-field LAD	22	41%
TTE: transthoracic esophagectomy; LAD: lymphadenectomy			

Table V. Lymph node metastases in patients with pT1b adenocarcinoma of the esophagus.

	Therapy	Nb of patients	Frequency of LNM
van Sandick 2000 [7]	THE or TTE	20	30%
Hölscher 1997	THE (TTE)	24	21%
Stein 2000 [10]	Merendino	6	0%
TTE: transthoracic esophagectomy; THE, transhiatal esophagectomy			

Conclusion

Because of the absence or very low rate of lymph node metastasis in mucosal adenocarcinoma of the esophagus endoscopic resection of small pT1a lesions (< 2 cm) seems to be appropriate. This is confirmed by the results of different series of endoscopic resection of mucosal esophageal adenocarcinomas [2]. If mucosal adenocarcinoma is too large for endoscopic resection or shows multifocality within the columnar cell lined lower esophagus a limited esophageal resection especially by Merendino operation is a good option. For all submucosal adenocarcinomas transthoracic en bloc esophagectomy and 2-field lymphadenectomy is the treatment of choice because of the high rate of lymph node metastasis. These patients have the chance to be healed by radical surgery and therefore limited resections with reduced radicality could miss the chance for cure of this stage of cancer.

In the future more detailed analysis of submucosal esophageal adenocarcinomas using molecular biomarkers will be performed [3,4]. This could lead to the definition of risk groups with more or less tendency to lymphatic metastasis. This could allow further refinement of therapeutic consequences.

References

1. Bollschweiler E, Baldus S, Schroder W, et al. High rate of lymph-node metastasis in submucosal esophageal squamous-cell carcinomas and adenocarcinomas. Endoscopy 2006;38:149-56.
2. Ell C, May A, Gossner L, et al. Endoscopic mucosal resection of early cancer and high-grade dysplasia in Barrett's esophagus. Gastroenterology 2000;118:670-7.
3. Stein H, Feith M, Mueller J, Werner M, Siewert J. Limited resection for early adenocarcinoma in Barrett's esophagus. Ann Surg 2000;232:733-42.
4. Gutschow C, Schröder W, Wolfgarten E, Hölscher AH. Merendino procedure with preservation of the vagus for early carcinoma of the gastroesophageal junction. Zentralbl Chir 2004;129:276-81.
5. Liu L, Hofstetter W, Rashid A, et al. Significance of the depth of tumor invasion in early (T1) esophageal adenocarcinoma. Modern Pathology 2005;18:110A-110A.
6. Westerterp M, Koppert L, Buskens C, et al. Outcome of surgical treatment for early adenocarcinoma of the esophagus or gastro-esophageal junction. Virchows Arch 2005;446:497-504.
7. van Sandick J, van Lanschot J, ten Kate F, Tijssen J, Obertop H. Indicators of prognosis after transhiatal esophageal resection without thoracotomy for cancer. J Am Coll Surg 2002;194:28-36.
8. Hagen J, De Meester S, Peters J, Chandrasoma P, De Meester T. Curative resection for esophageal adenocarcinoma: analysis of 100 en bloc esophagectomies. Ann Surg 2001;234:520-31.
9. Rice T, Blackstone E, Goldblum J, et al. Superficial adenocarcinoma of the esophagus. J Thorac Cardiovasc Surg 2001;122:1077-90.
10. Stein H, Feith M, von_Rahden B, Siewert J, Rahden B. Approach to early Barrett's cancer. World J Surg 2003;27:1040-6.
11. Oh DS, Hagen JA, T Chandrasoma P, et al. Clinical biology and surgical therapy of intramucosal adenocarcinoma of the esophagus. J Am Coll Surg 2006;203:152-61.
12. Altorki N. Three-field lymphadenectomy for esophageal cancer. Chest Surg Clin N Am 2000;10:553-60.
13. Lerut T, Coosemans W, Decker G, De LP, Moons J, Nafteux P, Van RD. Extended surgery for cancer of the esophagus and gastroesophageal junction. J Surg Res 2004;117:58-63.
14. Vallbohmer D, Marjoram P, Kuramochi H, et al. Towards the molecular characterization of disease: Comparison of molecular and histological analysis of esophageal epithelia. Ejc Supp 2006;4:48-48.
15. Brabender J, Marjoram P, Lord R, et al. The molecular signature of normal squamous esophageal epithelium identifies the presence of a field effect and can discriminate between patients with Barrett's esophagus and patients with Barrett's-associated adenocarcinoma. Cancer Epidemiol Biomark Prev 2005;14:2113-7.

Vagus-sparing esophagectomy and antrally-innervated stomach

J.M. Collard, R. Romagnoli, L. Goncette, C. Gutschow (Brussels)

Classic esophagectomy with truncal vagotomy

Basically, subtotal esophagectomy includes the division of both vagus nerves in the chest, because they run very close to the wall of the thoracic segment of the esophagus. This is particularly the case when all the tissues and lymph nodes in the posterior mediastinum are removed en-bloc with the esophageal tube [1,3].

We know that truncal vagotomy disturbs the functioning of all the organs of the digestive system. It impairs fundic relaxation, antral propulsive activity, pyloric relaxation, gallbladder contractility, and possibly results in diarrhea, dumping or gastric stasis, early satiety, increased antral exposure to duodenal contents, and even cholelithiasis [4-9].

Spontaneous recovery of both motor and secretory functions of the vagotomized stomach in relation to reorganization of the nervous plexuses within the gastric wall takes years to complete [10-12] so that in the mean time, quality of the alimentary comfort is far from satisfactory [13]. However, prolonged administration of a motilin-receptor agonist such as erythromycin enhances the spontaneous motor recovery process that takes place within the gastric wall, resulting in a better ability of the denervated stomach to accommodate, grind, and expel ingested food at early follow-up [14].

In order to avoid these side-effects, the concept of vagus-sparing esophagectomy was introduced years ago by Akiyama [15].

Vagus-sparing esophagectomy

Vagus-sparing esophagectomy precludes any lymph node clearance in the posterior mediastinum and along the lesser curvature of the stomach, as well. It should therefore be reserved for esophageal replacement in patients who undergo subtotal esophagectomy for either end-stage benign esophageal disease or high-grade dysplasia (HGD) arising in Barrett's [16,17].

Nowadays, when endoscopic peacemeal mucosectomy is more and more used to treat Barrett's HGD, resection of the whole length of the thoracic esophagus is to be considered in the presence of a long-segment Barrett's due to the possible co-existence of several invisible dysplastic histologic changes allover the metaplastic area. Another reason for considering esophagectomy (removal of full thickness of the esophageal wall) in a Barrett's patient with HGD is the risk for the presence of a deeper neoplastic lesion that cannot always be evidenced before treatment in spite of the use of more and more sophisticated endoscopic screening methods [16].

Sharp dissection of the esophageal wall under visual control by right thoracotomy or better, transhiatal stripping of the esophagus [15] allow safe separation of the nerves from the esophageal wall, so that the stomach is likely to keep most of its functions. After its downward stripping, the esophageal conduit is extracted outside of the gastric cavity through a small incision in the anterior aspect of the subcardiac area of the stomach (*Figure 1, left*). The gastroesophageal junction is divided by application of a linear stapler on its everted mucosal surface before the anterior subcardiac incision is sutured (*Figure 1, right*). Depending on the way the stripper is secured to the wall of the cervical esophagus (i.e., the mucosal coat or full thickness of the organ), the maneuver results in a single-piece mucosectomy or rather, in the resection of the whole esophageal tube. In the former instance, the muscle coat of the esophagus is left in the posterior mediastinum, which leads to position the esophageal substitute in the substernal space. On the other hand, when full thickness of the esophageal wall has been stripped, there is a need for the enlargement of the esophageal bed using large-balloon dilatation of the posterior mediastinal channel to give room to the esophageal substitute.

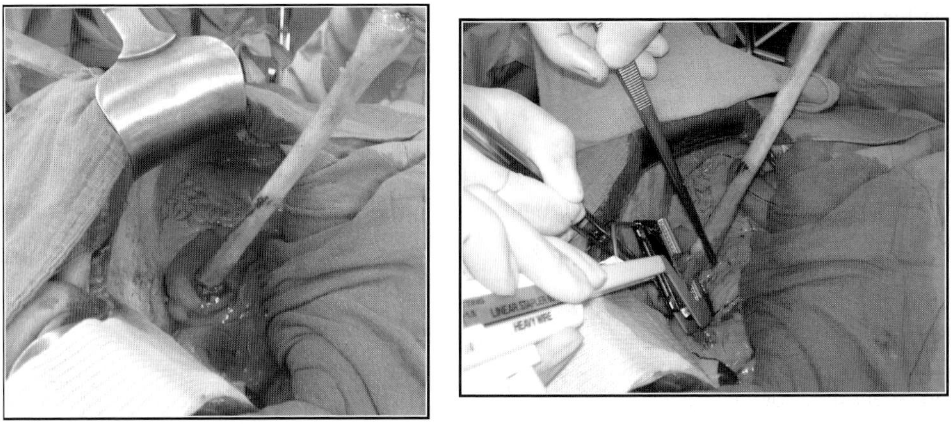

Figure 1. Extraction of the stripped esophagus through a subcardiac opening (left), and stapling division of the subcardiac area of the stomach (right).

Antrally-innervated whole stomach

Ten years ago, we described an original technique of gastric tailoring that allows both elevation of the whole stomach up to the neck as esophageal replacement and preservation of the vagal supply to the whole digestive apparatus except the gastric fundus [18,19].

After separation of the stripped esophagus from the stomach by stapling division of the gastric wall, the two-thirds of the lesser curvature proximal to the crow's foot are denuded by division of the terminal rami of the left gastric vessels flush with the gastric wall according to an original principle described previously [20,21] (*Figure 2*). Both nerves of Latarjet as well as the hepatic branches of the left vagus nerve within the lesser omentum are carefully identified and preserved. Such a dissection is similar to a proximal gastric vagotomy, an operation we were still performing a decade ago in patients suffering from chronic duodenal ulcer disease. No pyloroplasty is performed. The whole stomach is extracted outside of the abdominal cavity through the upper midline incision after division of both left gastroepiploic and short gastric vessels. The gastric pouch is inserted into a plastic bag, the fundus is sutured to the funnel of a Mousseau-Barbin's tube, and the antrally-innervated stomach is elevated up to the neck through either the posterior or the anterior mediastinum without any tension

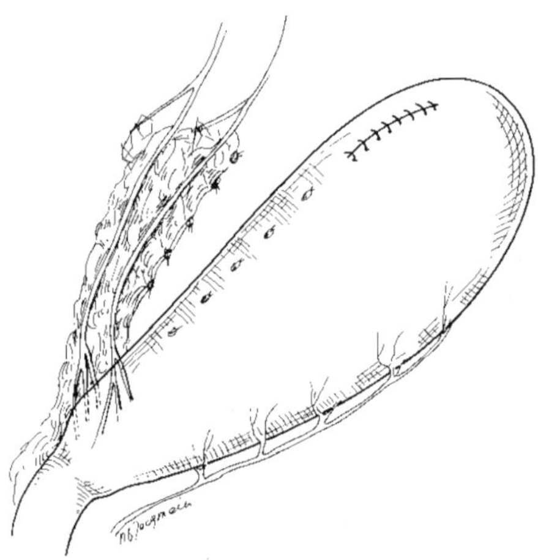

Figure 2. Denudation of the two-thirds of the lesser curvature proximal to the crow's foot flush with the gastric wall (black arrow) while respecting the two nerves of Latarjet in the lesser omentum.

on the gastric wall. A terminalized side-to-side semi-mechanical esophagogastrostomy is performed in the neck according to an original technique described previously [22].

Simple visualization of the antrum just before the elevation of the antrally-innervated stomach through the mediastinum at the operation reveals in most patients the presence of gastric contractions that sweep over the distal part of the stomach towards the pylorus, a phenomenon which is never noticed after bilateral truncal vagotomy.

High-amplitude peristaltic antral contractions occurring at a rate of about 3 cycles per minute are present on Barium swallow series (*Figure 3*) a few weeks post-operatively.

Intragastric manometry tracings also show the maintenance of a sustained motor activity in the antrum (*Figure 4*), which is quite different from the situation with the vagotomized stomach in which only flat curves are seen at early follow-up.

Gastric exposure to bile at 24-hour gastric bile monitoring with the Bilitec™ optoelectronic device usually is within the range of values obtained from healthy volunteers. In this respect, we showed in a previous study [9] that denervation of the antrum, pylorus and gallbladder together with the elevation of the gastric pouch up to the neck increase gastric exposure to bile significantly, unless a pyloroplasty is performed and a prokinetics such as erythromycin is given on a regular basis.

A drawback of the procedure is the maintenance of a normal intragastric acid profile with the percentage of time that intragastric pH is < 2 below the 5th percentile of controls. We know however that even after bilateral truncal vagotomy, acid secretion is not altered in a significant way in about 40% of patients, and that sooner or later, almost all the other patients with a decreased acid secretion just after the operation recover a normal intragastric acid profile at 24-hour gastric pH monitoring [11].

Although having a very good alimentary comfort, most patients have an early sensation of post-prandial fullness when overeating [4-6]. This symptomatology is likely related to

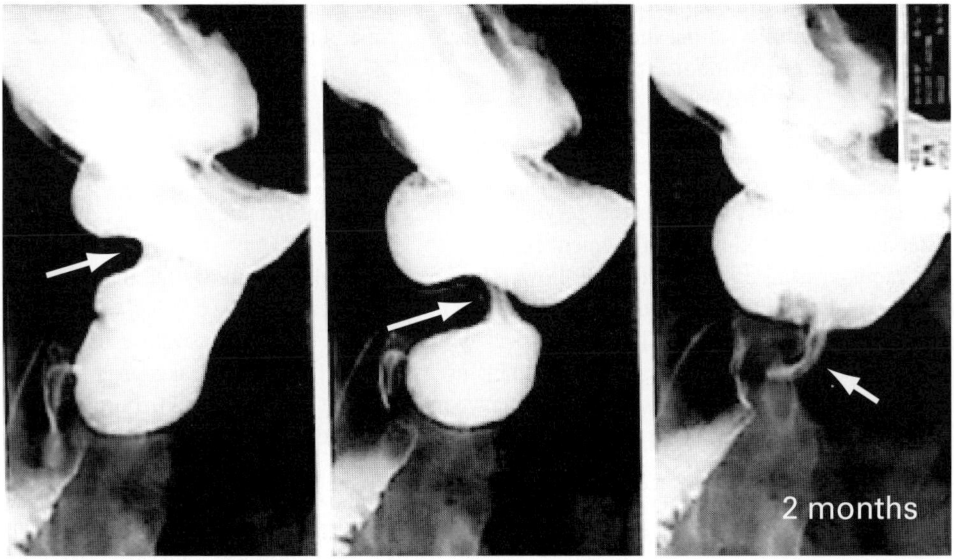

Figure 3. Upper G-I series showing a propulsive (white arrows, from left to right) antral contraction that punches the pylorus (right) 6 weeks post-operatively.

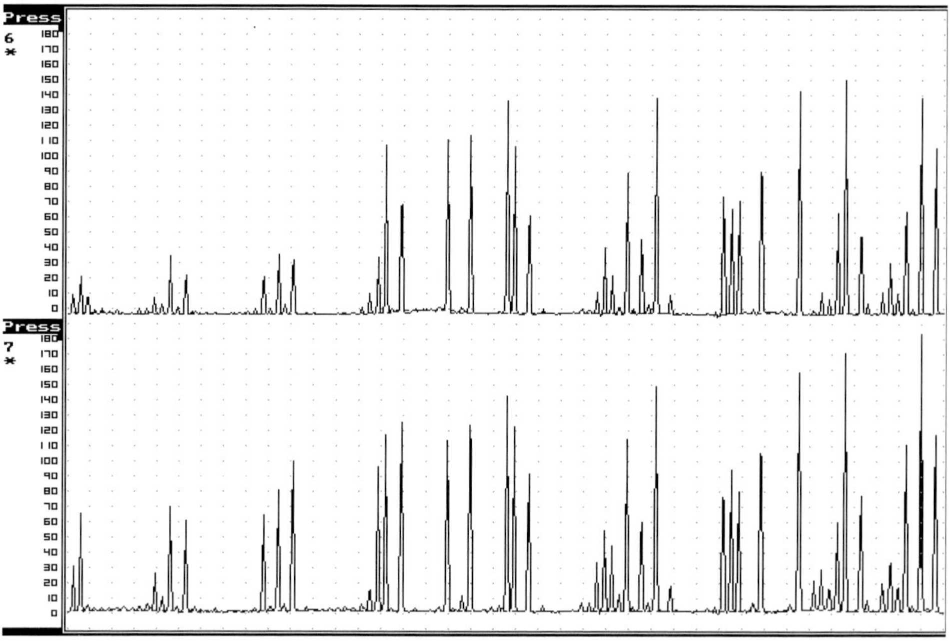

Figure 4. Manometric strips from 2 antral channels showing high-amplitude peristaltic contractions 6 weeks post-operatively. The distances between sides holes of the manometric probe and the pylorus are 2 cm (upper tracing) and 1 cm (lower tracing), respectively.

the denervation of the gastric fundus, a maneuver that impairs gastric wall relaxation at meals [6]. Another explanation for this residual sensation of post-prandial fullness could be the relative inability of the intrathoracic stomach to expand at mealtimes, cramped it is in the posterior mediastinum.

Colon interposition

Digestive continuity between the cervical esophageal stump and the stomach can be re-established with a long colon segment [23].

Vagus-sparing esophagectomy followed by colon interposition allows the maintenance of the vagal supply to the fundus together with a better protection of the cervical esophageal stump against acid reflux. The latter aspect is emphasized by the observation that about 40% of patients having a gastric transplant as esophageal substitute take proton pump inhibitors on a regular basis beyond three years after the operation [11]. Furthermore, metaplasia, either cardiac or intestinal, may develop in the cervical esophageal remnant over time [11].

As far as the alimentary comfort is concerned, Banki *et al.* [24] have interestingly shown that both the calorie consumption rate (number of calories ingested per minute) and percentage of meal consumed are far higher after vagus-sparing esophagectomy and colon interposition than after classic esophagectomy including division of both vagus nerves.

Advantages of the colon over the stomach as an esophageal substitute after vagus-sparing esophagectomy are to be weighted up with the fact that about 30 % of patients with a colonic graft may require revisional surgery to treat late mechanical complications such as anastomotic stricture or graft rebundancy [25] in the long run. In addition, the presence of severe atheromatous lesions in supplying arteries or of unfavorable congenital variations in the mesocolic vasculature may predispose to necrosis of the colic graft in the postoperative period [26].

In any event, performance of a vagus-sparing esophagectomy allows the maintenance of the vagal input to the organs of the digestive tract in patients who require an esophagectomy for benign or dysplastic disease of the esophagus. This technique meets functional requirements of an operation made on patients with a long-life expectancy.

References

1. Collard JM, Otte JB, Fiasse R, et al. Skeletonizing en bloc esophagectomy for cancer. Ann Surg 2001;234:25-32.
2. Collard JM. Exclusive radical surgery for esophageal adenocarcinoma. Cancer 2001;91:1098-104.
3. Collard JM, Romagnoli R, Hermans BP, Malaise J. Radical esophageal resection for adenocarcinoma arising in Barrett's esophagus. Am J Surg 1997;174:307-11.
4. Stoddard CJ, Smallwood R, Brown BH, Duthie HL. The immediate and delayed effects of different types of vagotomy on human gastric myoelectrical activity. Gut 1975;16:165-70.
5. Wilbur BG, Kelly KA. Effect of proximal gastric, complete gastric, and truncal vagotomy on canine gastric electric activity, motility and emptying. Ann Surg 1973;178:295-303.
6. Stadaas JO. Intragastric pressure/volume relationship before and after proximal gastric vagotomy. Scand J Gastroenterol 1975;10:129-34.
7. Ihasz M, Griffith CA. Gallstones after vagotomy. Am J Surg 1981;141:48-50.
8. Baxter JN, Grime JS, Critchley M, et al. Relationship between gastric emptying of a solid meal and emptying of the gall bladder before and after vagotomy. Gut 1987;28:855-63.
9. Gutschow CA, Collard JM, Romagnoli R, et al. Bile exposure of the denervated stomach as an esophageal substitute. Ann Thorac Surg 2001;71:1786-91.
10. Collard JM, Romagnoli R. Human stomach has a recordable mechanical activity at a rate of about three cycles/minute. Eur J Surg 2001;167:188-94.
11. Gutschow C, Collard JM, Romagnoli R, Salizzoni M, Hölscher A. Denervated stomach as an esophageal substitute recovers intraluminal acidity with time. Ann Surg 2001;233:509-14.
12. Collard JM, Romagnoli R, Otte JB, Kestens PJ. The denervated stomach as an esophageal substitute is a contractile organ. Ann Surg 1998;227:33-9.
13. Collard JM, Otte JB, Reynaert M, Kestens PJ. Quality of life three years or more after esophagectomy for cancer. J Thorac Cardiovasc Surg 1992;104:391-4.
14. Collard JM, Romagnoli R, Otte JB, Kestens PJ. Erythromycin enhances early postoperative contractility of the denervated whole stomach as an esophageal substitute. Ann Surg 1999;229:337-43.
15. Akiyama H, Tsurumaru M, Kawamura T, et al. Esophageal stripping with preservation of the vagus nerve. Int Surg 1982;67:125-8.
16. Collard JM. High-grade dysplasia in Barrett's esophagus. The case for esophagectomy. Chest Surg Clin N Am 2002;12:77-92.
17. Romagnoli R, Collard JM, Gutschow C, Yamusah N, Salizzoni M. Outcome of dysplasia arising in Barrett's esophagus: a dynamic view. J Am Coll Surg 2003;197;365-71.
18. Collard JM. The stomach as an esophageal substitute after total or subtotal esophagectomy. Thesis, Louvain Medical School, Brussels, Belgium, 1997:56-66.
19. Collard JM, Romagnoli R, Goncette L, Gutschow C. Whole stomach with antro-pyloric nerve preservation as an esophageal substitute: an original technique. Dis Esophagus 2004;17:164-7.
20. Collard JM, Otte JB, Jamart J, Reynaert M, Kestens PJ An original technique for lengthening the stomach as an esophageal substitute after oesophagectomy. Preliminary results. Dis Esophagus 1989; 2 : 171-174.
21. Collard JM, Tinton N, Malaise J, Romagnoli R, Otte JB, Kestens PJ. Esophageal replacement: gastric tube or whole stomach? Ann Thorac Surg 1995;60:261-7.
22. Collard JM, Romagnoli R, Goncette L, Otte JB, Kestens PJ. Terminalized semimechanical side-to-side suture technique for cervical esophagogastrostomy. Ann Thorac Surg 1998;65:814-7.
23. Nigro JJ, Hagen JA, Demeester TR, et al. Occult esophageal adenocarcinoma: extent of disease and implications for effective therapy. Ann Surg 1999;230:433-40.

24. Banki F,Mason RJ, DeMeester SR, et al. Vagal-sparing esophagectomy: a more physiologic alternative. Ann Surg 2002;236:324-35.
25. Jeyasingham K, Lerut T, Belsey RHR. Functional and mechanical sequelae of colon interposition for benign disease. Eur J Cardiovasc Surg 1999;15:327-31.
26. Sonneland J, Anson BJ, Beaton LE. Surgical anatomy of the arterial supply to the colon from the superior mesenteric artery based upon a study of 600 specimens. Surg Gynecol Obstet 1958;106:385-98.

Current satus and future directions for tumor vaccines in the clinical setting

M. Gibson (Baltimore)

Esophageal cancer, especially adenocarcinoma, is a disease with increasing incidence and high mortality. At diagnosis, approximately 50% of patients have advanced, incurable disease while of the remaining with locally advanced stages, at most 30% are cured with modern combined modality therapy. With the development of molecular medicine and tumor immunology, targeted therapies with small molecules and immunologic approaches with monoclonal antibodies and tumor vaccines are under clinical use and investigation for treatment of pre-malignancy and malignant neoplasms. These approaches provide an opportunity for improving treatment of esophageal cancer.

In order to investigate novel approaches to Barrett's esophagus and esophageal cancer, our group uses an animal model of surgically created duodenal-esophageal reflux (DER). With this model, we generated both Barrett's esophagus and adenosquamous cancer from which we generated three cell lines that appear histologically as squamous cell carcinoma (SCC) but retain certain molecular features of adenocarcinoma.

With the availability of these *in vivo* and *in vitro* models, and thus the ability to test new therapies for Barrett's esophagus and esophageal cancer, we proceeded to investigate a tumor vaccine approach to treatment of esophageal cancer. Our group pioneered the use of GM-CSF secreting whole-cell allogeneic tumor vaccines for the treatment of breast and pancreatic cancer. Based on the promising work in these diseases, we aimed to produce a similar vaccine for Barrett's esophagus and esophageal cancer. In this paper, we describe the creation of the animal model and vaccine, and the subsequent testing of the efficacy of this vaccine in a rat allograft model.

Methods

All procedures were prospectively approved by the Animal Care and Use Committee (ACUC) of Johns Hopkins University and animals received humane care in compliance with the "Guide for Care and use of Laboratory Animals", published by the National Research Council (National Academy Press, 1996). Animals were acclimatized in a central animal facility for 2 week before the experiments. Rats and mice were anesthetized with an intramuscular injection of ketamine and xylazine.

Surgical model of reflux induced esophageal tumors

Biliary reflux was induced in 10 week old, male Sprague Dawley rats, (200-250 gms, Harlan, Indianapolis, IN). The animals were allowed two weeks to acclimatize, and were housed at temperature of 20-22°C, humidity of 30-50% at 12 hour alternating light-dark cycles. The rats were fasted overnight, but allowed water *ad libitum* until the surgery. Briefly the esophagus was mobilized preserving the vagus nerves, and a loop of jejunum was then identified 4 cm from the ligament of Treitz. The gastroesophageal junction (GEJ) was divided and ligated, and an end-to-side anastomosis was constructed between the distal esophagus and jejunum (modified Levrat's model [1]). Once the animals awoke, they were allowed water *ad libitum*, and feeding recommenced the following day. Animals received appropriate analgesia during the peri-operative and post-operative periods. The experiment concluded 9 months post-operatively.

Harvesting of the tumors

Animals were anaesthetized as described before. Abdominal and thoracic viscera were exposed through a midline incision, and the tumor was assessed for size, and extent. The esophagus was mobilized from the neck down to and including the esophagojejunal anastomosis. The tumors were identified and carefully dissected away from the liver and adjoining structures. The esophagus was opened longitudinally to expose the lumen, and a small representative portion of tissue was then excised from the tumor mass and preserved in 10% formalin for histological examination. The tumors were then harvested and washed immediately with PBS solution to remove any food debris and contaminants and then stored in PBS at 4°C and transported to the laboratory for tissue culture.

Establishment of cell lines

- **Creation and propagation of JA, JB and Amy cell lines**

Tumors were harvested 9 months after surgical creation of reflux in rats. Tumors were mechanically minced and then enzymatically digested using collagenase. The disaggregated cells were then plated in appropriate growth media as a primary culture. The culture plates were checked for the presence of cancer cells everyday. After adequate growth, a single clone was picked using a cloning ring and transferred to 96 well plates. We froze and stored aliquots of the original lineage. Other cells continue to undergo passages (over 40) without changing phenotype [2].

Three new cell lines were created by *in vitro* propagation of two resected cancers that developed in the rat tumor model of esophageal cancer – the JA and JB lines from one case, and the AMY cell line from the other. We froze aliquots of the original then utilized these cells lines for creation of the vaccine.

Creation of tumor vaccine

To create the vaccine cells, we used electroporation to transfect a DNA expression vector, pCDNA3 (CONTROL) or mGM-pCDNA3.1 (with mGM-CSF), from Invitrogen Life Technologies, Carlsbad, CA into the cell lines. This approach is previously described by our group [3]. The efficiency of the transfection was checked by estimating the amount of GM-CSF secreted by the transfected cells using a Quantikine ELISA kit (R&D systems, Minneapolis, MN).

Allografts and vaccination of animals

Allografts developed from the tumor cell lines were established in rats. The rats were vaccinated according to the schedules described in the results section, and tumor growth was assessed by measuring the bi-dimensional size of the tumor. Inhibition of tumor growth was compared to tumor in non-vaccinated animals and plotted graphically. Tumor histology was evaluated by routine H&E staining.

Results

In vivo tumor and cell lines

We successfully established a surgically-induced gastroduodenal reflux model (*Figure 1*) which leads to pre-malignant lesions of Barrett's esophagus and progresses through dysplasia to carcinoma of the esophagus. Similar results are reported by other groups [4-8]. In our model, 75% of the animals developed Barrett's esophagus and 50% progressed to carcinoma. This model has the great advantage of producing both Barrett's metaplasia as well as carcinoma, which is the target of our vaccine. The tumors arose from the field of Barrett's esophagus and were adenosquamous in character, with a Barrett's component (*Figure 1*).

Three new cell lines were created by *in vitro* propagation of two resected cancers that developed in the rat tumor model of esophageal cancer – the JA and JB lines from one case,

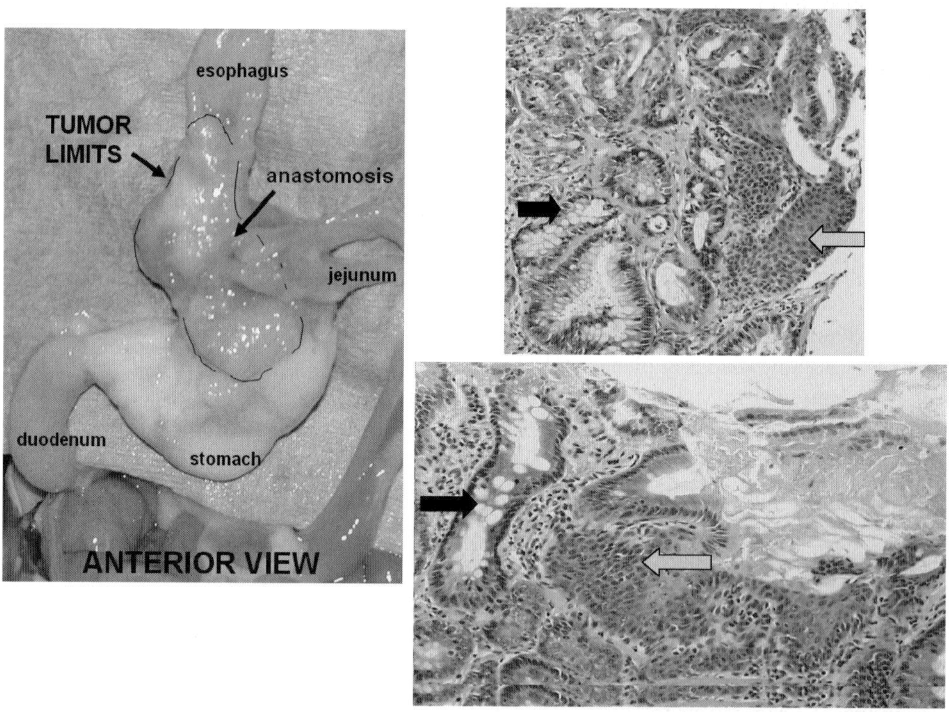

Figure 1. Surgical model of esophageal adenocarcinoma (grey arrow: normal squamous epithelium; black arrow: Barrett's columnar metaplasia with goblet cells). (See page XXXIII for colour figure).

and the AMY cell line from the other. We have demonstrated the ability of these cell lines to propagate long-term *in vitro* and to form tumors *in vivo* (i.e., xenografts) in athymic mice as a proof of malignant potential.

We froze aliquots of the original cells. With of to 40 passages, there has been no morphological change in any of the three cell lines. The cytospin histology of the JA and JB cell lines shows well differentiated squamous cell cancer while the cytospin of the AMY cell line showed rare presence of mucinous cells. The underlying histology of the JA and JB tumor which were established from the same tumor sample was adenosquamous while the AMY cell line was established from an adenocarcinoma.

To further characterize these cell lines, cytogenetics and gene profiling were done. Cytogenetic analysis confirmed a highly aneuploid cell population with derangement of key chromosomes which encode for a variety of oncogenes, thus confirming the neoplastic nature of these reflux induced tumors. The gene expression profile of these reflux induced tumors is similar to human esophageal cancer. This confirms it as an excellent model to study the processes involved in esophageal carcinogenesis and for devising newer chemopreventive and therapeutic strategies. The differentially expressed genes are deposited at the NCBI's Gene Expression Omnibus (http://www.ncbi.nlm.nih.gov/geo/) and are accessible through the GEO series accession number GSE1707.

Vaccine

We therefore developed a tumor vaccine for esophageal cancer in the rat reflux model by creating radiated cells from the JA and JB cell lines that are engineered to express GM-CSF. To establish the creation of stably transfected JA and JB cell lines, we tested the ability of the newly created vaccine cells to express GM-CSF. As shown in *Figure 2*, GM-CSF secretion was confirmed.

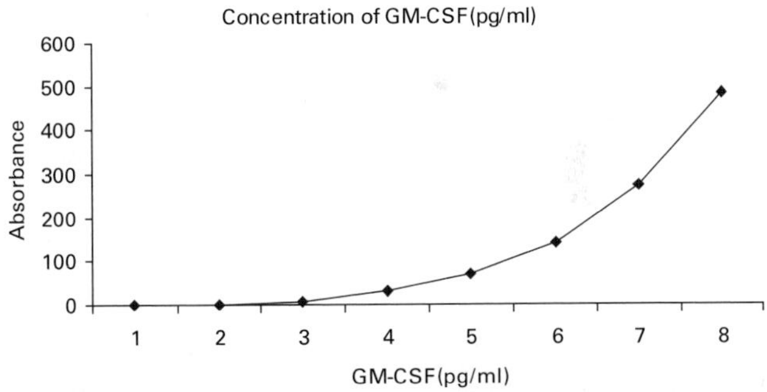

Cell line	JA cell line	JB cell line
GM-CSF (ng/ml/10^6 cells/24 hr)	4.61	4.35

Figure 2. ELISA of murine GM-CSF expression by rat esophageal cancer cells.

Efficacy of vaccine in rat allograft model

One of the drawbacks of the *in vivo* rat reflux model is the long duration needed for the carcinogenic progression to esophageal cancer (9 months to a year). The three cell lines (JA, JB, AMY) are now available to test novel chemopreventive and therapeutic agents and pathological processes involved in Barrett's esophagus and esophageal adenocarcinoma. This presents an opportunity for rapid allograft screening with subsequent confirmation of the hypothesis in the *in vivo* rat reflux model prior to designing human studies.

Following from these concepts, allografts developed from the tumor cell lines were established in rats. The rats were vaccinated 7 days prior to tumor implantation according to the following schedule and tumor growth was assessed sequentially at days 4, 7 and 10 prior to sacrifice at day 14. As shown in *Figure 3*,tumor size was substantially reduced in the vaccinated animals compared with the controls.

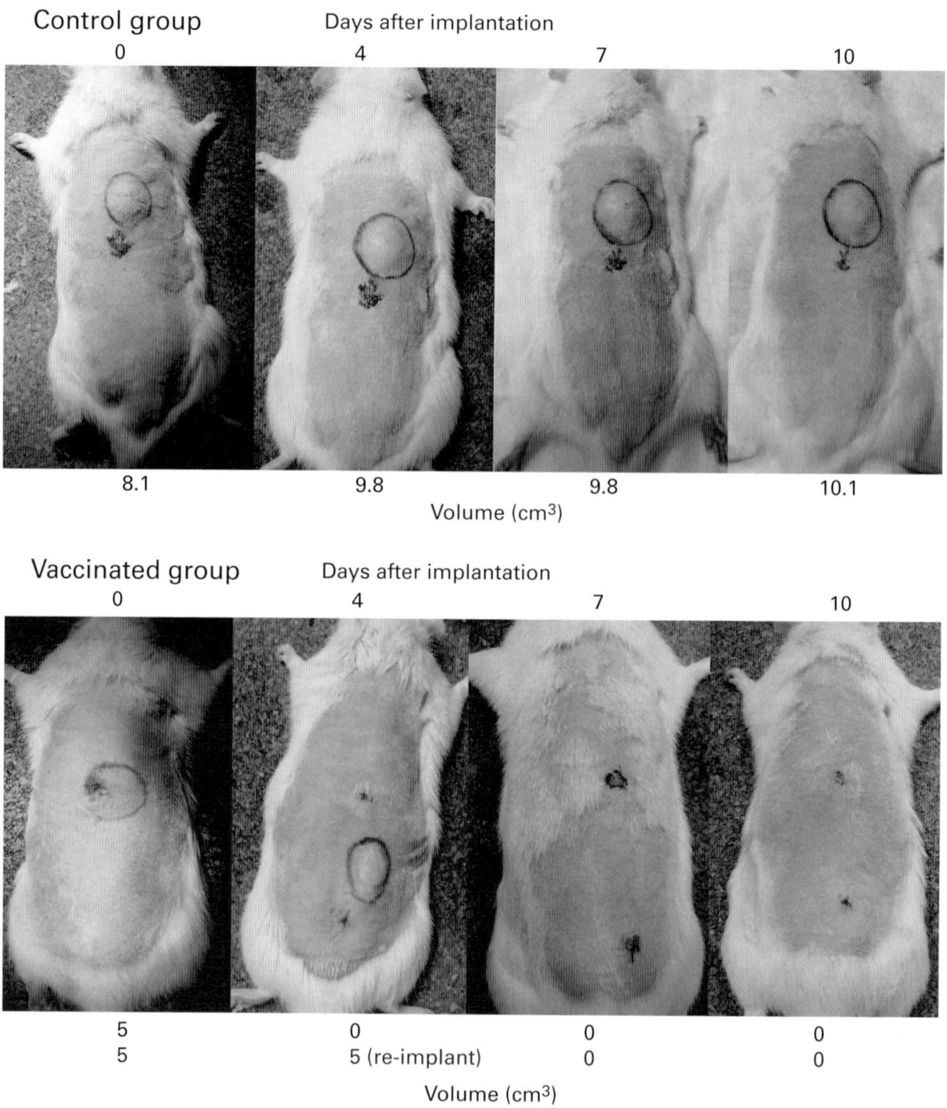

Figure 3. Tumor growth after vaccination. Note: for vaccinated group, animal #2 was re-implanted with tumor at a separate site at day 3 after initial tumor implantation (purple circle). (See page XXXIV for colour figure).

In most animals, significant tumor regression was seen by day 4, and by day 14 at sacrifice, nearly all tumors were gone. In one striking example tumor was not present at day 4. As such, this animal was re-implanted with tumor, and by day 7 this re-implanted tumor was also gone. This re-injection approach was confirmed in four additional rats. Histology of the implantation site after removal at day 14 was evaluated by H&E for both vaccinated and control animals. The control animal shows clear tumor growth, with an abundance of neoplastic cells and keratin pearls. The vaccinated animal shows macrophages, a lymphatic infiltrate and dead or dying tumor cells, confirming activity of the vaccine against the tumor (*Figure 4*).

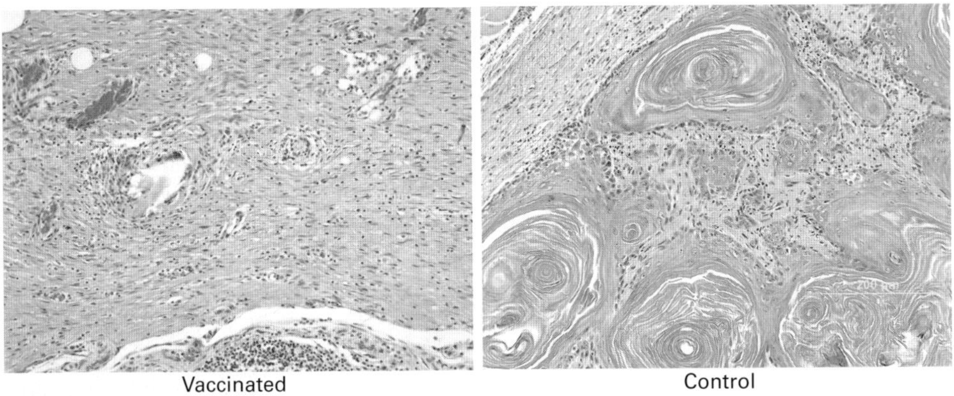

Figure 4. Histology of implantation site at day 14. (See page XXXIII for colour figure).

Discussion

In this project we aimed to create an animal model of esophageal cancer that would enable establishment of stable tumor cell lines for future use in *in vitro* and *in vivo* studies of this devastating disease. From this model we then wished to create a whole-cell, GM-CSF secreting tumor vaccine for treatment of esophageal cancer in these animal models. The overall goal of this work is to move this vaccine to use in humans for treatment of both Barrett's esophagus and esophageal cancer.

By using a surgical model of DER in rats, we established tumor at the GEJ with histology that included components of Barrett's esophagus as well as esophageal adenocarcinoma and SCC. Cells obtained from these tumors were then used to establish three stable cell lines—JA, JB and Amy—that have genetic profiles similar to those seen in esophageal cancers. Although established from adenocarcinomas, these cell lines displayed predominantly SCC features when grown *in vitro* and as allografts.

In order to investigate the activity of a tumor vaccine against these allografts created from the JA, JB and Amy cell lines, we created a whole-cell GM-CSF secreting tumor vaccine from the JA and JB lines. These cells stably expressed GM-CSF and were used to vaccinate animals that harbored allografts created from the JA and JB cell lines. Vaccination inhibited tumor growth and resulted in histologic changes consistent with immunologic infiltration and tumor cell death.

Increasing evidence demonstrates that all tumors possess tumor specific antigens capable of being recognized by antigen specific T-cells. These tumor specific neo-antigens most likely are the consequence of novel amino acid sequences generated by mutations or re-arrangements derived from genes that are silent in normal cells but become activated in tumor cells.

It is the tremendous diversity of the T-cell and B-cell receptors that endows the immune system with the ability to distinguish fine antigenic differences amongst cells. For the generation of an anti-tumor immune response, two criteria must be fulfilled. First, the tumor must present recently developed antigens or neo-epitopes not found on normal cells. Second, the immune system must be appropriately activated to respond to these recently developed antigens.

In development of this vaccine, rat tumor cells were genetically modified to express GM-CSF in order to attract professional antigen-presenting cells (APCs), such as macrophages or dendritic cells, to the site of the tumor. These APCs then take up the tumor cell proteins and process them by using their own cellular machinery to more effectively present them to helper and killer T cells (*Figure 3*). While multiple cytokines may be used, when vaccination was carried out with radiated tumor cells engineered to secrete multiple cytokines, GM-CSF produced the most potent, specific, and long lasting anti-tumor immunity [3].

Although this data is promising there are a number of limitations and drawbacks that must be considered and overcome prior to advancing this technology to further study in animals and humans. A major issue is the SCC histology of the *in vivo* generated tumors once they are passaged as cell lines and implanted as allografts. While clearly demonstrating Barrett's esophagus and adenocarcinoma features in the surgical model, these cells do not retain their adenocarcinoma features once harvested from the initial animal model. Given our wish to use this vaccine for treatment of Barrett's esophagus and adenocarcinoma, we will need to improve our model such that it more closely resembles adenocarcinoma. Although cytogenic and microarray analysis confirms that these cells harbor features of esophageal cancer, any vaccine cell will need to express epitopes shared with Barrett's esophagus and adenocarcinoma to be effective against these diseases.

One approach to this potential limitation is under ongoing study in our lab. For this project, we used the allograft model for convenience and proof of principle. Implanted tumors grow quickly such that data is rapidly available and hypotheses may be tested efficiently. Our other approach to vaccine development which may more closely resemble a true *in vivo* situation involves testing the vaccine in the rat surgical model of Barrett's esophagus and adenocarcinoma. These experiments are planned; however, it takes approximately nine months for tumor to grow in the surgical model. Furthermore, we still face the issue that the vaccine cells are derived from cell lines that express mainly SCC features. To that end, we are also attempting to develop additional cell lines that will maintain Barrett's esophagus and adenocarcinoma features *in vitro*. On the other hand, vaccines currently used in humans involve allogeic vaccines, suggesting that perhaps the vaccine cells and the patient's tumor do not have to so closely match for the vaccine to work.

In addition, to further enable introduction of this vaccine into humans, the vaccination approach and schedule must more closely resemble the real-life clinical situation. In these preliminary experiments, vaccine was given seven days prior to implantation of tumor. However, three situations are present in patients: Barrett's esophagus, locally advanced tumor which is resected and recurrent/metastatic tumor. For each model, the patients will receive vaccine after the disease is diagnosed. To address these questions, we are planning to carry out experiments in both the surgical and allograft model that give vaccine after establishment of tumor (by surgery or implantation).

Regarding eventual translation of this approach to humans, there are several barriers; however, work by our collaborators show that these may be overcome. One issue is the development of GM-CSF secreting whole-cell vaccines from human tumors. Our group successfully accomplished this with both breast cancer and pancreatic cancer. Of further concern is the safety, and eventually, efficacy of these vaccines. Work by Jaffee *et al.* supports that both can be done.

This group created a stable, GM-CSF secreting whole-cell vaccine from human tumor cells obtained at pancreatectomy. These cells were then used to generate a vaccine that was investigated for safety and efficacy in a phase I trial of 14 patients with locally advanced pancreatic adenocarcinoma treated with surgery followed by adjuvant chemoradiotherapy. Escalating doses of vaccine cells were given, and immunologic activity was assessed by evaluation of vaccination site histology and delayed type hypersensitivity reactions to tumor cells. A safe dose was achieved that induced vaccination site immune cell infiltration and measurable DTH reactions. Perhaps more intriguingly, patients that received the highest dose of vaccine sustained post-operative remissions much longer than are expected from historical controls. A randomized study is underway.

Conclusion

Given this study as clinical validation of the GM-CSF secreting whole cell tumor vaccine approach, we will continue to advance our studies of this in Barrett's esophagus and adenocarcinoma by the planned approaches described above. The overall goal is to produce a vaccine that will be used to treat established Barrett's esophagus and as well as resected esophageal cancer.

References

1. Levrat M, Lambert R, Kirshbaum G. Esophagitis produced by reflux of duodenal contents in rats. Am J Dig Dis 1962;7:564-73.
2. Sui G, Bonde P, Dhara S, et al. Epidermal growth factor receptor and hedgehog signaling pathways are active in esophageal cancer cells from rat reflux model. J Surg Res 2006;134(1):1-9.
3. Jaffee EM, Hruban RH, Biedrzycki B, et al. Novel allogeneic granulocyte-macrophage colony-stimulating factor-secreting tumor vaccine for pancreatic cancer: a phase I trial of safety and immune activation. J Clin Oncol 2001;19:145-56.
4. Attwood SE, Smyrk TC, DeMeester TR, et al: Duodenoesophageal reflux and the development of esophageal adenocarcinoma in rats. Surgery 1992;111:503-10.
5. Chen X, Yang G, Ding WY, et al. An esophagogastroduodenal anastomosis model for esophageal adenocarcinogenesis in rats and enhancement by iron overload. Carcinogenesis 1999;20:1801-8.
6. Miwa K, Sahara H, Segawa M, et al. Reflux of duodenal or gastro-duodenal contents induces esophageal carcinoma in rats. Int J Cancer 1996;67:269-74.
7. Pera M, Brito MJ, Poulsom R, et al. Duodenal-content reflux esophagitis induces the development of glandular metaplasia and adenosquamous carcinoma in rats. Carcinogenesis 2000;21:1587-91.
8. Buttar NS, Wang KK, Leontovich O, et al. Chemoprevention of esophageal adenocarcinoma by COX-2 inhibitors in an animal model of Barrett's esophagus. Gastroenterology 2002;122:1101-12.

Esophageal dilation in esophageal strictures

The Lausanne experience with treatment for benign esophageal stenosis using the Savary technique

E. Piotet, A. Escher, P. Monnier (Lausanne)

Benign esophageal strictures can be divided into two categories, according to their organic or functional origin. Functional strictures are the consequence of increased tonicity of the muscular wall while organic strictures mainly result from collagen deposits and fibrous tissue formation induced by mucosal injuries of diverse origins.

Endoscopy to obtain a biopsy specimen is mandatory for excluding neoplasm and assessing stricture characteristics. Length, precise location regarding upper and lower esophageal sphincters, spontaneous lumen diameter and mucosal appearance should be evaluated. Strictures are considered complex when they are greater than 2 cm in length or are angulated, irregular or do not allow the passage of a pediatric endoscope [1].

Endoscopic dilatation is the first-line treatment for benign esophageal strictures. Dilatations using a carved whalebone were first reported in the 17th century [2], and numerous dilators have since been developed. Mercury-filled Maloney dilators are flexible bougies without guide wires that are used for blind dilatation of simple strictures. Wire-guided dilators include the Eder-Puestow metal olives, which are now obsolete, the Savary-Gilliard polyvinyl-chloride bougies and the balloon dilators. The Savary-Gilliard technique was developed in the Department of Otolaryngology, Head and Neck Surgery, University Hospital of Lausanne in 1980, with the aim of decreasing the perforation rate, which then varied from 0.5 to 9%, depending on the dilatation system and the reported series [3,4]. Another widely used system is the through-the-scope balloon dilator, which exerts only radial forces during dilatation and can be advantageous in some instances.

We retrospectively reviewed the benign esophageal and pharyngeal strictures treated in our department to assess the efficacy and safety of the Savary-Gilliard technique.

Material and methods

Our database was reviewed to assess number and etiologies of the benign pharyngeal and esophageal strictures necessitating dilatation in our department between January 1, 1963 and December 31, 2005. Dilatations with the Savary-Gilliard dilators have been exclusively used in our clinic since 1980, rather than using the Maloney dilators or the Eder-Puestow olives, except for some cases of achalasia that were managed by balloon dilatation. The Savary-Gilliard set included a metallic guide-wire and polyvinyl chloride bougies, ranging from 5 to 18 mm in diameter. The procedure has been described in detail elsewhere [5], and was always performed under fluoroscopy.

Results of dilatation using this procedure were reported as the number of dilatations per stricture and the time interval between the different sessions over a 17-year period (January 1, 1989 to December 31, 2005). These two factors were directly related to the efficiency of dilatation. In our institution, patients without relief of symptoms or in whom a lumen of 15 mm in diameter could not be obtained after the first dilatation were included in a dilatation program. This consisted of repeated dilatations every 3rd week until permanent improvement was obtained. Patients for whom the first procedure was satisfactory were followed up and dilated only if dysphagia recurred. In case of gastroesophageal reflux disease (GERD)-induced strictures, the dilatation was followed by a proton pump inhibitor (PPI) treatment. Patients with achalasia were excluded from the analysis of results because of intermittent balloon dilatations.

Complications of dilatations were reported from January 1, 1980 to December 31, 2005. Severe complications were defined as potentially life-threatening situations and were assessed by reviewing the surgeon's endoscopy report. If the surgeon's report described any complications, then the patient's complete medical records were reviewed to determine any long-term effects of the complications.

Results

The retrospective analysis of our database showed a total of 1,349 benign pharyngeal or esophageal strictures requiring dilatation from 1963 to the end of 2005. There were 1,071 (79%) organic strictures of which etiologies are reported in *Table I*.

Non-organic or functional origins represented 21% of the data, with a total of 278 strictures. These were further divided into cricopharyngeal hypertonia (50%), achalasia (47%), and pylorus hypertonia after transhiatal esophagectomy (3%).

The total prevalence of benign esophageal strictures requiring dilatation among patients undergoing upper digestive endoscopy was 3%, 2.7% for organic and 0.3% for functional strictures, respectively.

A total of 1,120 dilatations using the Savary-Gilliard technique were performed, 1,094 (98%) for organic strictures and 26 (2%) for functional strictures.

The number of sessions per patient extended from 1 to 23 during the review period and was highly dependent upon the etiology of the stenosis, as shown in *Table II*. Time interval between dilatations varied from 7 days to 16 years, as reported in *Table III*.

Severe complications included esophageal perforation in 1 patient (0.09%), and massive bleeding was documented in 1 patient (0.09%). The mortality rate was 0.09%, with death occurring in 1 patient secondary to perforation. Our overall complication rate was 0.18%.

Table I. Repartition of benign organic strictures at CHUV from 1963 to 2006.

Etiology	Male	Female	Total
Peptic	290	166	456 (42.58%)
Iatrogenic	275	90	365 (34.08%)
- Post-RT ± CT, post-PDT	53	21	74 (6.91%)
- Post surgery	159	59	218 (20.35%)
- Post-surgery + RT	53	5	58 (5.42%)
- Post-sclerotherapy	7	2	9 (0.84%)
- Pill-induced	3	3	6 (0.56%)
Caustic	36	36	72 (6.72%)
Web	26	46	72 (6.72%)
Schatzki's ring	39	12	51 (4.76%)
Undetermined	15	7	22 (2.057%)
Pseudodiverticulosis	7	0	7 (0.65%)
Epidermolysis bullosa	3	4	7 (0.65%)
Ringed esophagus	4	1	5 (0.47%)
Pemphigoid mucosynechiant	0	4	4 (0.37%)
Candidiasis	3	0	3 (0.28%)
Lichen planus	0	2	2 (0.18%)
Submucosal fibrosis	2	0	2 (0.18%)
Scleroderma	0	1	1 (0.09%)
Post traumatic	0	1	1 (0.09%)
Myofibromatosis	1	0	1 (0.09%)
TOTAL	702	369	1,071
RT: radiotherapy; CT: chemotherapy; PDT: phototherapy			

Discussion

Results of dilatations

Our review revealed a wide range of variability in efficiency of dilatation as a function of the etiology of lesions. This was correlated to the morphologic features of each type of stricture, efficiency of dilatations depending upon the extent of involvement of the esophageal wall by fibrosis and inflammatory processes.

The group that responded poorest to dilatation included caustic, post-operative and post-radiation therapy strictures. During the 17-year period reviewed, the median number of dilatations per patient was 2 to 2.5 (see *Table II*), with a maximum of 23 dilatations for one patient. Median interval between dilatations was between 1.5 to 2 months (see *Table III*), reflecting the high proportion of patients who entered a dilatation program. According to our data, caustic and post-surgery and/or post-radiotherapy strictures were the most refractory to dilatation. This is in agreement with the data reported in the literature [1].

Table II. Number of dilations per stricture from 1989 to 2006.

Etiology (number of strictures)	Median	Mean	Range
Pill-induced (2)	1	1	1
Lichen planus (2)	1	1	1
Scleroderma (1)	1	1	1
Pseudodiverticulosis (3)	1	1	1
Myofibromatosis (1)	1	1	1
Web (10)	1	1	1-2
Undetermined (15)	1	1	1-2
Pylorus hypertonia (6)	1	1	1-2
Epidermolysis bullosa (3)	1	1.5	1-3
Neoplasic (298)	1	1.5	1-8
Peptic (54)	1	2	1-9
Mycotic (3)	1	3	1-7
Submucosal fibrosis (2)	1.5	1.5	1-2
Ringed esophagus (5)	2	1.5	1-2
Schatzki's ring (4)	2	3	1-6
Post-surgery (78)	2	2.5	1-20
Post-radiotherapy (48)	2	3	1-17
Post-surgery + radiotherapy (58)	2	3	1-23
Caustic (14)	2.5	3.5	1-11
Post traumatic (1)	3	3	3

Table III. Time interval between dilations of strictures from 1989 to 2006.

Etiology (total number of dilations)	Median	Mean	Range
Schatzki's ring (11)	4 years	4 years	2.5-6 years
Ringed esophagus (8)	5 months	20 months	2.5 months-4.5 years
Mycotic (9)	4 months	5.5 months	2.5-11 months
Neoplasic (434)	2 months	4 months	7 days-20 months
Peptic (102)	2 months	9.5 months	12 days-3 years
Post-surgery (198)	2 months	4.5 months	10 days-38 months
Post-radiotherapy (136)	2 months	4 months	9 days-7 years
Caustic (50)	1.5 months	9 months	14 days-16 years
Post-surgery + radiotherapy (176)	1.5 months	7 months	7 days-4 years

Caustic strictures are known for their extension in length and involvement of the entire thickness of the esophageal wall. Among the 73 caustic strictures reviewed by Brossard *et al.*, 60% were located in the upper esophagus, 48% were multiple and 49% measured more than 3 cm in length [6]. This results in tubulization of the scarred esophagus with increased difficulty for efficient dilatation. The outcome of caustic-stricture dilatations in our department was reported by Leuba *et al.* [7]. They found that when the length of the stenosis is greater than 3 cm in the cranio-caudal axis, management with dilatations is often insufficient, and indication for esophagectomy with coloplasty to restore normal oral intake must be discussed if there is no improvement of symptoms after a few dilatation sessions. Surgical management must be taken into consideration especially in young patients because of late cancerization.

Post-operative and post-radiotherapy strictures also often need repeat dilatations, and a combination of these two treatment modalities further increases the number of dilatations per stricture. The esophagus is known to be a fragile and radiosensitive organ, and late radiation injury is a common consequence of treatment of head and neck, lung, esophageal and breast tumors. Development of strictures is related to progressive obliterative endarteritis, ischemia and slowly developing fibrosis [8,9]. Some patients may be dilated once and then be asymptomatic, but most of them need multiple dilatations and inclusion in dilatation programs. Thereafter, the frequency of repeat dilatations is dictated by recurrence of dysphagia, with symptom-free intervals varying widely from days to several years. The circular involvement and the transmural fibrosis due either to peri-anastomotic inflammation, radiation or both, account for the tendency of the lesion to recur.

Another distinct group includes webs, which usually respond very well to dilatations. The median number of dilatations per stricture was one in this group, with a maximum of 2 dilatations per patient. A single dilatation is sufficient for complete resolution of symptoms in most patients.

Strictures related to dermatologic diseases, fungal infections, connectivitis or pill-induced strictures also tend to respond well to dilatation, but their small number in this sample does not allow us to draw any conclusions from the data.

A third group of strictures, in which response to dilatation is rather good but with frequent relapses, includes peptic strictures, Schatzki's rings and ringed esophagus.

GERD-related strictures accounted for 52% of the benign organic strictures before 1989, but dropped to only 18% after this period. The introduction of proton pump inhibitors (PPIs), commercialized in 1989, accounts for the fall in the prevalence of these lesions. It is now well recognized that the use of PPIs decreases the need for repeated dilatations in patients presenting with peptic strictures [10-12]. The majority of them respond well to treatment and can be dealt with by a single dilatation and PPI oral intake. For patients necessitating several dilatations, the median interval between procedures is 2 months (range 12 days to 3 years). This reflects the need for some patients to enter a dilatation program, whereas others have a long symptom-free interval and a late recurrence. This emphasizes the problem of patients' compliance to long-term drug intake, with the possible recurrence of stricture after years because of PPI cessation.

The few cases of Schatzki's rings and ringed esophagus in our series generally required more than a single dilatation (median, 2) and had long-term recurrence. Nevertheless, the symptom-free period after a single dilatation was 4 years for Schatzki's ring and 5 months for ringed esophagus, which was much greater than for the refractory strictures described previously. Moreover, patients do not have to enter dilatation programs following this procedure. This supports the efficacy of a single dilatation for treatment of these lesions, which, however, tend to form again with time [13]. When dilated, strictures of ringed esophagus tend to show longitudinal tears with little if any bleeding. This is a common feature of this condition, which could be due to a submucosal fibrosis, possibly induced by recurrent episodes of fungal infection.

Complications

Slight bleeding and mucosal erosions are frequently seen after esophageal dilatations, and these conditions resolve spontaneously without specific management. Nevertheless, two severe and potentially life-threatening complications may occur, namely esophageal perforation and hematemesis. Post-dilatation esophagoscopy should always be performed to rule out such lesions.

One case of massive bleeding was reported over the 26-year period of this series using the Savary-Gilliard technique, occurring in a patient treated with anticoagulants. Overall, the rate of severe hemorrhage was 0.09%.

Esophageal perforation represents the primary severe complication of dilatation, with rapid progression to sepsis, mediastinitis and death. Rapid diagnosis and aggressive treatment are required. In our 26-year review, transmural perforation occurred once because of faulty manipulation of the guide-wire. Overall, the perforation rate was 0.09%.

The single case of death secondary to dilatation occurred secondary to esophageal perforation. The overall mortality rate was thus 0.09%.

Our results show that the Savary-Gilliard technique for esophageal dilatation of benign strictures is safe, with only 0.18% of severe complications. With a perforation rate of 0.09%, we are at the lower limit of the 0.1 to 0.4% rate currently reported in the literature for esophageal dilatation in general [1,14,15]. The advantages of the Savary-Gilliard technique include the progressive flexibility of its guide-wire and the tapered bougies exerting constant pressure on the esophageal wall, which provides the surgeon with feedback concerning resistance during the procedure. Moreover, all of the dilatations in our department were performed under fluoroscopy. This may also account for the reduced rate of complications. In the literature, dilatations with the Eder-Puestow olives are associated with higher perforation rates, ranging from 0.4 to 0.9% [16,17]. The large gradient of pressure provoked by the form of these dilators and their extremely flexible guide-wire tip account for the higher perforation risk. This system is now obsolete. In the current literature, the perforation rate with the Maloney dilators is also reported to be higher than that with the Savary-Gilliard bougies. A study comparing perforation rates with Maloney, balloon and Savary dilators showed no perforation for the latter two procedures (156 and 90, respectively), and a 3.9 perforation rate for the Maloney dilators in 102 procedures [15]. Another prospective study of 300 patients dilated either with the Maloney, Savary-Gilliard, Eder-Puestow or balloon dilators, resulted in a single perforation, which occurred with a Maloney dilator used in the absence of fluoroscopy for dilatation of a Schatzki's ring [18]. Blind dilatation, as in the Maloney technique, increases the risk of misdirection of the dilator resulting in tracheal intubation, tearing or even perforation of the esophageal wall. Finally, a randomized study by Cox *et al.* showed better improvement on stricture diameter using the Savary-Gilliard or the Eder-Puestow bougies than with balloon dilators. Safety of both methods was similar [19]. Balloon dilators are also more expensive and cannot be used more than once. By contrast, Savary-Gilliard bougies may be reused indefinitely. At our institution, we are still using one of the same set of bougies that was used in 1980 when the technique was first developed. No problems with inter-individual contamination or infection have occurred.

Conclusion

Benign esophageal strictures treated in our department were primarily of iatrogenic origin (61%) since the decrease in prevalence of peptic strictures secondary to the introduction of PPIs in 1989. Dilatation with the Savary-Gilliard technique was safe, even for complex strictures, with only 2 cases of severe complication out of a total of 1,120 procedures. We advise the systematic use of fluoroscopy during dilatation as it probably contributes to this low complication rate. Long-term efficiency of dilatation varies and is highly dependent on the etiology of the stricture. Even in cases of complex strictures, the median of 2 to 2.5 dilatations per patient over the 17-year period reviewed, showed that the overall efficacy is good and provides a satisfactory quality of life for most patients.

References

1. Ferguson DD. Evaluation and management of benign esophageal strictures. Dis Esophagus 2005;18:359-64.
2. Spiess AE, Kahrilas PJ. Treating achalasia: from whalebone to laparoscope. JAMA 1998;280:638-42.
3. Gotberg S, Afzelius LE, Hambraeus G, et al. Balloon catheter dilatation of strictures in the upper digestive tract. Radiologe 1982;22:479-83.
4. Luna LL. Endoscopic treatment of esophageal strictures. Endoscopy 1983;15:203-6.
5. Monnier P, Hsieh V, Savary M. Endoscopic treatment of oesophageal stenosis using Savary-Gilliard bougies: technical innovations. Acta Endosc 1985;15:119-29.
6. Brossard E, Ollyo JB, Savary M, Monnier P. Le rôle de la dilatation dans la prise en charge thérapeutique des sténoses caustiques de l'œsophage. Med Chir Dig 1993;22:179-80.
7. Leuba D, Ollyo JB. Corrosion de la voie digestive supérieure : bilan, traitement et résultats. Acta Endosc 1991;21:665-8.
8. Laurell G, Kraepelien T, Mavroidis P. et al. Stricture of the proximal oesophagus in head and neck carcinoma after radiotherapy. Cancer 2003;97:1693-700.
9. Silvain C, Barrioz T, Besson I, et al. Treatment and long-term outcome of chronic radiation esophagitis after radiation therapy for head and neck tumors. Dig Dis Sci 1993;38:927-31.
10. Barbezat GO, Schlup M, Lubcke R. Omeprazole therapy decreases the need for dilatation of peptic oesophageal strictures. Aliment Pharmacol Ther 1999;13:1041-5.
11. Swarbrick ET, Gough AL, Foster CS, Christian J, Garrett AD, Langworthy CH. Prevention of recurrence of oesophageal stricture, a comparison of lansoprazole and high-dose ranitidine. Eur J Gastroenterol Hepatol 1996;8:431-8.
12. Marks RD, Richter JE, Rizzo J, et al. Omeprazole versus H2-receptor antagonists in treating patients with peptic stricture and oesophagitis. Gastroenterology 1994;106 :907-15.
13. Ibrahim A, Cole R, Qureshi WA, et al. Schatzki's ring: to cut or break, an unresolved problem. Dig Dis Sci 2004;49:379-83.
14. American Society for Gastrointestinal Endoscopy. Esophageal dilation. Gastrointest Endosc 1998;48:702-4.
15. Hernandez LJ, Jacobson JW, Harris MS. Comparison among the perforation rates of Maloney, balloon and Savary dilation of esophageal strictures. Gastrointest Endosc 2000;51:460-2.
16. Knutsen H, Fausa O. Dilatation of esophageal stenoses. Tidsskr Nor Laegeforen 1990;110:1711-3.
17. Yamamoto H, Hugues RW Jr, Schroeder KW, Viggiano TR, DiMagno EP. Treatment of benign esophageal stricture by Eder-Puestow or balloon dilators: a comparison between randomized and prospective nonrandomized trials. Mayo Clin Proc 1992;67:228-36.
18. Tucker LE. Esophageal stricture: results of dilation of 300 patients. Mo Med 1992;89:668-70.
19. Cox JGC, Winter RK, Maslin SC, et al. Balloon or bougie for dilatation of benign esophageal stricture? Dig Dis Sci 1994;39:776-81.

A gastroenterologist's approach for dilating benign esophageal strictures

R.K.H. Wong (Washington)

In approaching the problem of benign strictures, the clinician must first diagnose the etiology of dysphagia. There are two modalities to identify the problem: barium esophagram or a "swallowing study" to obtain a "road map" of the esophagus and/or an endoscopy which is excellent for identifying mucosal lesions and to obtain tissue for histological diagnosis. Most would agree that a barium study should be obtained in the following situations:

- complex strictures which may be long, tortuous, and narrow;
- proximal esophageal lesions where one suspects a Zenker's diverticulum or transfer problems in the oropharynx;
- a negative endoscopy in which the diagnosis is still questionable;
- possibility of a motor disorder of the esophagus.

The difficulty with dilating strictures relates to the degree of fibrosis or collagen deposited at the site of the stricture. The fibrotic response to inflammation is probably related to the type of injury and the duration of exposure (*Figure 1*). Strictures resulting from exposure to radiation, lye, or acute acid as seen with NG tubes are extremely difficult to dilate. A Shatzki's B-ring which has little fibrosis is simple to fracture, while peptic strictures will vary in dilation difficulty depending upon the extent of fibrosis.

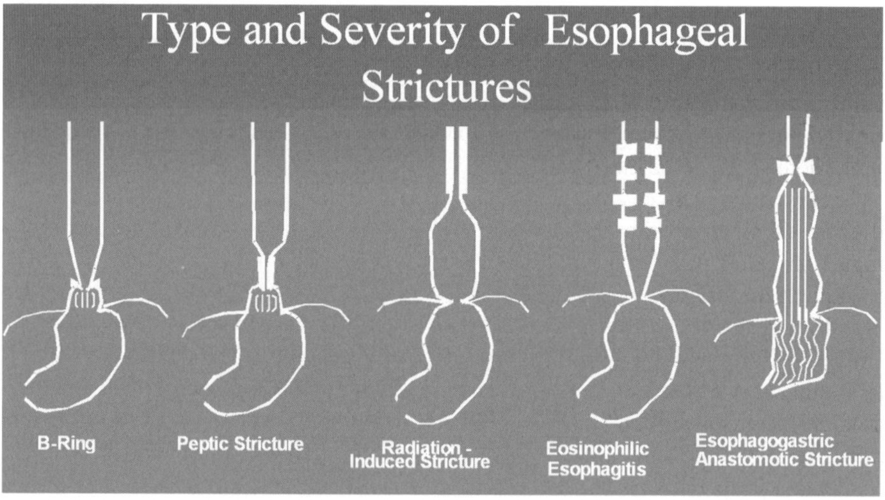

Figure 1. The severity of a stricture relates to the injurious agent, the duration of exposure and ultimately the extent of fibrosis.

Benign strictures have multiple etiologies (*Table I*) with the incidence of peptic strictures decreasing significantly with the advent of PPI's. Eosinophilic esophagitis strictures are diagnosed more frequently and seem to be an increasing reason for esophageal dilations. Other more unusual causes of benign strictures include infections such as Candida or strictures associated with skin diseases such as pemphagus vulgarus, or epidermolysis bullosum.

Table I. Types of benign strictures.

Peptic stricture – 70%
Schatzki's ring
Eosinophilic esophagitis ↑
Anastomotic stricture
Caustic strictures – NGT, scleroderma, lye, pill-induced, radiation, sclerotherapy, PDT
Skin lesions – Pemphigus vulgaris, epidemolysis bullosa
Infectious (Candida, CMV, HSV)
Achalasia

Table II. Characterization of strictures: simple *versus* complex.

Simple stricture	Symmetric and concentric ≥ 10-12 mm
Complex	≤ 10-12 mm Inability to pass endoscope Asymmetric Longer length

Typically a simple stricture is defined as one which is symmetric, > 10-12 mm and of short length while a complex stricture is asymmetric, < 10-12 mm, long, and tortuous (*Table II*). Esophageal dilators which are typically employed to dilate benign strictures include: Mercury filled dilators (Maloney, Hurst), polyvinyl thru the wire dilators (Savary-Gillard) and balloon thru the scope (TTS) dilators. Both longitudinal and radial forces are produced when employing Mercury filled and polyvinyl dilators while only radial forces are exerted with TTS balloon dilators. In spite of these differences in vector forces associated with a dilator, there seems to be no objective difference in dilation efficacy between dilators.

Mercury filled dilators are used to dilate simple strictures while the polyvinyl dilators and TTS balloon are used to dilate both simple and complex strictures. However, with long complex strictures, the polyvinyl dilator is most efficacious as wires can be inserted thru the length of the stricture while a TTS balloon may not be able to traverse the entire length of the stricture.

When performing a dilation, the "Rule of 3's" is commonly employed (*Table III*). This entails dilating a stricture to the point of mild to moderate resistance and then not going beyond 3 further sequential dilations. For the Maloney and polyvinyl dilators this means an increase of not more that 2 mm (6 F) in diameter. With the TTS balloon system, the incremental increase in balloon size is 3 F for each incremental increase in pressure. Each TTS balloon has 3 incremental pressure points which results in a total 9 F increase in the diameter of the balloon (3 mm) *versus* 6 F (2 mm) as noted with Maloney or Savary-Gillard dilators. Also, when using TTS balloons, one estimates the size of the stricture and then chooses which balloon size to employ, whereas when using Maloney dilators one sounds the esophagus to "feel" the tightness of the stricture before using the "rule of 3's". Hence,

Table III. Technique of dilation.

"Rule of 3"	Dilate to point of moderate resistance Then no more than 3 dilations in increments of 1 mm (2 F) Maloney or Savary dilators - 2 F increments
Balloon dilation - TTS	Between 36-54 F : 3 F increments Optimal duration of dilation unknown

when using TTS dilators, one must be cautious with the initial dilation to be certain that the initial balloon size is not too large which may result in an inadvertent tear.

Special attention concerning the technique of dilation (*Table IV*):

- patients should be coached ahead of time to relax during the dilation;
- the hand that advances the bougie should represent an extension of the dilator and the operator should sense anatomic structures that may resist advancement of the bougie such as the bite block, the teeth, the acute turn at the junction of the mouth and the oropharynx, the cricopharyngeus, possibly the lower esophageal sphincter and most importantly the obstruction;
- advancement of the dilator should be gentle and not forceful especially when the patient is retching as the stomach herniates into the esophagus during retching and acts as a distal obstruction. During retching, the tip of the Maloney dilator may reverse (make a U turn) when it comes into contact with the herniated stomach, causing the dilator to bow in the esophagus with continued advancement. This scenario may result in an esophageal tear, especially with larger size dilators;
- when employing a Savary-Gillard (SG) dilator, the neck should be straightened by positioning the neck so that it arches slightly backward. This maneuver will straighten the angle between the mouth and the oropharynx so that the overall direction of the vector force is in a straighter line. Likewise prior to dilation, the guidewire should be inspected for kinks and the SG dilator immersed in hot water for 3-5 minutes to soften the dilator allowing it to be more pliable so that it could be passed more easily thru the esophagus and to the obstructed area;
- following the dilation, the operator should have a good understanding and "feel" of how tight the obstruction felt so that comparisons concerning the efficacy of the dilation can be made during future dilations.

Table IV. Technique of dilation.

- In the old days… without sedation
- Talk to the patient - relax, think about somethong else, take slow deep breaths
- Deflate the stomach
- Hand is an extension of the dilator - should be able to feel any obstruction
- Gentle dilation - don't rush
- Stop during retching - stomach herniates into the distal esophagus ; acts as an obstruction and may cause the tip to the dilator flip up
- Use the finger tips of left hand to guide the dilator down pass the posterior pharynx - don't stimulate vomiting
- Teeth can be source of pseudo-obstruction

It seems that the greatest relief of dysphagia occurs when the esophageal lumen has been dilated between 13-15 mm (39 F-45 F). Prognostically for peptic strictures, a small lumen size, hiatal hernia > 5 mm, requirement for multiple dilations initially to relieve dysphagia, and persistent heartburn portend a poorer outcome and the need for frequent dilations (*Figure 2*). The risk of perforation varies between 0.1-0.4% and depends upon the complexity and etiology of the stricture. Radiation strictures are associated with more perforations and may be extremely difficult to dilate because of the large amount of fibrosis generated by the radiation. In some instance, there is complete lumen occlusion which may require laser dissection of the fibrosis with an ENT specialist in conjunction with a retrograde approach *via* a PEG orifice.

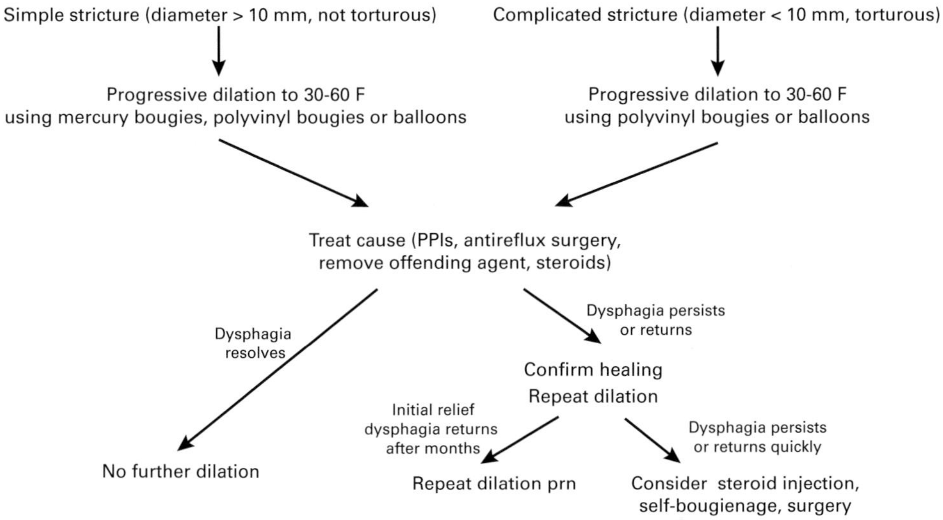

Figure 2. Management of benign esophageal strictures.

Medical therapy includes PPI's for peptic strictures which have decreased significantly over the last 10 years. In very difficult strictures (radiation, lye, anastamotic) several techniques have been utilized with mixed success:

- steroid injections with Kenalog 40 mg diluted to allow several injections during a single session. Multiple endoscopic sessions are required;
- teaching patients to do home dilations once the narrowed segment is dilated;
- placing a removable stent into the stricture which is removed at a later date.

For patients with eosinophilic esophagitis several therapies have been employed: oral steroids, inhaled steroids which are swallowed, montelukast; PPI's, food elimination diets and esophageal dilations.

The treatment of achalasia will vary with the expertise of the institution. However, with the advent of laparoscopy, laparoscopic Heller myotomies have become very popular and efficacious. A laparoscopic approach is reasonable in younger patients as pneumatic dilations are less efficacious than those performed in older patients (> 40 years). When performed, a laparoscopic Heller is usually accompanied with a Dor wrap and GERD is the most common long term side effect of surgery.

Pneumatic dilations for achalasia are most commonly performed with graduated balloon sizes (microvasive balloons, 3, 3.5 and 4 cm in diameter). Dilations begin with the smallest dilator with a single dilation performed per session. Patient's symptoms will guide the need for subsequent dilation and if available, esophageal emptying can be measured with a timed barium or an esophageal emptying study. Within a month, patients will usually know whether the dilation has been effective. Older patients, however, may not adequately sense improvement and an objective emptying study is important.

Recent studies indicate that follow up of achalasia patients is necessary to determine whether: dysphagia has recurred, esophageal emptying has decreased and esophageal dilation is progressing. This is important as extreme dilation of the esophagus may be associated with a fatal complication, aspiration pneumonia or esophageal cancer associated with esophageal stasis. Ultimately, an esophagectomy may be required as to prevent the above complications and maintain nutrition.

Bibliography

- Agnew SR, Pandya SP, Reynolds RP. Predictors for frequent esophageal dilations of benign peptic strictures. Dig Dis Sci 1996;41(5):931-6.
- Ahtaridis G, Snape WJ, Cohen S. Clinical and manometric findings in benign peptic strictures of the esophagus. Dig Dis Sci 1979;24(11):858-61.
- Attwood SE, DeMeester TR, Bremner CG. Alkaline gastroesophageal reflux: implications in the development of complications in Barrett's columnar-lined lower esophagus. Surgery 1989;106(4):764-70.
- Bell NJ, Burget D, Howden CW. Appropriate acid suppression for the management of gastro-oesophageal reflux disease. Digestion 1992;51:59-67.
- Cox JG, Winter RK, Maslin SC. Balloon or bougie for dilatation of benign oesophageal stricture? An interim report of a randomised controlled trial. Gut 1988;29(12):1741-7.
- Dakkak M, Hoare RC, Maslin SC. Oesophagitis is as important as oesophageal stricture diameter in determining dysphagia. Gut 1993;34(2):152-5.
- Dunne DP, Rupp T, Rex DK. Five year follow-up of prospective randomized trial of Savary dilation with or without intra-lesional steroids for benign gastroesophageal reflux strictures. Gastroenterology 1999;116:A152.
- Graham DY, Saeed ZA. Guidewire-assisted esophageal dilation. Gastrointest Endosc 1991;37(6):650-1.
- Guda NM, Vakil N. Proton pump inhibitors and the time trends for esophageal dilation. Am J Gastroenterol 2004;99(5):797-800.
- Hagiwara A, Togawa T, Yamasaki J. Endoscopic incision and balloon dilatation for cicatricial anastomotic strictures. Hepatogastroenterology 1999;46(26): 997-9.
- Heller SR, Fellows IW, Ogilvie AL. Non-steroidal anti-inflammatory drugs and benign oesophageal stricture. Br Med J (Clin Res Ed) 1982;285(6336):167-8.
- Kadakia SC, Parker A, Carrougher JG. Esophageal dilation with polyvinyl bougies, using a marked guidewire without the aid of fluoroscopy: an update. Am J Gastroenterol 1993;88(9):1381-6.
- Kochhar R, Makharia GK. Usefulness of intralesional triamcinolone in treatment of benign esophageal strictures. Gastrointest Endosc 2002;56(6):829-34.
- Kozarek RA, Patterson DJ, Ball TJ. Esophageal dilation can be done safely using selective fluoroscopy and single dilating sessions. J Clin Gastroenterol 1995;20(3):184-8.
- Mamazza J, Schlachta CM, Poulin EC. Surgery for peptic strictures. Gastrointest Endosc Clin N Am 1998;8(2):399-413.
- Marks RD, Richter JE, Rizzo J. Omeprazole versus H2-receptor antagonists in treating patients with peptic stricture and esophagitis. Gastroenterology 1994;106(4):907-15.
- Ott DJ, Gelfand DW, Lane TG. Radiologic detection and spectrum of appearances of peptic esophageal strictures. J Clin Gastroenterol 1982;4(1):11-5.
- Patterson DJ, Graham DY, Smith JL. Natural history of benign esophageal stricture treated by dilatation. Gastroenterology 1983;85(2):346-50.
- Pungpapong S, Raimondo M, Wallace MB. Problematic esophageal stricture: an emerging indication for self-expandable silicone stents. Gastrointest Endosc 2004;60(5):842-5.
- Raijman I, Siddique I, Rachal LT. Endoscopic stricturoplasty in the management of recurrent benign esophageal strictures. Gastrointest Endosc 1999;49:AB172.

- Ramage JI, Rumalla A, Baron TH. A prospective, randomized, double-blind, placebo-controlled trial of endoscopic steroid injection therapy for recalcitrant esophageal peptic strictures. Am J Gastroenterol 2005;100(11):2419-25.
- Repici A, Conio M, De Angelis C. Temporary placement of an expandable polyester silicone-covered stent for treatment of refractory benign esophageal strictures. Gastrointest Endosc 2004;60(4):513-9.
- Richter JE. Peptic strictures of the esophagus. Gastroenterol Clin North Am 1999;28(4):875-91.
- Saeed ZA, Winchester CB, Ferro PS. Prospective randomized comparison of polyvinyl bougies and through-the- scope balloons for dilation of peptic strictures of the esophagus. Gastrointest Endosc 1995;41(3):189-95.
- Scolapio JS, Pasha TM, Gostout CJ. A randomized prospective study comparing rigid to balloon dilators for benign esophageal strictures and rings. Gastrointest Endosc 1999;50(1):13-7.
- Spechler SJ. American gastroenterological association medical position statement on treatment of patients with dysphagia caused by benign disorders of the distal esophagus. Gastroenterology 1999;117(1):229-33.
- Spechler SJ. AGA technical review on treatment of patients with dysphagia caused by benign disorders of the distal esophagus. Gastroenterology 1999;117(1):233-54.
- Spechler SJ. Comparison of medical and surgical therapy for complicated gastroesophageal reflux disease in veterans. The Department of Veterans Affairs Gastroesophageal Reflux Disease Study Group. N Engl J Med 1992;326(12):786-92.
- Vollan G, Stangeland L, Soreide JA. Long term results after Nissen fundoplication and Belsey Mark IV operation in patients with reflux oesophagitis and stricture. Eur J Surg 1992;158(6-7):357-60.
- Wilcox CM, Alexander LN, Clark WS. Localization of an obstructing esophageal lesion. Is the patient accurate? Dig Dis Sci 1995;40(10):2192-6.
- Wilkins WE, Ridley MG, Pozniak AL. Benign stricture of the oesophagus: role of non-steroidal anti- inflammatory drugs. Gut 1984;25(5):478-80.

Endoscopic lumen restoration for complete pharyngo-esophageal obstruction following chemoradiation therapy for head and neck cancer

H.W. Boyce (Tampa)

Many remarkable advances in medical diagnosis and therapy have occurred over the past two decades. Most have been of benefit to one or more of a wide array of illnesses. These innovations in pharmacology, biochemistry, serology, imaging methods, surgical technique, endoscopic diagnosis and therapy have in some instances resulted either directly or indirectly in harmful side effects. The purpose of this presentation is to review experience over the past twenty years with a condition resulting from physician oversight, enhanced by the direct result of modern radiation/chemotherapy and an indirect effect of the success of percutaneous endoscopic gastrostomy (PEG). The increasing frequency of total pharyngoesophageal obstruction and the magnitude of its deleterious result upon patients, who have already endured the anxieties and side effects of therapy for head and neck cancer, including proximal esophagus, deserves emphasis. Hopefully, recognition of this potentially irreversible and disastrous sequela by otolaryngologists, surgeons, medical and radiation oncologists, gastroenterologists and other physicians may help in its prevention.

The problem at hand is benign total pharyngoesophageal lumen occlusion following radiation/chemotherapy for head and neck cancer, i.e. squamous cell carcinoma of the tongue, pharynx, larynx, cervical esophagus and less often, other sites. The typical scenario is that of a patient who received a percutaneous endoscopic gastrostomy prior to, or soon after, radiation and chemotherapy. During therapy, as expected, the usual mucositis and other therapy-related inflammation develops and results in odynophagia and dysphagia. This inflammatory response is not a complication and is a regular concomitant of successful cancer therapy. The patient complains of the symptoms of oropharyngeal pain, odynophagia, dysphagia, and receives appropriate standard symptomatic therapy with the exception of encouragement of per oral intake and consideration for early pharyngoesophageal dilation. When the dysphagia presents, or progresses to aphagia soon after completion of the course of radiation therapy, the patient should be completely evaluated and early per oral dilation considered. When evidence of lumen stenosis is detected by barium contrast study, after termination of radiation/chemotherapy, a plan for dilation therapy should be instituted. Instead of this approach, some patients are reassured by their therapists who state, "don't worry, your swallowing will improve in a few more weeks".

In the years before PEG was available, the combination of dysphagia and weight loss were much more ominous for the patient's overall health and nutrition and served to create sufficient concern to provoke prompt evaluation and therapy. The presence of dysphagia after therapy often led to early dilation and preservation of lumen patency sufficient for adequate oral intake unless there was also a concomitant loss of pharyngeal neuromotor function as a consequence of radiation therapy. The increasing frequency of this sequela, i.e. total or near total lumen occlusion with aphagia, is the basis for this presentation. Dysphagia or aphagia occurring under these circumstances must be treated early and adequately after radiation/chemotherapy regardless of the patient's healthy appearance that has been assured by enteral nutrition *via* PEG. In our series, the average delay in referral of patients for evaluation for endoscopic lumen restauration (ELR) was 8.2 months (range 2 weeks to 27 months) after onset of aphagia.

The outcomes of treatment following delayed dilation vary from superbly gratifying successes to sad failures. Lumen restoration procedures can, and should be attempted, especially in those patients with no evidence of residual or recurrent malignancy. The lumen obstruction may be caused by a very thin web-like membrane across the lumen, a dense fibrotic scar up to 2.5 cm in length, or in rare instances, an extremely narrow (1 to 2 mm) opening that prevents oral intake or passage of saliva.

Evaluation for a lumen restoration procedure:

- complete historical/physical evaluation;
- careful, small volume barium contrast videofluoroscopy using thin barium to determine the degree of lumen occlusion and to assess neuromotor function of the oropharynx. Neuromotor function evaluation cannot be completed if total hypopharyngeal occlusion has occurred;
- endoscopy of pharynx to assess structural abnormalities and degree of occlusion using guide wire probing with fluoroscopy;
- attempt to pass 0.038" or smaller guide wire under fluoroscopic control via the pharyngeal lumen if barium study confirms any degree of patency. If lumen access is achieved, wire guided antegrade Savary dilations should begin. If total obstruction is determined, a radiographic film is taken to document the proximal margin of the occlusion using the level of the maximum antegrade extent of wire passage without a bend in the wire tip;
- if lumen is totally occluded on barium study and wire passage fails, the PEG tube is removed and retrograde endoscopy *via* PEG stoma is performed to determine the distal

extent of occlusion. Again, a radiograph is obtained for documentation showing the transendoscopic guide wire tip extended to the distal point of obstruction;

- once proximal and distal levels of lumen occlusion are determined, a plan for attempting an endoscopic lumen restoration procedure is presented to the patient;
- ELR should be performed only by a physician with extensive experience with both endoscopy and dilation techniques.

Lumen restoration between hypopharynx and esophagus usually can be accomplished by combined antegrade – retrograde endoscopic procedures with fluoroscopy to assist with axis orientation from two directions. Accessories used to establish an opening between pharynx and esophagus have included biopsy forceps, rigid suction cannulus, blunt tipped probes, large gauge needles on a long stainless steel tube, and the rigid (reverse) end of a flexible guide wire. A broad spectrum antibiotic is given intravenously at the time of ELR and this is continued later *via* PEG tube for a total of 10 days. The patient remains in the hospital for two days and the second retrograde dilation is performed prior to discharge.

Once the strictured segment is penetrated, a flexible guide wire is passed and a strong silk suture (#3 or 4 silk, NOT #3-0 or 4-0!) is tied to a loop fashioned in the guide wire tip and pulled from mouth through the PEG stoma. Retrograde dilation is then performed using a series of small diameter Tucker (spindle-shaped) dilators attached to each other by loops of silk suture on the end of each dilator, usually of sizes 12, 14 and 16 French for the first session. After completing the initial dilation, the proximal end of the suture is retrieved from the pharynx using a transfer catheter through the nostril and then looped over the ear, tied firmly to the distal end of the suture and taped loosely to the upper chest. The next retrograde dilation is done after retrieving the suture through the mouth, tying its distal end to the first Tucker dilator and the proximal end to the last dilator. The suture is pulled retrograde over the index finger in the posterior pharynx used as a fulcrum to protect the larynx and epiglottis. The suture is retrieved as before and the ends tied to secure a continuous loop *via* gastrostomy and nostril. This technique is repeated every 3 to 5 days up to size 22 or 24 French. By this stage, a 0.038 inch or similar guide wire usually can be passed antegrade with fluoroscopy and Savary dilations started. After several sessions of gradually larger Savary dilations, the Savary, or other suitable wire can be passed with ease. The indwelling suture can then be permanently removed with assurance that lumen patency can be achieved.

A program of serial dilations is continued at 2 to 3 week intervals until lumen dilation is increased to 15 to 17 mm, usually over 2-3 months. At this level of dilation, a program of neuromotor swallowing rehabilitation is initiated under direction of a speech pathologist with expertise in swallowing disorders.

In our experience, successful lumen restoration after total lumen occlusion has been possible in 7 patients able to resume a modified regular or soft diet, 3 patients on liquids only (2 still undergoing initial dilation therapy) and 2 patients who have completed initial ELR only able to swallow saliva. Failures have been due to inability to gain access across an occluded segment so that either dilation could not be initiated or after successful dilation, inadequate pharyngeal motor function was demonstrated. In 2 patients, ELR failed on the first attempt and succeeded on the second.

Lumen restoration is necessary before residual pharyngeal neuromotor function can be assessed. When patients have been aphagic for weeks, months or years, the determination of adequate neuromotor function is not possible with certainty until multiple careful attempts at swallowing rehabilitation over a matter of weeks have been made.

If total loss of pharyngeal motor function is confirmed after a totally occluded lumen had been dilated to 17 mm or 51 French diameter over several weeks, the risk of aspiration is high and the prognosis is poor. During efforts at swallowing rehabilitation, it may become evident that pharyngeal dysmotility due to radiation therapy is a major problem. During the period after lumen restoration and adequate stricture dilation, regurgitation of gastric contents creates a significant risk for aspiration pneumonia in those with pharyngeal dysmotility. Once the severity and permanency of pharyngeal dysmotility is recognized, the proper decision to be made is clear to all concerned. The pharyngoesophageal stricture should be allowed to close completely. If the patient remains cancer-free and in good health on gastrostomy feedings, a prolonged though physically and socially uncomfortable, but productive, life is possible with aphagia.

In this series, 7 of 12 patients had successful ELR with return to a modified regular or soft diet and PEG tubes were removed. Following completion of the initial ELR procedure, 2 patients were able to swallow saliva only and were considered a high risk for aspiration due to pharyngeal dysfunction. Two recent patients have had successful lumen restorations and are presently undergoing serial dilations and PEG tubes continue as the primary route for nutrition. One is able to swallow small volumes of clear liquids and the other full liquids. A third patient is taking a soft diet. His PEG tube remains, but sadly, he has been found to have liver metastases. One patient had successful ELR and several dilations, but could not continue with our program due to transportation issues. He was subsequently treated by gastroenterologists in another community who elected to discontinue dilation and place a Polyflex stent. Within several weeks, this stent produced pressure necrosis of the anterior esophageal and posterior tracheal walls resulting in an esophagotracheal fistula. Patients with total pharyngoesophageal obstruction following radiation-chemotherapy for head and neck cancer deserve an attempt at ELR. This technique offers the best opportunity for restoring the ability for peroral nutrition with a low risk if an adequate level of oropharyngeal neuromotor function returns with a swallow rehabilitation program. There were no complications related to ELR in this series.

Zenker's diverticula

Zenker's diverticulum: endoscopic *versus* open approach

J.-M. Collard, L. Goncette (Brussels)

Pathophysiology and clinical expression

Although already suspected from clinical features in the 60's by Belsey in the UK [1] who recommended the routine performance of a cricomyotomy, it's not before the late 80's and early 90's that the critical role of the cricopharyngeus muscle in the genesis of Zenker's diverticulum was demonstrated both histologically by Lerut and Geboes in Belgium [2] and manometrically by Cook in Australia [3].

Histologic changes within the cricopharyngeus muscle (fibrosis, inflammation, ratio of type I to type II muscle fibers, etc.) alter the ability of Killian's mouth to open widely on deglutition so that increased hypopharyngeal pressure is required for food bolus to reach the cervical esophagus lumen. As a consequence, a mucosal pouch develops progessively through the muscle coat of the hypopharynx just proximal to the cricopharyngeus muscle in front of the spine.

From a clinical standpoint, the involvement of the cricopharyngeus muscle in the genesis of the disease is quite obvious in patients who seek consultation for dysphagia in relation to the presence of a cricopharyngeal barr or a very small diverticulum on barium swallow study. In contrast, it is much more difficult to figure out the initial implication of the muscle in those other many patients who present with a very large diverticular pouch, although having a very short history of disabling dysphagia. Bearing in mind the accepted mechanism of pouch formation, the lack of acute symptomatogy at a time when the pouch is at its initial stage in the latter patients is more than intriguing and remains to be elucidated. It is likely that the patient adapts himself to progessive, subtle changes in the ease with which he can swallow till swallowing problems become so disabling that medical assistance is needed. Notwithstanding this, a strong clinical argument that supports the existence of an underlying functional disorder is the possible recurrence of the diverticulum many years after its resection without concomitant myotomy, yet this is an uncommon observation because most patients are very old at the time of the operation and die before experiencing clinical recurrence (*Figure 1*).

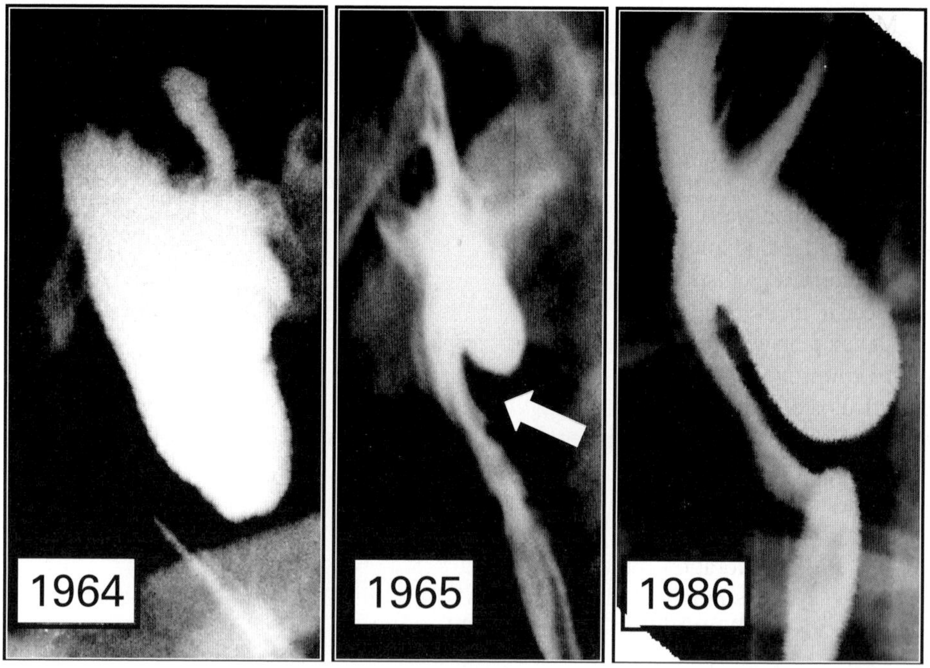

Figure 1. Radiographs showing a large diverticulum before resection without myotomy (left), a small pseudo-pouch caused by the imprint of the cricopharyngeus muscle (arrow) one year later (center), and the reappearance of a large diverticulum 22 years after the operation (right).

Although the hypopharyngeal pouch itself does not represent the disease, but is a consequence of a cricopharyngeal disorder, stasis of ingested material in its lumen adds to the lack of opening of Killian's mouth to explain symptomatology. Another factor that may account for symptoms is the forward compression of the posterior wall of the cervical esophagus by the pouch so that the esophageal lumen is collapsed. It thus appears that there are two distinct mechanisms that may generate dysphagia, i.e. dysfunction of the cricopharyngeus muscle (early stage of the disease) and a mass effect (advanced stage of the disease).

In this setting, adequate treatment of Zenker's diverticulum must include widening of Killian's mouth and suppression of intraluminal stasis. This can be achieved by either endoscopic division of the common wall between the diverticulum and the cervical esophagus, or transcervical cricomyotomy plus diverticulopexy.

Endoscopic division of the common wall

As early as 1917, Mosher in the UK [4] introduced the concept of transoral approach to Zenker's diverticulum using grasping forceps to disrupt the common wall between the diverticulum and the cervical esophagus. Later on, Dohlman in Canada [5] and Van Overbeek in the Netherlands [6] improved the technique using diathermic or laser coagulation.

Main merits of the endoscopic approach are:

- short duration of the operation;
- short-acting, light general anesthesia;
- magnified overview of the diverticular mucosa (taking of biopsy samples of any visible lesion within the pouch);
- real myotomy of the upper esophageal sphincter (the cricopharyngeus muscle is included in the common wall);
- early oral feeding after operation;
- very short hospital stay;
- no scar in the neck.

Developments in minimal access surgery and instrumentation in the early 90's allowed us to improve these conventional sutureless techniques of transoral esophago-diverticulostomy by both cutting and stapling the common wall between the diverticulum and the cervical esophagus by means of an endostapler [7].

Main merits of the stapling technique over the conventional sutureless methods are:

- excellent haemostasis of the wound edges (stapling);
- absence of contamination of peridiverticular tissues by the digestive contents (stapling);
- lower risk of perforation at the bottom of the common cavity (the course of the knife ends a few millimeters proximal to the distal end of the anvil);
- cheap technique (no need for a laser beam source).

As reported by Peracchia *et al.* [8], division of the common wall decreases both intrapharyngeal bolus and upper sphincter resting pressures significantly.

We described some technical tricks that are very useful to cut the common wall over its whole length [9] (*Figure 2A*). So, sawing the tip of the anvil of the endostapler minimizes the size of the residual spur at the bottom of the common cavity as also does endoscopic traction (stitch or forceps) of the wound edges for the placement of a second or a third cartridge of staples in very large diverticula. Moreover, the stapling procedure itself permits the bottom of the diverticulum to be pushed downward and the common wall to be stretched, providing a cut length somewhat greater than which has been estimated pre-

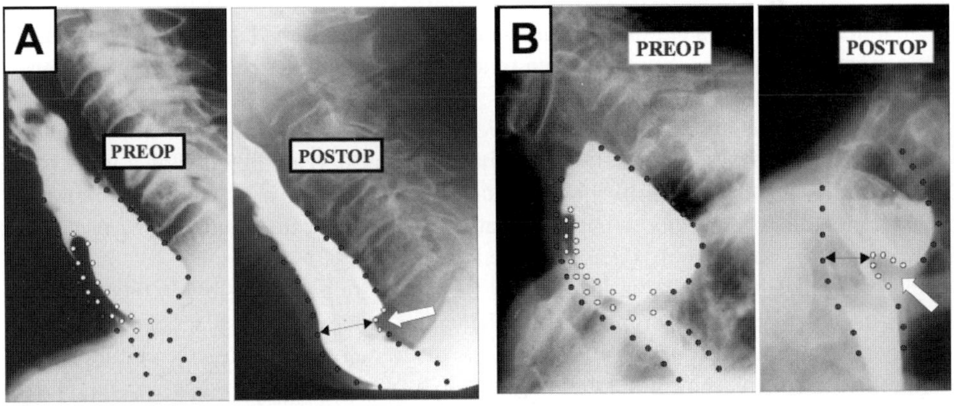

Figure 2. A. Complete stapling division of the common wall. **B.** Residual spur in a patient without residual complaints after stapling division of the common wall. Note however the large diameter of the cervical esophagus in spite of the presence of a residual spur.

operatively. Despite this however, a rather long spur may persist after the procedure in some patients (*Figure 2B*), i.e. those probably having peridiverticular fibrosis that reduces plasticity of the pouch and its realignement with the wall of the distal part of the cervical esophagus once the diverticuloesophagostomy has been done.

Surprizingly however, some of these patients may be relieved from their pre-oprative symptoms despite the presence of a residual spur after the operation. One possible explanation for this intriguing situation might be that according to the law of Poiseuille ($R = pi\ r^4\ (p_1 - p_2)\ /\ 8\ n\ L$), a minimal change in the radius (r) of a tubular structure results in an amazingly increased rate of flow (R).

In small (< 3 cm) diverticula (placement of one cartridge of staples impossible), shortness of the common wall precludes doing a complete cricomyotomy so that the short cut does not produce sufficient widening of Killian's mouth. This is in accordance with the common principle that for widening the diameter of any soft tubular structure, the longer the cut length the greater the gain in diameter (*Figure 3*).

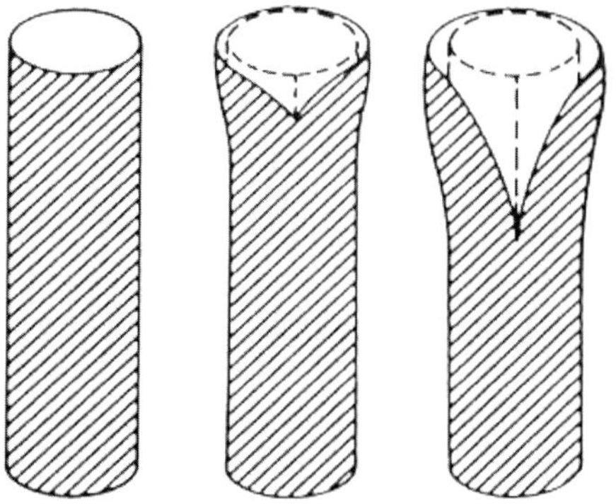

Figure 3. Illustration of the general principle for widening any soft tubular structure: the longer the cut length the greater the gain in diameter.

Another reason for not approaching a small diverticulum endoscopically is that endoscopic identification of the opening of the pouch into the esophageal lumen may be difficult. Indeed, the two lips of the doubble-lipped diverticuloscope (Collard-Weerda diverticuloscope; Karl Storz, Tuttlingen, Germany) can collapse this opening into a simple slit by stretching the oropharyngeal wall. This can even lead to catching of the lower lip of the diverticuloscope in the slit and perforation of the small diverticulum.

In this respect, the review of our own experience of both endoscopic and open procedures for Zenker's diverticulum [10] (*Figure 4*) showed that the clinical results were similar in patients with a more than 3 cm pouch whereas they were significantly worse after endoscopic management than after open treatment in those other patients with a less than 3 cm diverticulum.

The current relevance of all these considerations on small diverticula is emphasized by the fact that we now see fewer large diverticula than 20 years ago, i.e. at a time when transcervical operation for Zenker's diverticulum was carrying a bad reputation amongst general practitioners, usually telling their patients "keep your diverticulum because of the risk of loosing your voice if you are operated on".

Let's also keep in mind that the endoscopic procedure is not feasible in those patients in whom narrowness of the oropharyngeal channel together with the presence of prominent incisor teeth preclude proper positioning of the diverticuloscope across the common wall. In this respect, the placement of three fingers side by side between the superior and inferior incisor teeth is a rather reliable test for the preoperative evaluation of both the oro-pharyngeal anatomy and the likelihood of managing the diverticulum endoscopically.

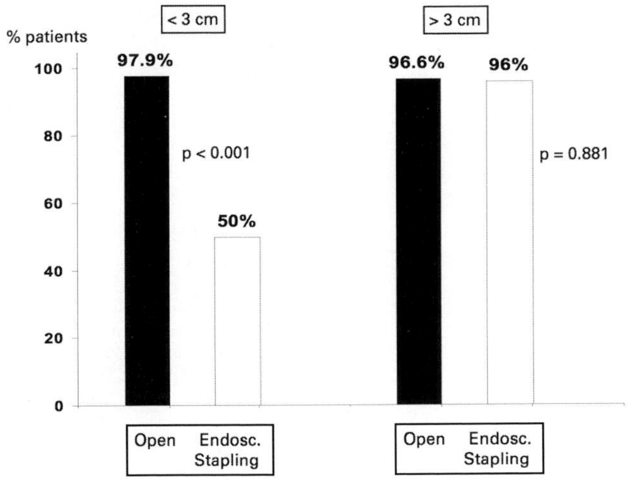

Figure 4. Symptomatic outcome (% patients with no or occasional symptoms) after open (black columns) and endoscopic (blank columns) treatments according to whether diverticulum was < 3 cm (left) or e 3 cm (right).

Cricomyotomy-diverticulopexy

Proper pouch dissection must be carried out to the collar of the diverticulum for complete exposure of the cricopharyngeus muscle.

Division of this 1 cm- in- length muscle must be extended over the first 3 to 4 cm of the muscle coat of the cervical esophagus to get sufficient enlargement of Killian's mouth.

Great care must be taken to avoid any inadvertent opening of the esophageal mucosa. In this regard, separation of the two coats of the esophageal wall from each other, although easy in most patients, may sometimes be very difficult due to the presence of severe peridiverticular fibrosis.

Myotomy of the cricopharyngeal muscle and of the proximal part of the esophageal muscle coat are the only manoeuvres to be done in the presence of either a cricopharyngeal barr or a 1-cm diverticulum. In the latter instance, the diverticular mucosa realigns itself with that of the proximal esophagus so that no pexy is needed (*Figure 5A*).

Pexy of the diverticulum must be done on the posterior pharyngeal wall rather than on the prevertebral fascia in order to maintain upward lifting of the pharyngolaryngeal block on deglutition (*Figure 5B*).

Drainage of the neck using aspirative drains is forbidden in order to avoid any succion of the denuded esophageal mucosa and subsequent fistulization.

Although very uncommon, giant diverticula are eventually to be resected because they take up too much room in the neck after dissection of the very large pouch and myotomy have been completed.

Choice of surgical technique

Cricopharyngeal barrs and 1-cm diverticula can only be treated by transcervical myotomy.

Large (i.e. > 3 cm) diverticula may be treated by either endoscopic stapling division or transcervical myotomy-pexy, the patient being offered, according to our own experience, the same chances at a favorable clinical outcome.

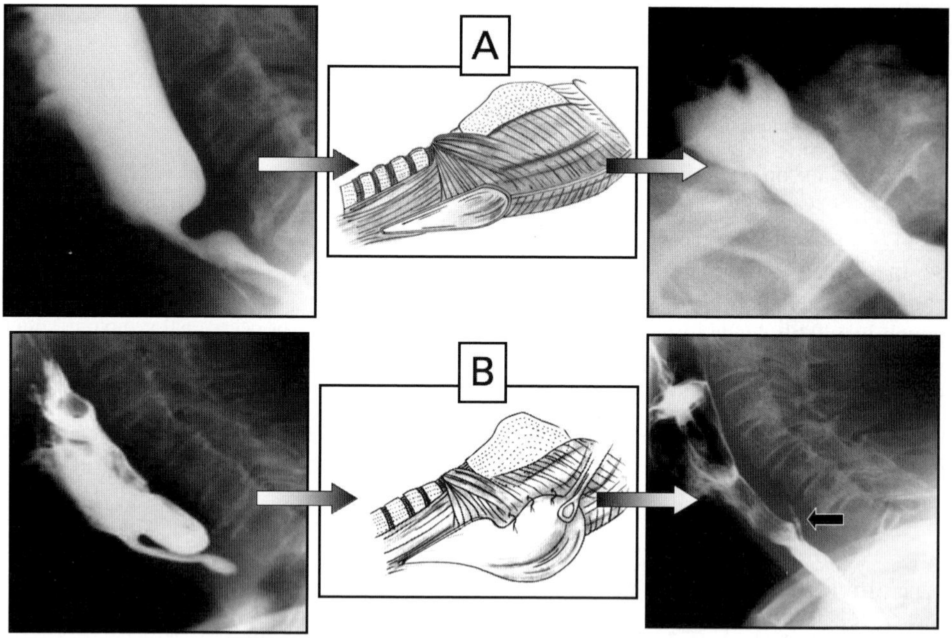

Figure 5. A. transcervical myotomy without pexy for a cricopharyngeal barr. B. Transcervical myotomy-pexy for a small diverticulum. Note the collapsed diverticular lumen behind the posterior pharyngeal wall (black arrow).

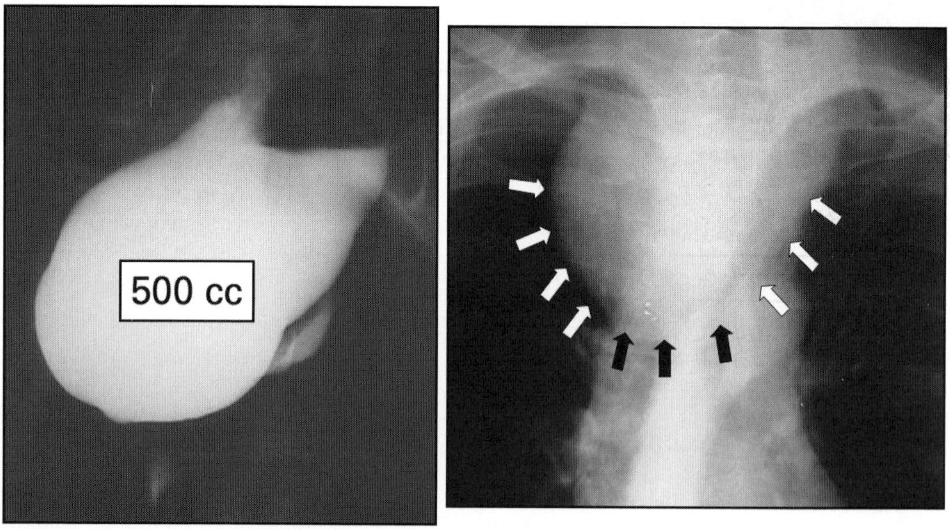

Figure 6. Giant diverticulum that was treated by endoscopic stapling division using 4 cartridges of staples.

Medium-size diverticula (i.e. from 1 to 3 cm) are best treated by transcervical myotomy-pexy than by transoral stapling division for all the aforementioned reasons.

Giant diverticula (i.e. > 6 cm) (*Figure 6*) are best treated by transoral stapling division placing several cartidges of staples on the long common wall while exerting appropriate traction on the wound edges after the first cartridge has been applied.

The endoscopic stapling technique is also best indicated in patients with a history of previous neck surgery due to the risk of injury to the left recurrent nerve if the diverticulum would be dissected by cervicotomy.

Incomplete endoscopic division of the common wall (*Figure 7*) is another indication of choice of the endoscopic approach. In such a situation indeed, trancervical dissection of the pouch inevitably leads to opening of the esophageal lumen at a point where tissues are of very poor quality with the subsequent high risk for the development of an external fistula. Should the transcervical approach be used and opening of the esophageal lumen occur, the covering of the mucosal defect with the posterior wall of the diverticulum is to be recommended [11].

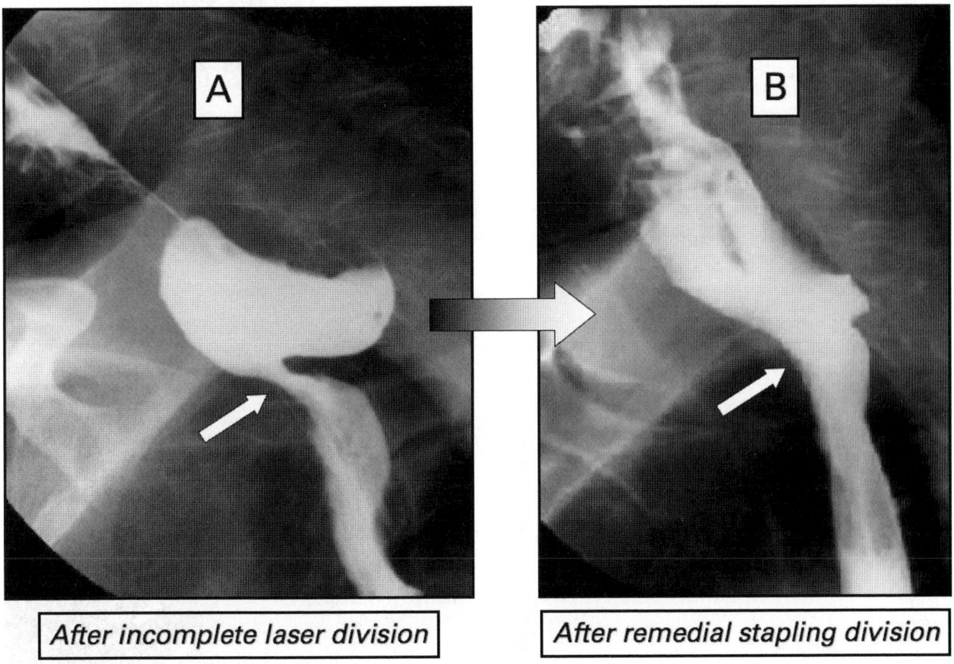

Figure 7. A. Incomplete endoscopic laser division of the common wall (patient still symptomatic post-operatively). **B**. Remedial endoscopic stapling division (patient totally asymptomatic post-operatively).

Conclusions

Optimal management of Zenker's diverticulum must combine myotomy of the cricopharyngeus muscle and muscle coat of the proximal esophagus, and suppression of any stasis within the pouch.

A good surgeon must be capable of performing all the available techniques, the size of the common wall between the diverticulum and the esophagus is the key-parameter to make the choice of the most appropriate procedure to be applied to a given patient.

References

1. Belsey R. Functional disease of the esophagus. J Thorac Cardiovasc Surg 1966;52:164-88.
2. Lerut T, Guelinckx P, Dom R et al. Does the musculus cricopharyngeus play a role in the genesis of Zenker's diverticulum? Enzyme histochemical and contractility properties. In: Siewert JR, Hölscher AH, eds. Diseases of the Esophagus. Berlin: Springer Verlag, 1988:1118-23.
3. Cook IJ, Gabb M, Panagopoulos V, et al. Pharyngeal (Zenker's) diverticulum is a disorder of upper esophageal sphincter opening. Gastroenterology 1992;103:1229-35.
4. Mosher HP. Webs and pouches of the esophagus, their diagnosis and treatment. Surg Gynecol Obstet 1917;25:175-87.
5. Dohlman G, Mattson O. The endoscopic operation for hypopharyngeal diverticula. Arch Otolaryngol 1960;71:744-52.
6. van Overbeek JJ, Hoeksema PE, Edens ET. Microendoscopic surgery of the hypopharyngeal diverticulum using electrocoagulation of carbon dioxide laser. Ann Otol Rhinol Laryngol 1984;93:34-6.
7. Collard JM, Otte JB, Kestens PJ. Endoscopic stapling technique of esophago-diverticulostomy for Zenker's diverticulum. Ann Thorac Surg 1993;56: 573-6.
8. Peracchia A, Bonavina L, Narne S, et al. Minimally invasive surgery for Zenker diverticulum. Arch Surg 1998;133:695-700.
9. Collard JM. Endoscopic approach to hypopharyngeal diverticulum. In: Peters JH, Demeester TR, eds. Minimally invasive surgery of the foregut. St-Louis, MS: Quality Medical Publishing, 1994:73-82.
10. Gutschow C , Hamoir M, Rombaux Ph, Goncette L, Otte JB, Collard JM. Management of pharyngoesophageal (Zenker's) diverticulum: which technique? Ann Thorac Surg 2002;74:1677-83.
11. Collard JM. Personal technique.

Open *versus* endosurgical approach for Zenker diverticulum: the critical role of cricopharyngeal myotomy

L. Bonavina, D. Bona, G. Saino (Milan)

The first successful resection of a Zenker diverticulum was performed by Wheeler in 1885. This procedure was subsequently abandoned because of a high rate of leakage from the suture line and was replaced by a two-stage operation. It was recognized only during the second half of the last century that correction of the functional obstruction caused by the upper esophageal sphincter (UES) is an important component of the surgical procedure [1,2]. Mosher in 1917 first attempted to divide endoscopically the septum between the esophagus and the pouch using punch forceps, but this procedure was soon abandoned. The concept of creating a common cavity endoscopically was restored to favor by Dohlman [3], who introduced diatermy, and by Van Overbeek [4], who introduced laser. Recent developments in minimally invasive surgery have led to the use of endoscopic stapling devices to divide the septum and relieve outflow obstruction at the pharyngoesophageal junction [5,6].

Patients and methods

Three-hundred-twelve patients underwent surgery for symptomatic Zenker diverticulum in our institution between 1976 and 2001. During this 25-year study period, a variety of surgical procedures were performed (*Table I*). The outcomes of the two most common techniques, i.e., stapled open resection plus cricopharyngeal myotomy, and transoral endostapling, form the basis of this report. The first cohort of patients consists of 108 consecutive individuals who underwent stapled diverticulectomy and cricopharyngeal myotomy over the period 1982-1992. The second cohort includes 132 individuals who underwent transoral endostapling over the period 1992-2001.

Table I. Surgical procedures performed in 312 patients with Zenker diverticulum.

Resection + myotomy	161*
Transoral septum stapling	131**
Pexy + myotomy	12
Myotomy	4
Resection	3
Invagination	1

* Including 108 stapled resections after 1982; ** after 1992

Pre-operative workup included barium swallow, upper gastrointestinal endoscopy, and esophageal manometry in most patients. At endoscopy, the length of the diverticulum was measured from the UES to the bottom of the pouch. The remaining esophagus was examined for the presence of associated disease. A thin guide-wire inserted at the end of the endoscopic examination assisted in positioning the manometric catheter when necessary. More recently, pharyngo-esophageal transit scintigraphy was performed pre- and post-operatively in individuals undergoing the endosurgical approach. The patients were kept on a clear liquid diet the day before the operation. Whenever necessary, especially in elderly individuals, intravenous antibiotics, intensive respiratory physiotherapy, and nutritional support were administered before surgery.

Technique of open diverticulectomy and cricopharyngeal myotomy

The operation can be performed under general anesthesia, local anesthesia, or C5-C6 superselective spinal anesthesia. The patient is positioned supine on the operating table with a small pillow under the shoulders. The head is hyperextended and slightly turned to the the right side. The neck is draped from the chin to below the clavicles. A skin incision centered at the level of the cricoid cartilage is made along the anterior border of the left sternocleidomastoid muscle. The subcutaneous tissue and the platysma are divided. The pharynx and cervical esophagus are exposed by retracting the sternocleidomastoid and carotid sheath laterally, and the larynx and thyroid gland medially. The omohyoid muscle, the middle thyroid vein, and the inferior thyroid artery are divided. Care is taken not to injury the recurrent laryngeal nerve which runs in the tracheoesophageal groove. The diverticulum is identified, grasped with Duval forceps, and retracted cephalad. The loose connective tissue surrounding the pouch is dissected to identify its neck on the posterior pharyngeal wall. The transverse fibers of the cricopharyngeal muscle can be seen just below the neck of the diverticulum. At this point, right-angle forceps can be used to develop a dissection plane inferiorly between the muscolaris and the mucosa, and the myotomy is performed using curved scissors for a length of about 5 cm on the cervical esophagus. The edges of the muscle are gently separated using a swab to expose the underlying mucosa. A Foley catheter inserted through the mouth and progressively withdrawn with the balloon inflated may be useful to distend the pharyngoesophageal junction during division of the muscle layer. The diverticulum in then transected using a TA 30 linear stapler (Tyco). A nasogastric tube is routinely placed. The neck wound is closed leaving a penrose drain. A gastrographin swallow study is routinely performed between on post-operative day 2 before resuming a soft diet.

Technique of transoral endostapling

The operation is routinely performed under general endotracheal anesthesia. The surgeon is sitting behind the patient's head. The hypopharynx is entered with a modified Weerda diverticuloscope (*Storz*) which is gently advanced right behind the endotracheal tube. Once in place, the instrument is held in place using a chest support. A 5 mm wide-angle 0° telescope is inserted and connected to a cold-light source and to a video-camera in order to obtain a magnified vision of the operative field on a television screen. The two self-retracting valves of the diverticuloscope, which can be approximated and angulated to fit the patient's hypopharyngeal anatomy, are then allowed to enter the diverticulum and the esophageal lumen, respectively. The septum between the esophagus and the diverticulum is therefore centered in the operative field. The depth of the diverticulum is checked using a graduated rod. This maneuver also allows to straighten the pouch and to elongate the common wall. A ETS 35 linear endostapling device (*Ethicon Endo-surgery*) is used to divide the septum. The anvil is placed in the lumen of the diverticulum and the cartridge into the lumen of the cervical esophagus. The instrument jaws are approximated across the septum along the midline before firing. With a single application of the endostapler, the posterior esophageal wall is sutured to the wall of the diverticulum, and the tissue is transected between three rows of staples on each side. Multiple stapler applications may be necessary according to the size of the diverticulum. Electrocoagulating endosurgical scissors may be used to complete the section at the distal end of the staple line. After removal of the stapler, the two wound edges retract laterally due to the division of the cricopharyngeal muscle. A nasogastric tube is generally not required. A gastrographin swallow study is performed on the first post-operative day. The patient is then allowed to drink and eat a soft diet and is discharged from the hospital.

Results

The main demographic and clinical data are reported in *Table II*. One patient died of pulmonary embolism during the post-operative period, giving an overall mortality rate of 0.4%. The morbidity in patients undergoing the open approach consisted of 2 leaks from the staple line treated conservatively and healed within two weeks; 1 transient left recurrent palsy, and 1 wound hematoma requiring surgical revision. With the endosurgical approach there were 3 conversions to open surgery within the first 2 years of experience. The reason was a difficult exposure of the common wall because of a limited head extension in 2 elderly individuals, and the occurrence of a mucosal tear during stapler insertion in the third patient. The hospital stay was markedly reduced in patients undergoing the endosurgical approach. Overall, 94% of patients undergoing the open approach and 93% of those undergoing the endosurgical approach were symptom-free after a median follow-up of 46 and 25 months, respectively. Pre- and post-operative manometric data in the two groups of patients are reported in *Table III*. Esophageal transit scintigraphy performed in a subgroup of patients (n = 15) undergoing the endosurgical approach showed a statistically significant increase of upper esophageal clearance of the liquid bolus (p = 0.02). Upper esophageal stasis of the radionuclide was similarly improved (p = 0.006).

Table II. Comparison of clinical features and outcome in patients with Zenker diverticulum who underwent open and endosurgical operation.

	Stapled resection + myotomy (n = 108)	Transoral stapling (n = 132)
Age (median/range)	62 / 30-83	64 / 37-92
Male/female ratio	2.7:1	3.5:1
Dysphagia (%)	100	100
Aspiration (%)	19	22
Hiatal hernia/reflux (%)	12	9
Weight loss (%)	17	32
Pouch median size (cm)	4	4
Regional anesthesia (n)	15	0
Mean operative time (min)	70	15
Post-op. mortality (%)	0.9	0
Leaks from staple line (%)	1.8	0
Recurrent nerve palsy (%)	0.9	0
Conversions	–	3 (2.3%)
Mean hospital stay (days)	8	3
Median follow-up (months)	46	25
Symptom-free (% patients)	94	93

Table III. Comparison of pre- and post-operative manometric data in patients undergoing surgery for Zenker diverticulum.

	Open (n = 24) Pre/post	p	Endosurgical (n = 43) Pre/post	p
Pharyngeal pressure (mmHg)	36.4/34.3	NS	47.9/42.4	NS
UES resting pressure (mmHg)	38/20	< .001	52.4/31.5	< .001
UES residual pressure (mmHg)	6.2/0.7	< .02	3.4/2	NS
UES length (cm)	3.1/2.4	< .01	2.5/2.3	NS

Discussion

It is currently believed that inadequate opening of the UES, resulting from fibrosis of the cricopharyngeal muscle, considerably increases hypopharyngeal intrabolus pressure and leads to formation of a pulsion diverticulum [7,8]. For this reason, surgical resection or suspension of the pouch performed without a concomitant myotomy may fail to relieve dysphagia and to prevent complications or recurrence of the pouch. Cricopharyngeal myotomy creates a weak area in the muscle over which pharyngeal pressure can be distributed during swallowing [9,14].

Treatment of Zenker diverticulum is indicated, regardless of its size, to relieve the disabling symptoms of oropharyngeal dysphagia and pharyngo-oral regurgitation, and to prevent the life-threatening complication of aspiration pneumonia and lung abscess, especially in the elderly population. The tendency of the pouch to progressively enlarge and the possible, although rare, development of a squamous-cell carcinoma represent additional arguments in favor of early treatment [15].

The results of this study show that both the surgical and the transoral procedure are safe and effective in the treatment of Zenker diverticulum. Although it may be unfair to compare the more recent series of transorally treated patients with the historical cohort of surgically treated patients, it appears that the endosurgical approach has some distinct advantages.

Unlike the traditional surgical approach, which varies depending on the preference of the individual surgeon, the endoscopic approach is focused on the UES. In fact, stapling the septum interposed between the pouch and the cervical esophagus allows the creation of a common cavity with simultaneous section of the UES. Compared to the conventional surgical operation, the advantages of endostapling include absence of skin incision, shorter operative time, minimal or absent post-operative pain, quicker resumption of oral feeding, and shorter hospital stay [16,17]. An additional advantage of this approach is expected in patients who had undergone surgery in the left side of the neck or who present with recurrent diverticulum after a conventional operation [18]. In such circumstances, the open approach may pose a major technical challenge to the surgeon and is associated with a high risk of leakage or recurrent nerve injury.

The endoscopic approach may prove difficult in patients with cervical osteoarthritis and in those with a reduced opening capacity of the mouth. The best indication to this procedure is represented by medium-sized diverticula in which at least two staple cartridges can be applied and an adequate cricopharyngeal myotomy be achieved. Diverticula smaller than 3 cm represent a formal contraindication to the endosurgical approach because the common wall is too short to accomodate one cartridge of staples and to allow complete division of the sphincter. This would result in an incomplete myotomy causing persistent dysphagia.

Although the pos-toperative outcome of these patients, who are often elderly and compromised, suggests a greater comfort and a quicker recovery compared to the conventional operation, it should be taken into account that the endosurgical approach requires a general anesthesia. Therefore, in patients with excessive operative risk, a conventional operation carried out under regional anesthesia still remains the procedure of choice [19].

At present, there is no evidence from high quality randomised controlled studies to establish which procedure is superior. It is clear that both operations relieve the outflow obstruction at the pharyngoesophageal junction, indicating that cricopharyngeal myotomy has an important therapeutic role in this disease independent of the resection of the pouch and of the surgical approach. Future trials may indicate the role of a tailored approach in the management of Zenker diverticulum [20].

References

1. Belsey R. Functional disease of the esophagus. J Thorac Cardiovasc Surg 1966;52:164-88.
2. Ferguson M. Evolution of therapy for pharyngoesophageal (Zenker's) diverticulum. Ann Thorac Surg 1991;51:848-52.
3. Dohlman G, Mattson O. The endoscopic operation for hypopharyngeal diverticula. Arch Otolaryngol 1960; 171:744-52.
4. Van Overbeek J, Hoeksema P, Edens E. Microendoscopic surgery of the hypopharyngeal diverticulum using electrocoagulation or carbon dioxide laser. Ann Otol Rhinol Laryngol 1984;93:34-6.
5. Collard J, Otte J, Kestens P. Endoscopic stapling technique of esophagodiverticulostomy for Zenker's diverticulum. Ann Thorac Surg 1993;56:573-6.
6. Narne S, Bonavina L, Guido E, Peracchia A. Treatment of Zenker's diverticulum by endoscopic stapling. Endosurgery 1993;1:118-20.
7. Cook I, Gabb M, Panagopoulos V, et al. Pharyngeal (Zenker's) diverticulum is a disorder of upper esophageal sphincter opening. Gastroenterology 1992;103:1229-35.
8. Shaw D, Jamieson G, Gabb M, Simula M, Dent J. Influence of surgery on deglutitive upper oesophageal sphincter mechanics in Zenker's diverticulum. Gut 1996;38:806-11.
9. Ellis H, Crozier R. Cervical esophageal dysphagia. Indications and results of cricopharyngeal myotomy. Ann Surg 1981;194:279-89.
10. Duranceau A, Rheault M, Jamieson G. Physiological response to cricopharyngeal myotomy and diverticulm suspension. Surgery 1983;84:655-62.
11. Bonavina L, Kahn N, DeMeester T. Pharyngoesophageal dysfunctions: the role of cricopharyngeal myotomy. Arch Surg 1985; 120:541-9.
12. Bonavina L, Bettineschi F, Fontebasso V, Ruol A, Nosadini A, Peracchia A. Cricopharyngeal myotomy and stapling: treatment of choice for Zenker's diverticulum. In: Nabeya K, Hanaoka T, Nogami H, eds. Recent advances in diseases of the esophagus. Tokyo: Springer Verlag, 1993:207-11.
13. Lerut T, Coosemans W, Cuypers P, et al. Cervical myotomy as therapeutic principle for pharyngoesophageal disorders. Dis Esoph 1996;9:22-32.
14. Mason R, Bremner C, DeMeester T, et al. Pharyngeal swallowing disorders. Selection for and outcome after myotomy. Ann Surg 1998;228:598-608.
15. Huang B, Krishnan K, Payne W: Long-term survival following diverticulectomy for cancer in pharyngoesophageal (Zenker's) diverticulum. Ann Thorac Surg 1984;38:207-10.
16. Peracchia A, Bonavina L, Narne S, Segalin A, Antoniazzi L, Marotta G. Minimally invasive surgery for Zenker diverticulum. Analysis of results in 95 consecutive patients. Arch Surg 1998;133:695-700.
17. Saetti R, Silvestrini M, Peracchia A, Narne S. Endoscopic stapler-assisted Zenker's diverticulotomy: which is the best operative facility? Head Neck 2006;28:1094-9.
18. Narne S, Bonavina L, Antoniazzi L, Cutrone C, Peracchia A. Safety and effectiveness of transoral stapling for recurrent Zenker diverticulum. In: Pinotti H, et al., eds, Recent advances in Diseases of the Esophagus. Bologna: Monduzzi, 2001:701-4.
19. Levard H, Laurent P, Boudet M, Perniceni T, Gayet B. Resection of Zenker diverticulum under regional anesthesia. Br J Surg 1997;84:120.
20. Sen P, Lowe D, Farnan T. Surgical intervention for pharyngeal pouch. The Cochrane Database of Systematic Reviews, 2005, Issue 3.

Achevé d'imprimer par Corlet, Imprimeur, S.A. - 14110 Condé-sur-Noireau
N° d'Imprimeur : 118091 - Précédent dépôt : avril 2008 - Dépôt légal : mars 2009 - *Imprimé en France*